Pediatric Transplant and Oncology Infectious Diseases

Pediatric Transplant and Oncology Infectious Diseases

William J. Steinbach, MD
Samuel L. Katz Professor of Pediatrics
Professor in Molecular Genetics and Microbiology
Chief, Division of Pediatric Infectious Diseases
Director, Duke Pediatric Immunocompromised Host Program
Director, International Pediatric Fungal Network
Duke University School of Medicine
Durham, North Carolina

Michael D. Green, MD, MPH
Professor of Pediatrics, Surgery and Clinical and Translational Science
Co-Director, Transplant Infectious Diseases
Division of Infectious Diseases
UPMC Children's Hospital of Pittsburgh
University of Pittsburgh School of Medicine
Pittsburgh, Pennsylvania

Marian G. Michaels, MD, MPH
Professor of Pediatrics and Surgery
Co-Director, Transplant Infectious Diseases
Division of Infectious Diseases
UPMC Children's Hospital of Pittsburgh
University of Pittsburgh School of Medicine
Pittsburgh, Pennsylvania

Lara A. Danziger-Isakov, MD, MPH
Professor of Pediatrics
Director, Immunocompromised Host Infectious Diseases
Division of Infectious Diseases
Cincinnati Children's Hospital Medical Center
University of Cincinnati
Cincinnati, Ohio

Brian T. Fisher, DO, MPH, MSCE
Associate Professor of Pediatrics and Epidemiology
Senior Scholar, Penn Center for Clinical Epidemiology and Biostatistics
Co-Director, International Pediatric Fungal Network
Chair, Infectious Diseases Subcommittee for the Children's Oncology Group
Division of Infectious Diseases
Children's Hospital of Philadelphia
Perelman School of Medicine at the University of Pennsylvania
Philadelphia, Pennsylvania

ELSEVIER

Elsevier
1600 John F. Kennedy Blvd.
Ste 1800
Philadelphia, PA 19103-899

PEDIATRIC TRANSPLANT AND ONCOLOGY INFECTIOUS DISEASES ISBN: 978-0-323-64198-2

Notice

Knowledge and best practice in this field are constantly changing. As new research and experience broaden our understanding, changes in research methods, professional practices, or medical treatment may become necessary.

Practitioners and researchers must always rely on their own experience and knowledge in evaluating and using any information, methods, compounds or experiments described herein. Because of rapid advances in the medical sciences, in particular, independent verification of diagnoses and drug dosages should be made. To the fullest extent of the law, no responsibility is assumed by Elsevier, authors, editors or contributors for any injury and/or damage to persons or property as a matter of products liability, negligence or otherwise, or from any use or operation of any methods, products, instructions, or ideas contained in the material herein.

Library of Congress Control Number: 2019953760

Content Strategist: Sarah Barth
Content Development Manager: Ellen Wurm-Cutter
Content Development Specialist: Meghan Andress
Publishing Services Manager: Deepthi Unni
Project Manager: Janish Ashwin Paul
Design Direction: Ryan Cook

Printed in the United States of America

Last digit is the print number: 9 8 7 6 5 4 3 2

To all the pediatric transplant recipients, children with cancer, and their families, who are the true inspiration for this textbook and who put their trust in us to help them through their illness. We also dedicate this book to the organ donors and their families, who give the ultimate gift and allow transplantation to be a reality.

To my wife, Dr. Susan Emmett, my children, Amelia and Aidan Steinbach, my parents, Dr. Charles and Katherine Steinbach, and my in-laws, Dr. John and Karen Emmett.

William J. Steinbach, MD

To my children, David, Erin, Molly, and Allison, my granddaughter, Lyla, and my wife, Jenny, who has been my partner and best friend for the past 36 years.

Michael D. Green, MD, MPH

To my parents, Dr. Milton and Lois Michaels, and my mentor, Dr. Ellen Wald, for their continued support and wisdom.

Marian G. Michaels, MD, MPH

To my husband, Ronnen Isakov, my children, Avital and Gavin Isakov, and my parents, Nancy and Nathan Danziger, for their limitless support.

Lara A. Danziger-Isakov, MD, MPH

To my wife, Megan Fisher, for her constant love, continuous support, and limitless encouragement, to my children, Makenzie, Bradan, and Luke, for sacrificing their time with Dad for this effort, and to my parents, Tim and Kathy, for encouraging us to reach our dreams.

Brian T. Fisher, DO, MPH, MSCE

CONTRIBUTORS

Chapter 1
Yeh-Chung Chang, MD, MSCE
Assistant Professor of Pediatrics
Division of Pediatric Infectious Diseases
Duke University School of Medicine
Durham, North Carolina

Andrew Barbas, MD
Assistant Professor of Surgery
Division of Abdominal Transplant Surgery
Duke University School of Medicine
Durham, North Carolina

Chapter 2
Jasmeen Dara, MD, MS
Assistant Professor of Clinical Pediatrics
Division of Pediatric Blood and Marrow Transplantation
University of California—San Francisco
San Francisco, California

Christopher C. Dvorak, MD
Professor of Clinical Pediatrics
Chief, Division of Pediatric Allergy, Immunology, and Blood and Marrow Transplantation
University of California—San Francisco
San Francisco, California

Chapter 3
Neil Patel, PharmD, BCOP
Department of Pharmacy
Children's Hospital of Philadelphia
Philadelphia, Pennsylvania

Abby Green, MD
Assistant Professor of Pediatrics
Division of Pediatric Infectious Diseases
Division of Pediatric Hematology/Oncology
St. Louis Children's Hospital
Washington University in St. Louis
St. Louis, Missouri

Chapter 4
Rebecca Pellett Madan, MD, MS
Associate Professor of Pediatrics
Division of Infectious Diseases
New York University Langone School of Medicine
New York, New York

Lara A. Danziger-Isakov, MD, MPH
Professor of Pediatrics
Director, Immunocompromised Host Infectious Diseases
Division of Infectious Diseases
Cincinnati Children's Hospital Medical Center
University of Cincinnati
Cincinnati, Ohio

Chapter 5
Marian G. Michaels, MD, MPH
Professor of Pediatrics and Surgery
Co-Director, Transplant Infectious Diseases
Division of Infectious Diseases
UPMC Children's Hospital of Pittsburgh
University of Pittsburgh School of Medicine
Pittsburgh, Pennsylvania

Michael D. Green, MD, MPH
Professor of Pediatrics, Surgery and Clinical and Translational Science
Co-Director, Transplant Infectious Diseases
Division of Infectious Diseases
UPMC Children's Hospital of Pittsburgh
University of Pittsburgh School of Medicine
Pittsburgh, Pennsylvania

Chapter 6
Gabriela M. Marón Alfaro, MD, MS
Associate Member
Department of Infectious Diseases
St. Jude Children's Research Hospital
Memphis, Tennessee

Hayley A. Gans, MD
Professor of Pediatrics
Division of Pediatric Infectious Diseases
Stanford University School of Medicine
Stanford, California

Chapter 7
Michele Estabrook, MD
Professor of Pediatrics
Division of Pediatric Infectious Diseases
Washington University in St. Louis
St. Louis, Missouri

Monica I. Ardura, DO, MSCS
Associate Professor of Pediatrics
Medical Director, Host Defense Program
Division of Infectious Diseases
Nationwide Children's Hospital
The Ohio State University
Columbus, Ohio

Chapter 8
Brian T. Fisher, DO, MPH, MSCE
Associate Professor of Pediatrics and Epidemiology
Senior Scholar, Penn Center for Clinical Epidemiology and Biostatistics
Co-Director, International Pediatric Fungal Network
Chair, Infectious Diseases Subcommittee for the Children's Oncology Group
Division of Infectious Diseases
Children's Hospital of Philadelphia
Perelman School of Medicine at the University of Pennsylvania
Philadelphia, Pennsylvania

Lillian Sung, MD, PhD
Professor
Division of Haematology/Oncology
Department of Pediatrics and Institute of Health Policy Management and Evaluation
The Hospital for Sick Children
University of Toronto
Toronto, Ontario, Canada

Chapter 9
Klara M. Posfay-Barbe, MD, MS
Professor of Pediatrics
Head of Pediatric Infectious Diseases
Children's Hospital of Geneva
University Hospitals of Geneva
Geneva, Switzerland

Natasha Halasa, MD, MPH
Associate Professor of Pediatrics
Division of Pediatric Infectious Diseases
Monroe Carell Jr. Children's Hospital at Vanderbilt
Vanderbilt University School of Medicine
Nashville, Tennessee

Chapter 10
Matthew S. Kelly, MD, MPH
Assistant Professor of Pediatrics
Assistant Professor of Global Health
Division of Pediatric Infectious Diseases
Duke University School of Medicine
Durham, North Carolina

Michael A. Silverman, MD, PhD
Assistant Professor of Pediatrics
Division of Infectious Diseases
Children's Hospital of Philadelphia
Perelman School of Medicine at the University of Pennsylvania
Philadelphia, Pennsylvania

Chapter 11
Joshua Wolf, MBBS, PhD, FRACP
Associate Member
Department of Infectious Diseases
St. Jude Children's Research Hospital
Assistant Professor
Department of Pediatrics
University of Tennessee Health Science Center
Memphis, Tennessee

Jeffrey S. Gerber, MD, PhD
Associate Professor of Pediatrics and Epidemiology
Division of Infectious Diseases
Children's Hospital of Philadelphia
Perelman School of Medicine at the University of Pennsylvania
Philadelphia, Pennsylvania

Michael J. Smith, MD, MSCE
Associate Professor of Pediatrics
Division of Pediatric Infectious Diseases
Medical Director, Pediatric Antimicrobial Stewardship
Duke University School of Medicine
Durham, North Carolina

Chapter 12
Ibukunoluwa C. Akinboyo, MD
Assistant Professor of Pediatrics
Division of Pediatric Infectious Diseases
Medical Director, Pediatric Infection Prevention
Duke University School of Medicine
Durham, North Carolina

Dawn Nolt, MD, MPH
Associate Professor of Pediatrics
Division of Pediatric Infectious Diseases
Doernbecher Children's Hospital
Oregon Health and Science University
Portland, Oregon

Chapter 13
Blanca E. Gonzalez, MD
Associate Professor of Pediatrics
Center for Pediatric Infectious Diseases
Cleveland Clinic Children's Hospital
Cleveland Clinic Lerner College of Medicine of Case Western Reserve University
Cleveland, Ohio

Marian G. Michaels, MD, MPH
Professor of Pediatrics and Surgery
Co-Director, Transplant Infectious Diseases
Division of Infectious Diseases
UPMC Children's Hospital of Pittsburgh
University of Pittsburgh School of Medicine
Pittsburgh, Pennsylvania

Chapter 14
Mehreen Arshad, MBBS
Assistant Professor of Pediatrics
Division of Infectious Diseases
Ann and Robert H. Lurie Children's Hospital
Feinberg School of Medicine, Northwestern University
Chicago, Illinois

Andrew Nowalk, MD, PhD
Associate Professor of Pediatrics
Clinical Director, Division of Infectious Diseases
UPMC Children's Hospital of Pittsburgh
University of Pittsburgh School of Medicine
Pittsburgh, Pennsylvania

Pranita D. Tamma, MD, MHS
Associate Professor of Pediatrics
Division of Infectious Diseases
Program Director, Pediatric Antimicrobial Stewardship
Johns Hopkins University School of Medicine
Baltimore, Maryland

Chapter 15
Daniel Dulek, MD
Assistant Professor of Pediatrics
Division of Pediatric Infectious Diseases
Medical Director, Peter F. Wright Immunocompromised Pediatric Infectious Diseases Service
Monroe Carell Jr. Children's Hospital at Vanderbilt
Vanderbilt University School of Medicine
Nashville, Tennessee

Victoria A. Statler, MD, MSc
Assistant Professor
Division of Pediatric Infectious Diseases
Medical Director, Pediatric Transplant/Immunocompromised Host Infectious Diseases Service
Norton Children's Hospital
University of Louisville School of Medicine
Louisville, Kentucky

Chapter 16
Flor M. Munoz, MD, MSc
Associate Professor of Pediatrics
Department of Pediatrics, Infectious Diseases
Texas Children's Hospital
Baylor College of Medicine
Houston, Texas

Philana Ling Lin, MD, MSc
Associate Professor of Pediatrics
Division of Infectious Diseases
UPMC Children's Hospital of Pittsburgh
University of Pittsburgh School of Medicine
Pittsburgh, Pennsylvania

Chapter 17
Lara A. Danziger-Isakov, MD, MPH
Professor of Pediatrics
Director, Immunocompromised Host Infectious Diseases
Division of Infectious Diseases
Cincinnati Children's Hospital Medical Center
University of Cincinnati
Cincinnati, Ohio

Tanvi Sharma, MD, MPH
Assistant Professor of Pediatrics
Division of Infectious Diseases
Department of Pediatrics
Harvard Medical School
Boston, Massachusetts

Chapter 18
Michael D. Green, MD, MPH
Professor of Pediatrics, Surgery and Clinical and Translational Science
Co-Director, Transplant Infectious Diseases
Division of Infectious Diseases
UPMC Children's Hospital of Pittsburgh
University of Pittsburgh School of Medicine
Pittsburgh, Pennsylvania

Thomas Gross, Jr., MD, PhD
Deputy Director of Science
Center for Global Health
National Cancer Institute
Rockville, Maryland

Upton D. Allen, MBBS
Professor
Pediatrics and Institute of Health Policy, Management & Evaluation
Senior Associate Scientist and Chief
Division of Infectious Diseases
The Hospital for Sick Children
University of Toronto
Toronto, Ontario, Canada

Chapter 19
William J. Muller, MD, PhD
Associate Professor of Pediatrics
Division of Infectious Diseases
Ann and Robert H. Lurie Children's Hospital
Feinberg School of Medicine, Northwestern University
Chicago, Illinois

Betsy C. Herold, M.D.
Harold and Muriel Block Chair in Pediatrics
Vice Chair for Research, Department of Pediatrics
Chief, Division of Pediatric Infectious Diseases
Professor, Pediatrics & Microbiology-Immunology
Albert Einstein College of Medicine and the Children's Hospital at Montefiore
Bronx, New York

Chapter 20
Debra J. Lugo, MD
Assistant Professor of Pediatrics
Division of Pediatric Infectious Diseases
Duke University School of Medicine
Durham, North Carolina

Danielle M. Zerr, MD, MPH
Professor and Chief, Division of Pediatric Infectious Diseases
University of Washington
Center for Clinical and Translational Research
Seattle Children's Research Institute
Seattle, Washington

Chapter 21
Alpana Waghmare, MD
Assistant Professor
Division of Pediatric Infectious Diseases
University of Washington
Center for Clinical and Translational Research
Seattle Children's Research Institute
Seattle, Washington

Janet A. Englund, MD
Professor
Division of Pediatric Infectious Diseases
University of Washington
Center for Clinical and Translational Research
Seattle Children's Research Institute
Seattle, Washington

Chapter 22
Diana F. Florescu, MD
Professor of Internal Medicine
Courtesy Professor of Surgery
Nebraska Medical Center
University of Nebraska
Lincoln, Nebraska

Erica J. Stohs, MD, MPH
Assistant Professor of Medicine
Associate Medical Director, Antimicrobial Stewardship
Nebraska Medical Center
University of Nebraska
Lincoln, Nebraska

Chapter 23
Benjamin L. Laskin, MD, MSc
Assistant Professor of Pediatrics
Division of Nephrology
Children's Hospital of Philadelphia
Perelman School of Medicine at the University of Pennsylvania
Philadelphia, Pennsylvania

Hans H. Hirsch, MD, MSc
Professor
Transplantation and Clinical Virology
Department of Biomedicine
University of Basel
Diagnostic Virology and Laboratory Medicine
Infectious Diseases and Hospital Epidemiology
University Hospital Basel
Basel, Switzerland

Chapter 24
William J. Steinbach, MD
Samuel L. Katz Professor of Pediatrics
Professor in Molecular Genetics and Microbiology
Chief, Division of Pediatric Infectious Diseases
Director, Duke Pediatric Immunocompromised Host Program
Director, International Pediatric Fungal Network
Duke University School of Medicine
Durham, North Carolina

Chapter 25
Rachel L. Wattier, MD, MHS
Assistant Professor of Pediatrics
Division of Pediatric Infectious Diseases and Global Health
University of California—San Francisco
San Francisco, California

William J. Steinbach, MD
Samuel L. Katz Professor of Pediatrics
Professor in Molecular Genetics and Microbiology
Chief, Division of Pediatric Infectious Diseases
Director, Duke Pediatric Immunocompromised Host Program
Director, International Pediatric Fungal Network
Duke University School of Medicine
Durham, North Carolina

Chapter 26
Jennifer E. Schuster, MD, MSCI
Associate Professor of Pediatrics
Division of Pediatric Infectious Diseases
Children's Mercy Kansas City
University of Missouri-Kansas City
Kansas City, Missouri

Brian T. Fisher, DO, MPH, MSCE
Associate Professor of Pediatrics and Epidemiology
Senior Scholar, Penn Center for Clinical Epidemiology and Biostatistics
Co-Director, International Pediatric Fungal Network
Chair, Infectious Diseases Subcommittee for the Children's Oncology Group
Division of Infectious Diseases
Children's Hospital of Philadelphia
Perelman School of Medicine at the University of Pennsylvania
Philadelphia, Pennsylvania

Chapter 27
Philip Lee, PharmD
Clinical Pharmacist for Pediatric Infectious Disease
Department of Pediatrics
Division of Pediatric Infectious Diseases
Albert Einstein College of Medicine and Children's Hospital at Montefiore
Bronx, New York

David L. Goldman, MD
Associate Professor of Pediatrics, Microbiology & Immunology
Director of Pediatric Infectious Diseases Fellowship
Albert Einstein College of Medicine and Children's Hospital at Montefiore
Bronx, New York

Chapter 28
John C. Christenson, MD
Professor of Clinical Pediatrics
Ryan White Center for Pediatric Infectious Diseases and Global Health
Riley Hospital for Children
Indiana University School of Medicine
Indianapolis, Indiana

Thomas G. Fox, MD
Assistant Professor of Pediatrics
Division of Infectious Diseases
Emory University School of Medicine
Atlanta, Georgia

Chapter 29
Sharon F. Chen, MD, MS
Associate Professor of Pediatrics
Division of Pediatric Infectious Diseases
Stanford University School of Medicine
Stanford, California

Hayley A. Gans, MD
Professor of Pediatrics
Division of Pediatric Infectious Diseases
Stanford University School of Medicine
Stanford, California

Chapter 30
Grant C. Paulsen, MD
Professor
Director, Pediatric Infectious Diseases Fellowship
Division of Infectious Diseases
Cincinnati Children's Hospital Medical Center
University of Cincinnati
Cincinnati, Ohio

Paul K. Sue, MD
Assistant Professor of Pediatrics
Division of Pediatric Infectious Diseases
University of Texas Southwestern Medical Center
Dallas, Texas

Chapter 31
Catherine Burton, MD, MSc, FRCPC
Assistant Professor of Pediatrics
Division of Infectious Diseases
Department of Pediatrics
University of Alberta
Edmonton, Alberta, Canada

Benjamin Hanisch, MD
Assistant Professor of Pediatrics
Division of Infectious Diseases
Children's National Health System
George Washington University School of Medicine
Washington, DC

Chapter 32
Ivan A. Gonzalez, MD, MSc
Associate Professor of Clinical Pediatrics
Director, Pediatric Infectious Diseases Training Program
Division of Pediatric Infectious Diseases
University of Miami Miller School of Medicine
Miami, Florida

Terri Stillwell, MD, MPH
Clinical Assistant Professor
Division of Pediatric Infectious Diseases
University of Michigan Medical School
Ann Arbor, Michigan

Chapter 33
Inci Yildirim, MD, PhD, MSc
Assistant Professor of Pediatrics and Epidemiology
Division of Infectious Diseases
Professor, Department of Epidemiology
Rollins School of Public Health
Emory University
Atlanta, Georgia

Elizabeth Doby Knackstedt, MD
Assistant Professor
Division of Pediatric Infectious Diseases
University of Utah School of Medicine
Medical Director Transplant/Immunocompromised Infectious Diseases
Primary Children's Hospital
Salt Lake City, Utah

Chapter 34
Erick F. Mayer Arispe, MD, MSc
Assistant Professor of Pediatrics
State University of New York
Downstate Medical Center and New York City Health + Hospitals/Kings County Hospital
New York, New York

Andi L. Shane, MD, MPH, MSc
Associate Professor of Pediatrics
Interim Chief, Division of Pediatric Infectious Diseases
Marcus Professor of Hospital Epidemiology and Infection Control
Emory University School of Medicine and Children's Healthcare of Atlanta
Atlanta, Georgia

PREFACE

Medicine is changing. The advent of paradigm-shifting advances in both hematopoietic stem cell and solid organ transplantation techniques have allowed a greater number of children than ever before to benefit from these lifesaving procedures. The rapid growth of newer chemotherapeutic classes and enhanced immunomodulation targeting innovative cellular pathways have accelerated cancer care and fostered the rapid overall expanse of the number of immunocompromised patients.

These revolutionary advances in immunosuppression come with a cost. Although the primary concern after transplantation or treatment for a malignancy will likely remain failure/relapse of the underlying indication or rejection of the transplant, severe infections in these immunocompromised patients are now a leading cause of death. The tenuous immunologic balance struck to prevent rejection or halt malignancy is always precariously weighed against the profound level of immunosuppression and increased susceptibility to infection seen in these patients. As medicine continues to push what is possible in new approaches to treatments of disease, this balance will only shift further toward greater concerns for infectious complications and mortality. Furthermore, the presentations of these infectious complications will vary as chemotherapeutic regimens and immunomodulation evolve. This ever-changing field requires transplant and oncology infectious disease physicians to stay at the forefront of knowledge for these therapies so that they can anticipate the infectious presentations that will invariably arise from them.

Pediatric medicine is also changing. Presentations of infectious diseases, diagnostic strategies, and treatment paradigms in adults are not always the same as those in children. Children undergoing transplantation and treatment for cancer often are immunologically naïve to important pathogens associated with infections in these populations and may not be old enough to have received their full complement of protective immunizations by the time that they are receiving care for these conditions. Children are also much more likely than adults to develop community-acquired viral and bacterial infections and are prone to more clinically significant disease. Treatments that are approved for the care of infections in adults may not have been approved or even studied in the pediatric population.

This textbook serves as the first edition dedicated toward the goal of elevating the subfield of pediatric transplant and oncology infectious diseases. The authors of each chapter were deliberately selected from a worldwide cadre of investigators and clinicians actively deciphering the mechanisms of disease and developing the latest approaches to optimal pediatric care.

William J. Steinbach, MD
Michael D. Green, MD, MPH
Marian G. Michaels, MD, MPH
Lara A. Danziger-Isakov, MD, MPH
Brian T. Fisher, DO, MPH, MSCE

FOREWORD

Today we recognize the importance of fever in a patient with neutropenia, whether the consequence of cytotoxic chemotherapy for cancer or a transplantation regimen, as the sign of a potentially life-threatening infection that prompts the need for immediate empiric broad-spectrum antibiotic therapy. This practice tracks back to the still seminal study that Gerry Bodey and colleagues reported in 1966 associating profound and prolonged neutropenia with the risk of infection.[1] During the past several decades, the numbers of patients at risk for fever and neutropenia have continued to increase, first with increasingly intensive combinations of cytotoxic chemotherapy regimens for leukemias and lymphomas and then for the solid tumors. The first bone marrow transplantation was performed in 1968, spawning the field of allogeneic, autologous, and now stem cell–based transplantation regimens. An additional risk group included solid organ transplantations (including kidney transplant and liver, heart, lung, and intestine). These patients also experience neutropenia and joined the ranks of immunocompromised hosts.[2] Many of these patients also had other alterations in the cellular and humoral immune system that made them vulnerable to a plethora of viral infections—especially herpesviruses such as HSV, CMV, VZV, EBV and HHV6, as well as respiratory and other infections. Serious infections with opportunistic fungi also emerged as important causes of infection, particularly in patients with prolonged neutropenia.

The treatment of childhood malignancies has improved dramatically over the past several decades, with survival rates approaching 90%.[3] That said, episodes of chemotherapy-related fever and neutropenia remain an important complication of these otherwise successful treatment regimens. Despite the overall success of the treatment of childhood cancer, the "holy grail" has always been the hope for more selective and specific cancer treatments that would not result in a compromised immune system and a heightened risk for infection; progress has been made with the development of tyrosine kinase inhibitors as well as other small molecules, monoclonal antibodies, and more recently, an expanding repertoire of immunotherapeutics (including checkpoint inhibitors, CAR-T cells), although some of these also result in a perturbation of the host's microbiome or other unique risks for infection.[4-6]

Cytotoxic therapy also results in alterations in humoral and cellular and innate immunity, breaches of the mucosal cutaneous barriers (including those related to IV catheters), and changes in the microbiome, and other changes in the host defense matrix.

Our understanding of the normal and abnormal immune system has become increasingly more sophisticated, aided by knowledge from other compromised hosts, especially those with HIV/AIDS. This was further refined by the elucidation of immune networks, including the delineation of the role of T-helper, suppressor, and regulatory cells, phagocytes, dendritic cells, mast cells and basophils, natural killer cells, and various cytokines and interleukins, interferons, and innate immune function receptors, along with genetically defined alterations that further define the risk for infection.

Nearly 80% of the microorganisms associated with infection in the febrile neutropenic patient arise from the endogenous microbial flora, highlighting the balance between aerobic and anaerobic organisms that presaged the evolving understanding of the microbiome and its role in the risk for infection as well as in modulation of host defenses, including the risk for graft-versus-host disease.[7,8] The gut microflora is increasingly recognized as a complex microenvironment, and anaerobes are essential in inhibiting adherence of new aerobes by altering metabolism and nutrient availability and by producing inhibitory toxins and fatty acids. Studies in germ-free mice also foreshadowed the relationship of the microbial flora with the immune system and prospect of graft-versus-host disease and with the response to various checkpoint inhibitors, awareness that the gut flora and microbiome can be associated with response to immunotherapy. There are also increasing data that the gut microbiome can affect the response to chemotherapy, including stem cell therapy, as well as modulate the immune system.[9]

Commensal organisms within the lumen of the gut also have profound influences on the immune system at the local level within the gut mucosa, both in draining mesenteric lymph nodes and systemically.[10] Some bacterial metabolites can enter the bloodstream directly, further altering the systemic immune system and thus altering granulopoiesis.[11] Indeed, dysbiosis in the setting of hematopoietic stem cell transplantation has been associated with differences in long-term survival, whereby individuals with lower diversity in microbiota have shortened survival and higher mortality rates compared with those with higher diversity.

Within this broad context it is also important to be cognizant of the changes in the patterns of infection that have occurred over the past decades. Gram-positive and gram-negative aerobic bacteria continue to play an important role in the infectious complications associated with immunosuppressive therapies, although the predominant organisms have varied over time and can also be institution specific. Although anaerobes remain infrequent causes of primary infection, they can be associated with mixed infections (especially cellulitis and fasciitis and perianal infections), although some, like *Clostridium septicum*, can also cause serious infections in neutropenic patients, even in the absence of fever. Important nosocomial infections—including *C. difficile*—occur within hospital settings as a consequence of antibiotics or certain chemotherapy agents that alter the microbial flora in the gastrointestinal tract and that are transmitted as the consequence of poor hand hygiene.

In addition to bacteria, fungi, viruses, and parasites are also causes of infection in immunocompromised hosts. Among the fungi, *Candida, Aspergillus, Mucor, Trichosporon, Fusarium, Scedosporium*, dematiaceous molds, and others are important, although they are still difficult to diagnose as causes of primary and secondary infections.[12-17] Fungal organisms are either endogenous (like *Candida*) or acquired fungi, like *Aspergillus*, mucorales, and others.[12,13]

Viruses are also important causes of infection in immunocompromised patients and have received increased recognition as primary or secondary causes of infection as diagnostic tools have improved. Among these are respiratory viruses, including influenza, parainfluenza, RSV, coronavirus, human metapneumovirus, and rhinovirus. Adenovirus has been a particularly serious cause of infection.[18,19] It is also important to note that co-infections with respiratory viruses and invasive fungal infections have been described.[20] Also important are the herpesviruses, from herpes simplex to varicella zoster, HSV-6, EBV, and CMV. The latter has been notable in having different presentations in different settings, especially in the early days of allogeneic bone marrow transplantation but also in HIV/AIDS.

Changes in diagnostic tools, from culture and Gram stain to sequencing and molecular diagnosis, along with various potential markers of infection, have been pursued over the years, although reliable predictive tools still require development.

Treatment options have also improved with the availability of new classes of antimicrobials. The principles of empiric, prophylactic, and therapeutic antimicrobial management have also continued to evolve as the result of single- and multiple-institution clinical trials.

The management of infectious complications in cancer and transplant patients requires a broad and deep knowledge of infectious diseases, immunology, chemotherapy, transplantation biology, and more. Thankfully, Bill Steinbach, Mike Green, Marian Michaels, Lara Danziger-Isakov, and Brian Fisher have assembled a comprehensive resource that addresses the rapidly evolving changes in this field in a science-based as well as a practical and accessible resource. Their book, *Pediatric Transplant and Oncology Infectious Diseases,* is a truly authoritative resource and guide for infectious disease, oncology, and transplantation providers and trainees.

Philip A. Pizzo, MD
David and Susan Heckerman Professor of
Pediatrics and of Microbiology and Immunology and
Former Dean, Stanford University School of Medicine and
Founding Director, Stanford Distinguished Careers Institute
Stanford University
Palo Alto, California

REFERENCES

1. Bodey GP, Buckley M, Sathe YS, Freireich EJ. Quantitative relationships between circulating leukocytes and infection in patients with acute leukemia. *Ann Intern Med.* 1966;64(2):328-340.
2. Rubin RH, Schaffner A, Speich R. Introduction to the Immunocompromised Host Society consensus conference on epidemiology, prevention, diagnosis, and management of infections in solid-organ transplant patients. *Clin Infect Dis.* 2001;33(suppl 1):S1-S4.
3. Hunger SP, Mullighan CG. Acute lymphoblastic leukemia in children. *N Engl J Med.* 2015;373(16):1541-1552.
4. Junc CH, Sadelain M. Chimeric antigen receptor therapy. *N Engl J Med.* 2018;379(1):64-73.
5. Druker BJ, Talpaz M, Resta DJ, et al. Efficacy and safety of a specific inhibitor of the BCR-ABL tyrosine kinase in chronic myeloid leukemia. *N Engl J Med.* 2001;344(14):1031-1037.
6. Longo DL. Imatinib changed everything. *N Engl J Med.* 2017;376(10): 982-983.
7. Kramer BS, Pizzo PA, Robichaud KJ, Witesbsky F, Wesley R. Role of serial microbiologic surveillance and clinical evaluation in the management of cancer patients with fever and granulocytopenia. *Am J Med.* 1982;72(4): 561-568.
8. Schimpff SC, Young VM, Greene WH, Vermeulen GD, Moody MR, Wiernik PH. Origin of infection in acute nonlymphocytic leukemia. Significance of hospital acquisition of potential pathogens. *Ann Intern Med.* 1972;77(5):707-714.
9. Gopalakrishnan V, Helmink BA, Spencer CN, Reuben A, Wargo JA. The influence of the gut microbiome on cancer, immunity, and cancer immunotherapy. *Cancer Cell.* 2018;33(4):570-580.
10. Koh AY. The microbiome in hematopoietic stem cell transplant recipients and cancer patients: opportunities for clinical advances that reduce infection. *PLoS Pathog.* 2017;13(6):e1006342.
11. Salva S, Alvarez S. The role of microbiota and immunobiotics in granulopoiesis of immunocompromised hosts. *Front Immunol.* 2017;8:507.
12. Arif S, Perfect JR. Emergence of the molds other than Aspergillus in immunocompromised patients. *Clin Chest Med.* 2017;38(3):555-573.
13. Ascioglu S, Rex JH, de Pauw B, et al. Defining opportunistic invasive fungal infections in immunocompromised patients with cancer and hematopoietic stem cell transplants: an international consensus. *Clin Infect Dis.* 2002;34(1):7-14.
14. Farmakiotis D, Kontoyiannis DP. Mucormycoses. *Infect Dis Clin North Am.* 2016;30(1):143-163.
15. Luplertlop N. *Pseudallescheria/Scedosporium* complex species: from saprobic to pathogenic fungus. *J Mycol Med.* 2018;28(2):249-256.
16. Polvi EJ, Li X, O'Meara TR, Leach MD, Cowen LE. Opportunistic yeast pathogens: reservoirs, virulence mechanisms, and therapeutic strategies. *Cell Mol Life Sci.* 2015;72(12):2261-2287.
17. Walsh TJ, Groll AH. Emerging fungal pathogens: evolving challenges to immunocompromised patients for the twenty-first century. *Transpl Infect Dis.* 1999;1(4):247-261.
18. Khanal S, Ghimire P, Dhamoon AS. The repertoire of adenovirus in human disease: the innocuous to the deadly. *Biomedicines.* 2018;6(1). doi:10.3390/biomedicines6010030.
19. Tebruegge M, Curtis N. Adenovirus: an overview for pediatric infectious diseases specialists. *Pediatr Infect Dis J.* 2012;31(6):626-627.
20. Shah MM, Hsiao EI, Kirsch CM, Gohil A, Narasimhan S, Stevens DA. Invasive pulmonary aspergillosis and influenza co-infection in immunocompetent hosts: case reports and review of the literature. *Diagn Microbiol Infect Dis.* 2018;91(2):147-152.

CONTENTS

SECTION 1 General Immunocompromised Host Infection Principles

1 **The Surgical and Immunosuppressive Basis for Infections in the Pediatric Solid Organ Transplant Recipient,** 1
Yeh-Chung Chang, MD, MSCE and Andrew Barbas, MD

2 **Immunologic Recovery and Basis for Infections in the Pediatric Hematopoietic Stem Cell Transplant Recipient,** 10
Jasmeen Dara, MD, MS and Christopher C. Dvorak, MD

3 **Cancer and Antineoplastic Therapies and the Risk of Infection in the Pediatric Cancer Patient,** 22
Neil Patel, PharmD, BCOP and Abby Green, MD

SECTION 2 Common Immunocompromised Host Infection Situations

4 **Infectious Disease Evaluation of Infants and Children Awaiting Solid Organ or Hematopoietic Stem Cell Transplant,** 34
Rebecca Pellett Madan, MD, MS and Lara A. Danziger-Isakov, MD, MPH

5 **Donor Screening and Donor-Derived Infections,** 40
Marian G. Michaels, MD, MPH and Michael D. Green, MD, MPH

6 **Prevention of Infections in the Hematopoietic Stem Cell Transplant Recipient,** 46
Gabriela M. Marón Alfaro, MD, MS and Hayley A. Gans, MD

7 **Prevention of Infections in the Solid Organ Transplantation Recipient,** 54
Michele Estabrook, MD and Monica I. Ardura, DO, MSCS

8 **Management Principles for Patients With Neutropenia,** 56
Brian T. Fisher, DO, MPH, MSCE and Lillian Sung, MD, PhD

9 **Vaccination Issues for Transplantation and Chemotherapy,** 63
Klara M. Posfay-Barbe, MD, MS and Natasha Halasa, MD, MPH

10 **Microbiome Implications in Transplantation and Oncology,** 71
Matthew S. Kelly, MD, MPH and Michael A. Silverman, MD, PhD

11 **Antimicrobial Stewardship in Immunocompromised Hosts,** 78
Joshua Wolf, MBBS, PhD, FRACP, Jeffrey S. Gerber, MD, PhD, and Michael J. Smith, MD, MSCE

12 **Hospital Infection Prevention for Pediatric Transplant Recipients and Oncology Patients,** 82
Ibukunoluwa C. Akinboyo, MD and Dawn Nolt, MD, MPH

13 **Safe Living After Transplantation or Chemotherapy,** 90
Blanca E. Gonzalez, MD and Marian G. Michaels, MD, MPH

SECTION 3 Specific Infections in Transplant Recipients and Oncology Patients

14 **Multidrug-Resistant Gram-Negative Infections in Transplant and Oncology Patients,** 97
Mehreen Arshad, MBBS, Andrew Nowalk, MD, PhD, and Pranita D. Tamma, MD, MHS

15 ***Bartonella, Legionella, Mycoplasma,* and *Ureaplasma,*** 103
Daniel Dulek, MD and Victoria A. Statler, MD, MSc

16 **Nontuberculous and Tuberculous *Mycobacterium,*** 109
Flor M. Munoz, MD, MSc and Philana Ling Lin, MD, MSc

17 **Cytomegalovirus,** 118
Lara A. Danziger-Isakov, MD, MPH and Tanvi Sharma, MD, MPH

18 **Epstein-Barr Virus and Posttransplant Lymphoproliferative Disorder,** 126
Michael D. Green, MD, MPH, Thomas Gross, Jr., MD, PhD, and Upton D. Allen, MBBS

19 **Herpes Simplex and Varicella-Zoster Viruses,** 134
William J. Muller, MD, PhD and Betsy C. Herold, MD

20 **Human Herpesvirus 6, 7, and 8,** 142
Debra J. Lugo, MD and Danielle M. Zerr, MD, MPH

21 **Respiratory Viruses,** 148
Alpana Waghmare, MD and Janet A. Englund, MD

22 **Adenoviruses,** 155
Diana F. Florescu, MD and Erica J. Stohs, MD, MPH

23 **BK and Other Polyomavirus Associated Diseases in Children,** 162
Benjamin L. Laskin, MD, MSc and Hans H. Hirsch, MD, MSc

24 **Aspergillosis,** 170
William J. Steinbach, MD

25 **Mucormycosis, Fusariosis, Scedosporiasis, and Other Invasive Mold Diseases,** 181
Rachel L. Wattier, MD, MHS and William J. Steinbach, MD

26 **Candidiasis,** 195
Jennifer E. Schuster, MD, MSCI and Brian T. Fisher, DO, MPH, MSCE

27 **Cryptococcosis and Other Rare Invasive Yeasts Infections,** 206
Philip Lee, PharmD and David L. Goldman, MD

28 **Histoplasmosis, Blastomycosis, and Coccidioidomycosis,** 214
John C. Christenson, MD and Thomas G. Fox, MD

29 ***Toxoplasma gondii,*** 227
Sharon F. Chen, MD, MS and Hayley A. Gans, MD

30 ***Nocardia* and *Actinomyces,*** 233
Grant C. Paulsen, MD and Paul K. Sue, MD

31 ***Pneumocystis* Pneumonia,** 241
Catherine Burton, MD, MSc, FRCPC and Benjamin Hanisch, MD

32 ***Strongyloides, Cryptosporidium,* and Other Parasitic Infections,** 247
Ivan A. Gonzalez, MD, MSc and Terri Stillwell, MD, MPH

33 **Gastrointestinal Viruses,** 253
Inci Yildirim, MD, PhD, MSc and Elizabeth Doby Knackstedt, MD

34 ***Clostridioides difficile* Infection,** 258
Erick F. Mayer Arispe, MD, MSc and Andi L. Shane, MD, MPH, MSc

Index, 263

1

The Surgical and Immunosuppressive Basis for Infections in the Pediatric Solid Organ Transplant Recipient

Yeh-Chung Chang, MD, MSCE and Andrew Barbas, MD

Balanced immunosuppression is essential to ensure acceptance of a solid organ transplant and an overall successful patient outcome. The fundamental purpose of immunosuppression is to modulate the immune system's ability to recognize the transplanted organ. However, an overly suppressed immune system increases the risk of certain infections in pediatric solid organ transplant recipients. The goal of balanced immunosuppression is to carefully walk the fine line between too little immunosuppression, which predisposes patients to organ rejection, and too much immunosuppression, which predisposes patients to opportunistic infections.

Although the focus on immunosuppression and its link to infection is warranted, there are other risk factors for infection in pediatric solid organ transplant recipients. Before transplant these may be similar between children and adults. Chronic disease alone is a key risk factor. Potential transplant recipients may undergo multiple rounds of antibiotic treatment for pneumonia, cholangitis, peritonitis, and urinary tract infection, thus increasing their chances of an antibiotic-resistant or opportunistic pathogen. Many potential recipients may also need hospitalization, thus increasing their exposure to multiple types of infections. Transplant candidates are often dependent on the use of central venous catheters, peritoneal dialysis catheters, hemodialysis catheters, ventricular assist devices or extracorporeal membrane oxygenation, all of which increase the risk of systemic invasion by various microorganisms.

Sources of infection after transplant broadly include donor-derived infections, infections acquired perioperatively, reactivation of latent infections, and other infections acquired throughout the patient's lifetime after transplantation, when there is the added effect of immunosuppressive medications. Postoperatively, poor wound healing is common, and there may be open chests or open abdomens that increase infection risk.

There are also unique issues in pediatric solid organ transplant recipients that contribute to the overall risk of infection. Pediatric recipients are more likely to have malnutrition, which can affect normal immune responses. The actual transplant surgical procedure can involve smaller vascular structures, with higher risk of complications (hematoma, thrombosis). The pediatric solid organ transplant recipient is often naïve to numerous infections, as there is less lifetime exposure to infectious agents. Compounding this is the fact that many children cannot complete the full primary immunization series before transplant. All of these factors contribute to an underdeveloped protective immunity. The following sections review the important surgical and immunologic risk factors for infection in more detail, with a focus on pediatric considerations when appropriate.

SURGICAL CONSIDERATIONS

Surgical infections in the pediatric solid organ transplant recipient are an important source of morbidity, particularly in the early period after transplantation. Surgical infections are broadly classified as either superficial or deep surgical site infections. The risk and nature of these infections differ by organ type.

Superficial Surgical Site Infections

Superficial surgical site infections refer primarily to wound infections in the skin from incisions made during the transplant procedure. Most commonly, these are caused by gram-positive organisms that colonize the skin. Antimicrobial prophylaxis administered before skin incision has been proven to reduce the incidence of these infections and has been adopted for transplant procedures.[1] Treatment of typical superficial surgical site infection includes antibiotic therapy with coverage of gram-positive organisms and local wound care. Local wound care may include exploration of any areas of induration and redness, which may harbor purulent drainage in the subcutaneous space. If such areas are found, treatment consists of reopening the skin and subcutaneous tissue, evacuating the subcutaneous fluid collection, sending any diagnostic samples for microbiologic cultures, and leaving the wound open to heal by secondary intention (granulation from the subcutaneous layer upward). Local wound care thereafter typically includes wet-to-dry dressing changes or the application of a negative-pressure dressing (wound vacuum-assisted closure).

Necrotizing wound infections represent a rare but severe form of wound infection that must be diagnosed and treated expeditiously, particularly in immunosuppressed individuals. These severe necrotizing infections are commonly polymicrobial, but can also be caused by group A *Streptococcus* and clostridial organisms. Presentation includes severe pain at the surgical site, high fevers, leukocytosis, and electrolyte abnormalities. These infections are characterized by rapid progression along soft tissue planes including fascia. Treatment requires intravenous antibiotic therapy and urgent operative debridement of involved tissues, which typically includes skin, subcutaneous tissue, and deeper fascia.[2]

Deep Surgical Site Infections. Deep surgical site infections occur in body cavities that are exposed during the surgical procedure. Most commonly, these infections are related to the development of fluid collections in these compartments, which are either primarily or secondarily infected. The causes of deep surgical site infections vary by the type of surgical procedure performed and are discussed by organ type. In many cases, catheter-based drainage of these infected fluid collections combined with antimicrobial therapy allows prompt resolution, but in some cases surgical debridement and drainage is required.

Heart transplantation. The most common deep space infection after heart transplantation is mediastinitis, which is characterized by a deep infection of the sternum. The incidence after heart transplantation is 2.5% to 7.5%, and risk factors include younger age (<1 year), epicardial pacing wires, and red blood cell transfusion.[3,4] Mediastinitis is typically a monomicrobial infection, with the most common etiology being both methicillin-sensitive *Staphylococcus aureus* and methicillin-resistant *S. aureus*. Treatment generally requires operative debridement of infected tissues, complex chest closure incorporating soft tissue flaps, and prolonged antimicrobial therapy.

Lung transplantation. After lung transplantation, deep space surgical infections most commonly occur in the pleural space. Fluid and hematoma can accumulate in the pleural space and become secondarily infected, developing into an empyema if the infection progresses. Infected pleural fluid is typically managed with chest tube drainage, but if an empyema develops, surgical debridement and drainage are warranted. The incidence of empyema is approximately 3% to 5% in the lung transplant population and is associated with a significant increase in morbidity and mortality.[5,6]

Kidney transplantation. Deep space infection after kidney transplantation arises from infected fluid collections in the surgical bed. Kidney grafts can be implanted in either an intraperitoneal or retroperitoneal location, depending on the size of the recipient. In younger/smaller recipients, the graft is typically placed in an intraperitoneal location, using the distal aorta and inferior vena cava as sites for vascular inflow and outflow, respectively. In this setting, fluid collections that arise thereafter are located in the peritoneal cavity. Fluid collections may consist of hematoma, lymphatic fluid, or, less commonly, urine from a urine leak between the transplanted ureter and recipient bladder. Most common among these are hematomas, which can serve as a rich source of nutrient media for microorganisms.

In older/larger pediatric recipients, the kidney graft is usually placed in a retroperitoneal position, using the external iliac artery and vein for inflow and outflow, respectively. The retroperitoneal space is a more confined, limited space and is thus usually easier to manage if fluid collections develop. The same types of fluid collections (hematoma, lymphocele, and urinoma) can arise in this space and are typically well managed with percutaneous catheter drainage.

Liver transplantation. Deep space infections after liver transplantation are common and can arise from multiple sources. The formation of a hematoma in the peritoneal cavity is very common after liver transplantation, owing to the coagulopathy that is common in both the pretransplant and early posttransplant period.

Biliary leakage is a primary source of infected fluid collections after liver transplantation. Owing to the relative scarcity of appropriately sized pediatric donors, many pediatric patients receive partial liver grafts consisting of a portion of an adult donor liver, either from a living or deceased donor. The most commonly used partial graft consists of the left-lateral section of an adult donor liver. The biliary drainage from this graft is via the left hepatic duct. Bile leaks can occur from the biliary anastomosis between the graft and a roux-en-Y limb of jejunum. More commonly, bile leaks arise from the cut surface of the liver, where the left-lateral section is divided from the remainder of the donor liver. Fortunately, most of these "cut surface" bile leaks are self-limited and well managed with surgical drains left at the time of transplant.

Multivisceral and intestinal transplantation. Infections in multivisceral and intestinal transplantation are common owing to the intensive induction immunosuppression administered and the exposure to enteric organisms related to bowel anastomosis. A multivisceral transplant typically consists of the donor liver, pancreas, and small intestine, retrieved from the donor as a single unit (en bloc). The vascular inflow for the graft is provided by an aortic conduit arising from the recipient infrarenal aorta, and the vascular outflow for the graft is via the inferior vena cava. In an isolated intestinal graft, the donor intestine is supplied by the superior mesenteric artery and the vascular outflow by the superior mesenteric vein, which are anastomosed to the aorta and inferior vena cava of the recipient, respectively.

Deep space infections after multivisceral or intestinal transplants may arise from enteric contamination or leakage at the sites of bowel anastomosis, most commonly involving gram-negative and anaerobic organisms. In general, two separate enteric anastomoses are required: one proximal and one distal. The proximal enteric anastomosis is usually constructed between the recipient stomach/proximal intestine and the graft jejunum. The distal enteric anastomosis is constructed between the graft ileum (or colon, if it is included) and the recipient colon. A diverting ileostomy is typically created to allow endoscopic access for the protocol biopsies necessary to monitor the intestinal graft for rejection.

The other primary sources of deep space infection after multivisceral or intestinal transplantation are infected hematomas that arise in the postoperative setting, similar to the other solid organ transplants discussed previously.

IMMUNOLOGIC OVERVIEW

COMPONENTS OF THE IMMUNE SYSTEM

There is a complex interplay within the diverse components of the immune system that helps protect hosts from infectious threats and foreign substances.[7,8] The first main component consists of the members of the innate immune system: neutrophils, macrophages, dendritic cells, natural killer cells, complement, and various signals such as cytokines and Toll-like receptors. The innate immune system provides constant surveillance against external pathogens. The second component consists of the acquired, or adaptive, immune system, including T cells and B cells, which help the immune system fine-tune the elimination of specific threats, and contribute to memory and tolerance. The acquired immune system helps regulate the overall immune response. The focus of this section is on alloactivation of the acquired immune system, specifically T and B cells, and related processes. The immune system is extremely intricate, and other immune mechanisms fall outside the scope of this chapter.

T cells are activated through a complex pathway of signals (Fig. 1.1), and more than one signal is required for full activation.[9] The major histocompatibility complex (MHC) on the antigen-presenting cell (APC) brings an antigen that binds to the T-cell receptor, known as signal 1. Additionally, a costimulatory signal, between B7 ligands

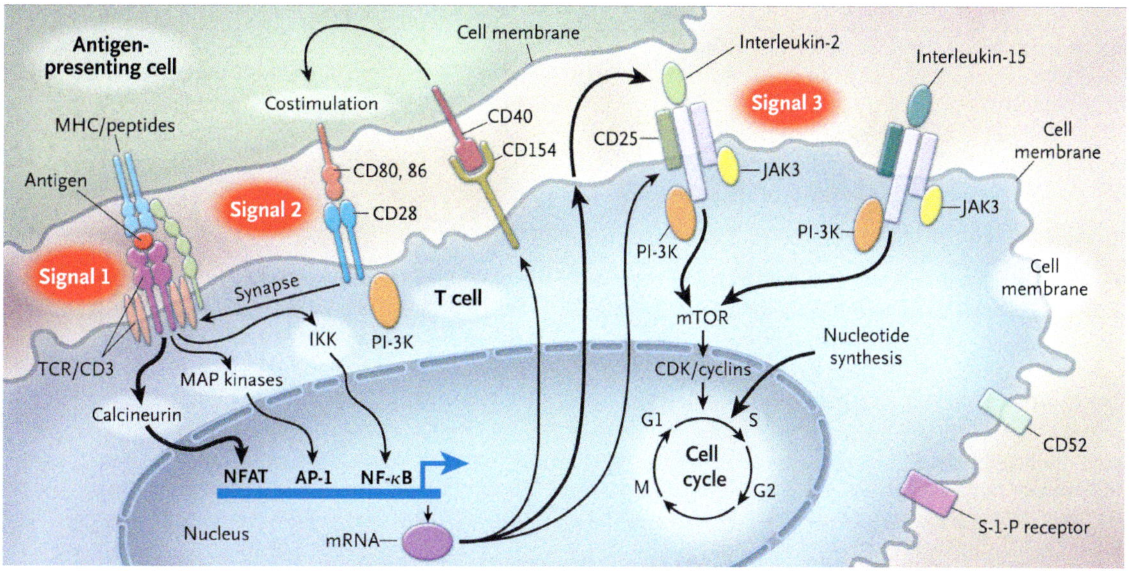

Fig. 1.1 This figure demonstrates the required signals for T-cell activation as well as the mechanistic targets for immunosuppressive agents. (From Halloran PF. Immunosuppressive drugs for kidney transplantation. *N Engl J Med.* 2004;351:2715-2729.)

(B7-1, or CD80; and B7-2, or CD86) on the APC and CD28 on the T-cell represents signal 2.[10] Lastly, an interaction between the cytokine IL-2, and its respective receptor on the T cell is represented by signal 3. The IL-2 receptor is made of three subunits, including alpha (CD25), beta (CD122), and gamma chains.

The normal process by which the host learns to recognize self from nonself includes the use of the MHC. There are two specific types of MHC complexes: class I and class II. Class I MHC is expressed by all nucleated cells and is composed of a polymorphic alpha chain, as defined by human leukocyte antigen (HLA) alleles and a highly conserved monomorphic beta-2 microglobulin chain. Nucleated cells constantly have turnover of their proteins, and the proteasome creates peptides, some of which bind to the MHC complex and are translocated across the cell membrane. The extracellular peptide–MHC is then shown to regulatory CD8 T cells, which are normally able to differentiate peptides that bear the intrinsic signature of the host, versus peptides that would indicate a foreign invader, such as a virus, or a malignant cell. Abnormal cells are then targeted for destruction. HLA alleles associated with the MHC class I complex include A, B, and C. In theory, the rise of polymorphisms in the HLA alleles helps with the immune response to a variety of infections and contributes to fitness on an individual and population level.[11]

The class II MHC complex is present only on APCs, macrophages, dendritic cells, and B cells. The class II MHC complex is bound to extracellular protein and is presented to CD4 T cells, which help potentiate the response to foreign invaders. HLA alleles most commonly associated with the MHC class II complex include DR, DQ, and DP.

Matching based on HLA alleles has been one of the primary strategies to ensure optimal clinical outcomes. Although a perfect match may not always be feasible because of the limited number of organs available or the shortened time frame for transplant, HLA mismatch can lead to increased risk of rejection and increased use of immunosuppressive drug regimens, which ultimately lead to increased risk for infection.

Other components of the immune system are worth mentioning here as they represent targets of current immunosuppressive therapies. Regulatory T cells are important in suppressing effector T-cell function through changing the cytokine makeup, competing for the same costimulatory signals, and directing cell-to-cell signals. Cultivating the work of regulatory T cells is necessary in reaching tolerance of the transplanted organ. B cells are also pivotal in their role in both fighting infection and other foreign agents through the secretion of antibodies and facilitation of opsonization. B cells undergo different types of differentiation; a key example is plasma cells that help produce the various immunoglobulin (antibody) types. Immunoglobulins bind to specific foreign antigens and help facilitate phagocytosis and the creation of immune complexes that neutralize pathogens and activate complement. B cells can also function as APCs, in regulatory roles, and as memory cells. They contribute to the development of rejection and are therefore often targets of immunosuppressive regimens.

Lastly, the role of complement cannot be underestimated.[12] The classic complement pathway is activated when C1q binds to the Fc portion of IgM or IgG, either in an antibody–antigen complex or on the surface of cells. Other pathways that lead to activation of complement include when the serum protein lectin binds to mannose, present on bacteria or viral-infected cells; and when complement spontaneously binds to cells recognized as foreign. The downstream target is the generation of C3b, which helps facilitate both opsonization (phagocytosis) and the creation of the terminal complement complex, which effectively punches holes in the cell membranes of pathogens and foreign cells.

Evolution of the immune system over time. The immune system of neonates and infants in the first year of life is not well developed. The fetal innate and acquired immune system is regulated in utero to better tolerate maternal antigens that may cross the placenta.[13] During the first year of life, although T cells are present, the response skews toward tolerance as the T cells begin to recognize self versus nonself. Although maternal antibodies do provide some immune protection for infants through the first 12 months of life, the weak response of the immune system to external threats leaves neonates and infants at high risk of serious infections. For those in this age group who receive an organ transplant, several considerations have been explored. The benefits of the immature neonatal and infant immune system have led to different strategies. ABO-incompatible liver and heart transplants are now being widely performed in young infants, with comparable results to ABO-matched transplants.[14] Many centers consider lighter immunosuppressive regimens in infants and young children. However, given that immunosuppression is still necessary, when infection occurs in younger patients, it can take longer for acquired immunity mechanisms to recognize foreign invaders and clinical symptoms may be more severe and take longer to resolve. There is also a theoretical risk that the immune system may recognize foreign threats as self during this period, leading to mistaken tolerance.

During the transition from infancy to adulthood, children are constantly bombarded by foreign antigens through inhalation, ingestion, and inoculation. This, in turn, strengthens both innate and acquired immunity. Furthermore, the administration of routine childhood vaccination helps generate robust responses to future potential threats. Children are also exposed to the sharing of diverse antigens in different environments, including day care centers, schools, and at home. During this period children may acquire herpesviruses, such as herpes simplex virus (HSV), cytomegalovirus (CMV), and Epstein-Barr virus (EBV), which stay latent in the host. The adolescent immune system is similar to that of adults and environmental factors continue to play a role in the evolving nature of immune responses in this population.

Fig. 1.2 outlines the common time line of posttransplant infections.[15] Note that donor-derived, typical bacterial and candidal infections tend to occur earlier (at <1 month after transplant), whereas most viral and other fungal infections tend to occur later (1 to 12 months after transplant). Patient-specific and regional epidemiologic risk factors are important considerations in the evaluation of every patient. To combat these different threats, most centers have established regimens of antimicrobial prophylaxis against fungal and viral pathogens stratified by specific age group, type of organ transplant, and donor/recipient serostatus.

REJECTION

One of the most common complications after solid organ transplant is organ rejection. There are different time frames of rejection, including hyperacute, acute, and chronic rejection. There are also many different types of organ rejection based on the arms of the immune system: cell-mediated and humoral. Both cell-mediated and humoral rejection can occur exclusively or simultaneously.[16]

Hyperacute Rejection

Hyperacute rejection occurs in vascularized grafts. The mechanism occurs through the action of antidonor antibodies that are already present in the recipient, leading to thrombosis in blood vessels and graft necrosis. These antibodies can occur in pediatric patients if they have been exposed to blood products or have undergone a previous transplant. Hyperacute rejection happens within minutes to hours after the transplant. Current testing methods for these antibodies include conducting flow, complement-dependent cytotoxicity, and virtual crossmatching before transplant.[17] In these assays, recipient serum is incubated with donor lymphocytes that carry different HLA antigens, and a positive reaction would indicate that there are donor-specific antibodies. Implementation of these screenings before transplant has led to countermeasures that have significantly decreased the incidence of hyperacute rejection.

Acute Rejection

Acute rejection occurs between 1 week and several months after transplant. Traditionally, this rejection has been separated into two categories: acute cellular rejection and acute humoral rejection. There are cases when one type of rejection is more dominant, but both acute cellular and acute humoral rejection can occur at the same time.

Acute cellular or cell-mediated rejection occurs when recipient T cells recognize donor tissue cells as foreign. As $CD8^+$ cytotoxic T cells mature in the host, they begin to recognize foreign antigens in the graft through the class I MHC molecule. The cytotoxic T cells then release perforins and granzyme, which induces apoptosis. Tumor necrosis factor alpha is also secreted by the cytotoxic cells, which then leads to an inflammatory cascade resulting in both upregulated and larger numbers of immune cells at the site of the foreign antigens, leading to injury of the transplanted organ.

Acute humoral rejection is becoming a significant cause of allograft rejection. Some studies have shown that it accounts for 15% to 20% of all rejection during the first year after transplant, especially in sensitized patients.[16] In humoral rejection, the role of B cells is important as they produce donor-specific antibodies and other cytokines, which lead to graft injury. Antibodies can be made to HLA class antigens, minor histocompatibility antigens, ABO antigens, and other non-HLA antigens. The complement system is activated and assists in creating further injury, as demonstrated by positive C4d staining in tissue specimens from affected organs.

The Banff criteria were created in 1991 to help diagnose and grade rejection for kidney transplants. For acute cell-mediated rejection, there is an emphasis on pathologic features, including interstitial inflammation, tubulitis, arteritis, and glomerulonephritis. The standardized criteria for diagnosing humoral rejection have focused on morphologic and immunohistochemical staining of tissue, as well as on serologic evidence of donor-specific antibodies. Subsequent revisions of the Banff criteria have incorporated molecular diagnostics into the diagnosis of antibody-mediated rejection.[18] There are similar guidelines for the diagnosis of T-cell rejection in liver, heart, and lung transplant patients. However, antibody-mediated rejection and intragraft markers vary according to organ type.

The main approach to the treatment of acute cellular rejection consists of high-dose corticosteroids. If the rejection proves refractory to corticosteroids, biologic agents such as anti-thymocyte globulin (ATG) or alemtuzumab (Campath) are used. Humoral or antibody-mediated rejection is difficult to treat. Plasmapheresis, in combination with intravenous immunoglobulin (IVIG), is the first-line treatment and can be followed by other agents, including rituximab, bortezomib, and complement inhibitors such as eculizumab.

Chronic Rejection

Chronic rejection is now one of the leading causes of graft rejection and failure; hyperacute rejection is becoming rarer because of the successful screening of donor-specific antibodies and more sophisticated immunosuppression regimens that have decreased the incidence of acute cellular rejection. A total of 20% of solid organ transplant recipients have graft loss by 5 years, and 50% lose their graft by 10 years after transplant as the result of chronic antibody-mediated rejection.[19] Outcomes have improved following the more advanced treatment of acute rejection, but outcomes of chronic rejection have not changed through out the years. This affects pediatric solid organ transplant recipients as these patients have ongoing morbidities, infections, and the adverse effects of immunosuppressive medications. In addition, many pediatric transplant recipients proceed with another transplant as graft dysfunction progresses, which further increases the risk of infection.

The mechanisms of chronic rejection can include either cellular, humoral, or both processes, but is most commonly antibody-mediated. Different rounds of inflammation stimulate the expansion of memory B and T cells, which then begin to develop de novo donor-specific antibodies. Diagnostic descriptions of chronic rejection vary by organ: chronic allograft nephropathy or interstitial fibrosis/tubular atrophy in kidney transplants, cardiac allograft vasculopathy in heart

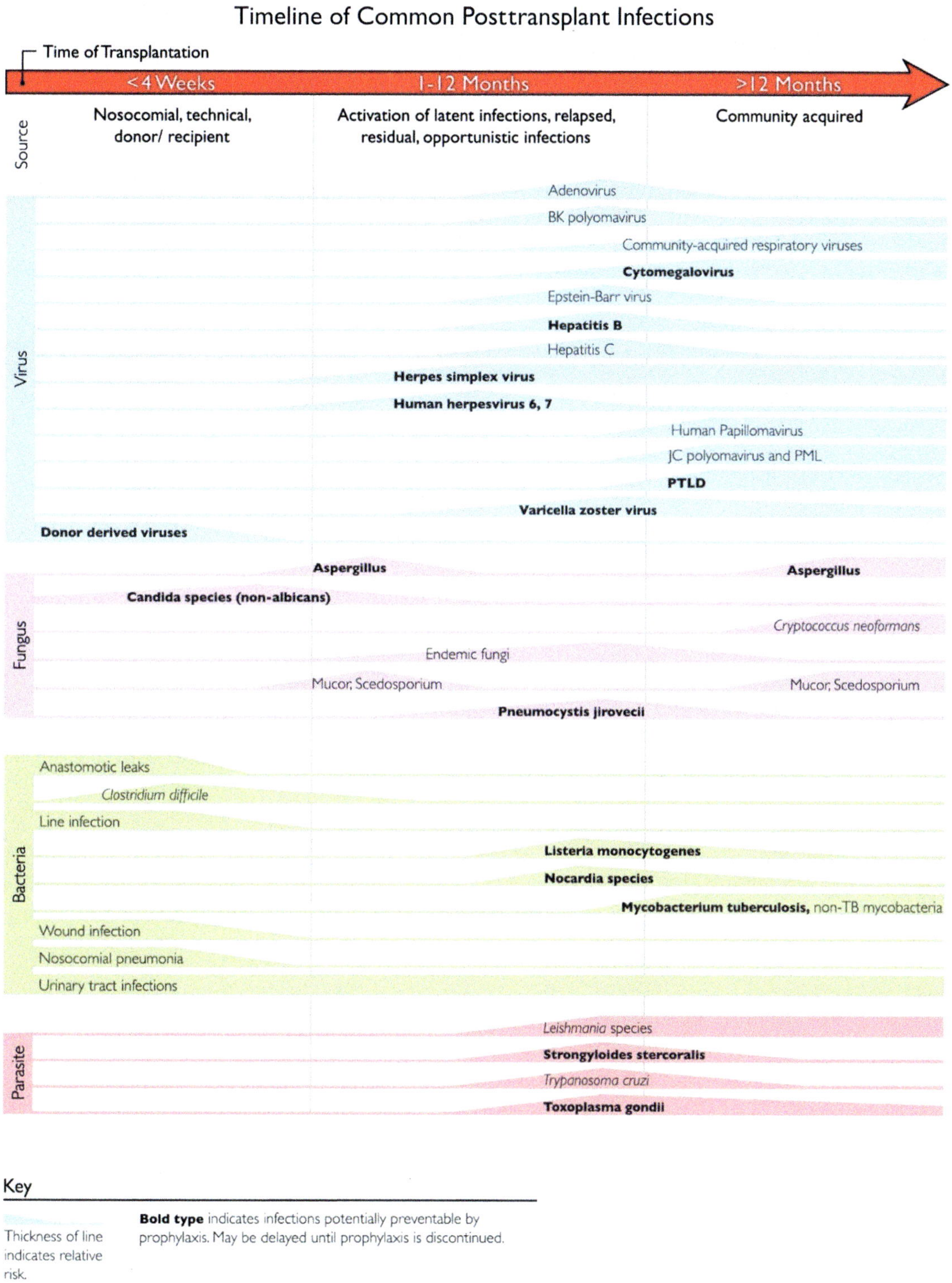

Fig. 1.2 This figure summarizes the normal timeline of infections in solid organ transplants. Increased thickness of lines denotes higher risk. (From Fishman JA, Avery RK. *Chapter 94: Late Infectious Disease After Organ Transplantation in Textbook of Organ Transplantation.* 1st edn. New York: John Wiley and Sons; 2014.)

transplants, bronchiolitis obliterans in lung transplants, and obliterative arteriopathy or interstitial fibrosis in liver transplants. It is thought that risk factors for chronic rejection include young age at the time of transplant, frequent infections, trauma, prior episodes of acute rejection, and medication nonadherence.[20] Complement is often not involved in this process, and C4d staining is negative in the tissue.[21] The long, indolent course of chronic rejection makes timely diagnosis of chronic rejection difficult. Many centers continue to screen transplant patients for donor-specific antibodies, but there is no universally accepted approach. More importantly, better therapies and further research are needed for chronic rejection as it remains difficult to treat.

CURRENT OUTCOMES

There is a fine balance between immunosuppression and infection in pediatric solid organ transplant patients. Overall, graft survival has increased over time as more immunosuppressive agents are now available and regimens are being optimized. There is some variation in clinical outcomes across the different types of organ transplants given distinct practices in immunosuppression. Nevertheless, infections remain a common complication in all pediatric solid organ transplants.

In pediatric kidney transplants, 10-year rates of patient and graft survival have reached 90.5% and 60.2%, respectively. There has been a significant improvement in early outcomes but limited improvement in long-term graft survival. Rates of acute rejection have fallen to 23%, but rates of infection remain at 39.6% within the first 2 years after kidney transplant.[22] Patient age younger than 18 years was associated with a higher risk of infection in another study comparing all kidney transplant recipients.[23]

In pediatric liver transplant recipients, using the latest data from the Studies of Pediatric Liver Transplantation (SPLIT) national consortium, patient survival rates at 3, 12, 24, and 36 months were 90.9%, 86.9%, 84.2% and 83.8%, respectively, whereas graft survival rates at 3, 12, 24, and 36 months were 85.5%, 80.2%, 76.0%, and 75.3%, respectively.[24] Rates of rejection at 3, 12, 24, and 36 months were 44.8%, 52.9%, 59.1%, and 60.3%, respectively. In this population, infection accounted for 28.4% of deaths and was a contributing factor in 39% of deaths.[24] Bacterial and fungal infections (not further specified) were the major infections causing death in this study.

Data from the International Society for Heart and Lung Transplantation showed that pediatric heart transplant recipients had a median survival of 22.3 years if they received a transplant in the first year of life, 18.4 years for recipients between 1 and 5 years, 14.4 years for recipients between 6 and 10 years, and 13.1 years for recipients between 11 and 17 years.[25] Rejection during the first year after heart transplant ranged from 22% to 36%, and 5-year incidence rates of rejection reached 48%.[26] Cardiac allograft vasculopathy affected 25% to 34% of patients 10 years after transplant. Infections caused 14% of all deaths in the first year after pediatric heart transplant, with bacterial causes in the early period, transitioning to viral and fungal causes of infection later in the first year after transplant.[25]

The majority of pediatric lung transplants are performed in children between the ages of 11 to 17 years, and combined heart–lung transplant outcomes are integrated into the lung transplant data. Overall median survival is 5.4 years for children after transplant, but if pediatric lung transplant recipients survive past the first year, overall median survival increases to 8.8 years after transplant.[27] Rejection rates at 1 year are 29%, and more than half of patients have bronchiolitis obliterans syndrome by 5 years after transplant. Non-CMV infection was the cause of death of 15.7% of patients at 1 month and 27.6% of patients between 1 and 12 months; this makes non-CMV infection the leading cause of death between 1 and 12 months after transplant in pediatric lung recipients.[27]

Data on pediatric intestinal transplant patients are limited, but for a population of both pediatric and adult intestinal transplants, 1-, 5-, and 10-year survival rates have been 76%, 56%, and 43%, respectively.[28] However, the risk of infection is high in this population, and up to 90% of patients develop a bacterial infection within the first year after transplant, and viral infections such as enteritis, CMV, and EBV infection are extremely common.[29]

IMMUNOSUPPRESSIVE MEDICATIONS

The next section describes the different classes of immunosuppressive medications (Table 1.1). In general, the approach to immunosuppression includes an induction regimen around the time of transplant and a maintenance regimen, with the goal of preventing rejection.

Induction Therapies

The purpose of induction therapy is to provide high-dose immunosuppression early in the post-transplant period to prevent acute rejection. There is no single standard approach to induction immunosuppression across different centers. Regimens may also differ according to type or organ and by patient-specific risk factors. Most commonly, biologic agents that deplete or disable T cells are used, and the effect of these agents can be long lasting. In other cases, induction therapy may consist of high-dose steroids alone.

Biologic Agents. The most commonly used agent for induction therapy is ATG. ATG is a polyclonal agent generated in rabbits (rATG or thymoglobulin) or horses (ATGAM). The antibodies are active against various T-cell markers, including CD2, CD3, CD4, CD8, CD11a, CD18, CD44, CD45, HLA-DR, class I heavy chains, and β_2-microglobulin. Typically after treatment, T-cell depletion results and effects can last for several weeks to months, greatly increasing the risk of infection. There is also risk of major infusion reactions. Many pediatric centers continue to use ATG for their induction regimens, although many other options are now becoming available.

Another agent that results in T-cell depletion is alemtuzumab (Campath), a monoclonal human antibody to CD52. CD52 is found on all T cells, B cells, and macrophages, dendritic cells, eosinophils, and natural killer cells and alemtuzumab causes profound depletion of these cells.[30,31] Effects can be seen up to 1 to 2 years after administration and, similar to ATG, alemtuzumab generates a high and prolonged risk of infection. Use of alemtuzumab shows a trend toward decreasing acute rejection, and reasons to use alemtuzumab include pursuing avoidance or early withdrawal of steroids and reducing calcineurin inhibitor (CNI) use.

The T-cell–depleting biologic agents (ATG and alemtuzumab) all have potential infectious and noninfectious adverse effects. The most common noninfectious adverse effects include early side effects, such as fever, chills, rash, and hypotension. Longer-term effects include the increased risk for infection, as well as potential for malignancy. Intense T-cell depletion significantly increases the risk of viral reactivation, including CMV, EBV, HSV, varicella, and polyomaviruses (such as BK virus), hepatitis B, and hepatitis C. These agents also predispose patients to increased risk of severe and prolonged infection with other viral agents such as respiratory viruses. Lastly, there is also an increased risk of fungal infections, including *Candida* species, endemic mycoses (*Histoplasma capsulatum, Blastomyces dermatitidis,* and *Coccidioides immitis*), and *Pneumocystis jirovecii*.

Basiliximab (Simulect) is a CD25 inhibitor that blocks the costimulatory signal through interleukin (IL)-2. CD25 is expressed only by activated T cells. Thus, use of basiliximab represents a more targeted approach without causing full T-cell depletion. Basiliximab is being used in both pediatric kidney and liver transplant patients. There have been conflicting data regarding its efficacy in pediatric patients, with one small study showing no difference between basiliximab and placebo,[32] and another study showing a comparable effect between basiliximab and ATG.[33] Basiliximab does not cause as much T-cell depletion as ATG or alemtuzumab and therefore has a more favorable safety profile with decreased infection risk. However, there is still an association with higher risk of herpesvirus infections including CMV and HSV.

Corticosteroids. Corticosteroids have been used in both induction and maintenance therapy and are also heavily used in the treatment of

TABLE 1.1 Summary of Immunosuppressive Medications

Category	Medication	Target	Common Adverse Effects
Induction			
Biologic agents	Anti-thymocyte globulin (ATG, rATG, ATGAM)	T cell markers	Fever, rash, leukopenia High risk of viral and fungal infections
	Alemtuzumab	CD52	Fever, leukopenia High risk of viral and fungal infections
	Basiliximab	CD25	Gastrointestinal side effects, fever, hypersensitivity (rarely)
Maintenance	Corticosteroids	Glucocorticoid receptors	Hypertension, peptic ulcers, osteoporosis, hyperglycemia, behavioral changes, poor wound healing High risk of viral and fungal infections, especially with high dose and prolonged use
Calcineurin inhibitors	Tacrolimus	FK binding proteins	Hypertension, nephrotoxicity, alopecia, leukopenia, neuropathy
	Cyclosporine	Cyclophilins	Gingival hyperplasia, hypertension, nephrotoxicity, hyperglycemia, neuropathy
mTOR inhibitors	Sirolimus	mTOR	Gastrointestinal effects, leukopenia, anemia, thrombocytopenia, hypertriglyceridemia, mouth sores
	Everolimus	mTOR	Gastrointestinal effects, leukopenia, anemia, thrombocytopenia, hypertriglyceridemia, mouth sores
Antimetabolite	Mycophenolate mofetil	Inosine monophosphate dehydrogenase	Bone marrow suppression, gastrointestinal side effects
	Azathioprine	DNA replication, purine synthesis	Bone marrow suppression, gastrointestinal side effects, pancreatitis
Biologic agents	Belatacept	CD80, CD86	Hypertension, diarrhea, edema
Rejection	Rituximab	CD20	Fever, hypersensitivity, lymphopenia, infection
	Bortezomib	Proteasome	Fever, gastrointestinal side effects, peripheral neuropathy
	Eculizumab	C5	Hypertension, tachycardia, cough, gastrointestinal side effects, infection (*Neisseria* species)

ATG, anti-thymocyte globulin; *ATGAM*, horse ATG; *mTOR*, mammalian target of rapamycin *rATG*, rabbit ATG.

rejection. They have both antiinflammatory and immunosuppressive effects. The mechanism of action is mediated through binding to cytoplasmic glucocorticoid receptors, which then translocate to the cell nucleus to affect the transcription of various genes, including the nuclear activating factor family.[34] This then leads to decreased production of cytokines, including IL-1, IL-2, interferon gamma, and tumor necrosis factor alpha. Globally, corticosteroids act on the immune system in various ways, including inhibiting lymphocyte proliferation and function and impairing the function of phagocytes. Corticosteroids are thus a powerful weapon and can be used to both prevent and treat acute and chronic rejection.

There are many well-known adverse effects of corticosteroids, including hypertension, weight gain, peptic ulcers, acne, hirsutism, stunting of growth, hyperglycemia, adrenal suppression, muscle breakdown, osteoporosis, behavioral changes, and encephalopathy (posterior reversible encephalopathy syndrome).[35] In addition, long-term use of corticosteroids can predispose transplant recipients to infections, including reactivation of latent viruses and fungal infections, such as *Candida* and *Aspergillus* species, endemic mycoses (*Histoplasma*, *Blastomyces*, and *Coccidioides*), and *Pneumocystis jirovecii*. Although these many adverse effects have driven the need to develop corticosteroid-sparing regimens, corticosteroids often remain the mainstay of immunosuppressive regimens after transplant.

Maintenance Therapies

The goal of maintenance immunosuppressive therapy is to prevent both acute and chronic rejection. The effect of maintenance therapy is less pronounced compared with induction therapy, but the effects can be additive over time.

Calcineurin Inhibitors. One of the mainstays of maintenance therapy is the CNIs: tacrolimus and cyclosporine. Tacrolimus, also known as FK506 or fujimycin (Prograf), was discovered in 1987 and is a macrolide that is produced by the fungus *Streptomyces tsukubaensis*. Cyclosporine, a cyclic undecapeptide, was discovered in 1976 and was extracted from the fungus *Tolypocladium inflatum* Gams. Tacrolimus binds to intracellular immunophilin proteins called FK-binding proteins, and cyclosporine binds to cyclophilins. These immunophilin-immunosuppressant complexes then bind to calcineurin, inhibiting its enzymatic activity. Normally, calcineurin dephosphorylates and therefore facilitates nuclear transcription of the transcription factor NF-AT, leading to transcription of multiple cytokines, including IL-2. Therefore, CNIs play a large part in inhibiting T-cell activation, although there is evidence to suggest that there is also inhibition of T-cell proliferation and general function.[36] The use of CNIs has led to increased length of graft survival.

Although CNIs have become a mainstay of immunosuppressive regimens after transplant, they have important systemic adverse effects. Nephrotoxicity was noted early in the use of cyclosporine and tacrolimus. Both CNIs can cause hypertension independent of their effects on the kidney, and both can also affect the bone marrow, leading to myelosuppression and cytopenias. Tacrolimus has also been implicated in the development of diabetes and tremors, more so than cyclosporine. Cyclosporine is more often associated with gingival hyperplasia and hirsutism. Both peripheral and central nervous systems can be affected during use of CNIs, and symptoms can include headaches, peripheral tremors, and at its worst, seizures, altered mental status, and encephalopathy.

In addition, CNIs are metabolized by the cytochrome P450 system. Natural occurring substances in grapefruit juice and other medications, including rifampin and azoles, can affect the metabolism of CNIs. Most protocols require frequent monitoring of serum levels of CNIs to ensure that pediatric patients have therapeutic, but not toxic, levels.

Generally, CNIs contribute less to infection risk compared with T-cell–depleting agents (ATG or alemtuzumab). At baseline, there is a small but modest increase in risk of CMV and BK virus infection with CNIs. However, those patients who are receiving tacrolimus maintenance therapy have lower overall incidence rates of CMV infection compared with other maintenance regimens; this may have more to do with lower rates of rejection, and thus, decreased need for corticosteroids and T-cell–depleting agents.[37] Lastly, although some CNIs possess some intrinsic in vitro activity against some fungal species, the immunosuppressive properties of these agents are more potent and outweigh their antifungal effectiveness.[37]

Mammalian Target of Rapamycin Inhibitors. Mammalian target of rapamycin (mTOR) inhibitors include sirolimus (also known as rapamycin or Rapamune), and everolimus. Sirolimus was isolated in 1972 from the fungus *Streptomyces hygroscopius*. These medications act on the mammalian target of rapamycin or mTOR pathway. mTOR is a serine-threonine kinase and forms complexes mTORC1 and mTORC2, which eventually lead to signals that control protein synthesis, cell cycle progression, cell growth, and proliferation.[38] The mTOR inhibitors lead to inhibition of T-cell proliferation and a deadened response to cytokines, such as IL-2.

Major adverse effects include stomatitis, diarrhea, cytopenias, lymphocele, poor wound healing, hypertension, rash, and interstitial lung disease. Like CNIs, mTOR inhibitors are also metabolized by the cytochrome system and drug levels are affected by other medications including azoles and rifampin. Therapeutic drug monitoring is usually advised for this class of immunosuppression.

It is often difficult to isolate the infectious risks of mTOR inhibitors as they are often used with other forms of immunosuppression. There is a trend toward a higher risk of HSV infection. Although some studies show that mTOR inhibitors are associated with a decreased risk of CMV or EBV infection, other studies do not show a significant difference.[39]

Antimetabolites. Major antimetabolite agents include mycophenolate mofetil (MMF or CellCept) and azathioprine (Imuran). MMF is the prodrug for mycophenolic acid, which inhibits inosine monophosphate dehydrogenase. This affects de novo guanosine synthesis. B and T lymphocytes are more affected than other cells because activated lymphocytes rely on a special isoform of inosine monophosphate dehydrogenase that has an increased affinity for mycophenolic acid. This leads to a cytostatic effect. The most common adverse effects are located in the gastrointestinal tract (up to 40% to 50%), but there can be leukopenia and neutropenia as well.[40] Azathioprine is one of the oldest immunosuppressive agents still in use in solid organ transplantation today. It was synthesized in 1957 as a 6-mercaptopurine prodrug. Once activated, azathioprine then terminates DNA synthesis by incorporating itself into actively replicating DNA strands, leading to breakage of the helix. It can also masquerade as inosine monophosphate and inhibit de novo purine synthesis. Major adverse effects of azathioprine include nausea, vomiting, diarrhea, cytopenias, rashes, and hair loss.[41] There is also some concern that both MMF and azathioprine increase risk of malignancy (lymphomas, skin cancer).

MMF has been linked to decreased rates of rejection and increased rates of graft survival compared with azathioprine. However, MMF has also been associated with increased rates of CMV, varicella, and BK virus infection. The association with BK virus infection is less clear as MMF is often used in concert with tacrolimus in the kidney transplant population, and it is difficult to distinguish the role of MMF versus the role of tacrolimus in BK infection.[42]

Biologic Agents. Belatacept (Nulojix) is composed of a recombinant cytotoxic T-lymphocyte antigen-4 (CTLA-4) linked to a modified Fc portion of human immunglobulin (IG) G1. The CTLA-4 then binds to CD80 and CD86, which prevents the interaction of CD80 and CD86 with CD28 on T cells, thus inhibiting one of the costimulatory signals. Most of the available data for belatacept have been derived from adults. One study showed similar efficacy between belatacept and current CNI regimens in terms of patient and graft survival, and there were improved cardiovascular and metabolic outcomes.[43] However, in this study, there was also a higher incidence of posttransplant lymphoproliferative disorder (PTLD), especially in EBV-seronegative patients. Other combinations of belatacept have been used, including in conjunction with alemtuzumab and sirolimus to use both a steroid and CNI-sparing regimen, and results have been comparable to current standard regimens.[44] This is a promising medication for adolescents as it can be used only in EBV IgG–positive patients and is associated with increased adherence to CNI regimens. The goal of belatacept use is to try to preserve renal function over time. Additional benefits include reduction of donor-specific antibodies and minimization/avoidance of steroids.

Standard Approach to Maintenance Therapy. Most current maintenance immunosuppressive regimens immediately after transplant include a CNI paired with an antimetabolite. A corticosteroid is often used initially and is tapered off slowly. As the patient becomes further removed from transplant and if there are no episodes of rejection, immunosuppression is slowly decreased over time. There have been some rare reports of achieving tolerance and lifting of all immunosuppressive agents, but currently most pediatric solid organ transplant recipients continue their immunosuppression into adulthood.

Rejection Therapies

Therapies used in rejection include corticosteroids, ATG, alemtuzumab as previous mentioned, as well as rituximab, bortezomib, eculizumab, and plasmapheresis in conjunction with intravenous immunoglobulin.

Biologic Agents. Rituximab (Rituxan) is an anti-CD20 chimeric monoclonal antibody that results in depletion of B lymphocytes. The goal of this therapy is to decrease the production of donor-specific antibodies. The main adverse effects of rituximab include infusion reactions (fevers, chills, hypotension, bronchospasm) and the loss of humoral immunity. Rituximab has been shown to help treat acute antibody-mediated rejection, and PTLD, but data in the treatment of chronic rejection in pediatric patients are lacking.[45] A myriad of infections have been seen in transplant recipients who have received rituximab, including a variety of bacterial infections, viral infections (hepatitis B, BK virus), and *Pneumocystis* pneumonia.

Bortezomib is a proteasome inhibitor that was originally approved for treatment of multiple myeloma and has a targeted effect on B lymphocytes. Initial studies seemed promising, but one recent trial did not show any improvement in late antibody mediated rejection.[46] Bortezomib has been associated with increased risk of HSV and varicella infection.

Eculizumab is a human monoclonal antibody against C5, which helps temper the complement cascade. Eculizumab has been used to treat refractory antibody-mediated rejection in both kidney and pediatric liver transplant patients.[47,48] It has also been used to prevent acute rejection in highly sensitized or ABO-incompatible transplants, but there have been a few breakthrough episodes of rejection. Lastly, eculizumab is helpful for treatment of thrombotic microangiopathy or atypical hemolytic uremic syndrome, which can occur after transplant. Given its effect on the complement system, use of eculizumab increases the risk of meningococcal infection. It is highly recommended that patients should be vaccinated with both meningococcal ACWY and meningococcal B vaccines before eculizumab administration. Because of reports of breakthrough meningococcal infection despite administration of all available meningococcal vaccinations, many centers also provide antibacterial prophylaxis (amoxicillin) in addition to vaccination when patients receive eculizumab, although this practice is not standardized.

Other Therapies. Other therapies include plasmapheresis and IVIG. The goal of plasmapheresis, or plasma exchange, is to draw off donor-specific antibodies, immune complexes, and activated complement factors, which helps limit the ongoing inflammatory cascade of injury. Multiple treatments are often required. IVIG provides antiinflammatory and immunosuppressive effects and also provides some humoral protection for the patient.

Standard Approach to Rejection Therapy. Before treatment of rejection, it is best to diagnose the type of rejection, which is best done through tissue biopsy. The standard approach to therapy is to start with high-dose corticosteroids. Other therapies (ATG, alemtuzumab, rituximab, plasmapheresis, IVIG) are added as necessary according to the type and severity of rejection and whether there is a lack of response to corticosteroid monotherapy. The amount of immunosuppression and cumulative effect of rejection therapy should prompt intensified monitoring of latent infections and consideration of antiviral and anti-*Pneumocystis* prophylaxis.

New Therapies. There have been many other therapies in various stages of development and trials.[49] FK778 (manitimus) is a derivative of a leflunomide metabolite and acts to inhibit de novo pyrimidine synthesis by acting on tyrosine kinase. However, trials have not been convincing enough to move its development forward. Tofacitinib is an oral Janus kinase 3 inhibitor that could prevent acute rejection, but it had a high rate of adverse events, including CMV infection, PTLD, anemia, and neutropenia. FTY720 (fingolimod) is a sphingosine receptor antagonist that traps lymphocytes in lymphoid tissues, not allowing them to exit. Adverse events with FTY720 use included bradycardia, gastrointestinal side effects, macular edema, and increased airway resistance. There are no ongoing plans to move forward with FTY720 in solid organ transplantation at this time. Tocilizumab is an anti–IL-6 monoclonal antibody that has shown promising results in treatment of chronic rejection, decreasing donor-specific antibody levels and stabilizing renal function.[50] Further studies are needed for these medications, especially in pediatric solid organ transplant populations.

CONCLUSION

The immune system plays an essential role in protecting human hosts from infection. Once a pediatric patient receives a solid organ transplant, modulation of the immune system is essential in preventing rejection. The field has advanced significantly since the early days of solid organ transplant. Multiple targets of the immune system and T-cell alloactivation have been discovered, resulting in more targeted immunosuppression and improved early outcomes. Yet improvements in chronic rejection have remained elusive and infection continues to affect a high number of pediatric solid organ transplant patients. In addition, long-term immunosuppression can lead to various adverse effects. Further research in the pediatric solid organ transplant population is needed, including newer drugs, protocols, and regimens. The ultimate goal in pediatric transplantation would be to balance the necessity of immunosuppression with the mitigation of adverse effects and infections, which would optimize outcomes in this patient population.

2

Immunologic Recovery and Basis for Infections in the Pediatric Hematopoietic Stem Cell Transplant Recipient

Jasmeen Dara, MD, MS and Christopher C. Dvorak, MD

Infections are one of the most frequent serious complications of hematopoietic stem cell transplantation (HSCT). The risk of infections corresponds to the complex interplay between organ dysfunction or tissue damage, exposure to pathogens, virulence of those pathogens, and the net state of immunosuppression. Although all of these factors are interrelated and each contributes to infection risk in some way, the time to recovery of the immune system is the most significant determinant of infection risk. The recovery of different components of the immune system is variable; therefore infection risk is often considered in time periods relative to transplantation. Traditionally, these periods have been considered fixed and are categorized as pre-engraftment (days 0 to 30), early post-engraftment (days 30 to 100), and late post-engraftment (days 100+) time periods (Fig. 2.1). Anchoring infection risk to these time periods can help establish a general construct for infection risk for bacteria, viruses, and fungi across the time periods. However, it is important that clinicians recognize that the timing of recovery for specific components of the immune system can vary considerably from one patient to another and thus fixed risk periods may not be ideal. For example, the duration of neutropenia corresponds with an increased risk of invasive fungal disease and is associated with the patient's indication for transplantation, extensiveness of prior therapy, stem cell source, cell dose, conditioning regimen, and graft failure or rejection if it occurs. It is more difficult to establish patient-specific or disease-specific immune recovery time periods; however, this knowledge will help guide the clinician through a more nuanced clinical assessment for a patient at a specific point in time after transplantation. This chapter aims to provide the clinician with the ability to assess infection risk using both the fixed time period approach as well as an individualized patient specific approach.

INFECTION RISK BY FIXED TIME PERIODS AFTER TRANSPLANTATION

Pre-Engraftment Period

The pre-engraftment period is often considered to correspond to days 0 to 30 after HSCT; however, this period can include days before neutrophil engraftment as well as days soon after. The infection risk in this early period is attributed to many factors, including neutropenia, the breakdown of mucosal barriers leading to subsequent microbial invasion, and acute graft-versus-host disease (GVHD) leading to further barrier breakdown and immunosuppression. Patients receiving myeloablative conditioning are most vulnerable in this early period owing to longer durations of neutropenia and mucosal barrier injury associated with myeloablative regimens. The majority of infections are monomicrobial and are most often the result of bacterial pathogens. The most common isolated organisms include coagulase-negative staphylococci, *Enterococcus* species, *Staphylococcus aureus*, or enteric gram-negative bacilli. The portal of entry for many of these organisms is either via a central venous catheter or translocation of a compromised mucosal barrier, often secondary to myeloablative conditioning regimens. Oral mucosal barrier injury can predispose specifically to viridans group streptococci; however, mucosal barrier injury can include any part of the alimentary tract from the oral cavity to the anus. *Clostridium difficile* infection is one of the most common causes of infectious diarrhea after HSCT given frequent exposure to precipitating factors such as chemotherapy and antibiotics.[1]

Invasive fungal disease, either yeast or molds, tends to occur in a biphasic pattern after HSCT with the first risk period presenting in this pre-engraftment phase. The most common fungal pathogens are *Candida* or *Aspergillus* species. More recent use of supportive care such as antifungal prophylaxis has led to a reduction of these events in the pre-engraftment period; however, breakthrough invasive fungal disease from genera other than *Candida* or *Aspergillus* may occur and, more rarely, resistance may occur.[1]

The next most frequently involved pathogens are viruses, which commonly include cytomegalovirus (CMV), herpesviruses, adenovirus, BK virus, respiratory viruses, and gastrointestinal viruses. Antiviral prophylaxis for some of these viral infections may delay or postpone the presentation into the early post-engraftment or late post-engraftment periods. CMV is the most common viral infection encountered in the posttransplant period. Antiviral prophylaxis has limited utility in the immediate posttransplant period owing to associated toxicities with current options. This differs from varicella zoster virus and herpes simplex virus, members of the herpesvirus family frequently encountered after transplant, for which institutions often use antiviral prophylaxis with acyclovir for the first year to prevent reactivation.[1,2] Other herpesvirus infections (Epstein-Barr virus, human herpes virus type 6, and, less commonly, human herpes virus type 7 and human herpes virus type 8) can also be identified in this period but far less frequently.[1] Although adenovirus and BK virus are not members of the herpesvirus family, these viruses can maintain a persistent asymptomatic state before transplantation and reactivation can occur in the early and late posttransplant periods. Lastly, hospital- and community-acquired respiratory (i.e., respiratory syncytial virus, rhinovirus, influenza) and gastrointestinal (i.e., norovirus, astrovirus) viral infections can be encountered in this early posttransplant period, most without any adequate treatment or prophylaxis, and can be devastating.[3]

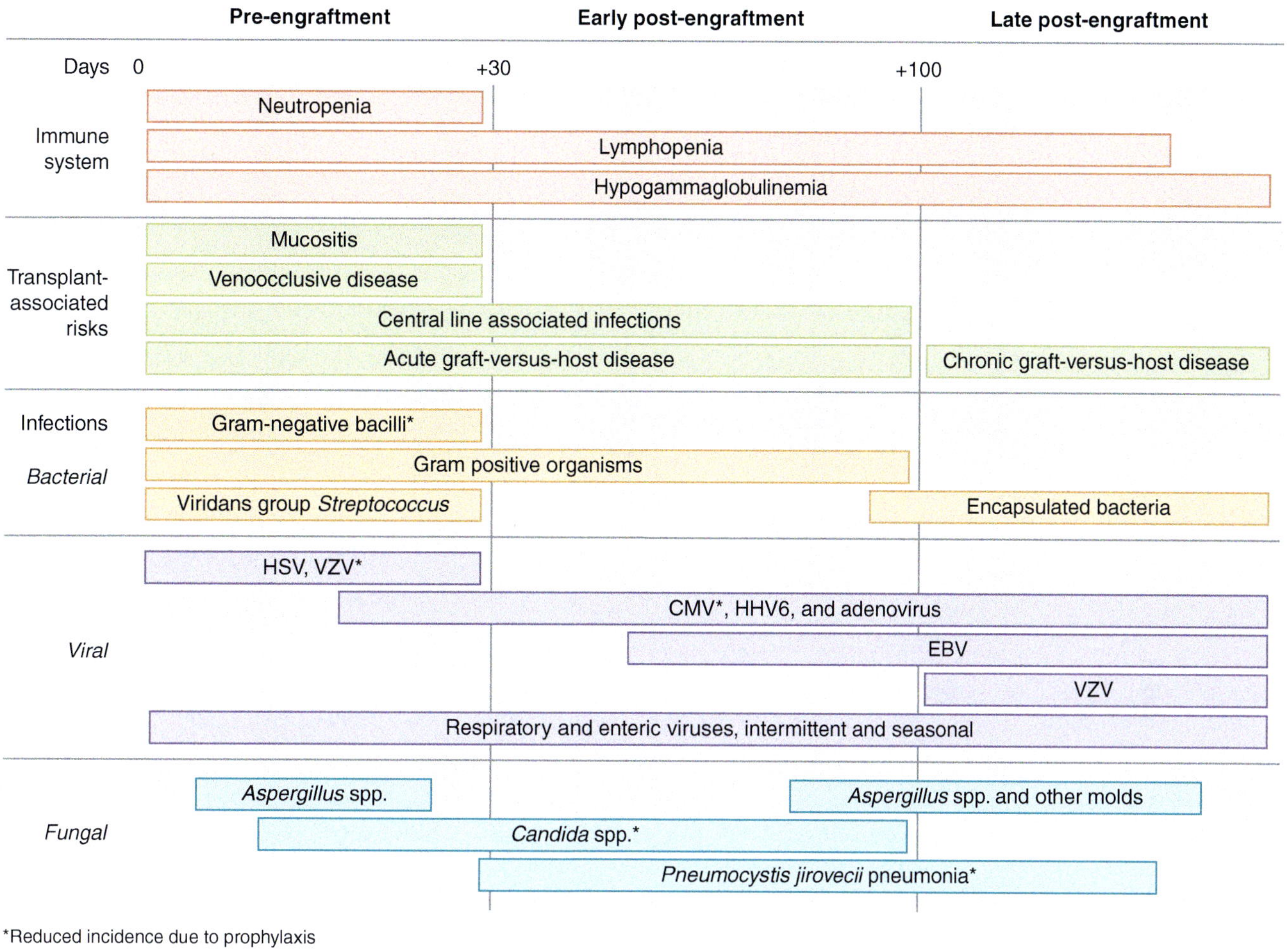

Fig. 2.1 Transplant infectious complications as identified in posttransplant immune reconstitution and risk factors. The asterisk indicates a reduced incidence as the result of prophylaxis. *CMV,* cytomegalovirus; *EBV,* Epstein-Barr virus; *HSV,* herpes simplex virus; *VZV,* varicella-zoster virus.

Early Post-Engraftment Period

In the early post-engraftment period, neutropenia has resolved, which is an important milestone for reduced vulnerability to bacterial and fungal pathogens. However, the clinician should still be alert to opportunistic infections from these pathogens owing to risk factors, such as continued need for central venous access, residual mucositis, intermittent neutropenia secondary to medication toxicity, or more rarely, graft loss. Persistent lymphopenia and slow T-cell reconstitution is primarily responsible for vulnerability to infections during this period. Poor T-cell reconstitution can be further delayed by the need for immune suppressive agents to manage HSCT complications such as acute GVHD. This combination of poor T-cell function and need for additional immune suppression predisposes children to an increased risk of latent viral reactivations, poor outcomes from typically self-limiting primary viral infections, and invasive mold disease. Additionally, this period is an important window of risk for *Pneumocystis jirovecii* pneumonia; therefore all patients continue prophylaxis through this period and often until T-cell reconstitution.[1]

Late Post-Engraftment Period

The late post-engraftment period starts 100 days after HSCT but varies in duration owing to the individual patient requirement for ongoing immunosuppression and delayed immune reconstitution. Patients may remain at high risk for infections because of prolonged immunosuppression secondary to treatment for chronic GVHD or autoimmune cytopenias. This results in delayed reconstitution of both cellular and humoral immunity. Bacteremia, sinusitis, upper respiratory tract infections, pneumonia, and meningitis are not infrequently caused by encapsulated bacteria (*Streptococcus pneumoniae, Haemophilus influenzae, Neisseria meningitidis*) during this period. Patients with chronic GVHD are particularly susceptible to these infections owing to poor opsonophagocytosis and hyposplenism, referred to as functional asplenia.[4] Therefore some institutions initiate antibiotic prophylaxis for functional asplenia to prevent overwhelming bacterial sepsis. In addition to encapsulated organisms, bacteremia during this period may also result from *Staphylococcus* species or gram-negative bacteria.[1] Factors that may predispose patients to bacteremia from these pathogens include the continued presence of central venous access or persistent mucosal barrier dysfunction. Although the peak of reactivation of latent viruses is in the early post-engraftment period, the risk persists through this late phase. For Epstein-Barr virus, reactivation can lead to the development of posttransplant lymphoproliferative disease, which typically presents between 3 and 5 months after transplant. Other atypical late post-engraftment infections may be due to *Nocardia* species, *Listeria* species, *Cryptococcus* species, and nontuberculous mycobacteria. Finally, the risk for *P. jirovecii* pneumonia can remain well after 100 days from HSCT, particularly if continued immune suppression is required.[1]

Approaches to Prophylaxis Relative to Infectious Risk Periods

In general, there are three methods to provide posttransplant antimicrobial prophylaxis: pharmacologic prophylaxis, immunoprophylaxis (immunoglobulin [IG] replacement therapy), and vaccinations. For each method, there are two approaches to guide initiation or duration of prophylaxis: a uniform time at risk approach or an individualized approach that takes into account ongoing immunosuppression and immune reconstitution. With the uniform time-at-risk approach, antimicrobial prophylaxis is continued until a designated time period elapses. An example would be the use of antifungal prophylaxis until day 100 (which may be extended for patients requiring immunosuppressive treatment for GVHD). Much of the data on the effectiveness for prophylaxis have evolved from trials designed with this simpler standardized time-at-risk approach. Although it has the advantage of consistency and ease of use, this approach likely results in overtreatment of some patients and undertreatment of others.

The second approach is individualization of the duration of time during which prophylaxis is provided or of the timing at which vaccinations are administered based on an assessment of an individual patient's cellular and humoral immunity. This system is much more cumbersome and has less evidence to support its use; however, it should theoretically result in earlier discontinuation of prophylaxis for some patients with adequate immune reconstitution and appropriately prolong prophylaxis for patients with immune defects that persist beyond an estimated risk period duration from transplantation. Examples of this approach include continuation of antifungal or antiviral prophylaxis until patients achieve functional cluster of differentiation (CD)4^+ T-cell reconstitution or discontinuation of IG replacement therapy when patients have adequate $CD19^+$ B cells, switched memory B cells, and evidence of IgM and IgA production. Whether a center uses the fixed time-at-risk approach or a more individualized approach will depend on the infrastructure of the transplant center and its ability to consistently apply a more nuanced approach to prophylaxis.

After HSCT and Ig replacement therapy is discontinued, recipients must be revaccinated. There are limited data on vaccine efficacy and ideal timing of vaccinations in HSCT recipients; however, it is accepted that there must be at least partial recovery of T and B cells before administration. Vaccination with polysaccharide antigen vaccines elicits T-cell–independent antibody responses and therefore typically fails to produce protective immunity in most allogeneic HSCT recipients within the first year after transplantation. However, conjugate vaccines evoke T-cell–dependent antibody responses and produce protective antibody responses within the first year after allogeneic HSCT even with patients receiving immunosuppression.[5] Therefore most revaccination guidelines are based on timing from transplantation, and HSCT recipients could undergo early revaccination with conjugate vaccines analogous to newborn vaccination schedules and achieve protective long term immunity. Vaccination with inactivated or toxoid-containing vaccines is recommended as early as 3 to 6 months after HSCT, whereas administration of live-attenuated vaccines is recommended at 24 months after HSCT. The delayed use of live-attenuated vaccines is based on concerns about transmission of vaccine-mediated disease and limited clinical data on safety or immunogenicity of earlier vaccination. The Advisory Committee on Immunization Practices to the Center for Disease Control and Prevention and the Infectious Diseases Society of America publish time-based guidelines on vaccination after transplantation, but vaccine schedules vary greatly among institutions.

TIMING OF IMMUNE RECONSTITUTION AFTER HEMATOPOIETIC STEM CELL TRANSPLANTATION

Immune reconstitution after HSCT involves the recovery of both hematopoietic and immunologic function. This occurs in several phases, resulting in recovery of specific components of the immune system at distinct time points (Table 2.1).

Innate Immune Recovery After Transplantation

The innate immune system can be divided into nonhematopoietic and hematopoietic compartments. The nonhematopoietic compartment includes physical barriers, such as the skin and mucosal surfaces, which can be damaged during transplantation by the pretransplant conditioning regimen. However, the damage is typically restored soon after transplantation. Repair can be inhibited by GVHD of the skin or mucous membranes. The skin and mucosal barriers can also be compromised by the presence of foreign material, such as a central venous catheter or a gastrostomy tube, for prolonged periods after transplantation.

Hematopoietic innate immune cells include neutrophils, macrophages, as well as natural killer (NK) cells. After myeloablative conditioning, patients undergo an aplastic phase, which is identified by severe neutropenia, anemia, and thrombocytopenia. The first laboratory sign of hematologic recovery is typically neutrophil recovery. Engraftment, classically defined as absolute neutrophil count greater than 500/μL, is typically achieved between 10 and 42 days and transplant, depending on the stem cell source (see Table 2.1). Hematopoietic growth factors, such as granulocyte colony-stimulating factor (G-CSF), can be used to accelerate recovery of granulocyte counts, minimize the duration of neutropenia, and decrease the risk for severe infections. The use of G-CSF after HCT is universal in the autologous setting but is more controversial in allogeneic graft recipients owing to a lack of benefit in reducing mortality. Most centers use G-CSF for recipients of umbilical cord blood (UCB) transplants, whereas its use in others is more variable as there are concerns that G-CSF may increase rates of GVHD or malignant relapse. However, administration of certain post-HSCT medications (such as ganciclovir or valganciclovir) may result in secondary neutropenia. Furthermore, the neutrophils may have abnormal function for up to 2 months after transplant.[6]

Monocytes are leukocytes that circulate peripherally until they eventually migrate into tissues where they develop into macrophages and dendritic cells. Monocytes, macrophages, and dendritic cells function through phagocytosis, a process that is particularly important for pathogen killing and tissue repair. However, mononuclear phagocytes also activate the adaptive immune system via antigen presentation and cytokine production. Posttransplant neutrophil recovery is occasionally preceded by the detection of peripheral monocytes; however, monocyte function may remain suboptimal for up to 1 year after transplant.[6] Although monocyte function is difficult to measure in clinical laboratories, based on data extrapolated from animal models, it is thought that tissue macrophages and dendritic cells are not significantly depleted as a result of transplant conditioning, and natural turnover results in their being gradually replaced by donor-derived cells for up to a year after HSCT.[6] Peripheral dendritic cells can also be detected at the time of neutrophil count recovery and a low dendritic cell count at engraftment may predict relapse, death, and acute GVHD.[7]

TABLE 2.1 **Comparison Between Stem Cell Sources**

	Auto-PBSC	Allo-PBSC	Allo-BM	Allo-UCB
Ease of collection	Recipient requires stem cell mobilization and central line apheresis	Donor requires stem cell mobilization and central line apheresis	Donor anesthesia	Very safe
Time to neutrophil engraftment (ANC >500)	Very fast (7-14 days)	Fast (14-21 days)	Slow (17-24 days)	Very slow (24-42 days)
T-cell reconstitution[a]	30 days	6-12 months	3-12 months	3-12 months
B-cell reconstitution[b]	60 days	4-12 months	3-12 months	2-6 months
Graft versus host disease	None	Common in mismatched grafts; increased risk of chronic GVHD compared with blood marrow	Less common	Uncommon or mild
HLA matching	N/A	Requires T-cell depletion for HLA mismatch	Requires HLA-identical match[c]	HLA mismatch well tolerated
HSC numbers	High	High	High (depending on host-donor weights)	Low

[a]T-cell reconstitution defined as CD4 count >200/μL. T-cell reconstitution is highly variable and dependent on T-cell depletion, HLA match, and the development of acute graft-versus-host disease.
[b]B-cell reconstitution defined as >200/μL.
[c]Mismatched blood marrow HSCT can be performed but less optimal.
ANC, absolute neutrophil count; *Auto-PBSC,* autologous peripheral blood stem cells; *Allo-PBSC,* allogeneic peripheral blood stem cells; *Allo-BM,* allogeneic bone marrow; *Allo-UCB,* allogeneic umbilical cord blood; *HLA,* human leukocyte antigen; *HSC,* hematopoietic stem cell; *N/A,* not applicable for autologous peripheral blood stem cells; *PBSC,* peripheral blood stem cells.
Data from Porrata LF, Litzow MR, Markovic SN. Immune reconstitution after autologous hematopoietic stem cell transplantation. *Mayo Clin Proc.* 2001;76(4):407-412; Wiegering V, Eyrich M, Winkler B, Schlegel PG. Comparison of immune reconstitution after allogeneic versus autologous stem cell transplantation in 182 pediatric recipients. *J Pediatr Hematol. Oncol.* 2017;2(1):2-6; and De Koning C, Plantinga M, Besseling P, Boelens JJ, Nierkens S. Immune reconstitution after allogeneic hematopoietic cell transplantation in children. *Biol Blood Marrow Transplant.* 2016;22(2):195-206.

NK cells are also key members of the innate immune system that influence adaptive function. Derived from the lymphoid lineage, NK cells have a unique function in the prevention of viral infections and antitumor immunity. NK cell reconstitution varies by graft source. NK cells recover in number and function in the first few weeks after allogeneic HSCT, much earlier than T- and B-cell reconstitution, which is likely related to the high IL-2 levels during the early posttransplant period.[8] Not only do NK cells appear early, they also acquire functional competence much earlier than other lymphocytes. Furthermore, NK cell activity after HSCT remains normal even in the presence of severe GVHD.[9]

Delay in neutrophil engraftment greatly increases morbidity, and failure of sustained neutrophil engraftment after a myeloablative-conditioning regimen requires urgent retransplantation. Engraftment failure can occur from inadequate hematopoietic stem cell quantity from poor collection or loss in postcollection processing, inadequate host support of infused cells, posttransplantation events such as infection or medications, or from host-versus-graft (immunologic) rejection. Engraftment failure is a very rare complication of autologous transplantation and is likely only present in the setting of poor cryopreservation of stem cells. For allogeneic HSCT, the risk of engraftment failure is dependent on a number of variables, including baseline host immunity, HLA disparity, type of conditioning regimen and stem cell source used, low stem cell dose, ex vivo T-cell depletion (TCD), ABO incompatibility, and disease status at transplantation. Patients with hematologic malignancies have a rejection risk of approximately 5%, whereas the risk may be greater than 10% in patients with nonmalignant conditions. Graft rejection is more common in haploidentical related and mismatched unrelated donor (URD) transplants and much less frequent in matched sibling donor transplantation. Generally, UCB transplant recipients have the highest risk of graft failure, whereas peripheral blood stem cell grafts have the lowest risk of graft rejection. The incidence of graft failure also varies considerably among institutions owing to differing approaches to conditioning.

Adaptive Cellular Immune Recovery After Transplantation

Often clinicians are reassured about a patient's infection risk once neutrophil engraftment is achieved. Although neutrophil recovery is an important milestone, patients continue to be vulnerable to opportunistic infection because of persistent cellular immunodeficiencies involving the adaptive immune system. The recovery of the adaptive immune system is much more nuanced, involving refinement and adjustment of T and B lymphocytes over the lifetime of an individual. After HSCT, T and B lymphocytes reconstitute slowly and develop both a cellular and humoral response. The cellular immune response to pathogens is initiated by antigen-presenting cells (e.g., macrophages and dendritic cells) but also requires the presence of functional T cells for activation. HSCT results in impairment of the adaptive immune response through loss of naïve T cells and reduced function of existing T cells. The recovery of the T-cell compartment initially relies on peripheral expansion of infused donor memory T cells, which leads to a narrow T-cell receptor repertoire. This process is driven by cytokines, such as IL-7 and IL-15, as well as by antigen stimulation and T-cell receptor (TCR) engagement.[9] Peripheral T-cell expansion is eventually followed by the production of naïve T cells in the thymus leading to a population of memory T cells with a diverse TCR repertoire. In patients receiving T-cell–replete grafts, peripheral expansion of infused memory T cells with a limited repertoire occurs initially until hematopoietic progenitors seed the thymus and produce T cells with a more diverse repertoire. In T-cell–depleted transplants, seeding of the thymus by hematopoietic progenitors is the primary route to T-cell reconstitution.

In either route, effective long-term and sustained T-cell lymphopoiesis is dependent on the presence of a functional thymus. Thymic dependence in generating a diverse T-cell repertoire after HSCT is a critical hurdle in patients without a thymus or with a poorly functioning thymus. Aging, recurrent or chronic infections, chemotherapy, radiation exposure, and GVHD can all lead to thymic atrophy and subsequent difficulty with T-cell reconstitution. Detection of recent thymic immigrants and T-cell polyclonality are typical methods used to determine thymic function. TCR excision circles (TRECs) are small circularized portions of DNA created through T-cell maturation in the thymus, which can be used as a surrogate marker for reconstitution of thymus-derived $CD4^+CD45RA^+$ naïve T cells. However, these are just markers for thymic output and, in general, it is difficult to completely assess the function of the thymus after transplantation.

Naïve T-cell populations are usually reduced for long periods after HSCT. The inability to reconstitute the naïve T-cell compartment for several years after HSCT, in the absence of GVHD, is likely a consequence of both thymic dysfunction and impaired peripheral naïve T-cell homeostatic mechanisms and survival. $CD4^+$ lymphocytes require a functional thymus for generation of $CD4^+CD45RA^+$ naïve T cells, whereas $CD8^+$ lymphocytes are predominantly derived by clonal expansion outside the thymus. Therefore $CD4^+$ T lymphocytes appear later than $CD8^+$ T lymphocytes leading to the inversion of the CD4/CD8 ratio found after transplant.[10] Inversion of the CD4/CD8 ratio is one of the earliest features of T-cell reconstitution after autologous or allogeneic transplantation from any graft source and can persist for up to several years after HSCT.[1]. $CD4^+$ T-cell reconstitution to a level of approximately 200/μL typically occurs around 3 months after HSCT but can vary considerably depending on the use of TCD methods, graft source (UCB), receipt of total body irradiation, or development of GVHD.[6]

The development of regulatory T cells (Tregs) may be important in determining outcomes after allogeneic HSCT. Tregs suppress the activity of effector T cells, thus reducing inflammation and promoting immune homeostasis after allogeneic HSCT.[11] The presence of donor Tregs enhances immune reconstitution and improves TCR diversity after transplantation.[11] Increased donor Tregs are associated with a decreased risk of GVHD, and many studies have shown that Tregs are significantly reduced in HSCT recipients with GVHD.[9] The relative predominance of effector T cells, compared with Tregs, leads to a proinflammatory milieu of cytokines. IL-6, characterized as both proinflammatory and antiinflammatory, is of particular interest in GVHD and moderates the differentiation of naïve T cells into either Tregs or effector T cells. IL-6 blockade promotes differentiation into Tregs and may mitigate the severity of GVHD.[9] Tumor necrosis factor alpha (TNF-α) is typically classified as a proinflammatory cytokine; however, it may also have antiinflammatory properties mediated through its effects on Tregs. TNF-α has been shown to increase expansion, stability, and possibly the function of Tregs, and may therefore have conflicting effects on both GVHD incidence (high is bad early after HSCT) and severity (low is bad later after HSCT).[12]

Adaptive Humoral Immune Recovery After Transplantation

The adaptive humoral immune response is mediated by antibodies and requires both functional T and B cells. In addition to the delayed recovery of T cells after HSCT, there is also impaired reconstitution of B cells. Impairment of B-lymphocyte number and function leads to absent Ig production and susceptibility to infections with encapsulated bacteria such as *S. pneumoniae* and *H. influenzae*. The B-cell compartment is the slowest to reconstitute. B-cell reconstitution depends on the intensity of conditioning. Typically, when myeloablative conditioning is administered, all B cells are genetically donor in origin but produced de novo from the bone marrow, and therefore do not retain immunologic memory from the donor. In reduced intensity conditioning, B cells may be of mixed host and donor origin, although data are lacking on whether the persistence of host B cells provides a bridge of immunologic memory. Typically, B-cell reconstitution occurs within 12 months but may take several years for complete development of memory B cells after allogeneic HSCT. Hematopoietic stem cells (HSCs) within the bone marrow undergo multiple stages of B-cell differentiation. Pro-B cells develop into pre-B cells and finally immature/transitional B cells. Transitional ($CD19^+CD21^{low}CD38^{high}$) B cells are the first B cells emigrating from the bone marrow and are elevated in the peripheral blood in the first months after HSCT before progressively decreasing. Transitional B cells emigrate to the spleen where they differentiate into IgM^+ memory or mature B cells. Mature B cells migrate to the primary follicle of the lymph node and spleen for antigen exposure and differentiation into switched memory B cells or plasma cells. Reconstitution of switched memory B cells occurs upon antigen exposure from pathogens, the environment, or vaccines and requires $CD4^+$ T-cell help for isotype switching. Therefore although naïve B cells reach normal levels by approximately 6 months after allogeneic HSCT, levels of IgM^+ memory B cells can remain low for up to 2 years.[13] Much like the TCR repertoire, B-cell antibody diversity is severely diminished and suffers prolonged recovery, which is worsened by GVHD and by the medications used to treat it.[14] Recovery of the B-cell count or specific antibody production is primarily of donor origin but can vary among types of allogeneic stem cell grafts, $CD34^+$ cell doses, donor ages, or recipient ages.[14]

After myeloablative conditioning, B cells are typically entirely of donor origin; however, plasma cells remain primarily of host origin in the first several months after transplant. Given the long-lived nature of plasma cells, it takes months to years to replace host plasma cells by newly produced donor plasma cells. Therefore institutions may consider continuation of Ig replacement therapy in HSCT recipients until there is adequate evidence of B-cell and plasma cell function as opposed to a predetermined period. Some considerations affecting discontinuation of Ig replacement may include absolute B-lymphocyte count, B-lymphocyte phenotyping, including percent of switched memory B cells ($CD27^+IgM^-IgD^-$), IgM and IgA production, and isohemagglutinin production.

AUTOLOGOUS HSCT AS A MODEL FOR IMMUNE RECONSTITUTION

Autologous hematopoietic stem cells can be given to rescue the bone marrow and immune system after high-dose chemotherapy toxicities, which can result in deep and prolonged bone marrow suppression. Infusion of autologous hematopoietic stem cells after high-dose chemotherapy can offer prolonged disease-free survival in hematologic malignancies, including Hodgkin and non-Hodgkin lymphomas, and distinct advanced pediatric tumors, such as brain tumors, neuroblastoma, and certain sarcomas. It requires the collection and storage of adequate HSC, preferably before alkylating agents or topoisomerase inhibitors. Immune reconstitution after allogeneic and autologous HSCT has some similarities; however, allogeneic HSCT carries a risk of graft failure as the result of immunologic rejection and involves a risk of GVHD, necessitating the use of immunosuppressive therapy to prevent and/or manage it. Autologous HSCT is therefore a model for immune reconstitution after transplantation because this method obviates known risk factors for impaired reconstitution, such as in vivo or ex vivo TCD, HLA disparity between donor and recipient, GVHD prophylaxis, occurrence of GVHD, and immunosuppressive therapy for GVHD.

Neutrophil engraftment occurs quickly after autologous transplantation, between 7 and 14 days (see Table 2.1). Although autologous HSCT recipients may have impaired thymic function owing to age-related involution, damage from chemotherapy, or injury from ionizing radiation, thymopoiesis is typically less affected, and there is a faster recovery of the naïve T-cell compartment compared with the allogeneic transplant recipients with similar conditioning regimens.[15] There is faster recovery of $CD3^+$ and $CD4^+$ T cells as well as increased B- and NK-cell counts in the first posttransplant year.[15] Normalization of T-cell number, lymphocyte proliferative responses to phytohemagglutinin, and IgM production occur in the majority of autologous HSCT recipients by 6 months after transplantation.[16]

Earlier immune reconstitution corresponds to a decrease in severity and incidence of infections after autologous compared with allogeneic HSCT. The most common infections in the first year after transplantation include catheter-related bloodstream infection, varicella zoster virus infection, and pneumonia, but the majority of these infections occur in the first 6 months after autologous transplantation. In most children, supportive care measures, such as protective isolation and prophylactic antimicrobials, can be discontinued at 6 months after autologous transplantation as the risk of infection also decreases after that time.[16]

Autologous transplantation of gene-modified hematopoietic stem cells, or gene therapy, is a novel approach to transplantation that involves the transfer of gene-corrected stem cells with ostensibly fewer immunologic complications and reduced toxicities from conditioning. Gene therapy is under investigation for a number of indications, including certain forms of severe combined immune deficiency in which patients lack the machinery necessary to produce lymphocytes. Patients who receive gene therapy for adenosine deaminase–deficient severe combined immune deficiency typically achieve immune reconstitution by 6 months after transplantation.

FACTORS AFFECTING IMMUNE RECONSTITUTION, AUTOREACTIVITY, AND ALLOREACTIVITY

The timing of immune reconstitution after HSCT, in particular after allogeneic HSCT, is affected by a number of variables, including HSCT procedure specific factors (e.g., HLA matching, source, conditioning regimen), pretransplant conditioning regimen, patient- and recipient-specific factors (e.g., age, sex, CMV status), and the presence and management of GVHD . The selection of a donor is a critical element contributing to the success of HSCT. There are several donor options, including identical twins (syngeneic, HLA-identical), the patient (autologous, HLA-identical), a sibling, relative URD (allogeneic HLA-matched, haploidentical, or mismatched), or UCB (allogeneic HLA matched or mismatched). Options for a donor depend on a number of variables with the goal of minimizing toxicities, decreasing risk of alloreactivity, and achieving adequate donor chimerism to lead to disease cure. These factors include the overall health and age of recipient and donor, disease progression, infection history, and clinical approach of the individual transplant center. There are many recipient and donor characteristics that could affect the timing of immune reconstitution and the subsequent infectious complications.

HLA Matching

Donor and recipient matching are performed on human leukocyte major histocompatibility complex class I (HLA-A, -B, -C), and class II (HLA-DR, -DQ, -DP) antigens as a key part of successful allogeneic HSCT. These six loci contribute to graft-versus-host, graft-versus-tumor, and graft rejection responses. HLA-matched sibling donors are preferred for most transplants as they offer the best chance of engraftment and fastest immune reconstitution; however, there is only a 25% chance of having a matched sibling if siblings are present and available for donation. Other considerations for matched siblings include sibling age, source of collection (bone marrow or peripheral blood stem cells [PBSC]), and the possibility of the sibling donor being a carrier for the disease being treated. For example, carriers for the *CYBB* gene (X-linked chronic granulomatous disease) can have aberrations in neutrophil oxidative burst capacity and have been found to be at increased risk of infection or autoimmunity in adulthood and therefore should not be used as matched sibling donors. Similar considerations may exist for other X-linked diseases as well as for certain metabolic conditions, such as Hurler syndrome, in which carriers have only half the normal enzyme levels.

For patients without an HLA matched sibling, HSCT can be performed using a matched URD, a mismatched URD (single or double antigen), an UCB, or a haploidentical donor. The risks of acute and chronic GVHD and transplant-related mortality increase with the number of HLA mismatches, particularly in patients lacking HLA-A–, -B–, or -DRβ1–matched donors; however, HLA-C, -DQβ1, and -DPβ1 are also important. For transplant of nonmalignant diseases, URDs should ideally be matched at all 12 alleles. For transplant of malignant disease, fully matched URDs may have higher rates of relapse and decreased graft-versus-tumor effects; therefore some degree of mismatch may be beneficial. Disparity at HLA-A, -B, -C, and -DRβ1 alleles are definite risk factors for survival after URD transplantation, whereas single HLA-DQβ1 or -DPβ1 mismatches appear to be somewhat better tolerated. In addition to characterizing a suitable donor, homozygous HLA antigen mismatches can further be characterized as favoring either rejection (host versus graft or graft versus host). Furthermore, the use of partially HLA-mismatched allogeneic HSCs requires testing for circulating donor-specific HLA antibodies, as the presence of donor-specific antibodies increases the risk of primary graft failure and should be avoided whenever possible. If there is no alternative donor available, the recipient can potentially be desensitized to donor-specific antibodies before transplantation using plasmapheresis, Ig, and rituximab.

Although disease-free survival after URD transplantation continues to improve over the past decade, URD PBSC transplants are associated with delayed immune reconstitution and recipients are more likely to develop GVHD compared with recipients of matched sibling transplants, particularly if recipients lack an HLA-A–, -B–, or -DRβ1–matched donor. This has led to the use of more aggressive and prolonged immunosuppression for prophylaxis of GVHD for HSCT recipients of URD PBSC grafts, which further delays immune reconstitution. Transplantation from an URD has been associated with increased risk of predominantly late infections. By 1 year after HSCT, the number of recipients in whom at least one late infection developed, particularly infections from viruses, was increased compared with those who received a transplant from a matched related donor.[9] This marked increase in late infections is the most important factor leading to increased nonrelapse mortality in URD transplantation.

Mismatched related (haploidentical) donors are often the only readily available donor for transplantation, which is essential in some diseases such as high-risk leukemias. However, recipients of unrelated or related mismatched donor HSCT have a higher rate of infectious complications than recipients of matched grafts, likely owing to the use of TCD methods.[17] CMV and aspergillosis account for 40% of nonrelapse mortality in high-risk leukemia patients who receive haploidentical transplantation.[18] More recent data show improved T-cell reconstitution with the use of posttransplant cyclophosphamide or the use of ex vivo combined $CD3^+$ and $CD19^+$ cell depletion in haploidentical HSCT, as these methods preferentially spare memory T cells.[19,20]

Stem Cell Source

There are several potential sources for donor hematopoietic stem cells, which include bone marrow, peripheral blood stem cells, and cord blood stem cells, and the choice of stem cell source may affect immune reconstitution following HSCT.

Bone Marrow. For more than three decades, blood marrow has been the most frequent source of stem cells for transplantation. It is a safe procedure; however, for the donors, it is associated with considerable discomfort, fatigue, and longer recovery time than PBSC collections. The percentage of stem cells ($CD34^+$ cells) among circulating total nucleated cells at steady state in bone marrow is approximately 18-fold higher than healthy donor peripheral blood.[21] After bone marrow infusion, innate immunity usually recovers over the first several months. Reconstitution of adaptive immunity takes place over the first 1 to 2 years and is slower than PBSC transplantation.[21]

Peripheral Blood Stem Cells. Mobilized PBSC have been widely used as a stem cell source largely because of the convenience of peripheral collection techniques. PBSC harvesting by single or multiple leukapheresis procurements avoids the risks associated with multiple marrow aspirations and general anesthesia and shortens donor recovery time. PBSCs are mobilized in the donor using G-CSF for several days before peripheral blood collection. This increases circulating $CD34^+$ stem cell concentrations approximately 16-fold from baseline and easily compensates for the low baseline counts.[21] The total numbers of T cells, monocytes, and NK cells contained in a PBSC allograft are more than 10 times higher than those in a blood marrow allograft. Despite this, there is no difference in the incidence of acute GVHD in patients who receive PBSC compared with blood marrow allografts. However, it is thought that the increase in T cells in PBSCs compared with blood marrow allografts results in an increased incidence of chronic GVHD in recipients of PBSC allografts. Migration of blood marrow–derived stem cells to the marrow niches is slightly better than PBSCs. However, neutrophil and platelet engraftment is significantly faster using PBSCs.[21] Additionally, recipients of PBSC transplants have higher naïve and memory T cells as well as T-cell proliferative responses to mitogens at 1 and 11 months after transplant compared with blood marrow transplant recipients.[22] Although there is no difference in outcomes in adult HSCT recipients, some studies suggest pediatric patients who receive PBSC, compared with blood marrow grafts, have higher rates of treatment-related mortality, treatment failure, and mortality related to increased incidence of GVHD.[23,24]

Umbilical Cord Blood. UCB has also been used as a stem cell source for more than 30 years. Umbilical cord stem cells allow for an increased level of HLA disparity; therefore cord blood transplantation (CBT) is an option for alternative hematopoietic stem cells when there are no available related or unrelated donors. This can be particularly important for racial or ethnic minorities who have limited URDs available in the National Marrow Donor registry. Furthermore, registry searches and screening can take several weeks. UCB has the additional advantage of immediate availability of cells and thus can be useful for urgent transplantation of certain malignant diseases. CBT has the advantage of lower rates of chronic GVHD compared with recipients of PBSC products. Although UCB contains significantly higher absolute numbers of T, NK, and B lymphocytes, most of the UCB T-cells are naïve T cells, resulting in prolonged time to engraftment, lack of transferred T-cell memory, and a high incidence of opportunistic infections, particularly in the first 3 to 4 months after transplant.[25] Early transplant-related nonrelapse mortality in CBT is primarily due to infectious complications, presumably related to the relative delay in neutrophil engraftment and $CD8^+$ immune reconstitution. Mortality from opportunistic infections in CBT can be predicted by age, CMV serostatus, HLA mismatch, and lower graft cell dose.[25] In addition to the high mortality associated with opportunistic infections, CBT is also complicated by an increased incidence of graft failure and relapse. T-cell reconstitution is dependent on thymopoiesis to produce long-term memory cells. Markers of thymopoiesis (recent thymic immigrants, TRECs, $CD4^+$ CD454RA+ T cells, and TCR repertoire diversity) are associated with CBT outcomes such as infections, disease, relapse, and overall survival.[9] Although UCB is enriched for hematopoietic stem cells, it is limited by the absolute quantity of stem cells that can be collected from a single donor. Given the association between stem cell dose and time to neutrophil engraftment, the use of double cord blood transplantation (dCBT), from two unrelated, partially matched grafts, has been used as a means to increase stem cell dose. After dCBT one of the grafts dominates long-term reconstitution while the other mediates short-term engraftment. Perhaps because of the increase in stem cell dose, there may be an increased risk of GVHD, and therefore, a benefit of graft-versus-leukemia (GVL) effect from dCBT. However, single-unit CBT was associated with better platelet recovery, a lower risk of GVHD, and a significant improvement in survival after dCBT compared with single-unit CBT has not been confirmed.[26] Despite the advances achieved with increasing cell dose in dCBT, there still remains a gap in the time to engraftment compared with blood marrow and PBSC grafts and this delay in engraftment is associated with an increased early transplant-related mortality, likely related to infectious complications.[26,27]

Stem Cell Dose

After stem cell collection, via either bone marrow harvest or peripheral blood apheresis, grafts are evaluated to determine the estimated stem cell dose. The total nucleated cell dose and $CD34^+$ cell dose are important factors contributing to the rate of engraftment. However, the dose required for rapid and stable long-term engraftment varies depending on the method of measurement and the source of stem cells. The dose of hematopoietic stem cells infused affects the rates of hematopoietic recovery after HSCT. Specifically, increased stem cell dose decreases the time to neutrophil engraftment. Despite improving the time to engraftment, it is unclear if increased stem cell doses improve overall immune reconstitution; however, the receipt of higher total nucleated cell doses has been associated with increased survival and decreased relapse.[28] However, the benefits of increasing stem cell dose need to be balanced against the associated increased risk of acute GVHD. Stem cell doses are also limited with certain types of stem cell sources, such as UCB.

Pretransplant Conditioning

The conditioning (or preparative) regimen is designed to provide myeloablation of the recipient marrow to allow for donor engraftment and immunosuppression to prevent rejection. Conditioning regimens may use chemotherapeutic drugs, serotherapy (antithymocyte globulin or alemtuzumab), and/or total body irradiation. The ideal conditioning regimen is based on clinical judgment that accounts for underlying disease, comorbidities, disease status, and donor and graft source. Conditioning regimens can be categorized as myeloablative, reduced intensity, or nonmyeloablative. Although the definitions are somewhat debated, myeloablative regimens consist of a single agent or combination of agents expected to destroy the hematopoietic cells in the bone marrow and produce profound pancytopenia. Reduced intensity or nonmyeloablative conditioning regimens consists of agents that do not fully eliminate the possibility of host hematopoietic recovery.

The use of myeloablative conditioning regimen results in long-lasting, likely irreversible, destruction of hematopoietic cells in the bone marrow and potential delays in immune reconstitution through thymic damage. The thymus is responsible for the generation of a diverse naïve T-cell receptor repertoire. After HSCT, the thymus is occupied by hematopoietic progenitors, which will later diversify and acquire an adaptive cellular immune response. Although myeloablative, reduced intensity, or nonmyeloablative regimens can damage the thymus, it is not known if the degree of damage varies by conditioning intensity.

Reduced intensity conditioning regimens have been developed as a means to achieve engraftment, allow for graft-versus-tumor effect, and limit chemotherapy-related toxicities. These regimens contain a varying degree of myelosuppression and immunosuppression and may include both chemotherapy, serotherapy, and radiation. One of the hypothesized advantages of reduced intensity conditioning is that it might lend to better immune reconstitution after transplantation owing to less damage of the thymus, allowing regeneration of naïve T cells derived from donor HSCs and perhaps also owing to proliferation of immunologically competent host T cells that survive the conditioning regimen. However, studies have shown conflicting findings and are difficult to interpret given the variability in protocols. Furthermore, donor lymphocyte infusions (DLIs) are frequently used after reduced intensity stem cell transplantation and may contribute to earlier recovery of some immune function via the transfer of memory T cells. Conversely, DLIs may induce GVHD, leading to further immune suppression.

Recipient- and Donor-Specific Factors

Donor Age. As the immune system ages, there is increased susceptibility to infections and cancer, decreased responsiveness to vaccines, and increased incidence of autoimmune disorders. The mechanisms underlying immunosenescence (the changes seen with an aging immune system) are complex and still being explored. Hematopoietic stem cells from aged donors have reduced engraftment capacity and potential for reconstitution. Consequently, increased donor age, even as young as 36 years, can affect HSCT outcomes.[29] Additionally, increasing donor age seems to be associated with a defect in hematopoietic stem cell function that skews that lineage potential away from lymphoid and toward myeloid precursors.[30]

The effect of donor age was best demonstrated in a retrospective analysis from the Center for International Blood and Marrow Transplant Research of more than 11,000 unrelated transplants performed from 1988 to 2011 that evaluated the effects of various donor characteristics (e.g., age, sex, CMV serologic status, ABO compatibility, race, and parity) on recipient outcome. After adjustment for patient disease and transplant characteristics, age and donor-recipient HLA match were the only donor traits significantly associated with overall survival. For every 10-year increment in donor age, there was a 5.5% increase in the hazard ratio for mortality. Older donor age was also associated with an increase in acute, but not chronic, GVHD.[31] Other studies have found that younger donors are also associated with lower incidences of serious complications, including secondary graft failure, posttransplant lymphoproliferative disease, obstructive lung disease, and relapse after allogeneic transplantation.[29]

Recipient Age. Age-related decline of the immune system's ability to regenerate a lymphocyte pool is an obstacle in stem cell transplantation, leading to increased susceptibility to infections and decreased efficacy of vaccines. Thymic involution and subsequently reduced exportation of naïve T cells is the most well described age-related change. The thymic microenvironment is in slow, but constant, change and eventually involutes with age. After total body irradiation and chemotherapy for conditioning there is significant damage to the thymic epithelial microenvironment, which results in reduced T-cell development.[32] Recovery of the thymic function after HSCT is largely dependent on the age of the recipient. In young patients, the long-term recovery of thymic function is unaffected and the epithelial compartment eventually recovers from chemotherapy. In comparison, thymic damage caused by cytoreductive conditioning can be particularly detrimental in older individuals whose thymus has already undergone significant involution. Although thymic aging can be observed as early as 1 year of age, significant impacts of aging on immune reconstitution are not apparent until after puberty.[33] Notably, the adult thymus still appears capable of regeneration at least up to middle age.[33]

Sex and Parity. Sex and parity are the most controversial of factors that can potentially affect stem cell transplant outcomes, especially when female donors are used for male recipients. This risk is thought to be due to the various Y chromosome–encoded T-cell epitopes, the HY minor histocompatibility antigens, the presence of which on male host tissues can be recognized by female donor T cells. This effect may be magnified in parous female donors to male recipients, who have developed memory lymphocytes against HY histocompatibility alloantigens. However, some nulliparous women also have allosensitization to HY antigens (via unclear mechanisms).[34] A large Center for International Blood and Marrow Transplant Research database multivariate analysis evaluating the effects of donor or recipient sex and parity showed no effect on the risk of acute GVHD; however, sex and parity were significantly associated with chronic GVHD.[35] For male recipients, nulliparous and parous female donors conferred an increased risk of chronic GVHD. For nulliparous and parous female recipients, parous female donors also significantly increased the risk of chronic GVHD.[31,35] There is no association between sex or parity and survival, relapse risk, or transplant-related mortality.[35]

Cytomegalovirus Status. CMV, a virus that establishes lifelong persistence, can reactivate during and after HSCT in the period after receiving conditioning while awaiting immune reconstitution. CMV has a bidirectional relationship with immune reconstitution. Delays in immune reconstitution lead to increased risk of CMV infection; however, CMV itself may have immune suppressive effects that can further delay immune reconstitution.

During the early posttransplant period when patients are most immunocompromised, seropositive recipients are at risk of CMV reactivation and increased transplant-related mortality. The risk is highest with CMV-seropositive recipients who receive grafts from CMV-seronegative donors; therefore CMV-seropositive donors are always preferred. Additionally, both UCB transplantation and haploidentical HSCT result in delayed immune reconstitution, and therefore pose additional risks of CMV reactivation and infection. The use of newer TCD methods (such as α/β TCD) and reduced intensity conditioning can somewhat mitigate the increased risk of CMV infection after haploidentical stem cell transplantation. CMV reactivation most often occurs in the first 100 days after transplant, but with concomitant chronic GVHD or in the setting of haploidentical transplantation, reactivation can occur much later. Studies suggest that recovery of both CMV-specific $CD4^+$ and $CD8^+$ T cells is essential for controlling CMV after HSCT.[36] Control of CMV is dependent on expansion of CMV-specific $CD8^+$ cytotoxic T lymphocytes (CTLs).[36] Evaluation of CTL function after allogeneic HSCT revealed that 50% of patients exhibited a detectable CMV-specific

CTL response by 3 months after allogeneic transplantation. Restoration of CTL response appeared to be dependent on $CD4^+$ recovery.[28] The factors influencing the recovery of CMV-specific $CD4^+$ and $CD8^+$ function after HSCT are poorly understood, but the use of high-dose steroids and type of stem cell source (bone marrow) have been associated with impaired $CD4^+$ and $CD8^+$ function 3 months after transplantation.[28]

Once CMV reactivates, the infection itself can further delay immune reconstitution and repopulation of a more diverse T-cell repertoire. One hypothesis for CMV infection to actively interfere with immune reconstitution is via infection of bone marrow stromal cells and reducing the homing of transplanted hematopoietic stem cells to bone marrow stroma, leading to graft failure.[37] Conversely, a unique association exists between CMV infection in transplant recipients with acute myelogenous leukemia (AML), wherein CMV reactivation is associated with protection from leukemic relapse, likely caused by the CMV-driven expansion of donor-derived memory-like NK cells and $\gamma/\delta\delta$ T cells.[28]

Graft-Versus-Host Disease.

In allogeneic transplant recipients, the presence of clinically significant GVHD is the most influential factor affecting the timing of immune reconstitution. Acute GVHD is an immunologic response against the host immune system, tissues, and organs and is primarily mediated by alloreactive donor T cells. Acute GVHD occurs in 20% to 60% of patients who receive allogeneic HSCTs and substantially contributes to transplant-related nonrelapse mortality. Development of acute GVHD is primarily influenced by HLA or less likely gender mismatches, the intensity of the conditioning regimen, CMV reactivation, and the stem cell source. The risk of GVHD can be partially mitigated by good donor selection, choice of conditioning regimen, TCD methods, and pharmacologic prophylaxis. Donor selection should always aim to minimize HLA disparity, with the possible exception of malignant diseases in which GVL responses (discussed later) may play a role, with preference for matched sibling donors, and perhaps male donors and nulliparous donors. With regard to conditioning regimens, myeloablative regimens are associated with a higher risk of GVHD than reduced intensity conditioning regimens, likely owing to increased tissue injury, particularly in the gastrointestinal tract. A certain graft source may also be preferred depending on these factors. For example, given the decreased risk of GVHD with bone marrow or UCB, bone marrow or CBT may be preferred in the setting of myeloablative conditioning, whereas peripheral blood stem cells are preferred in the setting of reduced intensity conditioning.

Impact of graft-versus-host disease prophylaxis on immune reconstitution. Prophylaxis of acute GVHD is centered around immunosuppression of the donor T cells, either pharmacologically or via ex vivo TCD. Pharmacologic prophylaxis does not have as profound an impact on immune reconstitution compared with ex vivo TCD methods; therefore pharmacologic prophylaxis may be preferred to TCD in the appropriate setting. GVHD pharmacologic prophylaxis regimens varies significantly among institutions but include agents such as antithymocyte globulin, alemtuzumab, cyclophosphamide, methotrexate, cyclosporine, tacrolimus, mycophenolate, and corticosteroids. Combination therapy, using more than one agent, is typically used as it is associated with a reduction in risk for acute GVHD compared with the use of single agents. Generally, the goal of GVHD prophylaxis is to maintain immunosuppression for the first 3 months after transplantation, but this duration may range between 4 weeks to 6 months after transplantation depending on the regimen used. In patients without GVHD, withdrawal of immunosuppression is associated with a reduced risk of relapse during the first 18 months; therefore shorter durations of GVHD prophylaxis are preferred for malignant disease.[38]

When antithymocyte globulin (ATG) or alemtuzumab (anti-CD52) is administered to the recipient in the pretransplant period, this is referred to as serotherapy or in vivo TCD. Serotherapy is considered instrumental in the prevention of rejection of the graft, especially from mismatched donors; however, owing to their long half-lives, ATG and alemtuzumab continue to be present at the time of donor product infusion and eliminate donor T cells, thereby offering prevention of acute GVHD. Despite the beneficial effects on prevention of graft rejection and GVHD, serotherapy adversely causes immunosuppression, delay in immune reconstitution, and increased risk of viral infections and reactivations, particularly with adenovirus.[39] Alemtuzumab has a longer half-life (15 to 21 days) than ATG (4 to 14 days) and therefore is associated with more prolonged T- and NK-cell recovery compared with ATG.[39]

Ex vivo TCD is an alternative approach to pharmacologic agents for GVHD prevention that requires manipulation of the donor product prior to administration to the recipient. Although the use of TCD methods may reduce the risk of GVHD in haploidentical stem cell transplant recipients, depending on the technique, it may be associated with significant risks, including delayed immune reconstitution, infectious complications and increased risk of graft failure and relapse. Ex vivo TCD includes methods such as $CD8^+$ cell depletion, $CD3^+/CD19^+$ cell depletion, TCR α/β T cell with $CD19^+$ cell depletion, or naïve TCD with or without T-cell add-back. Initial trials of ex vivo TCD using monoclonal antibodies admixed with the cells was associated with high risk of GVHD, leading to the additional treatment of T cells with complement or immunotoxins to eliminate T cells from the graft, which resulted in a 10% to 20% reduction of GVHD risk without pharmacologic prophylaxis. However, stringent TCD has been associated with increased risk of graft failure because donor lymphocytes, including both T cells and NK cells, are important mediators in engraftment. Therefore TCR α/β TCD methods that allow for repletion of donor γ/δ T cells and NK cells may help facilitate engraftment and prevent primary rejection. Finally, the use of $CD34^+$ positive selection is an approach that can exclude lymphocytes or immunologic components from the donor product that might be implicated in the pathogenesis of GVHD. This method has demonstrated substantial reductions in both acute and chronic GVHD while maintaining good disease control in patients with acute leukemia and myelodysplastic syndrome. Despite concomitant use of myeloablative conditioning regimens, $CD34^+$ selection shows good short-term (1 year) and longer-term (>1 year) toxicity outcomes, nonrelapse mortality, and overall survival.[40]

The mechanisms that predispose allogeneic stem cell transplant recipients to chronic GVHD are poorly defined; however, the most consistently documented risk factor for chronic GVHD is a history of acute GVHD. At this time, there is no specific immunoprophylaxis used to prevent chronic GVHD.

Impact of graft versus host disease on immune reconstitution. Although the pharmacologic agents administered to prevent or treat GVHD are a significant source of immune suppression, clinicians need to also recognize that GVHD in and of itself can result in delayed immune recovery. This is because acute GVHD represents an immunologic response against the host tissues, organs, and immune system, primarily mediated by alloreactive donor T cells.

Both the bone marrow, important for the development of hematopoietic progenitors, and the thymus, important for the maturation of hematopoietic precursors and T-cell development, are sites of alloreactivity during GVHD. Massive apoptosis and release of cytokines results in decrease in thymic output, delayed recovery of $CD4^+$ T cells, and restricted T-cell receptor repertoires.[41] Thymic epithelial cells are a direct target of alloreactive interferon γ–secreting donor T cells, which can lead to failure of donor-derived progenitors to differentiate via the classical central pathway.[42] The severity of acute GVHD-associated T-cell hypoplasia implies that GVHD abrogates not only thymic but also extrathymic T-cell reconstitution. After initial brisk proliferation of alloreactive T cells, antihost T cells undergo massive Fas-mediated apoptosis and lysis of grafted mature T cells.[43] Despite this, in younger patients (<25 years of age) with acute GVHD, thymic function generally recovers almost completely at 1 year and post-thymic T-cell lymphopoiesis typically resumes with resolution of GVHD and withdrawal of immunosuppression.[41] Owing to the severe and brisk destruction of lymphocytes and lymphocyte progenitors, advanced GVHD is the most significant independent predictor of subsequent (second, third, or fourth) infections. In addition to the impact on T-cell recovery, acute GVHD can have significant compromise of the skin and mucosal barriers of the alimentary tract that predispose to infection. The treatment of patients with acute GVHD with corticosteroids or other immunosuppressive drugs further increases the risk of infection.

By definition, chronic GVHD (cGVHD) presents after 100 days posttransplantation as a chronic inflammatory and sclerotic autoimmune-like condition that most frequently affects the skin, oral mucosa, liver, eyes, and gastrointestinal tract. The immunologic mechanisms underlying cGVHD are complex and differ from mechanisms underlying acute GVHD. Although donor-derived T cells are still considered to be the preeminent mediators of cGVHD alloreactivity, aberrant B cells clearly play a significant role in promoting autoimmunity and inflammation. The enhanced activity of T follicular helper cells in cGVHD appears to play a key role in the aberrant B-cell activity and the resulting autoimmune-like features of cGVHD.[44] It is thought that the alloreactivity and massive lymphoid apoptosis observed in acute GVHD might be responsible for the occurrence of autoimmunity in cGVHD.[43] This delay in immune reconstitution is primarily through thymic destruction and, in contrast to the damage seen in acute GVHD, is likely irreversible.[45] Patients with cGVHD are found to have low TRECs and shortening of telomere length, a measure of T-cell replicative capacity.[45] Furthermore, HSCT recipients in whom cGVHD develops are at increased risk of infections related to encapsulated organisms (particularly *Pneumococcus*), likely as the result of splenic dysfunction. This broad and profound immunologic dysfunction confers susceptibility to serious, often life-threatening, infections. In fact, chronic GVHD is the leading cause of late treatment-related deaths among HSCT recipients, and greater severity of cGVHD correlates with worse outcomes.[46]

Graft-Versus-Leukemia Effect. With HLA mismatched transplantation, donor T lymphocytes and NK cells may recognize neoplastic cells as foreign due to the expression of epitopes unique to the host. Cytotoxic T lymphocytes and NK cells subsequently become activated, lysing such cells. The T lymphocyte GVL or graft-versus-tumor effect is similar to that underlying GVHD. The first direct evidence of a pronounced antileukemic effect of GVHD was found in patients with AML with acute and/or chronic GVHD who had decreased relapse compared with patients with AML without GVHD.[47] Patients with AML who received syngeneic (twin sibling) grafts have an increased risk of relapse compared with allograft recipients without GVHD. Additionally, recipients of T-cell replete allografts have lower rates of relapse in the absence of GVHD compared with recipients of T-cell–depleted grafts.[47] However, this difference may not necessarily translate into prolonged disease-free survival in view of the morbidity and mortality associated with chronic GVHD.[21] Although cGVHD is associated with fewer relapses of leukemia, the severity of cGVHD does not further decrease the incidence of relapse. So, there may be a benefit to a mild degree of GVHD in patients with leukemia; however, avoidance of severe GVHD is still preferable. GVHD prophylaxis may be effective; however, an important concern is that such therapy would diminish the GVL effect. Furthermore, the association of GVHD with risk of relapse changes over time and HSCT recipients with GVHD have decreased risk of relapse after, but not before, 18 months after transplant.[38] The GVL effect could potentially be enhanced to prevent relapse. In patients without GVHD, withdrawal of immunosuppression might help to prevent relapse during the first 18 months after transplant but is likely not effective after 18 months.[38]

Despite this, GVL effects can be found independent of clinically significant GVHD and the immunologic mechanisms likely differ from those that underlie GVHD.[47] It is unclear whether GVL in the setting of absent or mild GVHD has an impact on the immune system. However, any impact appears to be relatively mild, given the lack of increased transplant-related mortality in patients with only mild GVHD. These findings have led to the investigation into other immunologic mechanisms involved in GVL effects, such as NK cells, killer cell immunoglobulin-like receptors (KIRs), and γ/δ T cells. KIRs are a particularly important moderator in the GVL effect. KIRs are surface receptors present on NK cells and a subset of T lymphocytes. Mismatching of the KIR ligand in the GVHD direction appears through NK-cell and cytotoxic T-cell activation, which result in a lower risk of relapse after allogeneic HSCT. This effect appears to be more evident in haploidentical transplantation using grafts depleted of T cells and in UCB transplantation.[48] Other mechanisms to augment the GVL effect include the use of donor lymphocyte infusions to induce sustained remissions. In the future, GVL effects may be enhanced through vaccine therapy or adoptive transfer of selective T cells to improve a portion of the immune response involved in GvL.[49]

ASSESSMENT OF IMMUNE RECONSTITUTION

There is no single marker for assessment of immune reconstitution after HSCT. This is primarily because recovery of a specific immune component of interest may require assessment of multiple laboratory values and will depend on the time period after HSCT under consideration. For example, neutrophil engraftment, assessed by frequent measurement of neutrophil counts, is classically used as a measure of innate immune system recovery. This is a common focus during the immediate early post-HSCT period. However, even when a patient is said to have achieved neutrophil engraftment (e.g., >500 neutrophils/μL), this result does not actually measure donor cell engraftment, as autologous reconstitution of neutrophils is possible after most conditioning regimens, nor does it inform on other recovery of other components of the innate immune system. Innate immune reconstitution can be further evaluated by measurement of NK cells. Recovery of the adaptive immunity is often of interest later after transplant and can include assessment of T-cell immunity via enumeration of T-cell subsets ($CD3^+$, $CD4^+$, $CD8^+$, and $CD4^+CD45^+RA$) and lymphocyte proliferative response to phytohemagglutinin. Although neutrophils are often measured frequently in the immediate post-HSCT period, the timing and form of measurement to assess recovery of other innate and adaptive function is variable by institution. Furthermore, it is not clear which level of a given test constitutes evidence of true reconstitution for a specific immune component.

Clinical research studies have used several markers at different time points of immune reconstitution, including absolute lymphocyte count, absolute $CD4^+$ count, CD4/CD8 ratio, T-cell subset testing by flow cytometry, Ig levels, rise in antigen-specific antibody titer after vaccination, lymphocyte mitogenic responses, quantification of TRECs, and T-cell receptor spectratyping or deep sequencing to assess the T-cell repertoire. Results from these studies have informed some general conclusions about laboratory values and general correlates of protection. For example, lymphocyte count 1 month after allogeneic HSCT is associated with better outcomes, including lower transplant-related mortality, higher relapse-free survival, and improved overall survival.[6] Additionally, a $CD4^+$ T-cell count below 200/μL at 3 months has been shown to be associated with increased infections, increased nonrelapse mortality, and decreased overall survival.[6] However, there remains an absence of clear guidance as to which immune function studies are clinically informative—and even if they are informative—and exactly when should they be performed. Because of the paucity of such data, institutions often develop their own approach for what laboratory tests to order, when to order them, and how to use the results for clinical decision making. This ultimately results in significant interinstitution variability. More data are needed to define the impact of different testing approaches on clinical outcomes so that centers can order these studies judiciously and harmonize their testing approaches.

IMPROVING IMMUNE RECONSTITUTION AFTER HSCT

Hematolymphopoiesis occurs in association with a complex network of cell types found in the bone marrow stroma, including nonhematopoietic (fibroblasts, adipocytes, and endothelial cells) and hematopoietic cells (macrophages and T-cells). Progenitor cell growth and differentiation depend on their interaction with stromal cells. Outside the bone marrow, lymphoid progenitors emigrate to the thymus to proliferate, mature, and differentiate. Several strategies have been proposed to enhance immune reconstitution after HSCT (Table 2.2), including cellular therapies, cytokines and hormones, sex steroid ablation, or enhancement of thymic tissue including the use of IL-7, thymosin α_1, growth hormone, keratinocyte growth factor, and sex steroid ablation. Of these, IL-7 has been most extensively studied in experimental and clinical trials. IL-7 acts directly on T-lymphoid precursors as a prolymphopoietic cytokine and has been shown to enhance thymopoiesis. A phase I trial of recombinant IL-7 in 12 adults undergoing T-cell–depleted allogeneic HSCT suggested that this approach improved T-cell recovery and T-cell repertoire diversity without increased GVHD or other toxicities.[50] Keratinocyte growth factor is a thymic epithelial cell (TEC) mitogen that stimulates proliferation and, when given before pretransplant conditioning, reduces TEC injury. Although keratinocyte growth factor has differential responses in various subsets of TECs, its efficacy can be enhanced in murine models by using p53 inhibition to restore cortical and medullary TECs and improve thymic function after HSCT.[9] Estrogen and testosterone have been implicated in the regulation of thymopoiesis, B-cell lymphopoiesis, and early lymphoid precursors. Androgen inhibition with leuprolide has been shown to reverse age-related thymic involution in animal models. Keratinocyte growth factor and androgen blockade may work in combination to protect TECs from conditioning-induced damage.[9] These mechanisms have been studied in murine models; however, the effects of keratinocyte growth factor and androgen blockage on immune reconstitution in human stem cell recipients is not yet elucidated.

TABLE 2.2 Strategies to Enhance Immune Reconstitution

Strategy	Mechanism
Reduced intensity conditioning	Decreased GVHD Decreased thymic damage
Increased cell dose	Improves engraftment Improves HPE Decreased GVHD
Stem cell processing T-cell depletion	Decreased GVHD
G-CSF and GM-CSF	Improves neutrophil and monocyte recovery
Low-dose IL-2	Improves HPE Improves thymopoiesis Increased CD4 T-cells and Treg counts
IL-15	Improves HPE Increased NK, NKT, and T cells
Thymosin-α_1	Improves thymopoiesis Increased CD4 recovery Early pathogen-specific T cells
IL-7	Improves thymopoiesis Enhances TCR-diversity Improved T-cell recovery
Keratinocyte growth factor	Improves thymopoiesis Prevent thymic damage
Cotransplanting MSCs	Supports engraftment of HSCs

G-CSF, granulocyte colony-stimulating factor; *GM-CSF,* granulocyte-macrophage colony-stimulating factor; *GVHD,* graft-versus-host disease; *HPE,* homeostatic peripheral expansion; *HSC,* hematopoietic stem cell; *IL,* interleukin; *NK,* natural killer; *NKT,* natural killer T lymphocytes; *Treg,* T regulatory; *TCR,* T-cell receptor.
Data from De Koning C, Plantinga M, Besseling P, Boelens JJ, Nierkens S. Immune reconstitution after allogeneic hematopoietic cell transplantation in children. *Biol Blood Marrow Transplant.* 2016; 22(2):195-206, Copyright © 2016 American Society for Blood and Marrow Transplantation; and Seggewiss R, Einsele H. Immune reconstitution after allogeneic transplantation and expanding options for immunomodulation: an update. *Blood.* 2010;115(19):3861-3868.

In the absence of thymopoiesis, homeostatic peripheral T-cell expansion is the most important mechanism of immune reconstitution. There are several cytokine-based therapies investigated to improve immune reconstitution through peripheral expansion, including low-dose IL-2– and IL-15–stimulated graft cells. Despite this, improvement of early T-cell immunity through homeostatic peripheral expansion is restricted to T cells with a limited T-cell receptor diversity, because the production of a diverse TCR repertoire requires antigen presentation in the thymus.[50]

A number of pretransplant and posttransplant cellular immunotherapies have been used to attempt to improve immune reconstitution, including chimeric antigen receptor T-cells, T regulatory cells, mesenchymal stem cells, adoptive NK cells, NK cells with γ/δ T cells, dendritic cell vaccination, DLIs, and virus-specific cytotoxic T cells.[49] Other methods can be applied at the time of transplantation, include the use of megadoses of donor hematopoietic stem cells or dCBT.[49] Donor lymphocyte infusions can be used for numerous indications, including as a means to improve postthymus lymphopoiesis; however, this is associated with a risk of producing severe GVHD. Because of high costs of production, regulatory burden, and complicated processing and production of other forms of cellular immunotherapies, these are not widely used in the HSCT setting. However, under the appropriate circumstances, they have the ability to treat life-threatening complications, such as relapse, viral reactivations, and GVHD, and could be used prophylactically in the case of NK cells and γ/δ T cells to prevent relapse and GVHD.

SUMMARY

Recovery of the innate and adaptive immune systems occurs gradually after autologous and allogeneic HSCT. Innate immunity usually recovers over the first several months, whereas adaptive immunity recovers over the first 1 to 2 years. Clinicians can consider infectious complications based on fixed time periods after HSCT receipt, such as during the pre-engraftment, early posttransplant, and late posttransplant phases. These periods are generally correlated with immune reconstitution, transplant-related toxicities, the development of GVHD, and receipt of immunosuppressive therapy, and can therefore be used to inform development of differential diagnosis for opportunistic infection. However, in reality, timing of immune reconstitution is affected by many variables, including the source of stem cells, degree of HLA match, the conditioning regimen used, manipulation of graft before transplantation, and the presence of GVHD, that will differ from patient to patient. Of these, the development of acute GVHD has the greatest impact on immune reconstitution, resulting in alloreactivity, apoptosis, and cytokine release. GVHD prophylaxis and treatment also results in delayed immune reconstitution. Therefore it is necessary to also understand the implications of the results of immune function testing for a specific patient and to adjust a differential diagnosis for opportunistic infections accordingly. Additionally, the duration chemoprophylaxis, immunoprophylaxis, and timing of vaccination schedules have traditionally been informed using the fixed time period after HSCT approach. However, increasingly centers are leveraging patient-specific immune function testing to inform cessation of these prophylactic interventions. Although the data to support the latter approach are limited, this approach seems to have logical merit. Several strategies have been evaluated to enhance posttransplant immune reconstitution without much success. Even so, newer cellular immunotherapies and graft manipulation techniques are likely to develop in the future to enhance immune reconstitution and decrease the risk of GVHD, allowing for the increased use of unrelated or related mismatched grafts.

3

Cancer and Antineoplastic Therapies and the Risk of Infection in the Pediatric Cancer Patient

Neil Patel, PharmD, BCOP and Abby Green, MD

Invasive infections are a common source of morbidity and mortality in children with cancer. The risk for infectious complications during therapy for cancer is inversely related to age: children with cancer are more commonly affected by infection compared with adult oncology patients, and infants are more vulnerable to infection than older children.[1] This is due to both environmental exposures that occur in childhood and the chemotherapy regimens used to treat pediatric cancer; the latter are more intensive in children than in adults with analogous malignancies.

Among pediatric oncology patients, children with acute leukemia are the group at highest risk for infectious complications. Fifty percent of pediatric patients with hematologic malignancies will have an infection at some point during therapy.[1] Children with acute lymphoblastic leukemia (ALL) have an infection-related mortality of nearly 5%, and among children with acute myelogenous leukemia (AML), infectious diseases are the cause of death in 5% to 10% of patients.[1,2] Mortality associated with invasive fungal disease in pediatric oncology patients is approximately 30%.[3]

Survival rates for childhood cancer are approaching 80%, which is vastly improved from prior decades. This is due in part to the refinement of chemotherapy protocols and the incorporation of novel, targeted therapeutic agents that have limited toxicity and extended survival. Additionally, supportive care regimens that optimize prevention and treatment of infectious diseases have substantially contributed to improved survival in pediatric oncology patients. However, with the improvement in overall survival come new infection-related complications that arise secondary to profound immunosuppression in the context of relapsed and refractory malignancy, unclear infectious risks of novel chemotherapeutics, and emergence of resistant organisms driven by increased use of anti-infective agents in this vulnerable pediatric population.

This chapter provides a paradigm for the assessment of infectious risk factors encountered by pediatric cancer patients based on specific cancer treatment regimens. Tailored supportive care recommendations are given for patients in the context of specific malignancies and chemotherapy regimens. Finally, risk factors and infectious pathogens common to specific pediatric oncology subpopulations are highlighted.

INFECTIOUS RISK ASSESSMENT IN ONCOLOGY PATIENTS

Not all pediatric oncology patients have the same risk for acquiring infectious diseases. Risk assessment can be evaluated at several levels, but the most superficial level is separation of hematologic (leukemia or lymphoma) from nonhematologic (solid) tumors. The treatment for hematologic malignancies requires therapy directed at the malignant and normal components of the immune system, leading to prolonged and profound immune deficits. In contrast, therapy for solid tumors largely consists of intermittent cytotoxic and myelosuppressive chemotherapy that only briefly disrupts immune function, predominantly by decreasing neutrophil quantity.

In general, the approach to infection prevention, diagnosis, and management in a pediatric oncology patient should incorporate the the intensity of chemotherapy that a child will receive (Table 3.1). Chemotherapy is the mainstay of cancer treatment in pediatric patients, and more intensive regimens are used for higher-risk malignancies. Increased intensity of chemotherapy results in more significant side effects, including bone marrow suppression, mucositis resulting in poor mucosal barrier integrity, and nutritional deficiency, all of which can contribute to an increased risk of opportunistic infection.

Myelosuppression leading to neutropenia is the most common hematologic toxicity of nearly all chemotherapy regimens. The majority of infectious complications, in particular bacterial infections and invasive fungal disease, occur in children with severe, prolonged neutropenia.[3,4] Life-threatening bloodstream infections (BSIs) are more likely to develop in patients with an absolute neutrophil count below 100 cells/μL.[5] Additional hematologic toxicities occur in children with lymphoid malignancies who experience prolonged periods of decreased lymphocyte count and function, and are therefore at risk for hypogammaglobulinemia. Patients with hypogammaglobulinemia are further predisposed to infections caused by viruses and encapsulated bacteria.[4]

Advances in prophylactic and empiric anti-infective therapy regimens have improved outcomes for high-risk pediatric oncology patients, particularly those with prolonged neutropenia. Details regarding specific recommendations for prophylactic and empiric treatment approaches during neutropenic periods are provided in Chapter 8: Management Principles for Neutropenic Patients. These approaches are aimed at reducing the risk of opportunistic bacterial and fungal infections during periods of neutropenia. However, the resulting burden of exposure to anti-infective agents can result in selective pressures leading to drug-resistant pathogens. This is compounded in children with cancer by the risk of acquiring drug-resistant pathogens from the health care environment by virtue of frequent and prolonged hospitalizations.[6] Understanding the prior anti-infective use and health care exposures for each patient is important for anticipation of infection or colonization with drug-resistant pathogens and may alter empiric treatment choices.

Several other factors pertinent to pediatric oncology patients result in immune compromise beyond neutropenia or lymphopenia. Therapy for most childhood cancers requires a central venous

TABLE 3.1 Infectious Risk Assessment by Oncologic Diagnosis

Malignancy	Typical Therapeutic Agents	Typical Regimen Duration	Location of Treatment	Expected Duration of Severe Neutropenia	Need for CVC Access?	Mucositis Risk	Additional Infection Risk Factors	Overall Risk of Infection
Leukemia								
ALL	*Conventional chemotherapy:* Steroids, anthracycline, asparaginase, vincristine, methotrexate, cyclophosphamide, cytarabine, *Mercaptopurine-targeted chemotherapy: + Ph+ ALL:* Imatinib, dasatinib Varied, usually in relapse protocols	6-9 months intensive followed by 2-2.5 years of low-intensity maintenance therapy	*Initial therapy:* Inpatient *Maintenance:* Ambulatory setting	Varied with each cycle, 7-28 days	Yes	Moderate (varies with each cycle)		High
AML	*Conventional chemotherapy:* Anthracycline, etoposide, cytarabine *Targeted chemotherapy:* Varied, usually in relapse protocols *HSCT:* For high-risk and relapsed patients	6-9 months of intensive chemotherapy	Primarily inpatient	14-21 days for each cycle	Yes	Moderate		High
CML	*Targeted chemotherapy:* Tyrosine kinase inhibitors	Lifelong	Ambulatory	None	No	None		Low
Lymphoma								
Hodgkin	*Conventional chemotherapy:* Steroids, varied cytotoxic and myelosuppressive agents *Targeted chemotherapy:* ± Brentuximab *HSCT:* Auto for relapsed disease *XRT:* ± Involved field	~6 months	Primarily ambulatory	<7 days per cycle	Sometimes	Minimal		Low-moderate
Non-Hodgkin	*Conventional chemotherapy:* Varied cytotoxic and myelosuppressive agents	~6 months	Mixed inpatient/outpatient	<7 days per cycle	Sometimes	Moderate		Moderate
CNS Tumors								
Embryonal	*Surgery* Conventional chemotherapy: Varied cytotoxic and myelosuppressive agents *HSCT:* Autologuous in some protocols *XRT:* axis	~1 year	Mixed inpatient/outpatient	<7 days per cycle	Yes	Moderate	CSF diversion catheters, surgical site infection	Moderate-high

Continued

TABLE 3.1 Infectious Risk Assessment by Oncologic Diagnosis—cont'd

Malignancy	Typical Therapeutic Agents	Typical Regimen Duration	Location of Treatment	Expected Duration of Severe Neutropenia	Need for CVC Access?	Mucositis Risk	Additional Infection Risk Factors	Overall Risk of Infection
Nonembryonal	Surgery *Targeted chemotherapy:* Various agents dependent on tumor type *XRT:* Craniospinal axis	Varied	Primarily ambulatory	Minimal	Rarely	Minimal	CSF diversion catheters, Surgical site infection	Moderate
Solid Tumors								
Sarcoma	*Conventional chemotherapy:* Alkylating agents, anthracyclines, platinums, dactinomycin, vincristine, etoposide *Surgery:* Resection of primary tumor *and/or* *XRT:* Tumor bed	6-9 months	Mixed inpatient/outpatient	<7 days per cycle	Yes	High	Poor nutrition, deconditioning, surgical site infection, endoprosthetic infection	Moderate
High-risk neuroblastoma	*Conventional chemotherapy.* Anthracycline, alkylating agents, vincristine, etoposide *Targeted chemotherapy:* Anti-GD2 antibody *Surgery:* Resection of primary tumor *and* *XRT:* Involved field *and* *HSCT:* Auto	1.5 years	Mixed inpatient/outpatient	~7 days per cycle	Yes	High		High

ALL, acute lymphoblastic leukemia; *AML*, acute myelogenous leukemia; *CNS*, central nervous system; *CSF*, cerebrospinal fluid; *CVC*, central venous catheter; *GD2*, glycolipid disialoganglioside; *HSCT*, hematopoietic stem cell transplantation; *Ph+*, Philadelphia chromosome positive; *XRT*, radiation therapy.

catheter (CVC) for administration of vesicant chemotherapy and frequent intravenous supportive care including total parenteral nutrition. The presence of a CVC compromises the innate immunity of the skin barrier and is an independent risk factor for BSI; this risk persists even after neutrophil count recovery. Approximately 25% of children with cancer have a BSI that is directly attributed to the CVC.[7] The type of CVC can determine risk for infections; there is a higher rate of BSI and specifically gram-negative rod infection with percutaneous CVCs compared with implanted access ports.[1,6]

Additional disruption of skin and mucosal barrier integrity can result from certain chemotherapeutic agents (Table 3.2), radiation therapy (XRT), and/or surgical procedures. Mucositis, or inflammation and ulceration of the mucosal lining of the gastrointestinal tract, can be caused by chemotherapy or XRT. Breaches in the mucosal lining of the mouth and intestines enable translocation of commensal organisms into the bloodstream. In the setting of neutropenia, translocation of organisms to the bloodstream is more likely to result in a BSI. Skin integrity is disrupted in pediatric oncology patients by surgical incisions, CVCs, gastrostomy tubes, and XRT-induced burns. Any breach in skin integrity serves as a nidus for skin and soft tissue infection, especially in patients undergoing myelosuppressive therapy. Surgical site infections are exacerbated in neutropenic patients by neutropenia-associated poor wound healing and can become sites of chronic or recurrent infection in children who require repeated treatment with chemotherapy.

TABLE 3.2 **Conventional Chemotherapeutics**

Chemotherapy Category	Chemotherapy Agent	Mechanism of Action	Immunosuppressive Effects	Drug-Specific Adverse Effects	Class-Specific Adverse Effects
Alkylating agents	Cyclophosphamide Ifosfamide	Nitrogen mustard: Cross-linking DNA strands	Neutropenia Lymphopenia	Hemorrhagic cystitis Mucositis (dose related) Infertility CNS toxicity (ifosfamide)	Alopecia Anemia Nausea/vomiting Thrombocytopenia
	Procarbazine	DNA alkylation; Inhibit protein synthesis by transmethylation of methionine into transfer RNA	Neutropenia Lymphopenia	Secondary malignancy (highly carcinogenic) Male infertility Disulfiram reaction	
	Temozolomide	DNA alkylation via methylating metabolite MTIC	Neutropenia Lymphopenia	Hepatotoxicity	
	Carmustine Lomustine	Nitrosourea: alkylates DNA and RNA	Neutropenia (delayed onset at 4-6 weeks after administration)	Secondary malignancy	
Platinum analogs	Cisplatin, carboplatin, oxaliplatin	Forms DNA cross-links; binds to DNA bases and disrupts DNA function	Neutropenia (dose dependent)	Cisplatin: Nephrotoxicity Ototoxcity Electrolyte disturbances Carboplatin: Thrombocytopenia Oxaliplatin: Peripheral neuropathy	Anemia Nausea/vomiting
Antimetabolites	Clofarabine	Antimetabolite: Purine nucleoside analog	Prolonged neutropenia	Capillary leak syndrome Mucositis	Anemia Nausea / vomiting Thrombocytopenia
	Cytarabine	Antimetabolite: Pyrimidine analog	Neutropenia High-dose cytarabine: increased risk of alpha hemolytic streptococcal infection during intensive treatment of AML	Diarrhea Neurotoxicity Rash / desquamation	
	Gemcitabine	Antimetabolite: Pyrimidine analog	Neutropenia	Flu-like symptoms Liver function abnormality	
	Mercaptopurine	Antimetabolite: Purine analog	Neutropenia in patients with homozygous mutation for TPMT activity	Hepatotoxicity	
	Methotrexate	Folate antimetabolite; inhibits dihydrofolate reductase	Neutropenia with delayed clearance or inappropriate supportive care	Hepatotoxicity Mucositis Nephrotoxicity	
	Nelarabine	Antimetabolite: Purine analog; ara-GTP accumulates at a higher level in T cells	Neutropenia	Liver function abnormality Neurotoxicity Peripheral neuropathy	
Natural product	Anthracyclines: daunorubicin, doxorubicin, idarubicin Anthracenedione: mitoxantrone	Topoisomerase II inhibitor Inhibit DNA and RNA synthesis by intercalation	Neutropenia Lymphopenia	Alopecia Cardiotoxicity Mucositis (doxorubicin >> daunorubicin)	Anemia Nausea / vomiting Thrombocytopenia (except Vinca Alkaloids)
	Dactinomycin	Intercalates guanine–cytosine base pairs in DNA	Neutropenia	Diarrhea	

Continued

TABLE 3.2 Conventional Chemotherapeutics—cont'd

Chemotherapy Category	Chemotherapy Agent	Mechanism of Action	Immunosuppressive Effects	Drug-Specific Adverse Effects	Class-Specific Adverse Effects
	Etoposide	Topoisomerase II inhibitor	Neutropenia	Mucositis Nausea / vomiting Secondary malignancy (1-3 years after treatment)	
	Irinotecan	Topoisomerase I inhibitor	Neutropenia	Diarrhea mediated by toxic metabolite unconjugated SN-38	
	Topotecan	Topoisomerase I inhibitor	Neutropenia	Mucositis	
	Vinca Alkaloids: Vincristine Vinblastine Vinorelbine	Microtubule inhibitors	Neutropenia (vinorelbine >> vinblastine >> vincristine)	Peripheral neuropathy (vincristine >> vinblastine >> vinorelbine)	

AML, acute myelogenous leukemia; *Ara-GTP*, araguanosine-5′-triphosphate; *MTIC*, 3-methyl-(triazen-1-yl)imidazole-4-carboxamide; *RNA*, ribonucleic acid; *SN-38*, 7-ethyl-10-hydroxy-camptothecin; *TMPT*, tumor molecular targeting peptide.

Nutritional deficiency is common during chemotherapy administration in children and can further compromise a patient's immune function.[5] Malnutrition impairs immunity as the result of decreased production of complement, cytokines, and immunoglobulins. Not surprisingly, underweight patients receiving chemotherapy have a higher incidence of febrile neutropenia than their peers.[8]

A less commonly recognized immune dysfunction in this patient population is functional asplenia that can result from irradiation to the spleen. Patients with abdominal tumors or Hodgkin lymphoma (HL) may receive targeted or indirect XRT to the spleen. Splenic dysfunction results in an increased risk for infection with encapsulated organisms. The Infectious Diseases Society of America and American College of Immunization Practices recommend that asplenic patients, including those with functional asplenia, be immunized with pneumococcal polysaccharide and meningococcal vaccines.

Finally, there is a recommendation that children currently receiving cancer therapy not receive routine immunizations with the exception of the annual influenza vaccine. Although the influenza vaccine should be administered to pediatric oncology patients, it may not be effective in the setting of chemotherapy. Thus many children are unvaccinated or undervaccinated while they are undergoing cancer therapy, leaving them at risk for vaccine-preventable infections.

DISEASE-SPECIFIC INFECTIOUS RISKS

Hematologic Malignancies

Leukemia is the most common cancer diagnosis in children and constitutes approximately 35% of all childhood cancers.[4] ALL accounts for 75% of leukemia diagnoses in patients younger than 20 years of age and occurs most frequently in children 1 to 4 years.[9] AML accounts for 18% of childhood leukemia and occurs bimodally with equal frequency in patients 1 to 4 years and 15 to 19 years.[10] The remainder of leukemia diagnosed in children is made up of chronic myeloid leukemia (CML), juvenile myelomonocytic leukemia (JMML), and biphenotypic leukemia or mixed phenotype acute leukemia (MPAL).

The survival rate of patients with ALL is significantly better than that of those with AML; children with ALL have a 5-year survival of more than 85%, whereas children with AML have an estimated 65% overall survival at 5 years. Survival rates for subtypes of ALL and AML differ, and predicted survival can be used to roughly estimate the intensity of therapeutic regimen. Efforts toward tailored therapy have focused on decreasing the use of cytotoxic and myelosuppressive chemotherapy to avoid short- and long-term toxicities without diminishing survival benefit.[11] A dramatic example of subgroup survival difference is that of acute promyelocytic leukemia (APML), which has an overall survival approaching 95% largely due to the incorporation of targeted agents such as arsenic trioxide and retinoic acid. Hence, patients with APML incur significantly fewer infectious complications of therapy than children with other subtypes of AML.

Conversely, children with relapsed or refractory leukemia are treated with very high-intensity chemotherapy and ultimately may receive an allogeneic hematopoietic stem cell transplantation (SCT); thus these patients are at highest risk for infectious complications. Infection accounts for the majority of treatment-related deaths in children with relapsed and refractory hematologic malignancies.

Although ALL and AML are treated differently, the first phase of chemotherapy for all acute leukemia is called "induction," and the goal is to achieve a complete disease remission. For all children with leukemia, the induction phase is a high-risk period owing to the adverse effects from neutropenia compounded by other complications, such as tumor lysis syndrome, thrombosis, and bleeding. Although there has been a decrease in mortality associated with improvements in supportive care, infections still account for up to 30% of induction deaths in pediatric patients with leukemia.[12]

Acute Lymphoblastic Leukemia. Patients with ALL are risk-stratified by criteria set forth by the National Cancer Institute into low-risk, standard risk, high-risk, or very high-risk disease groups. Determinants of risk include age, white blood cell count at presentation, cytogenetics, immunologic subtype (B cell, T cell, or MPAL), and response to induction therapy. Patients with ALL are risk-stratified based on predicted survival, and risk assessments are used to guide the intensity of therapy. In general, patients with ALL receive 6 to 9 months of intensive chemotherapy followed by 2 to 2.5 years of low-intensity maintenance chemotherapy. Risk of infection is concentrated during the first 6 to 9 months of treatment and increases with intensity of treatment regimen. The addition of anthracyclines (e.g., daunorubicin) to induction regimens in high-risk and very high-risk patients contributes to neutropenia and mucositis, both significant risk factors for infection. Thus patients treated for high- and very high-risk ALL have more infectious complications than their lower-risk counterparts.

Intensive portions of therapy are most commonly delivered via an implantable venous access port, which further increases the risk for infection. To mitigate risk, implanted ports are often removed when a patient begins the maintenance portion of therapy.

ALL is most frequently diagnosed in children 1 to 4 years of age; thus pathogens common to this age group predominantly cause the infectious complications seen in young children with ALL, including upper respiratory infection, otitis media, and gastroenteritis.[8] BSI is common during periods of neutropenia, and the frequency of BSI is correlated with duration of neutropenia. Because duration of neutropenia becomes more prolonged in later phases of chemotherapy, BSI and fungal infections occur with increased frequency in the latter portion of intensive chemotherapy for ALL, especially in higher-risk patients.[8]

T-cell ALL, which is a small fraction of childhood ALL, historically had a worse prognosis than B-cell ALL and was thus treated with more intensive chemotherapy regimens. As the biology of T-cell ALL has been elucidated in recent years and treatment protocols have been refined, outcomes for T-cell and B-cell ALL have become increasingly similar. A notable distinction of T-cell ALL is the predilection for recalcitrant central nervous system (CNS) disease, necessitating CNS-directed therapy. The most recent treatment protocols use dexamethasone rather than prednisone for T-ALL, which provides increased potency and CNS penetration, though it is associated with significantly more infectious complications.[13]

Acute Myelogenous Leukemia. Therapy for AML requires repeated cycles of myelosuppressive chemotherapy leading to periods of severe neutropenia averaging approximately 2 to 4 weeks. Thus patients with AML have a high risk of bacterial and fungal infection. Children with AML have a 5–10% infection-related mortality and 20–50% incidence of bacterial infection.[14] Notable exceptions to this treatment regimen are children with APML and those with Down syndrome–associated acute megakaryoblastic leukemia, both of which have excellent prognoses and require far less intensive therapy. Children with AML usually have a CVC in place for the duration of treatment to accommodate their significant supportive care needs during periods of prolonged myelosuppression.

The most common serious infections in pediatric patients with AML are caused by gram-negative bacteria, viridans group streptococci, and fungi. Viridans-group streptococcal bacteremia occurs in nearly 1 in 4 children treated for AML[15] and accounts for approximately 15% of all infection-related deaths in pediatric patients with AML.[14] The incidence of gram-negative bacteria infection in children treated for AML has decreased in recent years, likely as the result of widespread use of quinolone prophylaxis during periods of neutropenia, as well as improved infection control measures relating to the care of CVCs and maintenance of the hospital environment. The most common gram-negative organisms isolated are *Pseudomonas aeruginosa*, *Klebsiella* spp., and *Escherichia coli*.[14,16] Fungal infections occur in approximately 3% of patients undergoing therapy for de novo AML, although this incidence increases in patients with relapsed and refractory disease.[16,17]

Chronic Myeloid Leukemia. Pediatric patients with CML are treated similarly to adults, and the mainstay of treatment is aimed at inhibition of the ABL tyrosine kinase, driven by the *BCR-ABL* fusion protein that results from the chromosomal translocation (9;22). The *BCR-ABL* translocation, named the Philadelphia chromosome, results in constitutive activation of the *ABL1* kinase that drives cellular proliferation. CML has become a chronic disease through the use of *ABL*-class tyrosine kinase inhibitors (TKIs), which keep the disease controlled even when used as monotherapy. TKIs used for pediatric CML include imatinib, dasatinib, and less commonly nilotinib. All are available as oral preparations; thus treatment does not require central venous access. Infectious complications of CML therapy are rarely reported. Although *ABL*-class TKIs have the potential to cause neutropenia or lymphopenia, largely because of their off-target effects, these laboratory abnormalities are rarely seen in pediatric patients. Children who experience dose-limiting hematologic toxicity of TKIs are managed by adjustment of dose or by switching to an alternative TKI. Adult patients treated with imatinib have an increased risk of hepatitis B reactivation, although this has not been reported in pediatric patients.

Down Syndrome. Children with Down syndrome (DS) have an increased risk of developing hematologic malignancies, most commonly acute leukemia. DS-associated leukemia tends to have a favorable prognosis, although treatment has historically been complicated by significant infection-related morbidity. Children with DS have much higher rates of infectious and other treatment-related complications than children without DS. Recent efforts aimed at decreasing the intensity of therapy have resulted in improved survival rates for children with DS-associated leukemia owing to fewer therapy-related complications. Importantly, a comparison of two sequential clinical trials for therapy of DS-AML published in 2004 and 2016 demonstrated infection-related mortality rates of 20% and 4.9%, respectively.[18] Although the incidence of infection has not significantly decreased, the profile of infectious diseases in children with DS has shifted to an increased proportion of viral infections compared with bacterial and fungal infections. Viral pneumonia and viral gastroenteritis are the most common infections documented in children with DS during leukemia therapy.[18] Importantly, children with DS may have atypical presentations of infection including without fever, and during lower-intensity treatment phases.[19] Supportive care practices specific to children with DS require vigilance regarding skin hygiene and a high index of suspicion for infection despite atypical presentation.

Infant Leukemia. Infant leukemia, defined as acute myeloid or lymphoblastic leukemia in a child younger than 12 months, is a rare cancer and occurs in fewer than 200 children in the United States annually. The prognosis for infants with leukemia is poor, and treatment is challenging given the excess toxicity observed in this young age group. Induction mortality is much higher for infants with acute leukemia compared with older children, and much of the therapy-related mortality observed in infants is due to infectious complications.[20] The majority of infections are caused by gram-positive organisms, followed by gram-negative bacteria and fungi.[20] Efforts to de-intensify therapy are more challenging than in other pediatric oncology populations because infant leukemia is very difficult to treat. However, similar to patients with DS, infants require maximal supportive care, including efforts to prevent infection, close monitoring, and a high index of suspicion for infectious complications.

Lymphoma. Lymphoma is classically categorized as either Hodgkin (HL) or non-Hodgkin (NHL) disease. HL occurs with a bimodal distribution with the first peak during adolescence and young adulthood (15 to 24 years), which makes it a common pediatric malignancy. HL is indolent and very sensitive to chemotherapy and radiation; survival rates exceed 90% in all age groups. Treatment involves several cycles of chemotherapy, typically administered over a period of less than 2 years. Each cycle can result in episodes of neutropenia generally lasting less than 7 days, and involved-field XRT for some patients. Infection rates are low among children and adolescents treated for HL owing to low treatment intensity, although some specific infectious risks arise during treatment for HL: (1) patients with splenic involvement may receive radiation to the spleen, resulting in splenic dysfunction and a higher risk of infection with encapsulated organisms; and (2) radiation is a common treatment modality for patients with HL and brings with it infectious risks factors beyond myelosuppression, including disruption of skin and mucous membrane barrier integrity.

NHL occurs with higher incidence than HL in all ages and, for the purposes of this chapter, should be conceptualized by prognosis/intensity of therapy rather than cell of origin. Lymphoblastic lymphoma (LL) arises from either T or B cells and pathologically appears identical to ALL, although it is categorized as lymphoma because of a low burden of bone marrow disease (<25%). LL is treated similarly to ALL with 6 to 9 months of intensive therapy followed by several years of maintenance chemotherapy, and thus it has infectious risks similar to those of patients treated for ALL. Mature B-cell lymphomas include Burkitt, diffuse large B-cell lymphoma, and primary mediastinal B-cell lymphoma. These high-grade mature B-cell malignancies are treated with repeated cycles of intensive chemotherapy that often result in severe mucositis, malnutrition, and brief (<7 days) but profound myelosuppression. Anaplastic large cell lymphoma is a T-cell malignancy that occurs in adolescents and young adults, and is treated with chemotherapy regimens similar to those used for mature B-cell NHL. In general, infectious complications in pediatric patients with NHL are infrequent, although common risk factors of myelosuppression, central venous catheters, and mucositis occur with increased frequency in late-stage NHL that requires higher intensity treatment.

Solid Tumors

Solid tumors can be categorized as either intracranial or extracranial and portend different infectious risks based on anatomic location. Solid tumors are risk-stratified by stage at diagnosis, and in general high-stage disease requires more intensive treatment. Solid tumors are treated with a combination of chemotherapy, radiation, and surgery; each treatment modality brings with it specific infectious risks. Indwelling foreign materials are common to treatment of solid tumors, including central venous catheters, intraventricular catheters, and surgical material including long-term endoprostheses.

Central Nervous System Tumors. Brain and spinal cord tumors are the most common type of pediatric solid tumor and account for up to 20% of all childhood malignancies.[21] CNS tumors are an exception to the paradigm that chemotherapy intensity is increased in higher-risk malignancies. Children with CNS tumors are rarely treated with intensive chemotherapy, even those with very poor prognoses. The mainstays of treatment for CNS tumors are surgery and XRT and, although adjuvant chemotherapy is used, it is infrequently given at doses or combinations that cause significant myelosuppression. Thus infectious complications of CNS tumors and their treatment relate to surgical complications, the presence of indwelling catheters and other foreign material, and neurologic dysfunction.

Infectious risks specific to children with brain tumors include surgical site infections, ventriculitis/meningitis related to CSF diversion catheters, and infectious complications of neurologic dysfunction. Few studies have focused on infectious complications in children with brain tumors but have shown that the short-term postoperative infection rate is approximately 20% and consists primarily of wound infections and CSF catheter infections.[22] This infection rate is consistent with neurosurgical infection rates in patients without brain tumors. CSF catheter infections are most often introduced at the time of surgical placement or revision, although, less commonly, they can arise as a retrograde infection from the distal end of the shunt. The latter scenario can occur from bowel contamination of a ventriculoperitoneal shunt or hematogenous seeding of a ventriculoatrial shunt. CNS tumors or resection efforts result in neurologic dysfunction to varying degrees. Infections arise in patients with neurologic dysfunction for many reasons; some examples include aspiration events leading to pneumonia, bladder stasis leading to urinary tract infections, and decubitus ulcer infections.

Of note, there are CNS tumors of embryonal origin—medulloblastoma, atypical teratoid rhabdoid tumors, and primitive neuroectodermal tumors—that tend to occur in younger children and are treated with myelosuppressive chemotherapy, often followed by autologous stem cell rescue.[21] In addition to the infectious risks noted earlier for other CNS tumors, these patients are also at risk for bacteremia, typhlitis, and additional opportunistic infections common to children undergoing periods of profound neutropenia.

Neuroblastoma. Neuroblastoma is the most common extracranial solid tumor in children. It arises from embryonal neural crest tissue and may present as a localized, low-grade tumor or as high-grade, widely metastatic disease. Staging is determined by histology, genetic aberrations, and metastasis. High-risk neuroblastoma (HR NBL) has poor outcomes and is treated with multimodality therapy, including cytotoxic and myelosuppressive chemotherapy, surgery, XRT, autologous SCT, and immunotherapy. Infectious risks vary throughout the treatment course, which lasts 1.5 to 2 years, and more than 50% of children treated for HR NBL have a bacterial or fungal infection at some point during therapy.[23] Most infections occur during neutropenic periods resulting from myelosuppressive chemotherapy. Current treatment protocols include four or five cycles of neoadjuvant chemotherapy that result in neutropenic periods averaging 5 to 7 days. Postoperatively, children undergo myeloablative chemotherapy followed by autologous SCT with a longer expected duration of neutropenia (7 to 14 days). However, neuroblastoma therapy is one of the most rapidly evolving fields in pediatric oncology, with a current emphasis on decreased dosing of conventional chemotherapy to limit late-onset toxicity, and a movement toward targeted therapies. As this shift occurs, the infectious risks associated with therapy for HR NBL will also change.

Sarcoma. The majority of sarcomas arise during childhood and adolescence. The most common types of sarcoma are osteosarcoma, rhabdomyosarcoma, and Ewing sarcoma, although a variety of other bone and soft tissue sarcomas occur in the pediatric age group. Treatment for sarcomas includes repeated cycles of chemotherapy leading to brief (~7 days) but profound neutropenia, and local control of the tumor, which may involve surgical resection or XRT. Advances in surgical techniques have led to increased use of endoprosthetic reconstruction rather than amputation of affected limbs. Although this approach preserves anatomy and some function, the risk of infection associated with allograft or prosthetic placement is high and constitutes the primary mode of reconstructive failure for pediatric patients.[24] Soft tissue infections occur in up to 50% of limb salvage procedures, and infection of the prosthesis occurs in 8% to 18% depending on prosthetic material, location, and immunologic and nutritional status of the patient.[24] Treatment of an endoprosthetic infection is complex and often requires a combination of surgical debridement and prolonged antimicrobial therapy. In rare cases, amputation is required to definitively manage endoprosthetic infections.

Children with bone and soft tissue sarcomas are treated with highly emetogenic chemotherapy which, combined with disability related to tumor location, frequently results in malnutrition and prolonged deconditioning. These factors increase the risk for and complicate infections that occur in patients with sarcoma. Supportive care in the form of nutritional support and physical therapy are paramount to infection prevention.

Wilms Tumor. Wilms tumor is the most common renal tumor of childhood. Staging is based on histology, location, metastasis, and surgical outcomes, and treatment intensity increases with higher-stage disease. Treatment consists of low-intensity chemotherapy that rarely causes profound neutropenia, surgery, and occasionally XRT. Infectious complications in children with Wilms tumor are rare.

Hepatoblastoma. Hepatoblastoma is a liver tumor that arises in infancy and early childhood. It is a chemotherapy-sensitive tumor with very good survival rates. Children are treated with a combination of surgical resection and adjuvant chemotherapy. If the primary tumor is unresectable, patients may undergo liver transplantation, which occurs in approximately 20% of cases.[25] For these children, infectious risks are largely those affected by solid organ transplantation (see Chapter 1). Infectious complications are uncommon in cases of hepatoblastoma without liver transplant.

INFECTIOUS RISKS ASSOCIATED WITH ANTICANCER THERAPIES

Children with cancer who are treated with conventional cytotoxic and myelosuppressive chemotherapy are at an increased risk of febrile neutropenia, invasive infections, and infection-related mortality.[14] The goal of conventional chemotherapy during the induction or neoadjuvant phase in many pediatric cancers is to rapidly eradicate tumor cells to a clinically undetectable state termed remission. Optimization of chemotherapy dose intensity has resulted in improved cure rates and survival; however, the side effects of conventional chemotherapy occur as a result of lack of specificity for cancer cells and an unavoidable impact on rapidly dividing healthy cells. Thus the design of chemotherapy doses and treatment schedules requires a balance between destroying cancer cells and sparing healthy cells to avoid significant morbidity and mortality.[26] Common side effects of conventional chemotherapy include myelosuppression and damage to mucosal barrier integrity, both of which significantly predispose patients to infection and associated morbidity and mortality.

Bone marrow suppression constitutes a dose-limiting toxicity of conventional chemotherapy consisting of neutropenia, thrombocytopenia, and anemia. Neutropenia is a driving factor for the development of opportunistic bacterial and fungal infections, and patients with febrile neutropenia require prompt evaluation and treatment with antibiotics.[27] Combination chemotherapy consisting of multiple myelotoxic drugs results in profound, and sometimes prolonged, neutropenia and thereby increases risk of infectious complications. Growth factor support has become the standard of care after chemotherapy administration in children with solid tumors as it significantly decreases the duration of severe neutropenia and incidence of febrile neutropenia.[28,29] Growth factor use can similarly reduce the duration of neutropenia after chemotherapy for acute leukemia. However, growth factor support has the potential to introduce abnormalities in bone marrow progenitor populations, which can skew disease evaluations and possibly potentiate hematologic malignancy. Thus growth factor agents are not often used in children with leukemia. The next section reviews chemotherapeutic agents commonly used to treat pediatric cancers.

Conventional Chemotherapeutic Agents

The mechanisms of action of common chemotherapy drugs used to treat pediatric cancer are outlined in Table 3.2. The cytotoxic and myelosuppressive effects of these conventional agents result from DNA damage or inhibition of DNA replication, subsequently leading to the death of rapidly dividing cells. The major toxicity of all conventional chemotherapeutic agents is that tumor cells are not specifically targeted, and thus both malignant and healthy cells are destroyed. The main categories of conventional chemotherapy drugs include alkylating agents, platinum analogs, antimetabolites, and natural products. A combination of chemotherapy from different pharmacologic classes results in optimal therapeutic endpoints, but comes with a wide range of adverse events. In addition to myelosuppression and mucositis, some of the common and significant toxic effects of these drugs are provided in Table 3.2.

Alkylating Agents. Alkylating agents are integral to the treatment of many pediatric cancers, including ALL, HL, NBL, sarcomas, and brain tumors. These drugs work by forming reactive intermediates that attach an alkyl group to DNA base pairs which interfere with DNA replication. Myelosuppression is a common dose-limiting toxicity of alkylating agents. The nadir for absolute neutrophil count occurs 6 to 10 days after administration of alkylators, with recovery after 14 to 21 days. Delayed and prolonged myelosuppression occurs with nitrosoureas, such as carmustine and lomustine, where the nadir in platelets and neutrophils starts 4 to 6 weeks after treatment with a slow recovery thereafter.

Platinum Analogs. Platinum analogs are a backbone of many pediatric solid and brain tumors given their antineoplastic activity resulting from covalent binding of platinum to nucleophilic sites on DNA, leading to intrastrand and interstrand cross-links and DNA breaks. Besides myelosuppression, nephrotoxicity and ototoxicity are common side effects. Platinum analogs are also highly emetogenic, necessitating nutritional monitoring and support. Appropriate hydration is necessary for prevention of renal damage, and dose adjustments may be necessary to mitigate excessive or prolonged nephrotoxicity.[30]

Antimetabolites. The antimetabolite class consists of analogs of folic acid, pyrimidines, and purines that ultimately inhibit DNA synthesis and replication. Methotrexate is the quintessential folic acid analog and is used in high doses (>1000 mg/m^2) for ALL, lymphoma, and osteosarcoma. Methotrexate inhibits dihydrofolate reductase, an enzyme required for reduction of folic acid to tetrahydrofolate or folinic acid. This inhibition leads to a reduced capacity for methylation reactions necessary for the synthesis of DNA bases. High-dose methotrexate can have significant adverse effects, including bone marrow suppression and mucositis. To alleviate these side effects, intravenous hydration necessary for drug clearance and pharmacologic rescue with reduced folate or leucovorin is administered after high-dose methotrexate in pediatric patients.

Pyrimidine and purine analogs include various drugs that inhibit synthesis of essential DNA precursors (e.g., mercaptopurine) or are converted intracellularly to nucleoside analogs and incorporated into DNA, leading to cell-cycle arrest and apoptosis. Nucleoside analogs such as mercaptopurine and cytarabine are specifically used in hematologic malignancies. Clofarabine, a pyrimidine analog, is approved for relapsed/refractory ALL, although it comes with significant toxicities and is usually not well tolerated. Nelarabine is a purine analog and has resulted in improved outcomes for patients with T-cell ALL but causes myelosuppression and peripheral neuropathy.

Natural Products. Chemotherapy derived from natural products can be divided into vinca alkaloids (e.g., vincristine), camptothecin analogs (e.g., irinotecan and topotecan), antibiotics (e.g., anthracyclines or dactinomycin), and epipodophyllotoxin derivatives (e.g., etoposide). These agents affect cell cycle progression or cause double-stranded DNA breaks, resulting in rapid death of dividing cells. Vinca alkaloids are frequently used to treat pediatric cancers and block the cell cycle during mitosis by disrupting microtubule formation. Vincristine, the most common vinca alkaloid, is not myelosuppressive, unlike many other conventional chemotherapeutics. Camptothecin analogs inhibit topoisomerase I, thus promoting genotoxic double-stranded DNA breaks and can cause dose-limiting neutropenia. Anthracyclines/anthracenediones are a major subset of antibiotic chemotherapy agents that are highly active for ALL, AML, lymphoma, and many solid tumor treatment regimens. Finally, epipodophyllotoxin derivatives like etoposide directly inhibit topoisomerase II, which results in double-stranded DNA breaks. Etoposide, which is widely used in pediatric cancer, has a dose-limiting toxicity of neutropenia. Most natural product chemotherapeutics result in neutrophil nadir at 10 to 14 days with recovery by 21 days.[34]

Autologous Stem Cell Transplant

Hematopoietic SCT may be allogeneic, in which the donor and recipient are two different subjects, or autologous, in which stem cells are harvested from a patient and reinfused into that same patient. The purpose of autologous hematopoietic SCT (auto-SCT), also called stem cell rescue, in patients with cancer is to enable delivery of high-dose cytotoxic and myelosuppressive chemotherapy that, without a replacement of the bone marrow, would lead to prolonged or indefinite bone marrow aplasia. Although this treatment approach is not effective for acute leukemia, the indications for auto-SCT in children have expanded over the last several decades and now include refractory lymphoma, high-risk neuroblastoma, and medulloblastoma. A variety of other solid tumors have been treated experimentally with auto-SCT with varying outcomes.

The conditioning regimens, or chemotherapeutic agents administered before SCT, are tailored to each patient's disease process. The goal of conditioning is to use high-dose chemotherapy and/or XRT to kill cancer cells. A nearly universal side effect of the agents and doses used for conditioning is the destruction of bone marrow stem cells, thus the requirement for auto-SCT. Once autologous stem cells are infused, the time to neutrophil engraftment ranges from 1 to 3 weeks. During this period of profound neutropenia, termed the pre-engraftment period, the majority of infectious complications occur. In addition to profound, prolonged neutropenia, auto-SCT recipients have additional risk factors for serious infection, including central venous access, mucositis, and poor nutrition. There do not seem to be significant differences in infection risk attributable to underlying oncologic disease or conditioning regimen.[44]

Most infectious complications arise in the pre-engraftment period of auto-SCT. Infections occur in 21% to 34% of patients before neutrophil engraftment.[14,44] Bacterial infections are most common, followed by viral infections. Invasive fungal diseases are rare but occur with more prolonged periods of neutropenia. Bacteremia and *Clostridium difficile* colitis are the most common bacterial infections in the pre-engraftment period, and gram-positive bacteremia is slightly more common than gram-negative bacteremia. Viral infections are largely due to herpesviruses. Stomatitis and other manifestations of Herpes Simplex Virus are the most common viral infections to complicate pediatric auto-SCT, although the incidence has decreased with routine use of acyclovir prophylaxis[44] in patients who are known to have positive Herpes Simplex Virus serologic testing. Varicella zoster virus (VZV) reactivation is much more common in adult transplant patients than in the pediatric population and is reported to occur at a rate of 1% to 2% in children undergoing auto-SCT. Based on the profile of infections that have historically occurred in pediatric auto-SCT recipients, preventative measures are now used to decrease infectious risk. Data regarding the effectiveness of specific prophylactic approaches are discussed in the following pathogen-focused chapters.

Novel Chemotherapeutics

Systematic assessment of combination chemotherapy regimens through clinical trials has significantly improved survival rates in pediatric oncology. However, pediatric cancer continues to be the second leading cause of death in children, largely because of relapsed and refractory malignancies, which still have dismal outcomes. Recent approaches to improve therapy for relapsed and refractory pediatric cancer have focused on targeted treatments using biologic agents for immunotherapy, cellular-based immunotherapy, and small-molecule inhibitors.[31] Novel chemotherapeutics are increasingly used in the field of pediatric oncology and have aided in the quest to achieve cure while limiting short- and long-term toxicity.

The development of targeted treatments relies on the discovery of molecular changes that drive the malignant progression of cancer. Growth factor receptors, kinases and downstream signaling molecules, and immune surveillance mechanisms are the targets of most novel anticancer drugs. In this section, we review targeted therapeutics currently used in pediatric oncology, their mechanisms of action, and common side effects, including specific risk factors for infectious complications. The specific mechanisms of action and toxicity profiles for novel agents are summarized in Tables 3.3 and 3.4.

Immunotherapy: Biologic Agents. Cancer immunotherapy using biologic agents aims to augment or reprogram the immune system to specifically eliminate cancer cells by recognizing molecules that are expressed by cancer cells but have limited or no expression in healthy cells.

Rituximab, the first chimeric monoclonal antibody approved for oncology patients, targets cluster of differentiation (CD)20-positive B cells through complement-dependent and antibody-dependent cytotoxicity. Although this therapy can be highly effective for destruction of CD20-positive malignant cells, rituximab also targets healthy B cells, resulting in hypogammaglobulinemia. The degree and duration of hypogammaglobulinemia are dependent on the dosing of rituximab, but it renders affected patients vulnerable to infections cleared by the humoral immune response. Patients with hypogammaglobulinemia may benefit from immune globulin (IgG) supplementation to maintain levels above 500 to 600 mg/dL.[32] The rituximab package insert carries a specific warning for the risk of hepatitis B virus reactivation resulting in fulminant hepatitis and hepatic failure. Screening of hepatitis B surface antigen and hepatitis B core antibody is necessary for adult patients before initiating therapy; patients with hepatitis B surface antigen and hepatitis B core antibody–positive results should consider prophylactic antiviral therapy throughout treatment with rituximab. In children, screening should include confirmation of hepatitis B vaccination before initiating therapy. Children at high risk for hepatitis B should be screened and managed similarly to adult patients. Fatal progressive multifocal leukoencephalopathy owing to reactivation of JC virus is rare but has been reported in adults and one pediatric patient, resulting in a black box warning for this drug.[33]

Another method of biologic therapy enables precise delivery of chemotherapy to tumor cells using an antibody-drug conjugate.

TABLE 3.3 Immunotherapeutic Agents Used in Pediatric Oncology

Immunotherapy	Target	Pediatric Cancer	Mechanism of Action	Immunosuppressive Effects and Infectious Complications	Adverse Effects
Rituximab	CD20	B-cell NHL	CD and ADCC	Hypogammaglobulinemia Hepatitis B reactivation (adults)	Infusion related reactions
Brentuximab vedotin	CD30	HL ALCL	Disrupt microtubules	Neutropenia Upper respiratory tract infections	Peripheral sensory and motor neuropathy
Gemtuzumab ozogamicin	CD33	R/R AML	DNA strand break	Bacterial and fungal infections Neutropenia	Hepatotoxicity Hypersensitivity reactions
Inotuzumab ozogamicin	CD22	R/R B-cell ALL	DNA strand break	Bacterial and fungal infections Neutropenia	Hepatotoxicity Hypersensitivity reactions Sinusoidal obstructive syndrome
Dinutuximab	GD2	High-risk neuroblastoma	CD and ADCC	Catheter-related bloodstream infection	Capillary leak syndrome Infusion related reaction Neuropathy/pain
Blinatumomab	CD19	R/R B-cell ALL	T-cell engager	Catheter related bloodstream infection	Cytokine release syndrome Infection Neurotoxicity
Ipilumumab	CTLA-4	R/R solid tumors	Immune checkpoint inhibitor	Infectious complications are secondary to immunosuppressive drugs used to treat immune-mediated reactions	Rash Fatigue Musculoskeletal pain Immune-mediated reactions: colitis, hepatitis, pneumonitis, nephritis
Nivolumab	PD-1		Immune checkpoint inhibitor		
Pembrolizumab	PD-1		Immune checkpoint inhibitor		
Tisagenlecleucel; axicabtagene ciloleucel	CD19	R/R B-cell ALL	CAR-T	Febrile neutropenia Hypogammaglobulinemia Bacterial, fungal, viral infections	Cytokine release syndrome Cytopenias Neurotoxicity

ADCC, antibody-dependent cellular cytotoxicity; *ALCL*, anaplastic large cell lymphoma; *ALL*, acute lymphoblastic leukemia; *AML*, acute myeloid leukemia; *CD*, cluster of differentiation; *CTLA-4*, cytotoxic T-lymphocyte-associated protein 4; *GD2*, glycolipid disialoganglioside; *HL*, Hodgkin lymphoma; *NHL*, non-Hodgkin lymphoma; *PD-1*, programmed cell death receptor 1; *R/R*, relapsed/refractory.

TABLE 3.4 Small-Molecule Inhibitors Used in Pediatric Oncology

Drug	Indication	Mechanism of Action	Immunosuppressive Effects	Adverse Effects
Imatinib	Pediatric Ph+ ALL, CML	TKI: *BCR-ABL*	Neutropenia (infrequent)	Diarrhea Fluid retention Headache Nausea Rash Vomiting QT prolongation (dasatinib and nilotinib)
Dasatinib	Ph+ ALL, CML			
Nilotinib	Ph+ ALL, CML			
Sorafenib	FLT3-ITD+ AML	TKI: FLT3/ITD	Neutropenia Lymphopenia	Cardiotoxicity Hand-foot skin reaction Hypertension QT prolongation
Crizotinib	ALCL (ALK+ lymphoma) ALK+ NBL	Anaplastic lymphoma kinase, among others	Neutropenia Lymphopenia	Hepatotoxicity Nausea QT prolongation Vomiting

ALCL, anaplastic large cell lymphoma; *ALK*, anaplastic lymphoma kinase; *ALL*, acute lymphoblastic leukemia; *FLT3-ITD*, FMS-like tyrosine kinase 3–internal tandem duplication; *ITD*, internal tandem duplication; *NBL*, neuroblastoma; *Ph+*, Philadelphia chromosome positive; *TKI*, tyrosine kinase inhibitor.

Brentuximab vedotin is an antibody-drug conjugate that targets $CD30^+$ malignancies, including HL or anaplastic large cell lymphoma (ALCL), and enables direct delivery of a potent microtubule-disrupting agent, monomethylauristatin, to cancer cells. Peripheral sensory and motor neuropathy, neutropenia, and upper respiratory tract infections are some of the most common adverse events that occur when brentuximab vedotin is added to conventional chemotherapy for the treatment of HL or ALCL.[34]

Like brentuximab vedotin, gemtuzumab ozogamicin is another targeted monoclonal antibody-drug conjugate that delivers a cytotoxic calicheamicin derivative to $CD33^+$ myeloid cells, resulting in double-stranded DNA breaks and cell death. Gemtuzumab ozogamicin is currently approved for patients with refractory or relapsed $CD33^+$ AML. Patients undergoing AML treatment with cytotoxic chemotherapy combined with gemtuzumab ozogamicin have a significantly increased risk of infectious complications, most commonly bacterial sepsis and BSIs, as the result of compounded myelosuppressive side effects.[35,36] Similarly, inotuzumab ozogamicin delivers calicheamicin to $CD22^+$ B cells and is in use as single-agent therapy in children with refractory/relapsed B-cell ALL. In a retrospective cohort study of pediatric patients with relapsed/refractory B-cell ALL who received single-agent inotuzumab ozogamicin, febrile neutropenia was reported in 16% and infections were reported in 29% of subjects.[37] Reported infections were caused primarily by bacteria and fungi.

One of the only antibody therapies that has been approved solely for pediatric cancer, namely high-risk neuroblastoma, is dinutuximab (formerly Ch14.18). This chimeric antibody targets glycolipid disialoganglioside, a marker present on neuroblastoma cells and normal cells of neuroectodermal origin. Dinutuximab, when given in combination with conventional chemotherapy, surgery, XRT, and additional immune-modulating drugs, significantly improved event-free and overall survival in children with HR NBL.[38] The most common side effects include pain associated with nerve damage owing to glycolipid disialoganglioside expression on nonmalignant cells of neural origin, life-threatening infusion-related reactions, capillary leak syndrome, and catheter-related infections.[38] Central venous access is essential for administration of multiple cycles of parenteral dinutuximab along with appropriate supportive care, thus catheter-related BSIs are common.

Blinatumomab represents a novel immunotherapeutic approach as a bispecific T-cell engager that binds to $CD19^+$ B cells and $CD3^+$ T cells, creating a cytolytic synapse. The cytotoxic T-cell immune response enables lysis of malignant and normal $CD19^+$ B cells. The therapy entails a continuous infusion over 28 days, necessitating a central line, which increases the risk for catheter-related BSI. Hypogammaglobulinemia is expected until drug clearance given the targeting of nonmalignant $CD19^+$ B cells.[39] Thus patients are predisposed to opportunistic pathogens similar to those patients treated with rituximab.

Another immunotherapy mechanism focuses on limiting tumor cell escape of immune surveillance by circumventing immune checkpoints. Immune checkpoints, regulated by molecules, including programmed cell death receptor 1 (PD-1) and cytotoxic T-lymphocyte–associated protein 4 (CTLA4), decrease T-cell activation and allow cancer cells to survive. By blocking these checkpoint receptors or ligands, T-cell suppression is reversed, resulting in an enhanced immune-mediated antitumor effect. Immune checkpoint inhibitors approved for use in several adult cancers (non-small-cell lung cancer, renal cell carcinoma, and melanoma) include nivolumab, pembrolizumab, and ipilimumab. Studies are underway to measure the safety and efficacy of immune checkpoint inhibitors in pediatric patients, specifically for relapsed and refractory disease.[40] The toxicities associated with this class of agents relates to the proinflammatory process that can have adverse effects on the skin, gastrointestinal tract, liver, and lungs. To dampen this response, treatment interruption is usually necessary, and in some cases, high-dose corticosteroids and/or tumor necrosis factor alpha blockers are recommended for the treatment of severe immune-mediated reactions. Although uncommon, bacterial pneumonia, bacteremia, invasive pulmonary aspergillosis, herpes zoster, and pneumocystis pneumonia have been reported in patients requiring immune suppression with prolonged courses of steroids and/or tumor necrosis factor alpha blockers (e.g.. infliximab) for treatment of significant organ toxicity incited by immune checkpoint inhibition.[41]

Cellular-Based Immunotherapy. A cellular-based approach to cancer immunotherapy leverages T cells engineered to express a chimeric antigen receptor (CAR-T cells) that specifically targets tumor antigens. Over the past decade, CAR-T cells targeting the B-cell surface molecule CD19 (CART19) have been a large focus of emerging therapeutics for hematologic malignancies, and specifically pediatric ALL. Approval of the first CAR-T cell therapy in pediatric ALL occurred in 2017 and has revolutionized the potential for cell-based immunotherapy targeting other pediatric cancers. Both tisagenlecleucel and axicabtagene ciloleucel are genetically modified autologous T-cell products. To derive these products, patients undergo leukapheresis to collect autologous T cells that are subsequently modified *ex vivo* to introduce expression of a CD19-directed CAR. In doing so, the patient's T cells are reprogrammed to recognize CD19 present on B-cell ALL, which directs T-cell–mediated cytotoxicity toward malignant cells. Because CD19 is present on healthy B cells, a side effect of CART19 therapy is hypogammaglobulinemia secondary to B-cell aplasia, which can be lifelong. Thus CART19 recipients require monitoring of immunoglobulin (Ig) levels and replacement with IgG.

Given the nature of relapsed/refractory disease for which patients receive CART19 therapy, prolonged cytopenias are common; thus patients frequently have infectious complications caused by bacterial, fungal, and viral sources. Infectious prophylaxis is necessary in patients preparing to receive CART19 who have had prolonged myelosuppression. Antibacterial (e.g., levofloxacin), antifungal (e.g., voriconazole), and antiviral (e.g., acyclovir) prophylaxis should be used to prevent infections with pathogens common to this population. Patient-specific infection history should guide each prophylaxis regimen. Severe infections, including bacteremia, herpesvirus infections, and invasive fungal disease, have been reported in patients receiving tisagenlecleucel.[42]

The evolution of cancer immunotherapy brings hope and improved outcomes for pediatric patients. The toxicity profile of these therapies is distinct from conventional chemotherapy owing to more targeted mechanisms of action thereby limiting, but not eliminating, adverse events, including infectious complications. Given the relative novelty of this field, more epidemiologic studies are needed to inform estimates of the infectious risk for each immunotherapeutic agent.

Small-Molecule Inhibitors. Small-molecule inhibitors, such as tyrosine kinase inhibitors (TKI), have significantly augmented survival rates for a variety of pediatric cancers. Here we review several of the TKIs commonly used for treatment of pediatric cancer, although many more are in use and are being evaluated for efficacy in childhood malignancies. The targets and activity of TKIs against pediatric cancers are summarized in Table 3.4.

Imatinib is the first TKI to be approved for treatment of cancer and has dramatically changed therapy for *BCR-ABL*–driven leukemia. As an inhibitor of the BCR-ABL fusion protein, imatinib is highly active against ALL and CML that harbor a *BCR-ABL* translocation. Dasatinib and nilotinib are second-generation *ABL*-class TKIs that are effective in the treatment of *BCR-ABL*–driven ALL and CML. When used as single-agent therapy in CML, ABL-class TKIs are not significantly associated with infectious complications, and myelosuppression is not common.[36]

Sorafenib is a multikinase inhibitor that targets the FLT3 tyrosine kinase. A subset of pediatric and adult patients with AML have an internal tandem duplication of FLT3, and FLT3 inhibition has shown some promise in treating these aggressive cancers. There are many adverse effects associated with sorafenib and other FLT3 inhibitors, including hand-foot skin reactions, cardiotoxicity, hypertension, and QT prolongation; however, infectious complications are not commonly attributed to FLT3 inhibitors. Sorafenib is used in combination with conventional chemotherapy to treat FLT3–internal tandem duplication AML, and the concomitant myelosuppressive chemotherapy places these patients at high risk for bacterial and fungal infections.

Finally, crizotinib has shown significant efficacy in ALCL as it targets a constitutively active anaplastic lymphoma kinase that drives ALCL. Crizotinib is associated with a significant rate of decreased neutrophil count with high doses; however, this is usually transient and mitigated by dose reduction or therapy interruption.[43]

As more novel agents become available to treat childhood cancer, the use of conventional chemotherapeutics will undoubtedly be diminished. The shift in infectious risk factors and infectious complications of cancer treatment will require vigilance in monitoring of patients. Continued assessment of the evolving epidemiology of opportunistic infections will be essential for ensuring appropriate prophylaxis and treatment of infectious diseases in children with cancer.

4

Infectious Disease Evaluation of Infants and Children Awaiting Solid Organ or Hematopoietic Stem Cell Transplant

Rebecca Pellett Madan, MD, MS and Lara A. Danziger-Isakov, MD, MPH

BASIC PRINCIPLES OF THE INFECTIOUS DISEASE PRETRANSPLANT EVALUATION

The pretransplant infectious disease evaluation represents the first step in a long continuum of infection prevention that extends into the posttransplant period. This evaluation is a critical element in the pretransplant process and should be performed as early as possible, ideally as soon as a child is considered for transplant. The overall objectives of infectious disease evaluation are to (1) identify and mitigate infectious complications that may result in delay of transplant; (2) identify risk factors that may affect perioperative management; (3) identify posttransplant prevention strategies for specific risks; and (4) begin the discussion of long-term strategies for safer living in the posttransplant period. The evaluation should be comprehensive and not limited to basic serologic screening. A key guiding principle is that pretransplant screening tests should be performed to address those infections that may increase the risk of posttransplant complications *and* that will prompt specific intervention either in the pretransplant or posttransplant period. A dedicated infectious disease evaluation before transplant is a critical opportunity to review all prior and current infections and antimicrobial use that are likely to affect the transplant course and management, including unrecognized or latent infections.

It is especially important that pediatric transplant candidates receive an infectious disease review that is family-centered and considers occupational and recreational exposures not only for the transplant candidate but also for all other household contacts. Household water sources and dietary habits should be reviewed to identify risk factors such as well water exposure or ingestion of uncooked meat or fish. Travel history and animal exposures should be reviewed and discussed. For families with pets, guidance for living with animals after transplant is available through the U.S. Centers for Disease Control and Prevention and should also be discussed.[1] Children who live in areas of higher tuberculosis (TB) prevalence and/or who live in households with adults with active TB infection are at high risk for acquisition of TB infection before and after transplant. TB risk factors should be reviewed for all household contacts, with additional TB screening and treatment measures for household contacts as indicated, as discussed in more detail in the following text.

Pretransplant infectious disease evaluation also provides an important opportunity to review and update immunizations for both the transplant candidate and household contacts. It is important to note that live attenuated vaccines for varicella, measles, mumps, and rubella are not contraindicated for household contacts of transplanted children, and ensuring that household contacts are fully immunized is a critical preventative strategy for children who receive transplants and who may be susceptible secondary to incomplete immunization or waning immunity after immunization.[2] This “cocoon” immunization strategy is essential for household contacts of pediatric transplant candidates and recipients during influenza season.

The risk of donor-derived infection should also be discussed as part of the infectious disease pretransplant evaluation. This is a complex and multifaceted conversation that may be best approached across multiple visits with both an infectious disease consultant and the primary transplant team. Although families and providers alike are often concerned about the potential risk of human immunodeficiency virus (HIV) and hepatitis transmission via donors who are considered to be at either routine or increased risk by U.S. Public Health Service criteria,[3] it is also important to discuss the risk of other donor-derived infections, both unanticipated and expected.[4] This includes infections for which donors may be screened (*Strongyloides stercoralis*, *Toxoplasma gondii*, *Trypanosoma cruzi*) but also for donor infections that may be unrecognized at the time of transplant. Risk and implications of donor-derived infections that are often anticipated, such as cytomegalovirus (CMV) and Epstein-Barr virus (EBV), should also be discussed, especially for transplant candidates who are presumed to be uninfected by these viruses based on pretransplant screening serology.

The first step in the pretransplant infectious disease evaluation of both pediatric solid organ transplant (SOT) and hematopoietic stem cell transplant (HSCT) candidates is a comprehensive review of how the child’s underlying disease affects their risk of infection before and after transplant. For transplant candidates with a history of malignancy, the status of the child’s disease should be documented (remission or relapse), and prior chemotherapy and radiotherapy regimens should be reviewed. Both HSCT and SOT candidates may have a history of exposure to immunosuppressive agents, such as glucocorticoids or anti-CD20 monoclonal antibody; therefore recent serum immune globulin levels and quantitative lymphocyte subsets should be reviewed as indicated. The presence of a foreign body, prosthetic material, or structural abnormality (central venous or hemodialysis catheter, prosthetic joint, vascular graft, ureteral stent, hemodialysis graft fistula) should be documented. Prior imaging should be reviewed to assess for lung nodules, calcified granulomas, or cavitary lesions that may prompt further investigation before transplant.

Review of the child's underlying disease is followed by a comprehensive review of all prior and current infections and bacterial colonization history. Pediatric transplant candidates with a history of malignancy may have a history of bacteremia or invasive fungal infection), and children awaiting HSCT for primary immune deficiency may have an extensive history of opportunistic infections. Kidney transplant candidates may have a history of urinary tract infection, and hemodialysis and peritoneal dialysis recipients are at higher risk for catheter-related bacteremia and peritonitis, respectively. Hardware-associated infections may develop in heart transplant recipients who require ventricular assist device support, and ascending cholangitis or peritonitis may develop in children with liver failure. Lung transplant candidates with cystic fibrosis may have a history of respiratory colonization with multidrug- or extensively drug-resistant organisms such as *Pseudomonas aeruginosa*, *Burkholderia cepacia*, and *Stenotrophomonas maltophilia*. Thus special attention should be paid to prior bacterial culture and susceptibility results, as well as to prior antimicrobial utilization. Baseline sputum cultures are recommended for lung transplant candidates to identify colonizing organisms and their antimicrobial susceptibility patterns.

For transplant candidates who have a poorly documented history of allergic reaction to a specific antimicrobial, this history should be clarified. Formal allergy consultation should be completed as needed before transplant. Dental history should also be reviewed, and ideally, candidates should undergo complete dental evaluation and appropriate intervention before transplant.

Infectious Disease Screening of the Pediatric Solid Organ Transplant Candidate

Screening tests that are routinely recommended for pediatric SOT recipients, including those that are used to assess for latent infection or vaccine-induced immunity, are outlined in Box 4.1. In interpreting serology results, the provider should consider the following variables: (1) the candidate's history of blood product or immune globulin infusion; (2) the candidate's age (serology results in infants may reflect passive transfer of maternal antibody); (3) the immunosuppressive agents administered before transplant, such as corticosteroids or anti-CD20 monoclonal antibody; and (4) the inherent limitations of some screening assays, such as the inability of some assays to detect acute infection.

HIV and Hepatitis Screening

Current policy of the U.S. Organ Procurement and Transplantation Network mandates screening for HIV, hepatitis C, and hepatitis B for all SOT candidates, independent of age.[5] This screening is typically performed by serologic testing. Serologic testing for hepatitis B should include hepatitis B surface antigen, hepatitis B core immunoglobulin (IgG), and hepatitis B surface antibody, although the latter is not mandated. False-positive results for hepatitis C antibody screening are well described, particularly in low-prevalence populations. Positive results for hepatitis C antibody screening should be confirmed by hepatitis C ribonucleic acid viral load and potentially additional screening methods, depending on the patient's risk factors.[6] HIV and hepatitis B nucleic acid amplification testing (NAAT) may also be used to confirm positive serologic test results.

Documentation of hepatitis B immunity by either qualitative or quantitative hepatitis B surface antibody is important for determining risk stratification and the possible need for hepatitis B prophylaxis should the candidate receive an organ from a donor who has positive hepatitis B core antibody test results with negative results for hepatitis B surface antigen.[7] For candidates who are found to be nonimmune to hepatitis B, a primary hepatitis B vaccine series or booster vaccine doses should be administered, and immunity should be reassessed upon completion of vaccination or before transplant, whichever occurs first.[8] Higher doses of vaccine may be required for transplant recipients receiving hemodialysis, although data are limited in this area for children. It is also important to note that administration of hepatitis B vaccine can result in transient detection of hepatitis B surface antigen; thus

BOX 4.1 Routine Screening Recommendations for Pediatric Solid Organ and Hematopoietic Stem Cell Transplant Candidates

Chart and History Review

- Document current and prior infections, including antimicrobial susceptibility patterns
- Document current and prior antimicrobial use, including suspected or documented allergic reactions
- Review travel history, animal exposures, occupational and recreational exposures for candidate and household contacts
- Review immunization history for transplant candidate and all household contacts

Serologic Screening[a]

- Human immunodeficiency virus (HIV) serology[b]
- Hepatitis B surface antigen,[b] hepatitis B core IgG,[b] hepatitis B surface antibody
- Hepatitis C IgG[b]
- Hepatitis A IgG
- Cytomegalovirus (CMV) IgG (CMV PCR from urine or saliva for infants)
- Epstein-Barr virus (EBV) EBV capsid IgG and IgM, consider anti-EBV nuclear antigen IgG
- Toxoplasma IgG for all heart transplant and allogeneic/stem cell transplant candidates, consider for non-heart SOT and autologous stem cell candidates
- Measles IgG
- Varicella IgG

Additional Screening Measures

- Review of tuberculosis risk factors and tuberculin skin test/interferon gamma release assay (with chest radiograph if indicated)
- Sputum Gram stain and culture for lung transplant candidates
- Herpes Simplex Virus (HSV) 1 and 2 IgG for hematopoietic stem cell transplant candidates
- Respiratory virus testing for allogeneic stem cell transplant candidates, if symptoms are present
- Syphilis screening for infants and at-risk adolescents
- Sexually transmitted infection screening for adolescents
- Pelvic examination with Pap smear and human papillomavirus screening for sexually active adolescent females

[a]Interpretation of infant serology results may be complicated by passive transfer of maternal antibody.
[b]HIV, hepatitis B, and hepatitis C serologic testing is required for all solid organ transplant candidates per U.S. Organ Procurement and Transplantation Network policy.
IgG, immunoglobulin G; *PCR*, polymerase chain reaction; *SOT*, solid organ transplant.

testing for hepatitis B surface antigen shortly after immunization is not recommended.[9] Hepatitis A serology and immunization history should be recorded, and hepatitis A vaccine should be administered as needed.

Herpesvirus Screening

CMV (IgG) and EBV (capsid IgG and IgM) serology studies are typically used for transplant candidates to stratify the risk for posttransplant complications and to determine the relative need for prophylactic (CMV) and preemptive monitoring (CMV, EBV) strategies. IgG antibody to EBV nuclear antibody may also be helpful in assessing humoral immune response to past EBV infection. Unfortunately, the utility of a positive CMV or EBV serologic result is limited in infants younger than 12 months whose positive serology results may reflect passive transfer of maternal antibody. CMV NAAT (or viral culture based assay) from urine or saliva is recommended for infants, although a negative test result does not definitively exclude prior infection (Box 4.1 and Table 4.1).[10] Infants with a negative CMV NAAT result from urine or saliva or a negative CMV urine culture should be considered CMV naïve upon receipt of a CMV-seropositive organ (Table 4.1). It may also be prudent to consider all infants who receive an EBV-seropositive donor organ to be EBV naïve (recipient seronegative) for risk stratification purposes (Table 4.1).

Studies to assess for latent infection with Herpes Simplex Virus (HSV) are not routinely indicated for pediatric SOT recipients. Small studies predating the widespread use of ganciclovir and valganciclovir prophylaxis (both of which are active against HSV) suggest that severe complications attributed to HSV are relatively infrequent in the pediatric SOT population, with the majority of complications reported as mucosal lesions that responded to antiviral therapy.[11] Transplant candidates in whom lesions develop that are suspicious for herpes should have direct testing of the lesion to confirm the diagnosis. In children who have a history of recurrent lesions but who have not had direct lesion testing, serology results may be informative. Serology testing for human herpesviruses 6, 7, and 8 is generally not recommended for pediatric SOT candidates.[12]

All pediatric heart transplant candidates should undergo serologic screening for *Toxoplasma gondii* secondary to the high risk of reactivation in the myocardium and the need for targeted posttransplant prophylaxis in seropositive recipients.[13] The need for pretransplant *Toxoplasma* screening in non-heart transplant candidates is less clear, as posttransplant prophylaxis specifically for toxoplasmosis is not routinely recommended for non-heart transplant recipients. However, documented *Toxoplasma* reactivation has been reported in noncardiac organ recipients,[14] and the true incidence of toxoplasmosis in this population may be underestimated. Thus knowledge of latent infection with *Toxoplasma* before transplant or of serologic mismatch with a *Toxoplasma*-seropositive donor may guide the decision to provide targeted prophylaxis or more intensive monitoring for non-heart transplant recipients who receive more intensified immunosuppression for graft rejection.

TABLE 4.1 Risk Stratification According to Infant Cytomegalovirus and Epstein-Barr Virus Serostatus

Donor	Recipient	Highest Risk Stratification[a]
Positive	Positive or negative	D^+/R^-
Negative	Positive	D^-/R^+
Negative	Negative	D^-/R^-

[a]Assume cytomegalovirus (CMV) D^+/R^+ stratification only if infant transplant candidate is found to have positive CMV urine culture result or positive CMV urine/saliva polymerase chain reaction result.

Immunization records for measles, mumps, rubella (MMR) and varicella should be reviewed. Documentation of measles and varicella IgG before transplant is helpful for assessing the risk of disease and the need for prophylaxis, should the candidate have documented exposure to any of these viruses. Non-immunity by serology may reflect lack of or incomplete prior vaccination or waning immunity after appropriate immunization. It should also be noted that commercially available enzyme-linked immunosorbent assays may lack the sensitivity to detect vaccine-induced, varicella-specific antibodies and also do not reflect cell-mediated immune responses to varicella.[15] Thus a negative varicella IgG result may not truly reflect susceptibility to disease. Keeping in mind these limitations, administration of MMR and/or varicella vaccines should be considered for transplant recipients who are found to be non-immune by routine serology. The risks and benefits of administration of live attenuated vaccines shortly before transplant are discussed in more detail later in the text.

The decision to screen pediatric SOT candidates for syphilis depends on the local prevalence of disease and the age of the candidate. Screening should be performed in infants (who may be at risk for congenital syphilis) and in sexually active adolescents (who may acquire syphilis through sexual intercourse) but is generally not indicated in children between these age intervals in the absence of specific risk factors. In the past, syphilis screening was typically performed by first testing with rapid plasmin reagin (RPR) or Venereal Disease Research Laboratory assay, followed by confirmation of a positive result with a treponemal specific assay. Both rapid plasmin reagin and Venereal Disease Research Laboratory testing are acceptable screening tests for pediatric transplant candidates. However, at many institutions, syphilis screening is performed as a reverse-sequence algorithm that begins with the detection of syphilis-specific IgG and IgM antibodies by enzyme or chemiluminescence assay.[16] Special care should be taken in interpreting results of reverse-sequence algorithm testing for infants (in whom positive screening results may again reflect passive transfer of maternal antibody), for patients who have a history of treated syphilis, and for individuals without risk factors who are suspected to have false-positive results.[17] Screening for *Mycobacterium tuberculosis* is recommended for all pediatric SOT candidates and is discussed in greater detail later, along with recommendations for screening of pediatric SOT candidates with specific risk factors.

Approach to Infectious Disease Evaluation of the Pediatric Hematopoietic Stem Cell Transplant Candidate

Results of serology screening for pediatric HSCT candidates should be interpreted not only in the context of recent blood or immune globulin product infusion but also in the context of the type of anticipated stem cell transplant. For example, CMV seropositivity in a HSCT candidate conveys a greater risk of CMV-related complications after transplant if the candidate receives a graft from a CMV-seronegative donor. Similarly, *Toxoplasma* reactivation is unlikely after autologous HSCT but is more likely to occur in a seropositive recipient of a seronegative allogeneic or umbilical cord transplant. In general, the basic screening recommended for pediatric HSCT candidates (both autologous and allogeneic) is similar to the evaluation recommended for pediatric SOT candidates (Box 4.1). Serology results should be evaluated before HSCT for HIV, hepatitis B, and hepatitis C, with viral load confirmation if serology results are positive. Hepatitis A serology should be evaluated for evidence of prior immunization or infection.

In addition to CMV and EBV serology, HSV-1 and HSV-2 IgG testing should be performed for pediatric HSCT candidates, as HSV seropositivity may affect the posttransplant antiviral prophylaxis regimen. As with pediatric SOT candidates, pretransplant testing is not recommended for human herpesviruses 6, 7, and 8. *Toxoplasma* serology screening should be performed for allogeneic/umbilical cord transplant candidates but may be less informative in autologous HSCT candidates, who are at lower risk for reactivation after transplant. All pediatric HSCT should be evaluated for *M. tuberculosis* exposure risk and infection; the approach to tuberculosis screening in this population is discussed in detail later.[18]

HSCT recipients are at risk for severe lower airway disease from respiratory viruses, especially before engraftment and during times of profound lymphopenia,[19,20] and some guidelines recommend deferral of HSCT in the setting of upper respiratory tract infection (URI).[21,22] Allogeneic HSTC candidates who were screened for respiratory virus infection by multiplex polymerase chain reaction from nasal wash samples were found to a have significantly increased risk of mortality if they had both URI symptoms and documented respiratory virus independent of the virus detected.[23] This study suggests that allogeneic HSCT candidates should undergo respiratory virus testing in the setting of URI symptoms and that careful consideration should be paid to possible deferment of transplant until symptoms have resolved.

Approach to Tuberculosis Screening in the Pediatric Transplant Candidate

Studies consisting of mostly adult transplant recipients suggest that the prevalence of posttransplant *M. tuberculosis* infection varies significantly by geographic region but is at least 20 times as frequent in SOT recipients and at least twice as frequent in HSCT recipients relative to the general population.[24-27] Children are at greater risk for progression from latent TB infection to active disease at the extremes of age (<5 years and adolescence), and young children are especially more likely to progress to disseminated and/or extrapulmonary disease in the setting of transplant.[28-33] Children with latent or active TB are likely to have acquired *M. tuberculosis* infection from a close contact with active infection. Case series of pediatric liver transplant recipients who received a diagnosis of TB found that the majority of infected children had household contacts with either latent or active TB.[28,31] Accordingly, a critical first step in screening the pediatric transplant candidate for TB is to perform a comprehensive screening of all household contacts for risk factors, as well as for signs and symptoms of active infection, prior tuberculin skin test (TST) or interferon gamma release assay (IGRA) screening, and treatment history.[18] TST/IGRA screening and/or chest radiography should be strongly considered for household contacts who have risk factors for TB.

All pediatric transplant candidates should be screened for TB risk factors and for signs and symptoms of active TB. Several consensus statements and guidelines recommend that all pediatric transplant candidates undergo screening with TST or IGRA and chest radiography,[18,27,34] although the positive predictive value of TST/IGRA screening depends on risk factors for TB and local epidemiology. In general, TST screening is recommended for children younger than 2 years.[35] Either TST or IGRA may be used to screen children who are at least 2 years old; IGRA is the preferred screening method for children who have a prior history of bacillus Calmette-Guérin (BCG) immunization,[35,36] and IGRA offers the advantage of reporting a positive mitogen control for assessment of anergy. A positive TST or IGRA result should prompt a renewed evaluation for active infection and, if active infection is excluded, a discussion of the risks and benefits of treatment for latent TB infection. It is important to note that a negative TST or IGRA result in a child does not exclude the possibility of TB infection, and the possibility of infection should be carefully considered in infants and children who are known to have household contacts with latent or active TB. This is of particular importance for pediatric transplant candidates who have diminished lymphocyte numbers or function at the time of testing secondary to ongoing immunosuppression. In immunocompromised children with negative TST/IGRA screening, careful evaluation for risk factors, infected household contacts, and evidence of active infection is critical.

Additional Screening Measures for Pediatric Transplant Candidates

Pediatric transplant candidates who were born in areas endemic for specific infections or who have specific travel or exposure histories may require additional testing on a case-by-case basis (Box 4.2). Candidates who were born in or who spent significant time in South America, Central America, or Mexico may have asymptomatic infection with *Trypanosoma cruzi* (the protozoan parasite that results in Chagas disease), especially those who spent time in rural areas. Testing for *T. cruzi*–specific antibodies is limited by the lack of validated testing options and the lack of a gold standard diagnostic assay, and *T. cruzi* polymerase chain reaction is insensitive for diagnosis of chronic infection.[37] Candidates with risk factors who have positive *T. cruzi* serology results by commercially available assay may require additional confirmatory testing. These cases may be reviewed with state departments of health or in consultation with the U.S. Centers for Disease Control and Prevention Chagas Reference Laboratory (Division of Parasitic Diseases Public Inquiries Line, 404-718-4745; after-hours hotline 770-488-7100; https:www//cdc.gov/parasite).

Serologic testing is also recommended for candidates at risk for *S. stercoralis*, which is endemic throughout tropical and subtropical areas, as well as the southeastern and Appalachia regions of the United States.[38] Candidates who have spent significant amounts of time in endemic areas may acquire asymptomatic, lifelong infection, which then reactivates to cause severe disease and hyperinfection after transplant.[39] Screening by *Strongyloides* IgG is more sensitive than stool screening, and positive test results should prompt preemptive treatment with ivermectin before transplant.[40] Repeat serologic testing 3 to 6 months after treatment may be helpful in assessing response to therapy and the potential need for retreatment. Empiric treatment may also be considered for candidates from endemic areas who are anticipated to undergo imminent transplant.[40]

Stool ova and parasite examination, as well as additional stool testing to evaluate for *Giardia* and *Cryptosporidium* spp., should be performed for transplant candidates who have unexplained gastrointestinal symptoms or who have risk factors for parasite infection, such as exposure to well water sources. Additional testing for malaria, *Schistosoma* spp., and *Leishmania* spp. may also be indicated depending on risk factors.

BOX 4.2 Targeted Screening for Pediatric Solid Organ and Hematopoietic Stem Cell Transplant Candidates With History of Travel or Residence in Areas Endemic for Specific Infections

- *Trypanosoma cruzi* IgG
- *Strongyloides stercoralis* IgG
- Stool ova and parasite screening, with additional testing for *Giardia* and *Cryptosporidium* spp.
- Blood parasite (malaria spp.) smear and antigen testing
- Urine ova and parasite screening with *Schistosoma* spp. serology
- *Leishmania* spp. serology
- *Coccidioides* spp. serology

IgG, immunoglobulin G.

Various screening and prophylactic approaches for endemic mycoses have been suggested for transplant candidates, primarily based on studies of adult SOT candidates.[41-45] A 5-year prospective surveillance study that monitored both SOT and HSCT recipients at 15 pediatric and adult centers for infections secondary to *Histoplasma capsulatum*, *Blastomyces dermatitidis*, and *Coccidioides* spp., found that infection with endemic mycoses was infrequent.[41] Histoplasmosis was the most commonly identified infection in this cohort (12-month cumulative incidence rate among SOT recipients of 0.1) and was the only infection diagnosed among pediatric recipients. HSCT recipients in this cohort were at even lower risk relative to SOT recipients. Given the reported low prevalence of posttransplant disease in endemic areas[42,45] and the limitations of testing in asymptomatic patients, routine screening and/or prophylaxis for histoplasmosis and blastomycosis is typically not recommended in pediatric transplant candidates. Strategies for universal serologic screening and/or prophylaxis have been suggested for adult transplant recipients in areas endemic for *Coccidioides* spp.[43,44,46] Although these studies did not include children, screening can be considered for children from endemic areas.

GENERAL APPROACH TO PRETRANSPLANT IMMUNIZATION

An advantage of infectious disease evaluation early in the pre-SOT evaluation process is that it may allow sufficient time to vaccinate children with incomplete immunization histories or subtherapeutic responses to immunizations. Multiple studies have reported incomplete immunization of pediatric SOT candidates,[47-49] which may reflect failure to prioritize immunization in the setting of chronic disease or misplaced concern that inactivated vaccines are unsafe in chronically ill children. For the pediatric SOT candidate, every effort should be made to complete the full, age-appropriate vaccine schedule before transplant, but transplant should not be delayed to allow for vaccine administration. Even for children who are fully immunized, pretransplant serology results may indicate the need for additional doses after vaccine failure or waning immunity.[2] Expedited immunization schedules allow children to complete their vaccine schedule before transplant and at an earlier stage of chronic illness, when vaccines may be more immunogenic. Although immunogenicity data to support these schedules are lacking, there are no data to suggest that an expedited vaccine schedule is unsafe. Most pediatric SOT candidates have chronic illness that increases their risk for pneumococcal infection; thus pediatric SOT candidates older than 2 years should receive the *Streptococcus pneumoniae* polysaccharide vaccine after completion of their conjugate pneumococcal vaccine series. Influenza vaccine should be administered yearly to all children awaiting SOT.

Administration of live attenuated vaccines to children awaiting SOT merits special consideration. As vaccines for varicella, MMR, and rotavirus are typically not administered after transplant, every effort should be made to administer these vaccines to pediatric SOT candidates who are not receiving immunosuppression.[8] Ideally, children should receive two doses each of varicella and MMR vaccines before transplant, with at least one dose of each after the first birthday. MMR vaccine can be given as early as 6 months of age, and although licensed for administration to infants 12 months and older, varicella vaccine can be given as early as 6 months of age. The second doses of varicella/MMR vaccines can be given as early as 4 weeks after the first dose. Of note, varicella and MMR vaccines can be administered on the same day. If the vaccines are not given on the same day, they should be given at least 28 days apart. It should also be noted that administration of varicella and MMR vaccines is typically deferred in the 4 weeks before transplant, as there is a theoretical but poorly documented risk of vaccine-strain viral reactivation and dissemination if given shortly before induction immunosuppression.

Vaccine administration for the pediatric HSCT is often more complicated, as inactivated vaccines may not be immunogenic in children who are receiving or have recently completed chemotherapy; live attenuated vaccines may be unsafe in this population, and vaccine doses are repeated after immune reconstitution. When time allows, vaccines such as inactivated influenza and pneumococcal vaccines should be administered to reduce the risk of infection before HSCT. There may also be a role for administration of vaccines to hematopoietic stem cell donors. Immunization of donors with vaccines such as those against influenza and pneumococcus may allow for passive transfer of vaccine-induced antibody from the donor to recipient and may provide some protection before full immune reconstitution and reimmunization of the recipient,[50] although this strategy may be limited by logistical and ethical concerns.

An important component of the pretransplant vaccination strategy for both SOT and HSCT candidates is to ensure that all household contacts are fully immunized, including annual influenza vaccine and vaccines against pertussis, varicella, MMR, and pneumococcus. Pertussis readily spreads among household contacts, and household immunization with the conjugate pneumococcal vaccine reduces nasopharyngeal colonization with vaccine-specific serotypes that have been associated with invasive pneumococcal disease. Immunization of household contacts for varicella and MMR helps reduced the risk of household transmission of these viruses to susceptible transplant patients and does not pose significant risk of vaccine strain transmission within the household. Rotavirus vaccine may be administered to household contacts of transplant candidates, provided careful hand hygiene measures are followed.

SPECIAL CONSIDERATIONS FOR EXTREMES OF AGE

Infant and adolescent transplant candidates require age-appropriate pretransplant infectious disease screening. Although most passively transferred maternal antibodies have waned by 9 months, maternal antibody may be detected as late as 15 to 18 months, depending on the sensitivity of the assay used. Aside from the required HIV, hepatitis B, and hepatitis C testing discussed previously, serologic tests should be sent from infants only if the results will affect peritransplant management, and IgG results should be interpreted in the context of possible maternal antibody transfer. Serologic testing for hepatitis A, varicella, and MMR in infants is generally of limited utility, as detected antibody is likely to be maternal and will not affect the eventual need for immunization. Since the majority of childhood immunizations are administered during infancy, it is critical to ensure that vaccines are administered whenever possible before transplant to provide protection against vaccine-preventable illness both before and after transplant.

Adolescent transplant candidates should be tested for sexually transmitted infections, including chlamydia, gonorrhea, syphilis, and trichomoniasis. For adolescents who did not receive their human papilloma virus vaccine series earlier in childhood, every attempt should be made to administer this series before transplant. Adolescent female transplant candidates who are sexually active should undergo pelvic examination with baseline Pap testing and human papilloma virus HPV screening. Adolescent transplant candidates require comprehensive counseling regarding safer sex practices and avoidance of tattoos and other blood-borne pathogen exposures.

Future Directions

Immunization to reduce the risk of vaccine-preventable diseases is a cornerstone of pediatric care; thus immunization of the pediatric

SOT candidate is generally encouraged whenever possible. However, data are limited regarding the immunogenicity of vaccines in both chronically ill children awaiting SOT and in transplant recipients who are committed to lifelong, but in some cases low-dose, immunosuppression. The safety of live attenuated vaccines after transplant remains an understudied area. Studies are needed to evaluate the magnitude and durability of immune responses to vaccines administered before transplant, as well as the immunogenicity and safety (for live attenuated formulations) of vaccines administered after transplant, so that evidence-based vaccine schedules may be determined. These studies may indicate the need for alternative vaccination strategies for children who receive transplants, including higher-dose vaccine formulations or more accelerated schedules. In addition, studies are needed to more fully evaluate the benefits of immunizing individuals before HSC donation.

With the emergence of multidrug-resistant and extensively drug-resistant bacterial organisms, studies are also needed to determine if transplant candidates should be routinely evaluated for colonization with resistance to determine how colonization with these organisms should affect peritransplant management.

5

Donor Screening and Donor-Derived Infections

Marian G. Michaels, MD, MPH and Michael D. Green, MD, MPH

Donors of cells or organs are important potential sources of infection in children undergoing hematopoietic stem cell (HSCT) or solid organ transplantation (SOT). In both settings, the donor may be a source of anticipated or unanticipated transmission of pathogens to the recipient. Parents and patients are often appropriately focused on the transplant itself as a lifesaving procedure and therefore do not always appreciate that there may be microbes that can be transmitted with the cells or organ that could affect the recipients as well. It is critical not only for the transplant team to be cognizant of the risk of donor-derived transmissions, but it is also equally important for the team to educate and inform recipients and their families about these potential risks. This chapter reviews the concept of transmission of donor-derived infections and the role of laboratory and historical screening to mitigate this risk. Some of the more common types of infections that can be transmitted are discussed in addition to data describing published experience with donor-derived infections in HSCT and SOT. Although some specific pathogens are covered in general terms, the reader is referred to the chapters on the specific pathogens for a more intensive discussion about the pathogen and preventive strategies to protect the recipient.

ANTICIPATED AND UNANTICIPATED DONOR-DERIVED INFECTIONS

As already noted, some donor-derived infections are considered "anticipated" and screening is now routinely performed on both potential stem cell and organ donors and transplant candidates to assess the risk for and inform the use of strategies to prevent or modify the outcome of donor-derived infections. However, this was not always the case. In the early era of transplantation, the concept that a latent virus, bacteria, or parasite could transfer with a stem cell product or organ was not always obvious. It was only with insightful attention and carefully conducted epidemiologic studies that this mechanism of transmission became clear.

The classic example of a pathogen associated with donor-derived infections that is now considered an anticipated transmission is cytomegalovirus (CMV). Early observations of infectious complications of both HSCT and SOT identified the high frequency and importance of CMV in recipients of these procedures.[1,2] Subsequent seroepidemiologic and virologic studies confirmed the role of the donor in both primary and secondary infections caused by this pathogen. For SOT, the greatest risk for CMV transmission and disease occurs when a CMV- naïve (e.g., seronegative) recipient acquires infection from the allograft recovered from a CMV- seropositive donor. This infection occurs at a time when the recipient lacks the ability to develop a robust T-cell response to contain the virus as the result of antirejection immunosuppressive therapies that also inhibit the normal antiviral response. In contrast, for HSCT recipients the donor cells are needed to develop the immunologic response. Hence, although it is well established that a CMV-seropositive donor can infect a naïve recipient, the scenario in which a seropositive recipient receives stem cells from a seronegative donor is also problematic with myeloablative procedures.[3] In this scenario, latent CMV can reactivate in the recipient who will be lacking a mature, educated CMV-specific T-cell population from the donor. The risk of CMV (native or donor-acquired) may be further exacerbated through the use of extrinsic immune suppression to prevent or treat graft-versus-host disease. Further studies highlighted how knowledge of the CMV serologic status of the donor and recipient reliably informed risk stratification for frequency and severity of CMV in both HSCT and SOT recipients.

Despite the ability to identify the presence of CMV in a potential organ donor, the high prevalence of chronic latent infection with this pathogen in the population of potential donors makes avoidance of such donors for SOT impractical. For example, data from United Network for Organ Sharing (UNOS) showed that approximately 60% of all donors have positive test results for CMV, leading to 57% of all CMV-seronegative recipients receiving an organ from a CMV-seropositive donor.[4] Because the condition of patients on the wait list could deteriorate while they await a CMV-seronegative donor and given the availability of effective preventative and therapeutic strategies, most centers use these donors despite recognizing and anticipating the risk of donor-derived transmission and infection. The risk/benefit assessment of using a donor with an anticipated risk versus waiting for a donor without a particular known infection must always be put in the context of overall patient outcome for each individual child on the transplant waiting list.

The model of donor-derived infection from CMV was subsequently extended to a number of other pathogens. Of particular importance in pediatric transplantation is Epstein-Barr virus (EBV). Similar to the situation with CMV, EBV can be transmitted with a donor organ and lead to important complications of EBV disease including posttransplant lymphoproliferative disorder (PTLD).[5] The mismatch state of organ donor-positive and recipient-negative status is again associated with the highest risk for disease in SOT recipients. Because the pediatric population is more often seronegative compared with adult candidates, primary EBV infection often acquired from the donor is a significant concern in the pediatric SOT population.[5] In contrast to the CMV in HSCT recipients, the risk for EBV disease and PTLD after HSCT primarily depends on the EBV status of the donor. This is because latent EBV infection within the recipient is often eradicated as part of the ablation protocols used to prepare the HSCT recipient for HSCT (Thomas Gross MD, PhD, personal communication, December 21, 2018). Although the donor would be expected to have adoptive immunity against this virus, EBV derived from the donor is a cause of early disease after HSCT before donor-derived EBV-specific cytotoxic lymphocytes can establish control over the virus to prevent illness, including PTLD. Similar to the scenario with CMV, protocols for monitoring recipients at risk for acquiring EBV in both populations have helped to modify EBV infection outcomes and even prevent disease in children undergoing these procedures. Accordingly, most transplant centers have protocols in place to test CMV and EBV serologic status in HSCT and SOT recipients and donors.

With confirmation that the donor can be the source of infection, ongoing observations have identified countless other pathogens that have been associated with donor-derived infections in recipients of HSCT and SOT procedures. This has included pathogens that were not known to be present in the donor and were subsequently shown to be associated with donor-derived infection on retrospective evaluation. Such events exemplify the term "unanticipated" donor-derived infection. These events are relatively rare considering the large number of transplants that occur but are potentially devastating to one or more recipients (in the case of SOT) when they happen.[6-8] In general, recipients of HSCT or living organ donation are at lower risk for unanticipated donor-derived infections compared with recipients of deceased organs as the transplants are set up in advance so that time is available for appropriate screening. In addition, living donors can be educated about avoiding infections, and if they are sick on the day of planned donation, donation can be delayed until a later date.

Unanticipated donor-derived infections have been attributed to all classes of pathogens, including bacteria (e.g., methicillin-resistant *Staphylococcus aureus*), viruses (e.g., human immunodeficiency virus [HIV], rabies), fungi (e.g., coccidiomycoses), and parasites (e.g., *Strongyloides* infection).[6-8] In contrast to CMV, for which a deliberate decision is made to use an organ despite a predictable risk of transmission to and infection in the recipient, these pathogens represent examples of unexpected transmissions because screening (see later text) was not routinely performed in donors, results came back only after transplant had occurred, or appropriate screening tests were not available. In some circumstances, routine screening had not been previously performed but repeated cases of donor-derived transmission led to incorporation of screening for such pathogens as part of standard of care practice, either locally, regionally, or on a national or international basis. For example, some centers now routinely screen donors from geographic areas that are endemic for *Strongyloides*; if the donor is seropositive, intervention with prophylactic ivermectin can prevent disease transmission.[9] In a similar manner, knowledge of donors with bacterial infections such as *Streptococcus pneumoniae* bacteremia or meningitis can be safely used provided the donor and recipient receive appropriate treatment.[10] Accordingly, most centers would use such an organ.[10] Multidrug-resistant bacteria can be somewhat problematic if susceptibility testing is not available and can cause serious recipient disease. Many centers would refuse to use a graft from a such a donor, particularly with a carbapenem-resistant bacterium.[10] However, an Italian transplant group demonstrated that appropriate treatment early after transplant could allow for safe and successful use of organs from infected donors with resistant bacterial pathogens.[11]

REGULATORY OVERSITE OF DONOR SCREENING AND REPORTING OF DONOR-DERIVED INFECTIONS

With the recognition of the importance of donor-derived infections, government agencies charged with oversite of HSCT and SOT have worked to address and mitigate the risk of these infectious complications. The World Health Organization Guiding Principles on human cell, tissue and organ transplantation encourage countries to have national health oversight of transplant programs to ensure safety of donors and recipients.[12] In the United States, the Health Resources and Services Administration (HRSA), (a branch of the Department of Health and Human Services, oversees the conduct and safety of bone marrow, cord blood, and organ transplantation through different organizations. The National Marrow Donor Program (NMDP; now known as "Be the Match") is contracted by HRSA to oversee the national HSCT program, including donor/recipient adverse events that encompass donor-derived infections.[13] In addition, HRSA has separate contracts with 13 cord banks in the United States through the National Cord Blood Inventory (NCBI) to collect and store cord blood units. UNOS is contracted by HRSA to manage the Organ Procurement and Transplantation Network (OPTN) which in turn is responsible for safety oversight including donor-derived infections in SOT recipients.[14-16] Both programs have developed policy-based requirements for the screening of donors and mandated reporting of suspected donor-derived infection transmission events in recipients in an effort to understand and minimize the risk of these infectious complication.[13-16] In addition to the screening and reporting requirements for HSCT recipients, the NMDP Donor Patient Safety Monitoring Advisory Group (DPSM) investigates infectious disease transmissions as well as all serious recipient infections occurring in these patients. For SOT, the ad hoc OPTN/UNOS Disease Transmission Advisory Committee (DTAC) reviews the mandated reports of potential disease transmission events that are submitted from either the transplant center or the organ procurement organization. Both groups work to review their experience in an effort to improve patient outcomes through enhanced education and relevant policy modifications.

Current policy requires donor and recipient laboratory (serologic, molecular diagnostic, and microbiologic) screening for both HSCT and SOT (Table 5.1). Included pathogens for both HSCT and SOT are those with strong evidence supporting transmission potential or those associated with a high risk for severe disease. Examples of such pathogens include HIV, hepatitis B virus (HBV), hepatitis C virus (HCV), syphilis, and CMV. Although EBV testing is required for an evaluation of a potential deceased organ donor, it is not currently required for potential stem cell donors or for living organ donors. This may be due to the fact that the majority of adults are EBV seropositive, whereas only about 50% of the adults in the United States are seropositive for CMV. Although donor screening protocols for many of the pathogens have been in place for decades, others have been more recently added based on more recently appreciated risks. For example, *Toxoplasma gondii* serologic testing had been part of routine screening for cardiac organ transplantation for years but was recently added in the United States for all deceased organ transplant donors after a review of OPTN/UNOS experience identified a higher-than-expected transmission risk to recipients of non-cardiac organs.[14] In addition, some screening tests may be required for HSCT but not SOT, or vice versa. Finally, OPTN/UNOS policy also includes differing requirements for the evaluation of a living versus deceased donor, including consideration of geographic risk factors when individualizing the evaluation of a potential living organ donor.[14,15] In this circumstance, policy requires each center to have a written plan for consideration of screening for pathogens with variable geographic risks (e.g., trypanosomiasis and West Nile virus).[15] Similarly, because screening for infection caused by *Mycobacterium tuberculosis* cannot reliably be performed on potential deceased donors, it is required only for screening of potential living organ donors.

In addition to laboratory-based screening, a medical and social questionnaire is obtained on all living HSCT donors and living organ donors to identify the presence of risk behaviors that may increase risk for unexpected infections associated with donor-derived transmission.[13,15] For deceased organ transplantation, the

TABLE 5.1 Laboratory Screening of Organs and Bone Marrow

Organism or Site Screened	Methodology	Deceased Organs	Living Donors	Living HSCT Allogeneic Donors[a] Cord Blood Testing Performed on Maternal Sample[b]	Comments
HIV 1, 2	Antibody or Ag/Ab combination test	All In addition, PHS IRD must also have NAT HIV test or HIV Ag/Ab combination	All[c]	All Can be NAT	Positive test result is contraindication to use with HSCT recipients. Organs can be used only through HOPE Act variance.
HTLV I, II	Ab	Not required	All[c]	All	
Hepatitis C virus	Both Ab and NAT	All Special consent process required if HCV positive	All[c]	All	Positive test result is contraindication to use in HSCT with exception of documented urgent need.
Hepatitis B virus	HBsAg, HBcAb	All Special consent process required if HBsAg or HB NAT positive	All[c]	All and should include NAT testing	Positive test result is contraindication to use in HSCT with exception of documented urgent need.
Cytomegalovirus	Ab	All	All	All	
Epstein-Barr virus	Ab	All	All	Not required	
Toxoplasma gondii	IgG Ab	All	Not required	Not required	
Syphilis screen	Screening or diagnostic test	All	All[c]	All	
Tuberculosis	Intradermal or interferon-gamma release assay	Not required	If suspected of having an increased risk for tuberculosis	Not required	Positive test results from any donor need to be reported.
Respiratory culture (bacterial and yeast)	Sputum Gram stain and results of bronchoscopy	Required for potential donors of lungs or head and neck VCA only	Not required	Not required	
Urine culture (bacterial or *Candida* species)	Urinalysis or microscopy Urine culture if indicated	Positive culture results reported to transplant programs receiving kidneys or genitourinary VCAs	Positive culture results reported to transplant programs receiving kidneys or genitourinary VCAs	Not required	
Bone marrow culture for bacteria or fungi		Not required	Not required	Not required but many centers obtain, particularly if cells manipulated before transplantation	
Other	Positive culture results from: Ascites, blood, cerebral spinal fluid, deep wound, genital, pericardial, pleural fluid				Positive culture results need to be reported.

TABLE 5.1 Laboratory Screening of Organs and Bone Marrow—cont'd

Organism or Site Screened	Methodology	Deceased Organs	Living Donors	Living HSCT Allogeneic Donors[a] Cord Blood Testing Performed on Maternal Sample[b]	Comments
Other	Positive results from other serologic, NAT, or antigen testing indicating presence of parasites, mycobacterial smears or cultures, virus, or fungi			West Nile virus testing of living donors required	Positive results need to be reported.

Testing for deceased organs donors must use U.S. Food and Drug Administration–licensed, approved, or cleared tests using a Clinical Laboratory Improvement Amendments–certified laboratory or laboratories meeting equivalent requirements as determined by the Centers for Medicare and Medicaid Services.

[a]Up to 30 days before or 7 days after collection.

[b]Up to 7 days before or after collection.

[c]As close as possible, but within 28 days of organ recovery.

Ab, antibody; *Ag*, antigen; *HbsAb*, hepatitis B surface antibody; *HBsAg*, hepatitis B surface antigen; *HCV*, hepatitis C virus; *HIV*, human immunodeficiency virus; *HSCT*, hematopoietic stem cell transplant; *HTLV*, human T-cell lymphotropic virus; *IgG*, immunoglobulin G; *NAT*, nucleic acid testing; *PHS IRD*, Public Health Service increased risk donor; *VCA*, vascularized composite allotransplant.

donor is not available to directly query for this information; therefore several policies and protocols are in place to help decrease the risk of unanticipated infections and to attempt to identify whether the donor has risks for specific infections that might be missed on laboratory screening. A uniform donor history questionnaire has been developed and adopted for screening of potential deceased organ and/or tissue donors wherein the history is obtained from a family member or friend by trained personnel. Areas of focus included in the uniform questionnaire include assessing potential infectious risks associated with geographic exposures (e.g., country of origin or recent travel), environmental exposures (e.g., contact with individuals who were homeless or incarcerated), as well as questions associated with having an increased risk for having a blood-borne pathogen (e.g., use of nonprescribed intravenous drugs or having sex in exchange for drugs or money or having sex with a sex worker). More recently specific queries have been added about prior diagnosis of emerging pathogens, including Zika, Ebola, West Nile virus, dengue, and Chagas. An important limitation to the effectiveness of the questionnaire is that with deceased donors, the family member or person queried may not be aware of all behaviors or exposures that may be associated with an increased risk of a potentially transmissible infection.

In contrast to deceased donors, OPTN/UNOS policy does not require the use of the uniform questionnaire for living organ donors but rather mandates inclusion of questions addressing the presence of the same risk factors asked for deceased donors.[15] Like living organ donors, potential HSCT donors undergo behavioral and exposure risk screening without using a uniform questionnaire. Rather, donor centers must obtain a donor medical history that meets NMDP requirements for a marrow or apheresis donor that address relevant risks associated with transmission of pathogens via blood products.[13] Although one anticipates accurate completion of questionnaires obtained directly from potential donors, some individuals may choose to not answer all questions honestly, particularly if certain behaviors were not shared when the donor is known to the recipient or their family. Accordingly, ensuring confidentiality for all potential donors is essential.

LESSONS LEARNED

Lessons From Donor-Derived Infections in HSCT and SOT Recipients

The available literature on unanticipated infections from HSCT is sparse compared with organ donation, largely owing to the ability to screen living donors and blood more fully for infectious agents compared with deceased organ donors. However, microbial contamination can occur during harvest or manipulation of HSCT cells.[17,18] Accordingly, close attention to sterile technique and steps to minimalize manipulation help to prevent donor cell contamination. Other infections are rare; however, unanticipated malaria was transmitted in the past decade despite negative blood smear results.[19] Likewise, West Nile virus was transmitted to a pediatric HSCT recipient from a donor with negative test results 3 weeks before stem cell collection but seroconverted when retested after the recipient developed the disease.[20,21] These case reports highlight the need for careful assessment of geographic risks with consideration for further testing at the time of stem cell harvest in addition to educating potential donors about mosquito avoidance. To date, a review of the literature did not identify published reports providing cumulative donor-derived infection event data derived from regulatory driven oversight, which would provide population-based estimates of risk and outcomes of these events.

Lessons From the Ad Hoc Disease Transmission Advisory Committee

As previously noted, in the United States, unanticipated organ donor transmissions are required to be reported to the OPTN/UNOS through its patient safety network.[17] Potential donor-derived transmission events (PDDTEs) are reviewed by the DTAC in a blinded fashion and characterized as proven, probable, possible, intervention without disease transmission (IWDT), unlikely, or excluded for both the whole event and for each individual recipient. Severity scores are given for those determined to have scores of proven, probable, or possible transmission or IWDT. Limitations to this system have been elucidated by Ison and Nalesnik, including variability in the type of information provided and a variability in reporting by geographic region, suggesting that some centers are more likely to recognize the potential for donor transmission compared with others.[6] Despite this variability, DTAC data provide a large aggregate of data allowing for general recommendations to the transplant community that can help inform policy changes as needed for patient safety.[6,8,22,23] Since 2013, approximately 300 cases have been reviewed each year with 35 to 47 proven or probable transmissions each year. A 10-year review of DTAC cases noted an overall low rate of proven or probable disease transmissions. From the January 1, 2006, through September 8, 2015, study period, 174,388 recipients received organs from 63,382 deceased donors. Of 1420 reported PDDTEs, 219 cases met criteria for proven or probable disease transmission.[24] This accounted for 254 (0.15%) recipients who had a donor-derived disease. Infection was the most commonly reported PDDTEs, with 154 of 967 (16%) of reported cases resulting in a proven or probable transmission to at least one recipient. Viruses affected the most recipients (N = 61 recipients), but fungal infections, particularly coccidiomycosis, caused the most deaths (N = 13 deaths).

Although the overall experience with donor-derived infections in SOT recipients has been increasingly well documented over the past 10 to 15 years, specific evaluation of potential transmissions from pediatric deceased donors and the impact of donor-derived disease transmissions to pediatric organ recipients has only recently been reported.[8] Green and colleagues reviewed the experience of pediatric-specific PDDTE tracked by DTAC between 2008 and 2013.[8] Organ transplants involving pediatric donors and recipients from birth to 17 years were analyzed to characterize potential disease transmission from pediatric donors to adult or pediatric recipients and to evaluate potential transmission from all donors to pediatric recipients. A total of 5238 pediatric deceased U.S. donors accounted for 17,456 organ transplants during the study period; 103 PDDTE reports arose from these donors (2%). PDDTEs were characterized by DTAC as proven/probable (15%), possible (13%), IWDT (9%), or unlikely and excluded (63%). Disease was transmitted to 22 of 54 potentially exposed (adult and pediatric) recipients with 6 attributable deaths. An infectious pathogen accounted for 13 of 15 of the proven/probable transmission events associated with pediatric donors, affecting 19 of 50 potentially exposed recipients resulting in 5 deaths. Four separate viral pathogens from 6 donors accounted for proven/probable transmissions to 11 recipients; the unanticipated transmission of CMV (donor and recipient identified as CMV-seronegative before transplant) was the most common pathogen. No pediatric donor transmitted HIV, HBV, or HCV. Bacteria, fungi, and parasites accounted for 3 (all staphylococci), 3 (zygomycetes and histoplasma), and 2 (both *T. gondii*) proven/probable transmissions from 7 donors, respectively. From the recipient side, 11 of 11,188 pediatric recipients of deceased and living donor transplants during the study period were associated with a proven/probable PDDTE (<0.1%) with infectious pathogens accounting for 9 of 11 proven/probable events. Infections were split among pathogen categories (bacteria 2, viruses 3, parasites 3, and fungi 1). The authors concluded that reported rates of PDDTEs involving pediatric donors were very low and similar to rates from all donors, with resulting proven/probable transmissions occurring in only 0.1% of exposed recipients but when transmissions did occur, they could be associated with fatal outcomes. Rates of proven/probable transmission to pediatric recipients from any donor (<0.1%) were also very low and similar to that of all recipients.

EDUCATING CANDIDATES ABOUT DONOR-DERIVED INFECTIONS BEFORE TRANSPLANT

Educating parents, caregivers, and candidates about the potential for donor-derived infections is important so that surveillance and preventive strategies are not a surprise to a family. Likewise, even though unexpected donor transmissions are rare, they can be impactful and should be explained before transplantation so that a family recognizes their possibility. In the United States, a policy clarifying informed consent for transmittable diseases was passed in 2018.[4] The policy highlights that informing candidates and their families should be a process that starts early in the discussion of transplantation risks and benefits and continues through the time that a donor has been identified and accepted for transplantation. Information should include the donor screening process but must also emphasize that it is not possible to screen donors for all transmissible diseases. Specific consents are required to accept a donor with HCV or HBV positive test results and should include the potential for false-positive results, treatment strategies, and the risk of waiting on the candidate list for a donor with negative test results. The HIV Organ Policy Equity (HOPE) Act enacted in 2013 allows for HIV-infected candidates to receive an organ from donors who test positive for HIV.[25] To date, this has affected adult recipients but can be applied to pediatric recipients at approved transplant centers. In addition, special consent is required for donors who fit 1 or more of 11 criteria put forward by the U.S. Public Health Service (PHS) for having an increased risk for HIV, HCV, or HBV even without positive test results.[26,27] Although the risk for transmission is remote, 27% of all deceased organ donors met classification of donors as PHS increased risk donors (IRDs) for HIV, HBV, or HCV by 2018. This has led to misconceptions about the risk of infection transmission, and efforts are currently in place to review and consider revision of these guidelines. Some of the increased PHS IRD designation is driven by the opiate epidemic and concurrent drug-related fatalities affecting potential adult donors more than pediatric donors; however, the misplaced fear attached to the PHS term "increased risk donor" has likely led to unnecessary avoidance transplanting these organs in the pediatric population.[28] As an illustration, in 2014, children received 11.6% of kidneys from 18-to 34-year-old deceased donors classified as standard risk compared with only 3.5% of donors of the same age group who were HCV-negative but classified as PHS IRD.[28] Accordingly, improved education may assist with better use of these organs.

The Importance of Recognizing Donor-Derived Infections

As previously mentioned, in the United States, policies applicable to both HSCT and SOT recipients require both transplant centers and organ procurement organizations to report suspected donor-derived infection transmission events to NMDP or OPTN/UNOS, respectively. By evaluating these potential transmission events, these organizations can identify potential opportunities to enhance safety through education and/or policy. In addition, for SOT recipients, the recognition of one child with a donor-derived infection can alert transplant centers caring for recipients of other organs at risk for infection with the same pathogen. As such, the transplant centers of other recipients may be able to intervene in a timely manner to prevent disease in their patients. Pediatric infectious diseases specialists caring for HSCT, and especially SOT, recipients should always be aware of and consider the possibility that infections after transplantation may be donor derived. This is especially true for infections that occur early after transplant with pathogens that have been associated with unanticipated donor-derived transmissions. The pediatric infectious diseases specialist should work with the transplant team to ensure that suspected cases are reported appropriately according to policy requirements relevant to their patient (e.g., HSCT versus SOT).

SUMMARY

Knowledge of the potential for transmission of infectious pathogens from donor stem cells or organs is critical to optimizing outcomes of stem cell and SOT recipients. The use of laboratory-based screening assays combined with historical and behavioral risk assessment helps protect recipients by allowing for appropriate recognition of potential risks associated with use of stem cells or organs from a given donor. Pediatric infectious diseases specialists caring for transplant recipients must understand these risks and work with transplant teams to recognize when avoidance is advisable and when treatment or prophylaxis strategies should be instituted. In addition, they can assist with appropriate education and counseling of candidates and their families about donor-derived infections in a way that puts the risks and benefits in perspective. Finally, reporting to appropriate agencies is central to the ongoing analysis of donor-derived infections to allow for a continuous optimization of decisions and evaluation of protective strategies to improve transplant recipient outcomes.

6

Prevention of Infections in the Hematopoietic Stem Cell Transplant Recipient

Gabriela M. Marón Alfaro, MD, MS and Hayley A. Gans, MD

Patients who undergo hematopoietic stem cell transplantation (HSCT) are at risk for developing bacterial, fungal, viral, and/or parasitic infections, particularly those who receive allogeneic transplants. Infections in these patients are associated with high rates of morbidity and mortality; therefore preventative strategies are of outmost importance.[1]

For the purpose of this chapter, the term HSCT includes receipt of blood- or marrow-derived hematopoietic stem cells, regardless of transplant type (allogeneic or autologous) or cell source (bone marrow, peripheral blood, or umbilical cord blood). However, the risk of infection between types of HSCT differs depending on factors such as the patient's net immunosuppression, the presence of tissue or organ damage, and the rate of immune reconstitution after transplant. Reconstitution is typically faster in autologous HSCT recipients than in allogeneic HSCT recipients and differs between the different types of allogeneic transplant. The differential impact on and recovery of the immune system by HSCT type is discussed in detail in Chapter 2.

Infections during the course of HSCT may be derived from the patient's microbial flora, a reactivation of a latent infection from either the recipient or donor, or from primary infection. Three periods of risk for infections in HSCT recipients have been traditionally described based on the time since transplantation. The three periods are pre-engraftment (from transplantation to neutrophil recovery, approximately day 20 to 30), early postengraftment (from engraftment to day 100), and late post engraftment (after day 100). During each of these periods, patients are at risk of developing bacterial, fungal, viral, and/or parasitic infections. Allogeneic HSCT recipients are considered to be at high risk for infection during all three periods (see Fig. 2.1), whereas autologous HSCT recipients are most vulnerable during the pre-engraftment and immediate postengraftment periods.

Measures to prevent infections during HSCT include determination of recipient risk, appropriate selection of donors, infection control measures, and targeted prophylactic and preemptive therapy. This chapter provides a general overview of infection risk and prevention in pediatric HSCT recipients, including guidance for a comprehensive infectious disease pretransplant evaluation. Specific infection control measures are addressed in Chapter 12, and prophylactic and preemptive approaches are addressed in pathogen-specific chapters (see Chapters 14 through 34.

PRETRANSPLANT EVALUATION

The pretransplant infectious disease consultation is an important component of infection prevention in HSCT recipients. The goal is to evaluate the donor and recipient for acute infections, relevant exposures, latent infections, and colonization with resistant organisms. The assessment should include a review of the history and laboratory results of both the donor and the recipient. The history should be accompanied by a detailed physical examination and comprehensive imaging of the recipient. Documentation of this information in a detailed pretransplant evaluation note can prove to be a valuable guide should concerns about infection in the posttransplant period develop.

Recipient Evaluation

History. Areas of focus for history taking in the recipient and donor are presented in Box 6.1. A primary goal of this clinical encounter is to elicit any symptoms that may be concerning for the presence of an active infection or recent exposure to an infectious disease that could preclude proceeding to transplantation in the recipient. An equally important goal is to review the recipient's medical history, social history, and laboratory results from both the recipient and donor to identify gaps in prior preventative measures (i.e., incomplete vaccination), document concomitant comorbidities, identify the presence of latent viruses or colonizing resistant organisms, and document possible social behaviors that may place the patient at risk for future infection.

Transplant Information. Details regarding the type of graft, conditioning regimen, and plans for graft versus host disease (GVHD) prophylaxis are important for understanding the risk of infections in HSCT candidates. Clear documentation of these elements in the pretransplant evaluation makes them easily available if complications arise during the course of transplant.

The type of graft and number of stem cells to be infused should be noted as each of these factors may affect the time to recovery of the immune system after transplant, which will alter infection risk. For example, recovery of neutrophils after an umbilical cord transplantation takes significantly longer compared with receipt of a peripheral stem cell product. Additionally, manipulation of the graft product can also alter infection risk. T-cell–depleted grafts can help reduce the risk of GVHD but will also delay complete immune reconstitution of T-cell function, which can increase the risk for viral or fungal infection in the postengraftment periods. T-cell depletion can be achieved by ex vivo manipulation of the graft product or in vivo administration of a lymphocyte depleting agent such as anti-thymocyte globulin at the transplant. The latter is referred to as serotherapy. Discussions of these graft-specific features with the primary transplant team and the family before transplant can help frame the risk for infection and guide decisions for prophylaxis approaches.

Conditioning regimens include myeloablative conditioning, reduced intensity conditioning, or nonmyeloablative regimens. The risk for toxicity increases with the intensity of the regimen. Myeloablative conditioning regimens are associated with profound immunosuppression and increased risk of mucositis that will predispose a child to bloodstream infections. Radiation-containing regimens increase the likelihood of mucosal and skin breakdown in the recipient. GVHD

BOX 6.1 Pretransplant Evaluation of HSCT Donors and Recipients

Evaluation

Donor and Recipient

Evidence of active infection
Infectious disease exposures (including tuberculosis, animals, foods)
History of transfusions
Travel history or residence in areas of the world with endemic infections
Vaccination history
Social history including sexual history, illicit drug use

Recipient

Type and intensity of previous chemotherapy and/or radiotherapy
Status of the underlying cancer (first or second remission, relapse)
Infectious complications during cancer therapy (bacterial, fungal, viral, others)
Colonization or infection with resistant organisms
Dental history
Structural abnormalities (cardiac defects, prosthetic biomaterials, hemodialysis access fistula)
Evidence of recent or current infection, including upper respiratory tract or gastrointestinal viruses infections
Documentation of all current foreign bodies

prophylaxis in HSCT is usually achieved using calcineurin inhibitor–based therapy (i.e., cyclosporine, tacrolimus), sometimes in combination with mycophenolate mofetil. The use of these immunosuppressant therapies increases the risk of infections and has been associated particularly with viral and fungal infections. Use of posttransplant cyclophosphamide for prevention of GVHD may also delay engraftment and count recovery.

When documenting the planned conditioning and GVHD prophylaxis regimens, attention should be given to the possibility of drug-drug interactions with anti-infective agents that might be used in prophylaxis or preemptive strategies. For example, the triazole antifungal class is often leveraged in prophylaxis pathways, but these agents can have significant interactions with many other drug classes, some of which might be used for conditioning or GHVD prevention. Therefore it is important to discuss these details with the transplant team in advance of the transplant.

Physical Examination. The recipient should undergo a complete physical examination, with an emphasis on sites that could become infected or serve as an entry for infection. These include the oral cavity, perirectal region, skin, central venous catheter sites and any foreign bodies, and the upper and lower respiratory tracts. Any signs of active infection should be noted followed by appropriate workup and management. Additionally, these signs of infection should be discussed immediately with the transplant team as they may preclude the ability to move forward with conditioning.

Pathogen-Specific Testing. Laboratory testing for evidence of past infectious exposures is performed to detect asymptomatic persistence of certain pathogens in the HSCT candidate and the donor. Some tests are recommended for all HSCT donors and candidates, whereas others depend on epidemiologic risk factors (Table 6.1). Serologic tests are typically used to investigate past exposures for a multitude of pathogens; however, in some cases, screening using polymerase chain reaction (PCR) assays is indicated (i.e., human immunodeficiency virus (HIV) and hepatitis C virus [HCV]). When relying on serology results to determine past pathogen exposures, the clinician must be aware of the possibility for false-positive detection secondary to passive receipt of antibodies (e.g., young infants, recent receipt of immunoglobulin or packed red blood cells). Alternatively, false-negative serology results may be present in patients with an underlying primary immunodeficiency disorder or those who are secondarily immunosuppressed. In these clinical scenarios, a greater reliance on PCR diagnostics may be necessary but does not always allow for the establishment of latent pathogen presence.

Imaging. Although most HSCT recipients undergo pretransplant imaging, there are no defined standard of care protocols for imaging. Some institutions request imaging of the chest, abdomen, and sinuses for all recipients before transplant; others take a targeted approach based on past infectious history (i.e., fungal infection or pneumonia) and the site of infection. Recipients undergoing autologous or allogeneic HSCT for lymphomas or solid tumors routinely undergo chest and abdominal computed tomography (CT) imaging as part of their disease evaluation. Observational studies suggest that pre-HSCT routine CT imaging of the abdomen may not be warranted in other recipients who are asymptomatic and without previous infectious findings.[2,3] CT imaging of the sinuses is not routinely recommended as pre-HSCT radiographic findings have not been found to correlate with subsequent development of clinical sinusitis after transplant.[4] Based on these data and to spare patients from unnecessary radiation, the decision to perform CT imaging should be based on a careful risk assessment, history, and physical examination.

Additional Evaluations. Consultation with other specialists may help detect or prevent infections in the recipient. Dental evaluation should be considered for all HSCT candidates to evaluate their oral health and perform any necessary dental procedures to decrease the incidence of oral mucosa–borne infections during periods of mucositis. Otolaryngologic evaluation should be considered in symptomatic patients or those with a history of sinusitis. A direct scope may detect existing infections or anatomic features that may increase risk for infections and identify patients who may need closer follow-up during their transplant course.

Donor Evaluation

History. Similar to history attainment for the recipient, the goal of the history obtained from the donor is to identify active infection or prior infectious disease exposures that would make the donor ineligible or pose a risk of infection transmission to the recipient. Many of the historical data to be captured for the donor are similar to those collected for the recipient (see Box 6.1). A standard approach to capturing this information is important so that no pertinent information is missed. A standardized checklist has been developed by an American Association of Blood Banks (AABB) task force and complies with all regulatory requirements. The checklist is available at the AABB website (http://www.aabb.org/tm/questionnaires/Pages/default.aspx) and can be used as a guide for collecting this information. Generally, the donor assessment should identify social risk factors (e.g., intravenous drug use, prior blood transfusions, pregnancies, abortions, and tattoos), document immunization history, and prior travel. Often the donor is not always available for interview by the clinical team; however, clinicians should familiarize themselves with the AABB donor screening tool to know which historical elements need to be assessed from the donors.

Pathogen-Specific Testing. Requirements from the U.S. Food and Drug Administration (FDA), state, and other regulatory bodies for donor screening are frequently updated.[5] In the United States, unrelated donors are required to comply with guidelines from the U.S.

TABLE 6.1 Recommended Microbiologic Laboratory Assessment of HSCT Donors and Recipients

Pathogen	Laboratory Test	Donor	Recipient	Notes
CMV	CMV IgG or CMV total Ab, CMV PCR	Yes	Yes	CMV PCR in recipient
EBV	EBV VCA IgM and IgG Ab, EBNA, EBV PCR	Yes	Yes	EBV PCR in recipient
HBV	HBsAg, HBs Ab, HBc Ab, HBV NAT	Yes	Yes	
HCV	HCV AB, HCV NAT	Yes	Yes	
HIV	HIV-1/2 Antigen and Abs assay, HIV NAT	Yes	Yes	
HSV 1/2	HSV1 AB, HSV2 Ab	N	Y	
HTLV-1/-2	HTLV-1/2 Ab	Yes	Yes	
VZV	VZV IgG	Yes	Yes	
WNV	WNV serology, WNV NAT	Yes	Yes	
Syphilis	RPR or syphilis Ab	Yes	Yes	
Toxoplasma	*Toxoplasma* serology, PCR	Yes	Yes	
Additional Screening Depending on Exposure History or Local Epidemiology				
Respiratory viruses	Respiratory virus PCR	No	Yes	
Chagas	*Trypanosoma cruzi* Ab	Yes	Yes	
Histoplasma	Histoplasma serology, antigens	No	Yes	
Blastomyces	*Blastomyces* Abs	No	Yes	
Coccidioides	*Coccidioides* Abs	No	Yes	
Malaria	Malaria screen, blood smear, PCR	Yes	Yes	
Strongyloides	*S. stercolaris* Abs	Yes	Yes	
Tuberculosis	Risk factor assessment, TST, IGRA	Yes	Yes	
Zika virus	Risk factor assessment, Zika PCR	Yes	Yes	
Ova and parasites	Stool test	No	Yes	
Additional Screening by Some Institutions				
Surveillance cultures	Perianal swab, nasal swab	No	Yes	For infection control purposes
Adenovirus	Blood and stool PCR	No	Yes	Active disease and risk of dissemination

Ab, antibody; *CMV*, cytomegalovirus; *EBNA*, Epstein-Barr virus nuclear antigen; *HBc*, hepatitis B core antibody; *HBsAg*, hepatitis B surface antigen; *HBV*, hepatitis B virus; *HCV*, hepatitis C virus; *HIV*, human immunodeficiency virus; *HSCT*, hematopoietic stem cell transplant; *HSV*, herpes simplex virus; *HTLV-1/-2*, human T-lymphotropic virus 1 and 2; *Ig*, immunoglobulin; *IGRA*, interferon-gamma release assay; *NAT*, nucleic acid testing; *PCR*, polymerase chain reaction; *RPR*, rapid plasma reagin; TST, tuberculin skin test; *VCA*, viral capsid antigen; *VZV*, varicella zoster virus; *WNV*, West Nile virus.

Food and Drug Administration, The Joint Commission, the AABB, the National Marrow Donor Program, and the Foundation for the Accreditation of Cellular Therapy. Some tests are required of all donors and some depend on exposure history (see Table 6.1). As in recipients, most are serologic tests to investigate past exposures, but PCR is used as indicated. Donor screening should be performed within 6 months before stem cell donation.[1] Specimens for laboratory testing of peripheral blood stem cells or bone marrow should be obtained up to 30 days before donation and within 7 days for testing of lymphocyte or umbilical cord blood donation. For umbilical cord blood donation, mothers are screened for Hepatitis B virus (HBV), human immunodeficiency virus (HIV), syphilis, human T-lymphocyte virus (HTLV)-1/2, cytomegalovirus (CMV), West Nile virus, and Chagas disease.

Close attention should be paid to donor serology results, particularly CMV, Epstein-Barr virus (EBV), HBV, HCV, and *Toxoplasma gondii* as these results may lead to prevention and management strategies as discussed in the sections Prevention of Viral Infections and Prevention of Other Infections.

Active Infections. Donors with any evidence of an active infection should be treated for that infection with some assessment of treatment effectiveness, either by clinical examination or laboratory follow-up results, performed before product harvest. Specific examples would include donors with active tuberculosis (TB) or malaria. For the former, the donor should be treated and donation deferred until the infection is deemed to be controlled. Donors with active malaria should receive treatment and have a documented negative follow-up test result before donation. In certain circumstances, an identified suitable donor is identified but that donor retains an infection that may pose a risk to the recipient. In these circumstances, the risk of infection transmission needs to be weighed against the need to proceed with transplantation. It is possible in such scenarios that the infection risk can be reduced to optimize the balance of benefit over risk. For example, a suitable donor who is either HBV or HCV positive can be treated with antivirals to reduce the transmission risk (see the following special considerations section).

Special Considerations and Contraindications to Donation. Some infections in the donor are considered contraindications to stem cell donation (Box 6.2). In other cases, the decision to exclude a potential donor should be made on a case-by-case basis, particularly when delaying transplant may lead to mortality.

Donors with antibodies to HBV or HCV are eligible to donate as transmission is not universal and recipients may have the ability to receive effective antiviral therapy. Unrelated donors with positive results for hepatitis B surface antigen or positive HBV DNA test results are generally not considered an option for seronegative recipients.

BOX 6.2 Contraindications to Stem Cell Donation

- Human immunodeficiency virus infection
- Acute cytomegalovirus or Epstein-Barr virus infection
- Acute hepatitis A infection
- Zika virus[a]
- Acute toxoplasmosis
- Active tuberculosis (until well controlled)
- Acute tickborne infection
- Active or past history of Chagas disease
- Acute or recent West Nile virus infection
- Active malaria[b]

[a]Donors are considered ineligible if in the prior 6 months they had a diagnosis of Zika virus infection, resided or traveled to an area with Zika virus activity, or had sexual contact with a man who fits any of these criteria. Umbilical cord blood donors are ineligible if the birth mother had a diagnosis of Zika virus infection at any point during the pregnancy, resided or traveled to an endemic area, or had sexual contact with a man with similar exposures.

[b]For donors with active malaria, collection should be delayed until after completing treatment and the confirmatory testing result is negative.

However, if another suitable donor is not available, a family may be willing to accept such a donor. Recipients with positive HBV or HCV serology may more readily consider donors with similar positivity, especially if no other donor options are available. Similarly, donors with confirmed HTLV-1 may be used even in seronegative recipients, provided the benefits outweigh the risks for infection. In any of these cases, the recipient must be made aware of the potential risks.

Imaging. Depending on history and physical examination findings, donors may be screened using chest radiography to rule out active infection including TB (see the section Tuberculosis).

VACCINATION

Pretransplant vaccination of HSCT candidates is an effective and important measure to prevent infections. Whenever possible and depending on the time to transplant, recipients should be immunized with the vaccines that are indicated based on age, vaccination history, and exposure history. However, often underlying conditions leading into the HSCT or limitations in time preclude the ability to completely vaccinate a recipient before transplant. Therefore additional focus on complete vaccination of all household contacts is recommended to provide indirect protection for the recipient.[6] Pretransplant immunizations are discussed in detail in Chapter 9.

PREVENTION OF BACTERIAL INFECTIONS

Active Infections. Whenever possible, any active bacterial infections identified in the recipient during the pretransplant evaluation should be treated with the intent of elimination or suppression before transplant. In some cases, the HSCT is still performed despite a diagnosis of infection in the pre-HSCT period. In this circumstance, the treatment for the infection may need to continue through high-risk post-HSCT periods.

Preventing Exposure. Health care workers and others in contact with HSCT recipients should practice appropriate hand hygiene practices to avoid exposing recipients to bacterial pathogens. Additional precautions are needed for patients colonized with highly contagious or resistant organisms and those presenting with specific clinical symptoms (diarrhea or respiratory diseases). Additional specific infection control processes (e.g., isolation procedures) are further described in Chapter 12.

Preventing Early Disease (0-100 Days After HSCT). There are currently no antimicrobial prophylactic regimens recommended as standard of care for pediatric HSCT recipients. A recent large, multicenter, open-label, randomized trial of pediatric HSCT patients administered levofloxacin in the neutropenic period did not demonstrate a statistically significant reduction in bacteremia in the HSCT study group.[7] However, some experts argue that secondary analyses from this study did reveal a statistically significant reduction in bacteremia risk and purport that the findings of this study represent a clinically important reduction in risk of bacteremia. The decision to use fluoroquinolone prophylaxis in HSCT recipients must be considered in light of certain risks. Recently, levofloxacin prophylaxis has been associated with breakthrough bacteremia with meropenem-nonsusceptible *Pseudomonas aeruginosa* strains.[8] If the decision is made to use fluoroquinolone prophylaxis, local epidemiologic data should be carefully monitored starting before and continuing after initiating a prophylaxis pathway. The monitoring should specifically focus on the rate of bacteremia and the emergence of resistance in bacterial pathogens at the particular institution. Use of broad gram-positive agents for prophylaxis, specifically glycopeptides, should not be routine. There are limited data documenting the benefit of these agents for prophylaxis and their use may promote toxicity, emergence of resistant microorganisms, and necessitate further escalation of antibiotic therapy in the setting of empirical fever and neutropenia. In one open-label randomized trial of HSCT recipients, the use of antimicrobial therapy for targeted destruction of intestinal anaerobic bacteria (metronidazole) significantly reduced the severity of acute GVHD, but there were no differences in overall survival.[9] Although a reduction in GVHD risk is attractive, the practice of metronidazole administration can have negative consequences on the microbiome, allowing for enterococcal domination and subsequent invasive infection.[10] Therefore routine gut decontamination for pediatric HSCT candidates, either with metronidazole or other nonabsorbable antibiotics, is not recommended. Further discussion regarding the implications of the microbiome in HSCT can be found in Chapter 10.

Viridans group streptococci are normal commensals of oral surfaces that may lead to potentially fatal infections in HSCT recipients, especially in those with chemotherapy-induced oral mucositis. Recipients should undergo all necessary dental procedures before HSCT to decrease the risk for oral infections during transplant.[11] Additionally, empirical treatment of any HSCT recipient with fever, neutropenia, and severe mucositis should include an agent active against viridans streptococci.[12]

Preventing Late Disease (More Than 100 Days After HSCT). Some HSCT recipients have functional asplenia related to immune suppressive therapies they receive for GVHD and thus are at increased risk for infection from encapsulated organisms. For example, *Streptococcus pneumoniae* infection risk is increased in allogeneic recipients with chronic GVHD for as long as GVHD treatment is administered.[13] Although there are no definitive guidelines for antibiotic prophylaxis in these patients, many experts advocate prophylaxis management approaches similar to those for children with asplenia.

Catheter-Associated Infections. Catheter-associated infections are frequently encountered in HSCT recipients, particularly during the preengraftment phase and in patients with skin compromise secondary to GVHD. These infections often result in a need for catheter removal and, much less commonly, in death.[14] As such, the use of central line–associated bloodstream infection (CLABSI) prevention bundles is strongly advised to reduce this risk of CLABSI. The use of bundles has been associated with a decrease in bloodstream infections in HSCT pediatric patients.[15] Prevention of CLABSIs is discussed in detail in Chapter 12.

PREVENTION OF INVASIVE FUNGAL DISEASE

Approaches to invasive fungal disease prophylaxis, preemptive therapy, and directed therapy are discussed in Chapter 8 and respective fungal pathogen chapters (Chapters 24 through 28). General principles for approaching patients with active infections before transplant and the approach for preventing infections in the posttransplant period are presented in the following text.

Active Infections. Candidates for HSCT who have invasive yeast or mold disease can safely undergo transplant if their infection is treated immediately and aggressively with effective antifungal therapy and there is evidence of infection control before the transplant. Complete resolution is not necessary before transplantation if the patient has received appropriate therapy and shows clinical improvement. Such patients should continue receiving an appropriate antifungal agent at therapeutic doses throughout the pre-engraftment and early postengraftment periods until clinical evaluation and serial imaging verify the resolution of the infection.[16]

Preventing Exposure. Invasive candidiasis is usually caused by dissemination of endogenous *Candida* species colonizing the patient's gastrointestinal tract. The risk for invasive candidiasis is higher during the early posttransplant period because of neutropenia, severe mucositis, and the presence of a central venous catheter.[17] Therefore measures to reduce CLABSI and chemotherapy-induced mucositis are necessary to decrease the risk of disseminated yeast infection.

Nosocomial invasive mold disease in HSCT recipients results primarily from respiratory exposure to and direct contact with fungal spores. Therefore efforts aimed at reducing such exposures can be paramount to limiting this risk. Measures for minimizing exposure to mold in HSCT candidates and recipients are discussed in Chapter 12.

Preventing Disease. Topical antifungal drugs applied to the mucosa may reduce colonization by yeasts and molds in the area of application but have not been proven to prevent invasive or disseminated yeast or mold infections, and their use for prophylaxis is unclear.

Fluconazole remains the first-line drug for prophylaxis of invasive candidiasis before engraftment in allogeneic HSCT recipients. The optimal duration of prophylaxis to prevent candidiasis is not defined but typically is continued through at least the engraftment period. Echinocandins are alternative prophylactic agents that may be particularly useful in patients known to be colonized with fluconazole-resistant *Candida* species.[18] Few HSCT recipients require continuation of antifungal prophylaxis in the postengraftment period unless there are other factors such as the presence of GVHD.[19] When GVHD is present, the risk for invasive mold increases and thus antifungal prophylaxis in this period often uses an agent with mold coverage such as voriconazole or posaconazole. The latter is limited by dosing data that are only available down to age 13 years. Prophylaxis with itraconazole is effective and an option in this setting; however, the use of itraconazole is limited by absorption and tolerability. In patients who cannot tolerate azole therapy, echinocandins are an option for prophylaxis that provides some mold coverage, specifically against aspergillosis. In patients receiving antifungal prophylaxis during periods of GVHD, the prophylaxis should continue throughout the duration of immunosuppression therapy for the GVHD.[20]

PREVENTION OF VIRAL INFECTIONS

The management of viral infections, including prophylaxis, preemptive therapy and therapeutic options, is discussed in detail in Chapters 17 through 23. The general principles for prevention of these infections are presented in the following text.

Active Infections. It is important to determine whether a recipient or donor is actively infected with a virus before transplant and to attempt eradication or suppression. Several active or acute viral infections preclude cell donation (Box 6.2). However, many viruses, such as the herpes and polyoma viruses, establish latency and thus the therapeutic goal is control of infection during very high-risk periods. Active HBV and HCV infection in the donor warrants antiviral therapy before transplant with the goal of a graft that is PCR negative at time of transplant.[21] If this is not feasible, then recipient counseling, immunization when applicable, and treatment are recommended.

Preventing Exposure. Given the high associated morbidity and mortality, viral infections are feared after transplant, especially during the pre-engraftment and early postengraftment periods, as well as in patients requiring additional immune suppression, such as those with GVHD. Unfortunately, treatment options for many viral pathogens are limited and thus prevention strategies are paramount to reducing morbidity and mortality. Prevention is most directly achieved through donor screening and restrictions, which includes the contraindications listed in Box 6.2 but also via specific strategies such as using seronegative donors when possible or leukocyte-depleted blood products or graft.[22,23] In addition, vaccination is a powerful prevention method that should be used pretransplant (see Chapter 9).

Preventing Disease. Understanding the recipient's susceptibility to viral reactivation is crucial to preventing disease; thus screening as outlined in Box 6.1 is invaluable. An overview of the common viruses is presented in the following text, but not all viruses are discussed. See Chapters 17 through 23 for details on specific viruses.

The herpesviruses pose a particular risk for morbidity and mortality in HSCT recipients because of their ability to maintain latency or persistence after primary infection, thereby allowing for reactivation upon immune suppression. Depending on the herpesvirus in question, the impact from reactivation can be reduced through either a prophylaxis or preemptive approach. The former approach allows for administration of antiviral therapy before detection of viral reactivation, whereas the latter approach institutes close laboratory monitoring for early detection of viral reactivation followed by prompt administration of antiviral therapy when virus is detected.[24]

CMV was the most common viral reactivation before the implementation of prevention strategies, causing disease including pneumonia that resulted in mortality of 85% of HSCT recipients.[22] Preventative and preemptive approaches for CMV have evolved over decades, and current strategies have been highly successful in preventing CMV disease manifestations and are universally recommended.[25] Controversy remains over whether to use a prophylaxis or preemptive approach for CMV in this patient population; some centers choose the former and some the latter. Recent data support a preemptive strategy in HSCT populations given similar outcomes for both strategies, the potential for increased drug toxicity with a prophylaxis approach, and the possible delay in development of CMV-specific T-cell reconstitution associated with routine prophylaxis, resulting in late-onset disease.[22,26] Regardless of whether a prophylaxis or preemptive approach is used, centers should establish risk stratification profiles for each HSCT recipient using donor and recipient serology status. The highest risk for CMV reactivation is among HSCT recipient-positive and donor-negative patients. This is reversed in the risk profile for solid organ transplant recipients. Ganciclovir or valganciclovir are the most active agents against CMV and used commonly for prevention. Given the potential for bone marrow– suppressive effects, these agents are typically reserved for therapy after engraftment. Other agents active against CMV include foscarnet and cidofovir, but each of these carries a risk for renal toxicity. High-dose acyclovir has been studied as a prophylaxis regimen but there are limited data to support the effectiveness of this approach. More recently, the novel agent letermovir has been approved for prophylaxis in adults undergoing HSCT.[26] This agent is promising as it was not associated with bone marrow suppression when given as a prophylaxis agent soon after HSCT. However, there are no pediatric-specific comparative data to support its use as prophylaxis in this age range. Furthermore, there are no data on letermovir as an agent for preemptive therapy.

Similar to CMV, EBV is a ubiquitous herpesvirus that establishes latency once infection has occurred. The most serious complication of EBV infection in immunocompromised populations, including HSCT recipients, is the progression of disease to posttransplant lymphoproliferative disorder (PTLD), a potentially fatal condition that can develop in the absence of adequate EBV-specific T-cell function.[27] The risk for PTLD is highest in the first 6 months after transplant and is dependent on the type of donor, T-cell depletion, use of anti-thymocyte globulin, EBV serology mismatch between donor and recipient, and functional spleen status.[23] Antiviral agents have no impact on the development of EBV-PTLD; thus they do not have a role in prevention. In addition, intravenous immunoglobulin administration has not been shown to be effective; therefore serial EBV screening and preemptive therapies at detection of EBV reactivation with rituximab or EBV-specific CTL remain the most viable options for prevention of PTLD. However, there have been no comparative studies to confirm that routine screening and institution of these preemptive therapies is effective or necessary for all patients with EBV reactivation.

Herpes simplex virus (HSV) and varicella zoster virus (VZV) also reactivate in the early (<100 days) posttransplant period and warrant prevention, typically accomplished with acyclovir or more bioavailable formulations such as valacyclovir.[23] Recent studies suggest brincidofovir as a potential alternative but pediatric data for this agent are limited.[28] HSV reaction in seropositive recipients is common (up to 80%), occurs early after HSCT (in the first 4 weeks after transplant), and carries the risk for disseminated disease.[23] Acyclovir is highly effective in preventing reactivation and therefore should be used in patients who are HSV immunoglobulin (Ig) G recipient positive during high-risk periods, including early posttransplant and during enhanced immunosuppressive periods, such as during GVHD.

Acyclovir prophylaxis is also effective in reducing the risk of VZV reactivation or herpes zoster. Before the use of antiviral prophylaxis, nearly 50% of seropositive HSCT recipients developed herpes zoster with significant mortality with a median time to reactivation of 5 months and cumulative 30-month risk of 80%. The highest risk is in individuals with chronic GVHD. In the age of VZV vaccination, most HSCT candidates are seropositive to VZV before transplant. Importantly, seropositivity secondary to vaccination confers lower rates of herpes zoster in the post-HSCT period compared with VZV seropositivity secondary to natural infection. Regardless of seronegative status before transplant, any exposure to primary varicella after HSCT poses a risk for primary varicella disease, which can be devastating in these immunocompromised hosts, especially in the presence of corticosteroid treatment. The risk period for primary varicella is slightly different than the risk period for reactivation, extending well into the second year after transplant. The differential risk window is likely a function of the fact that primary exposures to varicella are often in the community and not in the hospital.[23] Upon documented exposure of HSCT recipients to varicella, postexposure passive prophylaxis with VariZIG should be pursued. When VariZIG is not available, conventional intravenous immunoglobulin can be considered. The goal should be to administer immunoglobulin as soon as possible after exposure but ideally no longer than 10 days after exposure.

Other herpesviruses, including human herpesviruses 6, 7, and 8 (HHV6, HHV7, HHV8, respectively) can reactivate after HSCT.[29,30] However, the most prevalent is HHV6, reactivating in 30% to 40% of HSCT recipients. The risk of reactivation is associated with unrelated donor transplantation, GVHD, and EBV co-infection. The most significant clinical entities associated with HHV6 reactivation are encephalitis and bone marrow suppression leading to concerns for the graft.[30] Studies assessing the comparative effectiveness of prophylaxis or preemptive therapy for HHV6 are lacking; however, when clinicians administer antiviral therapy for HHV 6, ganciclovir and foscarnet are often first-line agents. Acyclovir has some in vitro activity for HHV 6 but is not frequently used in this setting. There are minimal data on the epidemiology and implications of reactivation of HHV7 and HHV8. At this time there are no routine recommendations for prophylaxis or preemptive therapies for HHV 6, HHV 7, or HHV 8.

Respiratory viruses are common infections that can cause significant morbidity and mortality in children after HSCT.[31] Unfortunately, nosocomial spread is documented, making acquisition in hospitalized children undergoing HSCT a possibility. Screening for the presence of respiratory viruses before HSCT in symptomatic patients is warranted (see Table 6.1) because children with positive results and symptoms before transplant were shown to have lower survival 100 days after HSCT.[32] Some centers perform respiratory virus testing in the pretransplant period even in the absence of symptoms. The utility of testing in asymptomatic individuals is not clear as current testing modalities such as PCR can detect virus long after symptom resolution and the implications of detecting virus at this stage are unknown.

The incidence of respiratory tract viruses is dependent on the specific virus and time of year, but overall rates are documented at 4% to 7%. The risk for progression to lower respiratory tract disease ranges from 10% to 50%. Mortality from respiratory viral infections is possible with any virus but appears to be most common with respiratory syncytial virus (RSV) and adenovirus (AdV) reported as 60% and 75%, respectively. In general, HSCT recipients have prolonged viral shedding, and combined with higher viral loads, supports increased risk for progression of disease.[31]

Most respiratory viruses lack preventative therapeutic options. Influenza virus is the only respiratory virus for which a vaccine exists. All HSCT candidates should receive the vaccine yearly but effectiveness of the vaccine in immunocompromised hosts is limited. Vaccination of household members can create a protective window around the patient and reduce exposure. Postexposure prophylaxis, typically with a neuraminidase inhibitor, is often recommended for influenza. As there are no other proven preventative therapeutics, a focus on reducing exposure to symptomatic individuals is extremely important. Many institutions are adopting limited visitation protocols during the respiratory viral season, have mandatory influenza vaccination for employees, and establish infrastructure for not allowing sick employees to come to work.

Once a child with an HSCT has an upper respiratory tract viral infection, there is often interest in preventing progression to lower respiratory tract disease. However, the therapeutic options for interrupting this progression are limited. The use of ribavirin has often been used for patients with respiratory syncytial virus (RSV) infection soon after HSCT, but data in children on effectiveness are limited. Recent increases in the cost of aerosolized ribavirin have led many clinicians to try oral formulations of ribavirin, which are much cheaper but have even less evidence to support their utility. Adjunctive therapies such as providing passive immunity with palivizumab or conventional immunoglobulin have been used but also have limited supportive evidence for effectiveness. There are numerous antiviral therapies under investigation that may be beneficial in the future as agents to be used in postexposure prophylaxis or preemptive therapy scenarios, but currently, none of these agents have been approved for use in routine clinical care.

AdV is distinct from other respiratory viral pathogens as it can establish latency and thus can reactivate infection in pediatric HSCT recipients. Reactivation of AdV can cause pulmonary and extrapulmonary organ dysfunction that can lead to significant morbidity and mortality.[33,34] Risk factors for AdV reactivation include T-cell–depleted products, lymphopenia, GVHD, and recent bacteremia. Given the high morbidity and mortality, some have advocated for preemptive strategies that include surveillance blood or stool testing with initiation of antiviral therapy once virus is detected. Cidofovir and more recently brincidofovir are the antiviral agents used in a preemptive approach. Of note, although many experts have supported this approach,[33] there are no comparative data to confirm that a preemptive approach is effective. The successful use of AdV-specitific cytotoxic T-lymphocytes for treatment of asymptomatic AdV infection and AdV disease has been reported in case reports and case series, but universal use of this approach for all asymptomatic AdV infections is likely not practical at this time.

Infection with HBV and HCV before HSCT can complicate the posttransplant period, but detection of infection in an HSCT candidate is not a contraindication for transplantation.[21] Pretransplant screening should include both viruses as detection before transplant can allow for steps to mitigate posttransplant complications. For HBV-infected recipients, this can include pretransplant immunization, administration of antiviral therapy before and after transplant, and selecting donors with resolved infection. However, if a donor does have history of HBV, the donor should be treated and tested before donation to ensure that the graft will be free of HBV.

Transplants in a patient with a history of HCV infection carry potentially more risk for posttransplant complications such as development of venoocclusive disease.[21] Patients with a presence of protective serologies and absent detection of virus do not need treatment. However, recipients who are HCV–ribonucleic acid (RNA) positive, including those with chronic infection, do require treatment. Donors should also be screened for HCV. Identification of infection in the donor is not an absolute contraindication for donation, especially if there are limited donor options for a recipient. However, given the high rate of HCV transmission from HCV-RNA–positive donors to HSCT recipients, treatment of the donor until HCV-RNA–negative status is achieved is the desired strategy to prevent transmission to the recipient. However, if HSCT is urgent, treatment of the recipient after transplantation is a viable option.

Polyoma viruses, including BK virus, are a challenge after HSCT, with reactivation causing hemorrhagic cystitis, nephropathy, and potentially disseminated disease leading to morbidity and mortality.[35,36] There is bimodal distribution of BK reactivation after HSCT. Early reactivation tends to occur in the pre-engraftment period and is associated with receipt of conditioning therapy, whereas late-onset BK reactivation occurs in the postengraftment period. Early reactivation incidence has declined, mostly as a result of less toxic conditioning regimens. Some reports have suggested a variety of uroprotective measures, including MESNA (2-mercaptoehtnaesulfonic acid sodium salt) and hyperhydration, diuresis and hyperhydration (delete medications) and prophylactic fluoroquinilones. However, there are no comparative data to support the effectiveness of any of these strategies.

PREVENTION OF OTHER INFECTIONS

Pneumocystis jirovecii (Formerly *Pneumocystis carinii*) Pneumonia

Allogeneic HSCT recipients should receive prophylaxis against *P. jirovecii* pneumonia (PCP) and continue until evidence of T-cell immune recovery.[1] A general guide for PCP prophylaxis duration is to administer prophylaxis for at least 6 months after an allogeneic HSCT, but the actual duration for each patient is based on the need for continued immune suppression such as in patients with GVHD. Early cessation of PCP prophylaxis in allogeneic HSCT recipients has been associated with PCP.[37] The utility of PCP prophylaxis in autologous HSCT recipients is not as clearly established; some institutions use universal prophylaxis and some reserve it for those receiving myeloablative conditioning regimens, graft manipulations, high-dose glucocorticoids, or recent treatment with a purine analog. As with allogeneic recipients, the duration of PCP prophylaxis in an autologous HSCT recipient should consider patient-specific factors, but prophylaxis is typically continued for at least 3 to 6 months after transplantation.

Trimethoprim-sulfamethoxazole (TMP-SMX) is the preferred regimen because it appears to be the most efficacious and has activity against other pathogens such as *T. gondii*. Breakthrough PCP infections occur more frequently with other agents.[1,38] Because of the concern of myelosuppression and the low risk of PCP during the first month after transplant, TMP-SMX is generally started after engraftment, although some institutions initiate earlier or do not discontinue prophylaxis if the patient was previously receiving it.

Tuberculosis

HSCT candidates should be evaluated for active or latent TB, including attainment of a complete history to document TB risk factors, TB exposures, and possible prior diagnosis of latent TB infection or active disease. Patient with a history consistent with TB exposure or symptoms may require further diagnostic evaluation. There is no current consensus about whether the tuberculin skin test or an interferon-gamma release assay (IGRA) should be the primary diagnostic tool in this setting.[1] Some institutions have increasingly used IGRAs in this clinical setting as the IGRA provides a control, which will inform whether a negative TB screen is the result of truly absent prior TB exposure or is a function of the patient's poor immune function.

Active Infection. Patients with active TB diagnosed before transplant should be treated with the goal of controlling the infection before transplantation.

Preventing Infection. Although specific effectiveness data on secondary prophylaxis in HSCT recipients are limited, it is often recommended for individuals during periods of increased risk for TB reactivation.[1,39] This would include HSCT candidates with positive tuberculin skin test (TST) results (regardless of prior bacillus Calmette-Guérin vaccination status) or IGRA results, patients with untreated latent TB infection, and those exposed to individuals with active pulmonary or laryngeal TB. Isoniazid prophylaxis is generally initiated after completion of the conditioning regimen owing to drug interactions, but if there are no significant interactions with isoniazid and the patient is at particularly high risk of developing TB disease, it can be initiated before conditioning[1]. Drug interactions, especially with the mold-active azoles, can lead to significant toxicity and concomitant administration should be avoided.

Cells from a donor with latent TB have not been shown to be a source of risk for the recipient; therefore screening donors for latent TB is not mandatory.[1] Potential donors with signs or symptoms of active TB should be evaluated for TB, and donation should be deferred until the TB is well controlled.

Toxoplasma Gondii

Toxoplasmosis is an uncommon but potentially fatal opportunistic parasitic infection in HSCT recipients. Most cases of toxoplasmosis are due to reactivation in allogeneic HSCT recipients.[1,40] Rare cases of donor-derived infections have been reported.[41]

Active Infection. Recipients with positive *Toxoplasma* serology results (IgG) should be tested for active infection (IgM serology and PCR). In addition, such patients should undergo evaluations for end organ disease, including an ophthalmology consult and cerebrospinal fluid testing if neurologic symptoms are present. If active *Toxoplasmosis* infection is diagnosed, transplantation should be deferred until the infection is well controlled.

Preventing Infection. Prophylaxis with TMP-SMX, which is frequently used for PCP prophylaxis, is also effective for preventing toxoplasmosis and should be preferred over other PCP prophylaxis agents (such as pentamidine) in recipients with positive *T. gondii* serology results. For patients who cannot take TMP-SMX, alternative regimens include pyrimethamine plus leucovorin, pyrimethamine plus sulfadiazine, pyrimethamine and sulfadoxine plus leucovorin, and atovaquone with or without pyrimethamine.[1] As these second-line prophylaxis approaches can be challenging, an alternative approach is to screen high-risk *Toxoplasma*-seropositive patients with quantitative PCR after transplant and start preemptive therapy only in those with a positive PCR assay.[1,42] The management of *Toxoplasmosis* in transplant patients is reviewed in Chapter 29.

Strongyloides Stercolaris

The most feared presentation of strongyloidiasis in the immunocompromised host is hyperinfection syndrome, which can manifest as disseminated disease with septic shock.[43,44] The clinical findings may be attributable to direct organ invasion by the filariform larvae or to secondary gram-negative bacteremia, pneumonia, or meningitis owing to hematogenous seeding from a primary gastrointestinal tract or lung source. Mortality rates up to 80% have been reported for hyperinfection syndrome.[43,44]

Transplant candidates with a potential exposure history, such as travel to or residence in endemic areas, should be tested before conditioning. Those with positive pretransplant screening test results for *S. stercolaris* or those with unexplained eosinophilia should receive empiric treatment before HSCT with ivermectin for 2 consecutive days with repeat treatment after 2 weeks.[1] Management of strongyloidasis is discussed in detail in Chapter 32.

7

Prevention of Infections in the Solid Organ Transplantation Recipient

Michele Estabrook, MD and Monica I. Ardura, DO, MSCS

Solid organ transplantation (SOT) has transformed the prognosis of many children with organ failure. An estimated 135,860 SOTs were performed worldwide in 2016. A total of 33,610 SOTs were performed in the United States, with children, the majority of whom were younger than 10 years, receiving 1878 of these transplants.[1,2] Despite advances in the field of transplantation, infections remain an important cause of morbidity and mortality in pediatric SOT recipients. Refinements in immunosuppressive regimens have led to the reduction of graft rejection episodes and prolonged graft and patient survival. However, the evolving armamentarium of immunosuppressive agents with differing mechanisms of actions on distinct components of the immune system has also contributed to the risk for and modified the clinical manifestations of transplant-related infections.[3] Indeed, the clinical diagnosis of infection in an SOT recipient may be complicated by lack of signs of inflammation, and conversely, transplant-associated entities, such as graft rejection, may mimic infection. As the number of pediatric SOTs increases,[4] it is important for pediatric providers to have knowledge of the risk factors for infection after SOT and use optimal prevention strategies.

The risk for infection is determined by the interplay of multiple factors before and after SOT, including the epidemiologic exposures and underlying conditions of both the recipient and donor, the type of transplanted graft and its associated immunosuppressive regimen, and the recipient's overall "net state of immunosuppression," which is defined by transplant, host, and pathogen-specific factors.[5] Young age at the time of SOT is an important variable that influences infection risk and type; it follows that younger patients are less likely to have encountered certain pathogens and thus lack immunity, but they are at high risk of developing infection from the donor or acquiring primary infection after SOT while receiving immunosuppression. Furthermore, the extent to which immunosuppressive regimens affect the developing immune system in children who require SOT in infancy has not been fully elucidated. The risk of infection and type of pathogen is also dependent on time elapsed since SOT; the greater the immune dysfunction, the greater the predisposition to infection and to severe disease.[5] In this chapter we review the multiple preventative strategies that may be used to help mitigate the risk of infection after SOT.

PRETRANSPLANT EVALUATION

The pretransplant evaluation of the candidate is essential in informing strategies to prevent infections after SOT (see Chapter 4). It screens transplant candidates for infections that may preclude transplant, identifies active infections that require treatment before proceeding with SOT, and determines the risk of latent infections that may require antimicrobial therapy or will dictate posttransplant monitoring. The pretransplant evaluation allows for the identification of unique exposures or risk factors for pathogens that cause opportunistic infections but are not routinely tested for, including certain parasites, arboviruses, and endemic fungi. This period is also the optimal time to provide vaccination to SOT candidates to increase their likelihood of adequate immunogenicity before receiving immunosuppressive agents, as well as vaccinating the child's household contacts (see Chapter 9). Lastly, patients and families should be counseled regarding strategies for safe living that can limit or at least reduce the risk of epidemiologic exposures to potential infections (see Chapter 13).

The pretransplant evaluation of the donor (see Chapter 5) identifies both latent and active infections that pose a risk of transmission to the organ recipient and guides monitoring and preventive strategies for the recipient after transplant. Unexpected transmission of infections from donors to pediatric recipients is infrequent and is associated with an attributable mortality rate of less than 1%.[6] Determination of risk factors for the designation of increased risk donor for human immunodeficiency virus, hepatitis B, and hepatitis C is important for informed decisions regarding use of those donor organs and posttransplant monitoring of the recipient.[7,8]

VACCINATION

Pediatric patients remain at risk for vaccine-preventable infections before and after SOT.[9,10] Current guidelines provide a context for vaccination that emphasizes the importance of optimizing vaccination before SOT and completing or reimmunizing after SOT in the setting of ongoing immunosuppression.[11,12] This may include an accelerated immunization schedule before transplant, according to the Centers for Disease Control guidelines. The safety and immunogenicity of live virus vaccination in select SOT recipients is an area of ongoing study.[13] Immunizations before and after SOT are covered in detail in Chapter 9.

PERIOPERATIVE ANTIMICROBIAL PROPHYLAXIS

In the first 30 days after SOT, infections related to the duration and complexity of the surgery and possible complications, the presence of devices, and the disruption of mucocutaneous barrier integrity are most frequent. In pediatric recipients, receipt of organs from adult donors causes a size discrepancy that may lead to an increased infectious risk from anastomotic complications or need for delayed abdominal or thoracic closure.[14,15] Implementation of infection control practices, including bundles to prevent surgical site infections, central line–associated bloodstream infections, urinary tract infections, and other health care–associated infections minimize potential risks.

Perioperative antibiotic prophylaxis is guided by the organ being transplanted and is considered the standard of care to prevent postoperative surgical site infections, which occur in 3% to 53% of SOT recipients.[16,17] Prophylaxis strategies need to take into account the incidence and local institutional epidemiology and susceptibility profiles of certain pathogens to inform patient management. General prophylaxis principles of using the narrowest, most efficacious agent for the shortest duration (24 to 48 hours) and optimizing pharmacokinetics/pharmacodynamics perioperatively should be used; however, there is a paucity of controlled evidence to guide optimal choice of antimicrobial and duration of prophylaxis. Additionally, much of the evidence is derived from adult studies and guidelines, which are limited with regard to pediatric-specific recommendations. The epidemiology and certain risk factors identified in adults may indeed be distinct in children given the differences in underlying conditions that caused organ dysfunction. Thus additional pediatric studies with robust methodologies and sufficient sample size are needed to confirm or revoke whether adult data should continue to be extrapolated to the management of pediatric SOT recipients. Lastly, certain scenarios may warrant modification of perioperative antimicrobial regimens. For example, in transplant candidates with a ventricular assist device or those with active bacteremia or candidemia who are receiving extracorporeal membrane oxygenation, the perioperative antimicrobial regimen should include coverage for the pathogen. Adjustments based on the pretransplant colonization status of the recipient may also be warranted when there is concern that bacteria or fungi may seed vascular suture lines, lead to loss of integrity at the graft anastomosis site, and cause direct damage to the allograft.[17] For example, in pediatric lung transplantation when a frequent indication for transplantation may be cystic fibrosis, pretransplant colonization in the recipient should be considered when choosing the perioperative antimicrobial prophylaxis, although optimal type and duration of prophylaxis is unknown. Finally, infections identified in the donor should also be considered when choosing appropriate perioperative antimicrobial agents.

When broadening the antimicrobial spectrum or prolonging duration of prophylaxis, consideration is needed regarding possible adverse effects, including the risk of contributing to the development of multidrug-resistant organisms (MDROs). The increasing burden of MDROs causing colonization and infection in the donor graft or recipient is an emerging challenge in SOT, and additional pediatric-specific data are needed to establish optimal management schemes (see Chapter 14). A robust institutional antibiotic stewardship program is vital in MDRO prevention (see Chapter 11). Whether the performance of active culture surveillance around the time of SOT on donors or candidate should be performed to inform prophylaxis is unclear; however, results of testing in adult SOT recipients have served to intensify infection control practices and decrease transmission risk.[18,19] Indeed, infection prevention practices are critical in preventing health care–associated infections in this vulnerable population (see Chapter 12).

POSTTRANSPLANT PROPHYLAXIS AND MONITORING

Ongoing antibiotic prophylaxis may be warranted after SOT in certain recipients. For example, in renal transplant recipients trimethoprim-sulfamethoxazole may be used for urinary tract infection prophylaxis. Results of pretransplant serologic testing in both the donor and recipient for herpesviruses that establish latency, including cytomegalovirus, Epstein-Barr virus, and Herpes Simplex Virus, are important determinants of individual risk for infection after SOT and help guide posttransplant interventions.[20] The interpretation of serologic testing in infant SOT candidates younger than 12 months is challenging. A false-positive result may reflect passive transfer of maternal antibodies or receipt of immunoglobulin or blood products. Thus, young infants should be stratified to the highest risk category. Young children are more likely to be naïve for these herpesviruses and so, upon receipt of a graft from a seropositive donor, are more likely to develop a primary infection with the associated complications. Viral prophylaxis strategies, preemptive treatment, and monitoring parameters are discussed and vary by institution depending on the organ transplanted, virus, and serological status of the donor and recipient.[20-25] Virus-specific immunologic monitoring assays hold promise in quantitatively and functionally interrogating the adaptive immune system and informing prophylaxis management in adults; however, additional pediatric data are needed to determine their utility in clinical practice.[26-29] Molecular-based screening of potential increased risk donors for human immunodeficiency virus, hepatitis B, and hepatitis C has the potential to reduce, but does not completely eliminate, the risk of donor-derived transmission of these infections.[30]

The prevention of other infections, including *Toxoplasma*, *Pneumocystis jirovecii*, mycobacterial, and fungal infections, are discussed in detail in the relevant chapters. The type of prophylaxis, duration, and monitoring are determined by type of organ transplanted, pretransplant donor and recipient screening, and relevant geographic exposure. It is important to note that the contemporary epidemiology of infections—for example. *P. jirovecii* pneumonia and cytomegalovirus—highlight the fact that prophylaxis strategies may modify the epidemiology and delay timing of infections after SOT, but they may not completely eliminate the risk of infection.[20,31] Lastly, prophylaxis strategies may need to be revised or reimplemented in the post-SOT period in response to therapies directed at graft rejection.

Adjunctive therapies may be used in an effort to reduce infection risk after SOT. Hypogammaglobulinemia after SOT has been associated with an increased risk of infections, particularly when total immunoglobulin G concentrations are less than 400 mg/dL.[32] However, whether immunoglobulin replacement mitigates this risk and leads to improved patient outcomes is less clear.[33-35] Pediatric SOT recipients are at risk for community-acquired respiratory viruses with associated complications, particularly with exposure to other young children, day care, and school.[36] With the exception of administering an annual inactivated influenza vaccine and using respiratory syncytial virus–specific humanized monoclonal antibody palivizumab for prophylaxis in select children younger than 24 months who will be profoundly immunocompromised during the respiratory syncytial virus season, prevention consists of good hand hygiene and awareness of safe living after transplant (see Chapter 13).

SUMMARY

The risk of infection peri- and post-SOT is a dynamic continuum that is dependent on multiple factors related to the child and donor, transplantation, immunosuppressive regimens, and epidemiologic exposures. Knowledge of these factors allows for the application of multiple preventative strategies, including antimicrobial prophylaxis, surveillance schemes, infection control, stewardship, and vaccination efforts that allow for mitigation, but not complete elimination of the infectious risk. Additional pediatric data are needed to optimize these preventative strategies in children after SOT.

8

Management Principles for Patients With Neutropenia

Brian T. Fisher, DO, MPH, MSCE and Lillian Sung, MD, PhD

Chemotherapy agents have been the cornerstone of cancer treatments since the 1960s when the first concerted attempts were made to treat cancer. Although these agents are effective at destroying cancer cells, they often indiscriminately destroy other healthy cells, such as epithelial cells and leukocytes, with rapid turnover. Not long after chemotherapy agents were initially used in cancer treatment, clinicians and researchers recognized the negative consequences of chemotherapy agents on white blood cell counts and the inverse association of the amount of circulating white blood cell counts with infection risk.[1] In particular, a decreasing granulocyte (neutrophil) count was linked to infection risk. These initial reports identified an increased risk for infection when the neutrophil count dropped below 500/mm^3 and associated the duration of the low neutrophil count, referred to as neutropenia, with the degree of infection risk. As infection onset during periods of neutropenia was often associated with a new-onset fever, the condition became known as fever and neutropenia (FN). Despites decades of advancement, FN continues to be one of the most common and important complications of cancer therapy in children. Not only does FN result in significant morbidity and mortality, it translates into increases in resource utilization and reduction in quality of life (QOL). Fortunately, in the past 2 decades there has been an increased focus on conducting research that has informed guidelines for optimal supportive care approaches with the goal of reducing the consequences of FN in children with cancer.[2]

EPIDEMIOLOGY

The initial studies linking a drop in neutrophil count with subsequent infection established 500 neutrophils/mm^3 as the threshold below which neutropenia was declared. In the contemporary literature, this threshold is often set at 200 neutrophils/mm^3. This definition of neutropenia should be used as a guide and not as an absolute. Additionally, the direction of the neutrophil count from one day to the next is also important when assessing infection risk. For example, a neutrophil count that is 200 neutrophils/mm^3 but decreasing from preceding days is likely more concerning than a count of 150 neutrophils/mm^3 that has increased steadily over successive days.

Generally, most chemotherapy regimens and hematopoietic stem cell transplant (HSCT) conditioning regimens cause myelosuppression that results in some degree of neutropenia, but a variety of factors are necessary to consider when interpreting the potential for infection during a specific neutropenic period. This includes malignancy type and location, patient age, chemotherapy regimen being administered, the presence of central line access, and the ability to administer granulocyte colony-stimulating factor (G-CSF) after chemotherapy. For example, children receiving induction chemotherapy for leukemia are at significant risk for infection. Part of the reason for this risk is the prolonged neutropenia that presents after some intensive and myelosuppressive induction chemotherapy regimens. The ensuing neutropenic period in the leukemia population is often not when G-CSF is used because of the concern for stimulating production of leukemia cells. Children with solid tumors, including brain tumors, can receive similarly myelosuppressive chemotherapies; however, their duration of neutropenia is often shortened by administration of G-CSF. Understanding nuances such as these can assist the clinician in determining in a more customized fashion the true risk of infection during a neutropenia period after chemotherapy for a specific patient.

Owing to the aforementioned variation in risk, the incidence of fever during neutropenia can range from 10% to 60%, with even higher rates among the highest-risk groups such as children with acute myeloid leukemia or relapsed acute lymphoblastic leukemia.[3,4] Of note, pediatric-specific evidence for antibacterial and antifungal prophylaxis is evolving. As such, prophylaxis use increases the incidence of FN and the epidemiology of causative agents is likely to change. Although prophylaxis may decrease rates of documented infection, the risk for resistant pathogens during breakthrough FN episodes is likely to increase.[5]

The distribution of pathogens identified during episodes of fever and neutropenia is wide, and despite significant diagnostic evaluations at presentation, many episodes are not linked to a specific pathogen. This presentation of FN is often referred to as fever of unknown origin. In the late 1970s, a descriptive study of a large cohort of pediatric and young adult patients with FN found that approximately 50% of patients had a microbiologically or clinically documented infection within 7 days from presentation.[6] Despite advancement in modern microbiologic techniques and technology, the rates of fever of unknown origin in pediatric FN events remain above 50%.[3]

Bacterial Pathogens

When an infectious pathogen is identified as the source of FN, bacteria are the most common causes. Although bacteria as a group have remained as the most common identified etiology of pediatric FN, the epidemiology of causative pathogens has evolved.[3,7,8] The first reports on the epidemiology of bacterial infections during neutropenia most commonly implicated gram-negative pathogens, specifically *Escherichia coli*, *Pseudomonas aeruginosa*, and *Klebsiella* species.[9] The transition from a gram-negative to a gram-positive bacterial predominance occurred in the latter 2 decades of the last century.[7] This shift in pathogen type is likely multifactorial, but is often assumed to be related to increased reliance on central venous catheters and chemotherapy regimens that cause mucositis, resulting in an increase in pathogens such as viridans group streptococci. It is anticipated that gram-positive organisms will continue to predominate into the future as more centers will likely use prophylactic antibiotic regimens that have broader gram-negative activity in high-risk patient groups.

TABLE 8.1 **Distribution of Bacterial Pathogens in Selected Pediatric Fever and Neutropenia Cohorts**

	AUTHOR YEAR				
Characteristic	**Pizzo et al.[6] 1982**	**Ariffin et al.[8] 2002**	**Castagnola et al.[3] 2007**	**Hakim et al.[10] 2009**	**Alexander et al.[5] 2018**
Study location	United States	Malaysia	Italy	United States	United States and Canada
Patient type	Leukemia, lymphoma, solid tumor	Any malignancy	Leukemia, solid tumor, or allogeneic HSCT	Any malignancy	Leukemia and HSCT (Control arm only)
Clinical scenario	Fever and neutropenia	fever and neutropenia	Fever and neutropenia	Fever and neutropenia	Neutropenia periods
Episodes observed (Total no. of patients)	1001 (324)	762 (513)	614 (NA)	337 (337)	399 (307)[a]
Episodes with bacteria isolated n (%)	188[b] (18.8%)	270 (35.4%)	97 (15.8%)	54 (16%)	86 (22%)
Gram-positive pathogens n (%)	106 (49%)	103 (38.1%)	57(58.8%)	31[c] (57%)	53 (61.6%)
Gram- negative pathogens n (%)	74 (39%)	167 (61.9%)	40 (41.2%)	23 (43%)	33 (38.4%)

[a]Limited to bacteremia events.
[b] Includes 8 events of anaerobic infections not included in either gram-positive or gram-negative rows.
[c]Includes 7 episodes of *Clostridium difficile* infection.
HSCT, hematopoietic stem cell transplantation.
Data from Fisher BT, Sung L. The febrile neutropenic patient. In: Cherry J, Harrison G, Kaplan S, Steinbach W, Hotez P, eds. *Feigin and Cherry's Textbook of Pediatric Infectious Diseases.* 8th ed. Philadelphia, PA: Elsevier Saunders; 2019:657-664.

Despite the general predominance of gram-positive bacteria, significant variation in the epidemiology of bacteria during FN exists between centers. Table 8.1 displays identified bacterial pathogens across various international pediatric oncology studies between 1982 and 2018.[3,5,6,8,10] The variation by geographic location likely results from practice variation, such as approach to chemotherapy protocols, diagnostic testing practices, and prophylaxis regimens. Most recently, a pediatric randomized controlled trial of levofloxacin during periods of prolonged neutropenia in children with acute leukemia and those undergoing HCT was completed. Although levofloxacin was found to be effective, the rate of breakthrough infection was still 22% in the leukemia group and 11% in the HSCT group. Gram-positive organisms, most frequently viridans group streptococci, accounted for more than 77% of the breakthrough events.[5]

Fungal Pathogens

Invasive fungal diseases (IFDs) are rarely the source of the initial onset of fever during a neutropenic period. More typically, the concern for IFDs increases after a prolonged period of FN despite broad-spectrum antibacterial therapy. There are published consensus criteria for defining proven and probable IFDs that have been helpful to standardize the definition of IFDs across research studies and to provide some diagnostic criteria for clinicians.[11] However, diagnosing IFDs by these published criteria can be difficult because invasive procedures are often needed to identify a fungal pathogen and patients with prolonged neutropenia cannot always tolerate such procedures. Therefore many published reports of IFD incidence as a source of FN may underestimate actual infection rates. Understanding these limitations, prospective multicenter data have documented a proven or probable IFD rate ranging from 3% to 5% of children hospitalized with fever and neutropenia.[12] The rates of IFDs when considering prolonged neutropenia regardless of fever have been reported to be much higher.[13] This highlights the fact that fever is not always present as a sign of IFD.

Candida species are the most common fungal pathogens identified during periods of FN. This is likely because *Candida* species commonly colonize the skin and intestinal tract and may become more dominant in the setting of prolonged exposure to broad-spectrum antibiotics. The skin and mucosal barriers are often compromised by the presence of central venous catheters and/or chemotherapy exposures that can allow for invasive of *Candida* isolates. Specific mortality data regarding invasive candidiasis in pediatric oncology patients and HSCT recipients are limited, but the attributable mortality of invasive candidiasis in all pediatric patients has been estimated to be 10%.[14]

Episodes of invasive mold disease are less common but are much more challenging to treat and have significantly higher rates of case fatality. In contemporary pediatric cases series, less than two-thirds of patients with an invasive mold disease IMD responded to therapy in the first 12 weeks and 30% of patients died within the same time period.[15,16] Among the mold pathogens, *Aspergillus* species are most common, followed by organisms of the Mucorales order.[15-17]

Viral Pathogens

The advancement in viral diagnostic methodologies has resulted in better estimates of viral infections during periods of FN. Much of the interest in testing for a viral pathogen is the possibility that finding an explanation for fever may reduce the need for further diagnostic testing. The yield of viral testing in patients with FN has been reported in multiple studies (Table 8.2).[18-22] The frequency of laboratory-confirmed viral respiratory infection ranged from 8% to 59%. Of note, the study reporting an 8% incidence of viral respiratory infection obtained viral respiratory specimens via mouth swabs and thus likely underestimated the true rate.[22] The range of infection rates for the remaining studies was 37% to 59%.

Although some authors have suggested these rates of viral detection support routine comprehensive viral testing at the time of presentation for FN,[19,22] the utility of routine viral testing is not clear. First, ideally

TABLE 8.2 **Frequency of Viral Respiratory Pathogens at Presentation for Fever and Neutropenia**

	AUTHOR YEAR			
Characteristic	**Long et al.[18] 1987**	**Arola et al.[20] 1995**	**Koskenvuo et al.[21] 2008**	**Torres et al.[19] 2012**
Study duration	5 years	17 months	5.5 years	21 months
Patient type	Leukemia, solid tumors	Any malignancy	Leukemia	Any malignancy
Clinical scenario	Suspicion of virus	Fever	Fever	Fever and neutropenia
Total patients (Episodes)	200 (not reported)	32 (75)	51 (138)	193 (331)
Testing methods	Culture, immunofluoresence	Culture, antigen, and antibodies	Culture, antigen, and PCR	PCR
Respiratory virus isolation rate	148 (N/A)	28 (37%)	61 (59%)	190 (57%)
Sterile site bacterial pathogen plus virus isolation	Not reported	None	13%	33%

N/A, not available; *PCR*, polymerase chain reaction.
Data from Fisher BT, Sung L. The febrile neutropenic patient. In: Cherry J, Harrison G, Kaplan S, Steinbach W, Hotez P, eds. *Feigin and Cherry's Textbook of Pediatric Infectious Diseases.* 8th ed. Philadelphia, PA: Elsevier Saunders; 2019:657-664.

the identification of a viral pathogen should inform clinical management decisions. However, identification of a virus does not necessarily exclude the possibility of a concomitant bacterial infection. The percentage of patients with both a viral and bacterial infection ranged from 13% to 33%.[19,21] Some clinicians are comfortable stopping antibiotics during the FN episode in the setting of a viral syndrome but only for low-risk patients with FN. Based on the possibility of both bacterial and viral infection, empiric antibiotics are often continued in high-risk FN episodes. Second, the sensitivity of viral polymerase chain reaction testing results in detection of virus well after clinical resolution, and thus viral detection by polymerase chain reaction may not always confirm the source of fever in a neutropenic patient. Finally, there are limited effective antiviral therapeutic agents available, and thus detection of some viruses will not inform targeted antiviral therapy. Considering these reasons collectively, viral testing should be limited to patients in whom positive results would allow for de-escalation of antibiotic therapy (e.g., in a low-risk FN episode) or initiation of an appropriate antiviral therapy (e.g., neuraminidase inhibitor for influenza). Of note, the hospital's infection prevention and control division may desire testing for symptomatic patients to inform appropriate isolation precautions that could limit hospital transmission of viral pathogens.

EVALUATION

Initial Risk Stratification

Early comparative studies highlighted the effectiveness of early initiation and continuation of empirical antibiotic and subsequently empirical antifungal therapy to reduce the morbidity and mortality associated with FN.[23,24] These studies served as the foundation for standards of care for FN management that have been applied for decades across all episodes of FN. However, use of empirical broad-spectrum antibiotics and antifungal agents for prolonged periods in all patients is not ideal as it presents risks for medication toxicities, prolongs hospital stays, and potentiates evolution of resistance. As not all FN episodes carry the same risk for infection, it is important to stratify each FN episode into risk groups for true infection. Such risk stratification can inform evidence-based decisions for more discriminant use of anti-infective agents and other health care resources.

Identifying which children are at a lower risk of complications can allow for a reduction in the intensity of anti-infective therapy and monitoring. Conversely, identifying children at higher risk of complications can allow for prophylactic approaches, rapid escalation of therapy, or closer observation. Fortunately, there have been substantial research efforts to identify criteria for stratifying FN episodes into low and high risk. Often, these studies leverage a composite of factors to derive risk prediction models or rules. More than 25 such risk prediction studies have been conducted in pediatric cancer.[3,5] These studies have been heterogeneous and have included different pediatric cancer populations and different clinical endpoints (such as bacteremia, serious infection, death, and intensive care unit admission), thereby reducing the ability to combine the individual study data into a composite analysis. However, review of the individual studies can be informative.

There have been six prediction models derived from pediatric cohorts that (1) focused on identifying patients at low risk for infection using data elements evident on a single FN assessment and (2) have been validated.[25] Selection of a single schema that can be applied across all clinical scenarios has not been possible, potentially because of heterogeneity in clinical settings and resources. Therefore clinicians should review each of the validated low-risk stratification schemas, choose which schema matches their clinical setting, and determine if the application of that schema is feasible for their center. The choice of strategy should be determined by an institution's ability to implement more complex rules and the timeliness of receipt of required components of the rule, such as C-reactive protein. Whichever schema is chosen, centers should establish a quality improvement infrastructure to routinely monitor their process for identification of low-risk FN episodes and outcomes of these episodes to ensure the chosen prediction model is safe and continues to have local applicability. Of note, these prediction models were derived in cohorts of children with cancer and chemotherapy-induced FN and thus their applicability to FN episodes in the post-HSCT period is not known.

Initial Investigations

Regardless of risk stratification, when a child with FN initially presents to the health care center, timely triage and assessment are important. An evaluation for the cause of fever should be conducted and should include a careful history and physical examination. It is important to establish an updated interim social history that includes, but is not limited to, recent exposure to other symptomatic people, recent travel, new animal exposures, visitors from other regions, changes in diet, adherence to preventative measures, and any sustained local trauma (e.g., fall with skin abrasion). The physical examination should be equally thorough and warrants particular attention to the mouth to evaluate for mucositis and oral infections, central venous catheter tunnel and exit sites, and the entire skin surface, including the perianal area.

The standard evaluation should include blood cultures from each lumen of the central venous catheter if present. The utility of adding a peripheral blood culture at the initial evaluation of FN continues to be controversial.[26] The value of peripheral blood cultures has been addressed in nine studies,[26,27] The estimate of the proportion of true bacteremia episodes detected by peripheral blood cultures alone, when central venous catheter culture results are negative, was 12% (95% confidence interval 8% to 17%), revealing that peripheral cultures consistently increase identification of true bacteremia compared with central cultures alone. Increased yield is likely related to timing or volume. However, contaminant identification from a peripheral culture is similar with an estimated rate at 13% (95% confidence interval 8% to 20%). Based on these data, the potential benefits of a peripheral culture include increasing the detection of bacteremia and providing data for a more accurate designation of central line–associated bloodstream infection. Conversely, the downsides of a peripheral blood culture include patient discomfort and anxiety and the potential to identify contaminants, leading to unnecessary antibiotic therapy. There are no data to inform whether peripheral blood culture results alter the outcomes of FN episodes. Centers need to consider the potential advantages and disadvantages of a peripheral blood culture and establish their own standard of care so that a consistent strategy can be implemented.

The importance of obtaining a urinalysis and/or a urine culture at the presentation of FN to evaluate for a urinary tract infections (UTIs) is also controversial. Typically, a UTI is suspected on the basis of pyuria or nitrites present on urinalysis. However, in this population, the presence of neutropenia negates a patient's ability to mobilize neutrophils to the urinary tract and thus pyuria is not an expected sign to measure by diagnostic testing.[28] Therefore the usefulness of a urinalysis would be reliant on nitrite testing, which is not ideal as nitrites are present only with pathogens capable of converting nitrates to nitrites and may be absent in younger children with UTIs.[29] This makes the urinalysis a limited diagnostic tool in the setting of FN. A urine culture can be helpful to identify a causative pathogen for the FN episode and this identification may help direct antibiotic therapy. However, attaining a urine culture can be difficult, especially in younger children. Therefore many experts recommend that if a clean-catch or mid-stream urine sample can be easily and reliably obtained, then urinalysis and urine culture should be obtained at the onset of FN. Otherwise, these diagnostic tests should be omitted from the initial evaluation of FN, assuming the patient does not have in a previous history of UTIs or suspicious signs or symptoms. Antibiotic administration should not be delayed to obtain a urine sample.

Finally, the role of routine chest radiographs as a routine component, even in the absence of respiratory symptoms, of the diagnostic workup in pediatric FN has been assessed in six observational studies.[2] The two most recent of these studies included children with FN after chemotherapy and HSCT and found rates of pneumonia that were less than 3% in children without respiratory symptoms. Furthermore, the incidental findings on chest radiographs in the few patients with pneumonia did not alter clinical care. Therefore routine chest radiographs should not be performed in children with FN who do not have localizing respiratory symptoms. A chest radiography should be performed in children who have concomitant respiratory symptoms at FN presentation.

MANAGEMENT OF BACTERIAL INFECTIONS

Initial Antibiotic Therapy

As noted previously, the early epidemiology and comparative studies of FN identified significant risk for infection during this period and benefit from initiation of empiric combination broad-spectrum and intravenous antibiotic treatment. However, the recommended approach to FN has evolved through significant investigation over the past 4 decades and the prior "one-size-fits-all" approach for antibiotic administration in the setting of FN has proven to be unnecessary. This evolution in practice was first apparent in adults with FN and more recently has been changing among children with FN. In general, management decisions for FN are now dependent on risk stratification. Additional factors beyond risk stratification that can affect management decisions include prior infection history, clinically evident sites of infection, patient and institution bacterial resistance patterns, drug availability, and acuity of illness.

Consideration for Patients With High-Risk Fever and Neutropenia

For patients with high-risk FN, broad-spectrum intravenous antibiotic therapy is still recommended to provide good coverage for gram-negative organisms given their virulent nature. Additionally, empiric antibiotics for high-risk FN should include coverage for viridans group streptococci and *P. aeruginosa* as these are somewhat common causes of bacteremia and pose risk for severe infection. The original empiric antibiotic regimens for FN consisted of parental administration of two agents with antipseudomonal coverage. However, the role of combination antibiotic therapy versus monotherapy for FN has been assessed in multiple studies. In two separate meta-analyses, monotherapy was compared to a combination dual aminoglycoside-containing regimen in patients with FN.[30,31] Both analyses demonstrated that monotherapy was not inferior and was less toxic than combination therapy. In the pediatric setting, a systematic review of randomized trials concluded that no significant differences in failure rates, infection-related mortality, or overall mortality were observed with monotherapy compared to combination therapy, even among studies restricted to high-risk FN.[32] A more specific pediatric meta-analysis compared monotherapy antipseudomonal penicillin monotherapy and antipseudomonal penicillin plus an aminoglycoside and found that monotherapy was not inferior to combination therapy.[33] Collectively, these data debunk the prior belief that combination gram-negative antibiotic therapy is necessary for high-risk FN.

There are numerous possible monotherapy regimens that have been evaluated and thought to be reasonable options in children with FN, including antipseudomonal penicillins such as piperacillin-tazobactam, antipseudomonal cephalosporins such as cefepime, and carbapenems such as meropenem or imipenem. Ticarcillin–clavulanic acid was an additional available antipseudomonal penicillin but is no longer manufactured. In the systematic review of randomized trials,[32] five studies were identified that compared antipseudomonal penicillin monotherapy to fourth-generation cephalosporin monotherapy and found no difference in treatment failure, infection-related mortality, or duration of fever. Two pediatric-specific evaluations found that treatment failure, mortality, and adverse effects were similar when antipseudomonal penicillins were compared to antipseudomonal cephalosporins or carbapenems.[34,35] Interestingly, although treatment failure rates were similar across groups in this study, cefepime was associated with increased all-cause mortality when compared to other β-lactam antiiotics.[35] However, this finding was not replicated in other studies, and in one meta-analysis the point estimate for mortality actually favored the cephalosprin compared with antipseudomonal penicillin.[36] Consequently, cefepime remains a first-line therapeutic option for empiric therapy of FN. Ceftazidime monotherapy lacks adequate gram-positive coverage and thus should not be used if these organisms are of concern, such as in patients with high risk for viridans group streptococci.

Routine empiric glycopeptides (such as vancomycin) should not be used. A meta-analysis of 14 randomized trials demonstrated that addition of a glycopeptide to empiric therapy did not lead to more success (if addition of a glycopeptide in the study control arm was not considered failure) but was associated with more adverse effects.[33] Empiric glycopeptides should be reserved for patients in clinically unstable condition or those who have a signs or symptoms suggestive of a gram-positive infection, such as central venous line tunnel or exit site infection.

Considerations for Patients With Low-Risk Fever and Neutropenia

Each institution should develop a tailored strategy to limit therapy intensity in patients with low-risk FN that will help limit unnecessary antibiotic exposures that can result in toxicity, reduce resource utilization, improve convenience, and optimize QOL. Although there has been an effort to identify a group of patients with FN who do not require any empiric antibiotics, this approach has not had widespread adoption. Rather, the two strategies commonly considered are outpatient management and enteral antibiotic administration. These two strategies are often used together and in adults with low-risk FN, outpatient management with enteral antibiotics is recommended in specific scenarios.[37] Over the past several years, data have emerged suggesting that enteral and outpatient management of children with low-risk FN is also appropriate provided that suitable selection of patients and monitoring are achieved. A recent survey of pediatric hematology and oncology physicians showed that many North American clinicians have adopted outpatient management in some circumstances.[38]

The advantages of outpatient management compared with inpatient management include better QOL for children, as well as reductions in health care utilization,[39] health care–associated infection, and acquisition of resistant organisms.[39,40] Outpatient management can be initiated at the onset of FN or after a brief period of hospitalization (step-down management). In a systematic review of pediatric randomized trials,[32] four studies were identified in which patients were randomly assigned to inpatient versus outpatient management; no differences in outcomes were observed. The point estimates favored outpatient management in the mortality analysis, and no infection-related deaths were observed in the 124 randomly assigned low-risk children treated as outpatients. This finding was replicated in a meta-analysis of observational trials in which no infection-related deaths were observed among the 953 children treated as outpatients.[34] It is important to emphasize that outpatient management requires the establishment of infrastructure, training, and personnel to allow the safe implementation of ambulatory management of FN.

The second approach to reduced intensity of therapy for low-risk FN is the use of enteral antibiotic regimens. Enteral antibiotic administration is attractive because it facilitates outpatient management, is usually less expensive, and does not require intravenous access, and thus reduces the risk of central venous catheter–associated infections. Specific considerations unique to children include the requirement for suspension formulation in children who cannot take pills or tablets and refusal of oral administration of enteral formulations in some children, especially younger children. In a systematic review of pediatric randomized trials,[32] eight studies randomly assigned pediatric patients with FN to intravenous versus enteral therapy in the same setting (inpatient or outpatient). There was no significant difference in treatment failure, and no infection-related mortality was observed among the 470 patients randomly assigned to receive enteral empiric therapy. To augment these data, more information about the safety of oral administration was obtained from a meta-analysis of prospective pediatric trials in which enteral antibiotics were started within 24 hours of FN onset.[41] No infection-related deaths were observed among the 676 children given enteral antibiotics. Thus enteral antibiotic administration may be appropriate if the child can tolerate this route of administration reliably and does not have severe mucositis or diarrhea. Typical enteral antibiotic therapy options used in pediatric FN include fluoroquinolone monotherapy, fluoroquinolone and amoxicillin-clavulanate, and cefixime.[42] Even for children with low-risk FN managed as inpatients, enteral administration may be advantageous as it reduces nursing resources and may facilitate early discharge (step-down management).

Modification of Empiric Antibacterial Therapy

After initiating empiric antibiotics for FN, the empiric regimen should be modified to ensure appropriate coverage for any identified microorganisms or clinical focus of infection. If an organism is identified and is considered the source of the febrile episode, some experts have advocated that it is appropriate to narrow coverage to target that pathogen, whereas others support continuation of the empirical therapy regimen. Unfortunately, there are no published pediatric data to guide this decision and many centers often continue broader empirical therapy regardless of the sensitivity profile of the identified pathogen. In patients in whom empiric glycopeptides or dual gram-negative coverage was initiated at presentation, reassessment should be performed at 24 to 72 hours, and these additional antibiotics should be discontinued unless there is a specific microbiologic reason for their continuation. For children with persistent fever, vigilance for an undetected source of infection is important and continued evaluation may include repeat blood cultures from the central venous catheter, although the optimal frequency of cultures (for example, daily or every second day) is not known. Modification of antibiotic treatment for persistent fever alone, including the addition of empiric vancomycin, is not necessary in children whose conditions remain clinically stable.[43] Children whose conditions deteriorate warrant broadening of empiric antibacterial therapy as infection with a resistant organism is possible. Thus broadening should include coverage for resistant gram-positive, gram-negative, and anaerobic organisms.

Cessation of Empiric Antibacterial Therapy

Current pediatric FN guidelines recommend continuation of empiric antibiotic therapy until all of the following criteria are met: blood culture results are negative, the child is clinically well, fever has resolved, and there is evidence of bone marrow recovery.[2,25] A specific threshold defining neutrophil count recovery is not clear, although most clinicians consider a rising absolute neutrophil count sufficient. One randomized trial of pediatric low-risk patients found that cessation of antibiotics on day 3 irrespective of count recovery versus continuation of antibiotics was associated with similar outcomes.[44] However, *Enterobacter* spp. bacteremia occurred in one child in the early cessation group. Consequently, it may be reasonable to discontinue antibiotics on day 3 in low-risk children with FN who are afebrile with negative culture results if careful monitoring is in place.

In high-risk patients, the optimal duration of antibiotic therapy is unknown in the setting of persistent profound neutropenia without bone marrow recovery. The initial pediatric FN study of 33 high-risk pediatric patients suggested that cessation of empiric antibiotics on day 7 may be associated with bacteremia and poor infection outcomes compared with continuation for 14 days.[23] However, this study was conducted in the 1970s and it is not known whether these results are generalizable to the current era. A recent adult randomized trial of cancer patients and HSCT recipients with high-risk FN compared early cessation of empiric antibiotics with continuation of antibiotics until count recovery. Patients were enrolled only if they were afebrile for at least 72 hours and clinically well at the time of randomization. Patients with early cessation of antibiotics had an overall reduction in antibiotic exposures, similar rates of adverse events, and similar overall mortality. A similar study in children has not yet been performed but would prove informative as the continuation of antibiotics until neutrophil recovery in high-risk patients results in prolonged hospitals stays and increased resource use. Until such a study is completed, many experts recommend continuation of empiric antibiotics for at least 14 days for high-risk FN in the absence of evidence of neutrophil recovery. Whether this strategy is optimal in the setting of antibacterial prophylaxis (see "Prophylaxis Strategies" in later text) is not known.

INVASIVE FUNGAL DISEASE MANAGEMENT

Evaluation for Invasive Fungal Disease

Children at high-risk for IFD were identified in a systematic review of risk factors for IFD in pediatric oncology and HSCT patients.[13] Patients at high-risk for IFD are those with acute myeloid leukemia (AML), high-risk acute lymphoblastic leukemia, relapsed acute leukemia, and children undergoing allogeneic HSCT. All other patient groups should be categorized as IFD low-risk. However, IFD is still a possibility in low-risk groups of patients receiving chemotherapy (e.g., standard-risk acute lymphoblastic leukemia) or undergoing autologous HSCT, and thus clinical awareness of IFD is still important in these low-risk groups. The primary risk period in high-risk patients is during episodes of prolonged neutropenia. However, even in the absence of neutropenia, IFD is still a possibility in these patient groups, particularly in association with steroid exposure or during periods of graft-versus-host disease in HSCT recipients.

In terms of evaluation, a systematic review of fungal biomarkers in children receiving cancer treatments[45] concluded that galactomannan has little value as a surveillance diagnostic tool during prolonged FN as it has poor positive predictive value. However, it is important to note that these studies were not performed upon identification of a suspicious lung nodule and the value of galactomannan in children in this setting is unknown. Serum beta-D-glucan and fungal polymerase chain reaction assays should not be used as diagnostic tests during prolonged FN owing to poor diagnostic properties in children and lack of standardization in the case of polymerase chain reaction.

Recommendations for imaging for the evaluation of IFD during prolonged FN (≥96 hours) despite broad-spectrum antibiotics have been derived from a systematic review in pediatric patients.[2,32] It is recommended that lung computerized tomography be performed in children with prolonged FN who are considered at high-risk for IFD because the lungs are the most frequent site of infection and characteristic radiographic signs can be observed. Abdominal imaging, even in the absence of localizing signs or symptoms, may be useful as findings on imaging consistent with, IFD were observed in many patients. The ideal abdominal imaging modality is not known, but ultrasonography is readily available, is not associated with radiation exposure, and usually does not require sedation and, as such, is likely preferable over computerized tomography or magnetic resonance imaging for abdominal assessment. Sinus imaging results were frequently abnormal in prolonged FN but abnormalities did not appear to distinguish between those with and without sinus IFD. Thus routine sinus imaging for prolonged FN is likely not warranted in the absence of localizing signs or symptoms.

The optimal timing for imaging to evaluate for IFD is not known. Some centers perform imaging at the time the patient meets criteria for prolonged FN, whereas others wait until blood counts recover. The former approach allows for early detection of possible IFD, but many argue that unless a diagnostic procedure is going to be performed, detecting possible IFD at that time will not change management because empiric antifungal therapy will be started anyway. Those advocating for waiting until blood count recovery hypothesize that the presence of neutrophils allows for increased ability to detection IFD lesions if present. These two approaches have not been compared in a systematic way, and thus centers need to decide which approach is most acceptable for their institution.

Empiric Antifungal Therapy

Patients at high-risk for IFD should start empiric antifungal therapy in the event of persistent or recurrent fever lasting 96 hours or longer after initiation of broad-spectrum antibacterial agents during a neutropenic period. Empiric antifungal therapy should consist of either caspofungin or liposomal amphotericin B as these two therapies were similarly effective, and liposomal amphotericin B was slightly better and less nephrotoxic than amphotericin B deoxycholate.[2] Empiric antifungal therapy may be discontinued at resolution of neutropenia if the patient is clinically well without evidence of an IFD.

In terms of patients at low risk for IFD, one prospective study compared empiric antifungal therapy to withholding empiric antifungal therapy in neutropenic children with persistent fever in this population. No benefit with respect to fever resolution or IFD was detected with empiric antifungal therapy.[46] Thus in patients at low risk for IFD with prolonged FN, empiric antifungal therapy may be withheld.

Preemptive therapy is an area of great interest. A randomized trial of 149 children with persistent FN who were at high risk for IFD compared empiric versus preemptive antifungal treatment.[47] Preemptive therapy was associated with significantly shorter duration of antifungal treatment (6 vs. 11 days; $P < .001$) with similar rates of IFD, mortality, and IFD-related mortality, suggesting that preemptive therapy may be a reasonable approach in pediatric patients at high risk for IFD.

PROPHYLACTIC STRATEGIES

Antibacterial Prophylaxis

There has been considerable interest in antibacterial prophylaxis for periods of neutropenia, resulting in a many published trials. A 2005 large meta-analysis of predominantly adult randomized trials found that antibiotic prophylaxis significantly decreased the risk of death, infection-related mortality, and bacteremia.[42] Fluoroquinolones were the focus of many of the studies in this meta-analysis because of their broad-spectrum activity, preservation of gastrointestinal tract anaerobic flora, high fecal concentration, systemic bactericidal activity, tolerability, and favorable side effect profile. Despite the established benefits of prophylaxis, adult FN guidelines questioned their routine use because of uncertainty regarding the overall balance of benefits and harms.[37] The benefits of prophylaxis must be weighed against potential negative consequences, including *Clostridium difficile*–associated diarrhea, bacterial resistance, and adverse effects including musculoskeletal toxicities. The Children's Oncology group undertook a large randomized trial to determine whether prophylactic levofloxacin during neutropenia decreased the risk of bacteremia in children with acute leukemia or those undergoing HSCT.[5] A total of 624 patients, 200 with acute leukemia and 424 undergoing HSCT, were enrolled to this trial. Among the 195 patients with acute leukemia, the risk of bacteremia was significantly lower in the levofloxacin group compared with the control group (21.9% vs. 43.4%, $P = .001$). Among the 418 patients undergoing HSCT, the risk of bacteremia was not significantly lower in the levofloxacin group (11.0% vs. 17.3%, $P = .06$), although the clinical significance of this reduction in bacteremia can be argued. In terms of secondary endpoints, FN was less common in the levofloxacin group (71.2% vs. 82.1%, $P = .002$), thus demonstrating that levofloxacin was effective as prophylaxis in children with expected neutropenia. There were no significant differences in severe infection (3.6% vs. 5.9%, $P = .20$), *C. difficile*–associated diarrhea (2.3% vs. 5.2%, $P = .07$), or musculoskeletal toxicity at 2 months (11.4% vs. 16.3%, $P = .15$) or 12 months (10.1% vs. 14.4%, $P = 0.28$) between the levofloxacin and control groups. However, a *C. difficile* positive assay result was less frequent in the levofloxacin group (7.8% vs. 14.0%, $P = .02$). Total days and any exposure to antibiotics used to treat FN were fewer in the levofloxacin group ($P < .0001$ for both). Thus levofloxacin prophylaxis should be used for children with acute leukemia receiving intensive chemotherapy and should be considered for HSCT patients, particularly those undergoing allogeneic HSCT. Despite the lack of harm detected in the targeted outcomes from this large pediatric trial, the study does not address the long-term impact of resistance. It is likely that with continued use of levofloxacin in this setting at a given hospital, that the hospital antibiogram may reveal increasing levofloxacin resistance, resulting in increased rates of breakthrough infection. Centers that use levofloxacin prophylaxis should initiate a monitoring system to monitor rates of breakthrough bacteremia. If rates return to preprophylaxis rates, then the benefits of prophylaxis may no longer be present.

Antifungal Prophylaxis

Because IFDs are relatively difficult to diagnose and treat, there has been considerable interest in determining the efficacy of different prophylactic approaches in patients at high risk for IFDs. Fluconazole prophylaxis was compared with placebo in two randomized controlled trials of mostly adult allogeneic HSCT recipients.[48,49] Fluconazole decreased the occurrence of IFD owing to a reduction in invasive candidiasis. Because children undergoing allogeneic HSCT are at risk for molds in addition to yeasts and because fluconazole does not provide any coverage against molds, there has been great interest in exploring the role of prophylactic antimold coverage. However, thus far agents with antimold activity, including micafungin, voriconazole, and amphotericin B formulations, have not proven to have clinically significant advantages over fluconazole prophylaxis in the HSCT population. Furthermore, some agents such as itraconazole showed a higher rate of toxicity leading to withdrawal, and agents such as amphotericin B led to infusion-related toxicities and renal toxicity.

Posaconazole is an antifungal agent with broader antimold activity than voriconazole and thus represents a potentially better prophylactic option. In a randomized trial of adolescent and adult patients with AML or myelodysplastic syndrome and prolonged neutropenia, posaconazole prophylaxis, when compared with fluconazole or itraconazole, reduced the rate of proven or probable IFD. Furthermore, overall survival was significantly better in posaconazole-treated patients.[50] However, only 16 adolescents between the ages of 13 and 18 years were included, and thus the generalizability of the results to children is limited. Furthermore, administration of posaconazole to children younger than 13 years is challenging because of the lack of dosing information and the requirement to administer the drug orally with adequate food intake, which can be a challenge for children receiving intensive chemotherapy.

The Children's Oncology Group recently completed two antifungal prophylaxis randomized trials. One study compared fluconazole and caspofungin in children with AML; the second study compared either fluconazole or voriconazole to caspofungin in pediatric allogeneic HSCT recipients. Results of both studies are expected in the near future and may influence standard of care for antifungal prophylaxis. Until these study results are available, most experts support the use of fluconazole as a prophylaxis agent during neutropenia periods for children at high risk for IFD.

9

Vaccination Issues for Transplantation and Chemotherapy

Klara M. Posfay-Barbe, MD, MS and Natasha Halasa, MD, MPH

Vaccination has repeatedly been acknowledged as one of the most important tools for reduction of mortality worldwide and one of the most cost-effective ways to decrease health care–related costs. Immunocompromised children are at higher risk of complications caused by vaccine-preventable pathogens; however, it has been recurrently demonstrated that they are undervaccinated.[1,2] This can be linked to several factors, such as an overlooked priority in an already very sick child, uncertainty about the proper timing for vaccines, false impression about the effectiveness of immunization in immunocompromised hosts, young age at the beginning of hospital care, or the fear of side effects, especially for live-attenuated vaccines. Current guidelines provide a framework to approach vaccination before and after transplantation and during chemotherapy. However, evidence on vaccination in the immunocompromised hosts, especially in the pediatric population, is often lacking, and if available the quality of evidence is grades II or III.[3-5] When available, data are mainly from adult studies and are limited with regard to pediatric-specific recommendations. Additionally, there are few prospective randomized controlled trials to determine vaccine efficacy, optimal timing of vaccine administration, predictors of vaccine immunogenicity, or correlates of protection in these vulnerable pediatric populations.[6] Consequently, despite published recommendations, immunization of these at-risk hosts is variable and often suboptimal and needs to be improved.[3,7]

Routine childhood vaccines are provided mostly by the primary care physician; however, for transplant recipients and oncology patients, there can be variability in where these patients receive their vaccination (e.g., transplant centers physicians or with oncology centers). Therefore ensuring appropriate communication and documentation between both groups is paramount to optimiz vaccine administration and to avoid missing opportunities for vaccination.

GENERAL CONSIDERATIONS

Vaccination History

Vaccination history should be evaluated early in the transplant process, and when feasible, prior to transplantation. Serology testing to document antibody response can be considered in cases of uncertain vaccination history, uncertain but if done should be before immunosuppression to assist with the catch-up vaccination program.

Vaccine Administration Before Immunosuppression

As a general rule, vaccination and updating vaccination should be performed when feasible before planned immunosuppression and transplantation. This is obviously easier in solid organ transplant (SOT) recipients, as well as in older children for whom booster doses could be sufficient. For optimal efficacy the window period vaccination is 2 weeks for inactivated vaccines and 4 weeks for live vaccines before the initiation of immunosuppression.

Protective Titer Levels

Although there is a clear benefit of full vaccination before treatment, the waning of antibodies and subsequent insufficient protection is unpredictable. Hence, it is useful to measure antigen-specific serology levels at least 2 weeks (preferably 4 weeks) after vaccination. Many factors affect the ability to produce protective antibodies, including the type of primary disease, type and level of immunosuppression therapy, concomitant infections, organ failure, genetic factors, and previous immune status.

Window of Time Between Intravenous Immunoglobulins, Blood Products, and Vaccine Administration

Receipt of intravenous immunoglobulins or other blood products does not significantly affect the immune response to inactivated or toxoid vaccines. In contrast, they can interfere with the response to live attenuated vaccines, especially measles, mumps, rubella (MMR) and varicella-zoster (VZV) vaccines, as they may contain significant amounts of specific antibodies that limit the expansion of vaccine virus production after vaccination and, accordingly, the immunologic response. The window of time for delaying vaccines—ranging from 3 to 11 months—depending on the dose of intravenous immunoglobulins and/or which specific blood products are given.[8]

Donors and Contacts of Immunocompromised Host

Donors should be up-to-date for currently recommended vaccines based on age, vaccination history, and exposure history according to the most current vaccine guidelines. However, administration of live attenuated vaccines should be avoided within 4 weeks before stem cell harvest or organ donation.[9] Vaccination of the donor for the benefit of the recipient is not routinely recommended at this time.[9]

Health care workers and close contacts, such as family members who are in frequent contact with immunocompromised patients, should be fully immunized.[3] The pretransplant evaluation period is the ideal time to review immunization and to ensure that all caretakers and siblings are up-to-date and fully immunized, including for influenza during season and hepatitis A and B. When both inactivated or live attenuated vaccines for the same disease are available, the inactivated form is preferred to avoid prolonged shedding and risk for the candidate.[3]

Live attenuated influenza vaccine can be given if it is the only available option with good use of infection prevention precautions for a 2-week period after vaccination. However, it is contraindicated in the case of household individuals who live with hematopoietic stem cell transplantation (HSCT) recipients within 2 months after transplant or

We would like to include special acknowledgments to Drs. Einas Batarseh and Lubna Hamdan for their assistance and participation in drafting and editing this chapter.

those with active graft-versus-host-disease (GVHD). In case of administration, close contact between the immunocompromised patient and household members should be avoided for 7 days.[9]

Close contacts of immunocompromised hosts should not receive smallpox or oral polio vaccine. However, other live vaccines are encouraged in this group to prevent patients who have undergone transplantation from having contact with wild-type viruses (e.g., MMR and varicella). If a close contact develops cutaneous lesions after varicella vaccine, they should avoid contact with the immunocompromised host until the lesions clear.

In addition, although infants in the household can receive rotavirus vaccines, the immunocompromised patient should avoid handling diapers for 4 weeks after vaccination. Pets should also be fully immunized.[3]

SOLID ORGAN TRANSPLANTATION

Pretransplantation Vaccination

Pretransplant assessment of SOT candidates always includes reviewing their vaccination and vaccine-preventable disease histories. For infections that are well recognized, such as typical chickenpox, a history is generally sufficient to establish seropositivity. However, for other diseases, such as measles or pertussis, recall of disease is often misleading. The main concept is that candidates should be up-to-date with vaccinations for their age at the time of transplantation according to local recommendations and epidemiology.[3,7] Both inactivated and live attenuated vaccines should be administered as early as possible to increase the likelihood of better immunologic response, which may be diminished by end-stage organ disease. Ideally, vaccines should be given at least 2 weeks (inactivated vaccines) to 4 weeks (live attenuated vaccines) before SOT to allow for immune response.[3,9] Vaccine titers should be monitored at least at the time of assessment but ideally should be repeated just before SOT if there is a significant time gap between the two events to evaluate risk or document protection. Specific serologic results that could be measured include the following vaccines: tetanus, *Haemophilus influenzae* type b for children younger than 5 years of age, *Streptococcus pneumoniae*, hepatitis A, hepatitis B, varicella, MMR, and when relevant, rabies.

In children without prior vaccination or with an incomplete vaccination history, it can sometimes be difficult to prioritize which vaccine should be given first. It is worth highlighting that several vaccines can be given at the same time, including live attenuated vaccines. Live attenuated vaccines must be given either at the same time or 1 month apart. There is no such rule for inactivated vaccines, which can be given either on the same day or on any consecutive days. The age of the child, the number of vaccine doses already received, and the season should be considered when prioritizing which vaccine to administer first, as well as additional risk factors, such as outbreaks or local epidemiology. Nevertheless, these factors should all boil down to evaluating the risk of infection for the candidate.

For inactivated vaccines, influenza vaccine (when in season), pneumococcal vaccine, and hepatitis A and B vaccines should be prioritized. Next, a combination vaccine, including tetanus, diphtheria, pertussis, polio with or without *H. influenzae* type b, as well as meningococcal vaccine should be next. Other inactivated vaccines, such as human papillomavirus (HPV), rabies, tick-borne encephalitis, and so forth can be administered as a third tier.

For live-attenuated vaccines, the combination vaccine MMR should be the first priority or rotavirus vaccine (depending on age), as no specific treatments are available for the viruses they protect against and there is a high risk of severe outcome if disease occurs after transplantation. MMR can be given as early as 6 months of age for patients at risk of transplantation. A second dose is usually administered as early as 4 weeks after the first dose. If vaccination was started before 1 year of age and the second dose was also administered before the first year of life, a third dose should be given.

Varicella vaccine should be given if the child is seronegative; this can be administered on the same day as MMR vaccine or with an interval of 1 month. It is usually recommended after the first year of life because of possible interference with maternal antibodies but can be administered at 9 months of age if SOT is considered, with a second dose at least 4 weeks later. If seroconversion did not occur, a third dose should ideally be given before SOT if time allows.

Rotavirus vaccination of infants awaiting SOT is more controversial and data are lacking. In theory it could be given before SOT to infants younger than 6 months old. However, prolonged viral stool shedding, particularly with the first dose, is well recognized and therefore may not be ideal in an upcoming SOT setting.

Posttransplant Vaccination

General Considerations. At least 3 months after SOT when the child's condition is clinically stable and with baseline low immunosuppression, it is important to repeat the specific serologic tests for vaccine-preventable diseases. At this time, antibody waning or loss of seroprotection should be noted and a new plan for giving booster doses established. This process should be repeated regularly—for example, yearly at follow-up visits.

The optimal time to start immunizing after SOT is unclear. However, the type and amount of immunosuppression may modify the capacity to elicit protective vaccine responses. Therefore it is important to check seroconversion at least 4 weeks after immunization for those vaccines for which assays are available and protective levels are known. Although specific antibody levels may not be sufficient for ensuring full protection, they are used as surrogate markers.

Inactivated Vaccines. Most centers give inactivated vaccines 3 to 6 months after SOT if immunosuppressive drugs are stabilized at a low level, to ensure the best possible immune response (Table 9.1). The decision to vaccinate should be based on the necessity (antibody titers below the protective threshold, exposition to disease, local epidemiology), the age, and the evaluation of the capacity for immune response. This chapter reviews the available data on select inactivated vaccines.

Pneumococcal Vaccine

Invasive pneumococcal infection is more frequent in immunocompromised children. Two vaccines are currently available: a 23-valent polysaccharide vaccine (PPV23), which cannot be given to children younger than 2 years, and a 13-valent protein-conjugate vaccine (PCV13). Both vaccines are proven to be safe and immunogenic in SOT.[10] However, for children older than 2 years, the current recommendations include giving a PPV23 at least 2 months after first completion of the PCV13 dosing.[7,11,12]

Waning of antibody titers have been described over time. It is possible to measure specific seroresponses, which helps to evaluate the vaccine response and the maintenance of protective antibody titers. Current recommendations differ by age: children younger than 2 years should receive the PCV13 according to guidelines. For those 2 to 5 years, guidelines differ by previous doses received. For those who are unvaccinated or have an incomplete schedule (<3 doses), 2 doses of PCV13 should be given with a second dose 8 weeks or more after the first dose. For those with an incomplete schedule of 3 doses, 1 dose of PCV13 should be given. For those with an age-appropriate complete schedule, 1 dose of PCV13 should be given. For children older than

TABLE 9.1 Currently Available Vaccines and Current Recommendations in Most Countries. Before and After SOT.

Antigen	Before SOT	After SOT
Inactivated, Engineered Vaccines		
Diphtheria	Yes	Yes
Tetanus	Yes	Yes
Pertussis	Yes	Yes
Polio	Yes	Yes
Haemophilus influenzae type b	Yes	Yes
Streptococcus pneumoniae, conjugated vaccine	Yes	Yes
Neisseria meningitidis, quadrivalent preferably	Yes	Yes
Hepatitis A	Yes	Yes
Hepatitis B	Yes	Yes
Influenza	Yes	Yes, yearly
Human papillomavirus	Yes	Yes
Rabies	At risk*	At risk*
Japanese encephalitis	At risk*	At risk*
Tick-borne encephalitis	At risk*	At risk*
Typhoid (Vi)	At risk*	At risk*
Cholera	At risk	At risk*
Anthrax	No	No
Live Attenuated Vaccines		
Measles	Yes	No†
Mumps	Yes	No†
Rubella	Yes	No†
Varicella-zoster	Yes	No†
Zoster (not for children)	—	—
Rotavirus	Yes	No
Influenza	Inactivated preferred	No
Polio (oral)	Inactivated preferred	No
Yellow fever	At risk*	No
Typhoid (Ty21a)	Inactivated preferred	No
Bacille Calmette-Guérin	No†	No
Smallpox	No	No

*At risk depends on the local epidemiology, travel to specific at risk countries, and the age group.
†Depends on the country's usual recommendations.
SOT, solid organ transplant.

5 years, PPV23 should be given. The data for PPV23 show that it could be repeated with an interval between doses of at least 5 years.[3]

Influenza Vaccine

Morbidity and mortality related to influenza virus can be prevented in SOT patients with the use of influenza vaccine. Live attenuated influenza vaccines should not be used in SOT patients. Studies have shown that influenza vaccine may be poorly immunogenic in the early posttransplant period and in younger children. However, a study in adult SOT recipients showed that vaccination as early as 1 month is both safe and immunogenic.[13] The possible benefits of vaccination outweigh its minimal risks; because of this influenza vaccine is usually recommended before discharge, which may be as early as 1 month after SOT (during high influenza activity), and revaccination 3 to 6 months later can be considered if it is still influenza season.[3,13] For children younger than 9 years old, 2 doses of influenza vaccine are recommended for those vaccinated for the first time.

Several studies have looked at different strategies to increase immunogenicity and efficacy with influenza, but data are still insufficient to recommend one strategy over another. Booster doses 5 weeks after the standard vaccination seemed to be safe and induced more increased antibody titers compared to single dose in adult SOT recipients.[14] Another strategy is to administer high-dose inactivated influenza vaccine (IIV), which in pediatric SOT recipients appeared to be safe with acceptable side effects and with a higher percentage of titer increase.[15] Others have tried using adjuvanted influenza vaccine to increase immunogenicity. However, several groups have reported increased anti–human leukocyte antigen antibody production in patients receiving adjuvanted influenza, but the clinical relevance of this fact seems unclear.[16] Protective hemagglutinin inhibition titers can be measured after vaccination but are not performed routinely and are reserved to research settings in most centers.

Hepatitis B Vaccine

Being immunized before SOT against hepatitis B with protective titers reduces the risk of acquiring hepatitis B from anti–hepatitis B core antigen-positive donors.[17] SOT recipients with missing or incomplete vaccination against hepatitis B should be immunized with high-dose vaccines.[7] The seroconversion rate is between 40% and 70%, but it is important to document it. Primary nonresponders can benefit from a repeat series of high-dose vaccination.[18,19]

Furthermore, antibody waning is frequent; therefore anti–hepatitis B surface antigen titers should be monitored regularly (every 6 to 12 months after SOT) and booster doses (1 to 3) should be administered if titers are below 10 IU/mL.[3]

Although it is rare in children, patients with chronic hepatitis B should be considered for vaccination 2 to 6 months after liver transplant to possibly eliminate the lifelong requirement for hepatitis B immunoglobulins, even if the rate of seroconversion is low.[7]

Hepatitis A Vaccine

Unlike the recommendation for adults for whom only liver transplant recipients or persons at high risk of exposure (travel or residence in high-risk area) are immunized, all SOT children should be immunized against hepatitis A.[3] Immunogenicity of the vaccine after SOT is lower than in the healthy population and accelerated antibody waning has been described. Therefore serological monitoring is necessary and booster doses should be given when the patient is not seroprotected, especially when exposure is expected. Data are not available on the long-term effectiveness of repeated hepatitis A vaccination.

Pertussis Vaccine

Pertussis outbreaks are reported worldwide and the pre-SOT vaccination is often suboptimal, putting patients at risk for pertussis in the post-SOT setting.[20] Serologic measurements to evaluate specific seroprotection against pertussis are difficult to provide in a routine setting. Therefore proof of clinical protection is difficult to assess. Sometimes, tetanus-specific antibody titers are used as surrogate markers. Others have measured seroresponse to pertussis toxin or filamentous hemagglutinin after SOT, but seropositivity rates were variable and usually relatively low, not clarifying which test is the most relevant clinically.[21] Finally, waning of pertussis seroresponse has also been reported in the healthy population, but the benefit of repeating pertussis vaccines in addition to what is usually recommended is unknown.

Human Papillomavirus Vaccine

The relative risk of HPV-related cancer in pediatric SOT patients is debated. Nevertheless, immunizing SOT patients against HPV may decrease the overall risk of cancer and decrease the risk for HPV warts, a significant issue in SOT patients.

Three vaccine formulations are available: (1) a quadrivalent vaccine providing protection against HPV-6, -11, -16, and -18; (2) an adjuvanted bivalent vaccine protecting against HPV-16 and -18; and more recently, (3) a 9-valent HPV vaccine protecting against HPV-6, -11, -16, -18, -31, -33, -45, -52, and -58. The quadrivalent HPV vaccine, which also protects against virus strains causing 90% of genital warts, was preferred in the SOT population[7] but will likely be replaced by the 9-valent vaccine. Missing or incomplete vaccination against HPV can be started 3 to 6 months after SOT as a 3-dose series.

Meningococcal Vaccine

Young children and adolescents are particularly at risk for invasive meningococcal disease. In addition, anatomically or functionally asplenic patients—such as some SOT patients—are also at an increased risk for disease. However, there are no available data on the incidence or morbidity linked with meningococcal disease in pediatric SOT. Several vaccines are available, such as against a single type of *Neisseria meningitidis* (type B or C) or as a quadrivalent (conjugated or polysaccharide) vaccine against A, C, W135, and Y. Usually, a quadrivalent vaccine (single dose at age 11 with a booster dose 2 months later) and a monovalent vaccine against serogroup B are recommended. Vaccination at a younger age may be introduced in the near future. Immunogenicity is poorly studied owing to the difficulty to establish standardized correlates for protection. However, in a small study in pediatric liver and kidney transplant recipients, titers did increase and remained elevated for at least 18 months after vaccination.[22]

Live Attenuated Vaccines. Currently, three live attenuated vaccines against viral diseases are available routinely: varicella, MMR, and rotavirus vaccines (see Table 9.1). These diseases are linked with a higher risk of morbidity and mortality in SOT patients.[4] In addition, in many countries, some of these diseases, such as varicella, measles, and rotavirus, are endemic or present as regular outbreaks. Therefore vaccination before SOT is ideal. However, pediatric SOT recipients are often too young to start or complete their vaccination before surgery. Live attenuated vaccines were until now not recommended after transplantation in SOT patients, but owing to new data, these vaccines may be administered in some well-identified patients, such as for varicella in children who are renal or liver transplant recipients, those who are receiving minimal or no immunosuppression, and those who have no recent graft rejection.[9,23]

Measles-Mumps-Rubella Vaccine

The only available vaccine against measles is live attenuated and is combined either with a mumps and rubella vaccine or with mumps, rubella, and varicella vaccine. At this point, vaccination is not recommended after SOT by most transplant societies, but several centers administer MMR vaccine either in a research setting or in an outbreak setting.

In 2018, under the guidance of the International Pediatric Transplant Association, a consortium of experts reviewed all available data on MMR vaccination and made recommendations to consider MMR vaccination for SOT patients who are at risk owing to outbreaks or who live in an endemic country and are clinically well at least 1 year after transplant and more than 2 months back to baseline immunosuppression after rejection, with steroids dose less than 2 mg/kg per day or total cumulative more than 20 mg; tacrolimus level less than 8 ng/mL for two consecutive readings; or cyclosporine level less than 100 ng/mL for two consecutive readings. In addition, they should have absolute lymphocyte counts above 1500 for children 6 year or younger and above 1000 cells/μL for children older than 6 years; CD4 above 700 cells/μL for children 6 years or younger; and above 500 cells/μL for children older than 6 years; and normal serum immunoglobulin G for age.[24] Hopefully, these recommendations will be integrated in future guidelines. Protection against the mumps or rubella is usually lower after vaccination and is reported to be between 43% and 100%.[25-27] For all antigens, serologic follow-up after vaccination to administer booster doses when waning or when antibody loss is documented should be implemented regularly.

Varicella-Zoster Vaccine

VZV is still endemic in many countries with regular outbreaks in children. Because SOT patients are at a higher risk for complications, such as disseminated disease or pneumonia, antiviral agents such as acyclovir are used to prevent a poor outcome. Vaccination is currently not recommended after SOT by most transplant societies, but evidence is accumulating that suggests it could be used in selected patients.

A few studies are available reporting on seroprotection after VZV vaccine in more than 100 well-selected pediatric SOTs. Seroresponse varies between 32% and 100% in studies with very different patient populations and study protocols.[23-26,28,29] In these publications, VZV vaccination was considered safe with a few (mild) breakthrough diseases. In some studies, cell-mediated immunity was also evaluated after vaccination and a significant postvaccine increase was reported.[23]

In 2018, the expert consortium reviewed all available data for VZV and recommended considering VZV vaccination in selected patients. Data on combination MMR-varicella vaccine are lacking in SOT. Therefore it is not currently recommended to administer the combined vaccine jointly. In general, when both vaccines are considered, it is suggested to start with VZV as a treatment option in case of unwanted viral replication.

Rotavirus Vaccine

The live attenuated rotavirus vaccine is usually recommended to infants as young as 6 weeks as a series of vaccines (2 or 3 doses depending on the vaccine). It has not been studied in SOT and is currently contraindicated. It is likely that within the next few years new data will be available and recommendations on live attenuated vaccines after SOT will be revised.

ONCOLOGY PATIENTS

The optimal timing of immunizations before, during, and after chemotherapy in children with malignancy is still debatable. Whether it is advisable or not to vaccinate depends on the possible adverse effects of the vaccine and on the possibility of providing an adequate immune response and the risk of exposure. Both the underlying cancer diseases and the chemotherapeuticals, radiotherapy, blood products, and monoclonal antibodies used affect their poor responses. In addition, multiple new therapies, including monoclonal antibodies, are available to treat cancer. However, the clinical trials assessing postvaccine immune responses are lacking. In addition, most trials assessing vaccine responses are in hematologic malignancies, with few vaccine studies in children with solid tumors.

A major drawback with chemotherapy is immune suppression, and as a result it can take up to 6 to 12 months after the end of treatment for patients to recover their immune function.[30] Moreover, there is evidence of waning of vaccination immunity after chemotherapy. It was found that the presence of protective antibody titers after chemotherapy depends on several factors, including type of vaccine as it was higher for hepatitis B virus (HBV, about 50% of patients) but lower for MMR (between 20% and 40%) and polio-diphtheria-tetanus (between 10% and 30%) vaccines, and the intensity of chemotherapy regimen and primary malignancy.[30] Thus recommendations and options include checking vaccine titers after chemotherapy has been completed and revaccination if titers are not found to be protective, or administering booster vaccinations 6 months after stopping chemotherapy without checking titers.[30] Further research to address the gaps of knowledge regarding the timing of vaccination in oncology patients is needed.

Generally, vaccination during periods of intensive chemotherapy, such as for induction or consolidation chemotherapy for acute leukemia, is not generally recommended. Inactivated vaccines can be given during periods of maintenance chemotherapy, according to local vaccine recommendations for age but are not considered valid doses and patients should receive booster doses starting 3 months after chemotherapy and 6 months for patients using anti–B-cell antibodies, unless there is a documentation of a protective antibody level.[7] If vaccines are given, the administration of indicated inactivated vaccines 2 or more weeks before chemotherapy is preferred.

Inactivated Vaccines

In principle, inactive vaccines based on toxoid, protein subunits, bacterial antigens, or immunogenic proteins obtained with recombinant technology are not contraindicated during chemotherapy.[30] This category includes vaccines for tetanus, diphtheria, pertussis, poliomyelitis, hepatitis B, influenza, *Haemophilus*, pneumococcus, and meningococcus.[30] The main issue with administering these vaccines during chemotherapy is potential suboptimal responses.

Pneumococcal Vaccines

Invasive infections by capsulated bacteria may represent severe complications during chemotherapy, especially in leukemic patients in whom an impairment of pneumococcal immunity has been reported.[30] There is limited experience on the use of vaccinations for pneumococcus, *Haemophilus*, and meningococcus[30]; thus evidence-based guidance is lacking with the exception of vaccinating before splenectomy.[30] Recommendations for children newly diagnosed with hematologic or solid malignancies aged 2 to 5 years indicate they should receive 1 dose of PCV if they have received 3 doses of PCV before age 24 months and 2 doses of PCV (8 weeks apart) if they have received an incomplete schedule of 2 of fewer doses of PCV before age 24 months. PPV23 should be administered to children 2 years and older at least 8 weeks after the indicated dose(s) of PCV.[7] This strategy is known as prime and boost.

Influenza Vaccines

Influenza is one of the community-acquired respiratory infections that can cause a significant morbidity in pediatric oncology patients, including hospitalization and secondary bacteremia.[30] In addition, influenza infection has also been associated with delayed chemotherapy, which can negatively affect the ultimate disease outcome. Emphasis should be directed to the importance of administering the annual IIV to children with malignancies except those receiving anti–B-cell antibodies or intensive chemotherapy such as for induction or consolidation chemotherapy. In addition, IIV can be administered at 3 months or earlier after chemotherapy, but the response rate may be low. Live attenuated influenza vaccine is not indicated in patients before or during chemotherapy and may be given starting 3 months or later after chemotherapy as recommended for other live vaccines. Strategies such as the administration of 2 doses of standard IIV and/or higher doses of influenza vaccine need further attention.

Human Papillomavirus Vaccines

Long-term survivorship after cancer is increasing, which has then been associated with secondary malignancies, including cancers related to HPV infections. Despite the lack of clinical trials of the immunogenicity and efficacy of HPV vaccines, HPV vaccination in childhood survivors after cancer should be given with either the quadrivalent HPV or 9-valent HPV.

Hepatitis A and B Vaccines

The efficacy of vaccination for HBV and hepatitis A virus (HAV) early after the diagnosis of pediatric malignancy has been evaluated.[30] This measure is generally adopted in countries with a high prevalence of HBV or HAV infection, in which vaccination is not routine because of limited health resources.[30] These studies showed that vaccination of seronegative patients for HBV and HAV in the early phase of chemotherapy reduces the risk of contracting hepatitis and confers protection to immune-compromised patients, although at a lower rate than in healthy populations or in patients not undergoing therapy.[30]

Live Vaccines

As a general rule, live vaccines should be avoided during chemotherapy, especially when there is profound leukopenia, full-dose steroid therapy, and during induction therapy.[30] Diseases such as measles and varicella can lead to DNAemia in the active period of the disease in cancer patients who receive chemotherapy or radiotherapy. Therefore

MMR and varicella vaccines should be administered when the disease is in remission (3 months after the drugs are discontinued at the earliest) or before chemotherapy, or at least 6 months later in children receiving anti–B-cell antibodies.[9]

HEMATOPOIETIC STEM CELL TRANSPLANTATION

Vaccines administered in the posttransplant period may have diminished immunogenicity and efficacy for a variety of reasons, such as immunosuppressive medications, underlying disease, rejection or GVHD; the primary disease of the patient; the type of ablative therapy before transplant; and many other factors.[31] It has been demonstrated that antibody titers to vaccine-preventable diseases (e.g., tetanus, polio, MMR, and encapsulated organisms) decline between 1 and 4 years after HSCT if the recipient is not revaccinated.[32] Therefore, despite prior history of vaccination in this population, HSCT recipients should be revaccinated routinely after transplant, regardless of the source of the transplanted stem cells.[33]

Timing to Start Vaccination

Immune reconstitution starts with engraftment of neutrophils but lymphocyte recovery, which is necessary for vaccine response, may require several months. Most recommend starting revaccination with inactivated vaccines 6 to 12 months after transplantation, and after 24 months for the live attenuated vaccines if patients do not have GVHD and are not taking immunosuppressive agents.[4,7]

Research is still needed to investigate reasons to delay vaccinations after transplant, but there has been some agreement on the criteria used to decide vaccination delay (Fig. 9.1.) In addition, owing to increased morbidity and mortality from vaccine-preventable diseases (e.g., pneumococcal and influenza diseases) in the early transplant period, some studies have investigated giving inactivated vaccines are early as 2 months after HSCT. Fig. 9.2 demonstrates vaccination schedules in post-HSCT recipients 6 and 12 months after HSCT.[34]

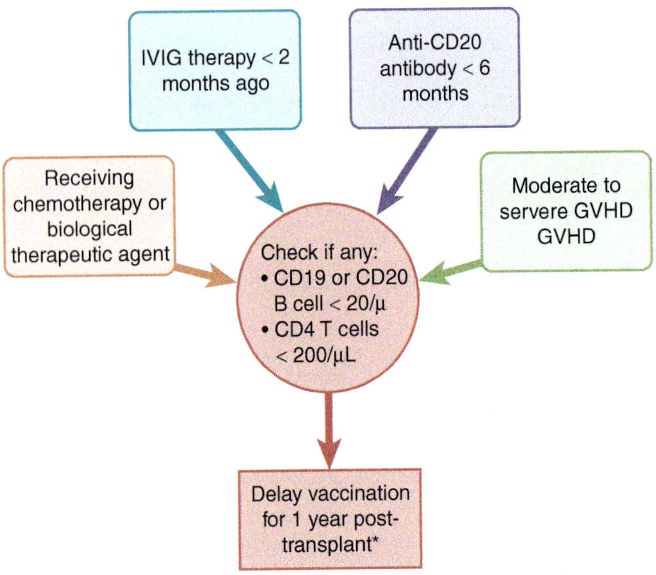

*Patients with primary immunodeficiency disorders (PID), vaccinations are always delayed at least 1-year post transplant.

Fig. 9.1 Approach to delay vaccination until 12 months after hematopoietic transplant. *IVIG*, immunoglobulin.

Pneumococcal Vaccine

Pneumococcal infections can be very severe in HSCT recipients, especially those with chronic GVHD. Historically, the full PCV series is recommended starting at 6 months post-HSCT; however, some studies have administered PCV three months post-HSCT, but then revealed waning and lower antibody titers compared to those who received PCV later (9 months). Current U.S. recommendations recommend 6 months after HSCT followed by PPSV23 for those without chronic GVHD. For those with chronic GVHD fourth dose of PCV is recommended[9]; however, European recommendations include starting 3 months after HSCT.[35]

Influenza Vaccination

There is an ongoing controversy regarding the guidelines for the timing of influenza vaccine administration in the United States versus the timing in the European guidelines. The U.S. guidelines state to start 6 months after transplant, whereas the European recommendation indicates that influenza vaccines can be given as early as 3 months after HSCT with a second dose of vaccine 3 to 4 weeks after the first dose, especially in recipients who received transplants less than 6 months earlier.[35] Current studies are investigating the utility of administering 1 of 2 doses of high-dose and/or standard-dose IIV.

Tetanus Toxoid, Diphtheria Toxoid, Pertussis, and Poliovirus

Reimmunization with repeated doses of inactivated poliovirus vaccine, diphtheria toxoid, and tetanus toxoid effectively restores immunity, and the most robust immune responses are seen when vaccination begins at 6 months after HSCT, although some studies have started as early as 6 weeks after HSCT. Because this population is considered as "never vaccinated," they should receive a full series of toxoids, diphtheria-tetanus vaccine, and not vaccines usually used for booster doses for adults. Despite the fact that DTaP (note these are higher antigen doses) is not licensed for individuals older than 7 years, some experts will use this vaccine instead of Tdap because DTaP has higher antigen doses.

Meningococcal Vaccine

MenACWY-D (Menactra), MenACWY-CRM (Menveo), and MenACWY-TT (Nimenrix) are three currently available quadrivalent meningococcal vaccines, and data are insufficient to determine the optimal time for vaccination. Recent studies have shown that 2-dose quadrivalent meningococcal vaccines series may produce protective responses in pediatric HSCT recipients. Meningococcal group B vaccine (Bexsero) is recommended for patients older than 9 years old with anatomic or functional asplenia condition (i.e., GVHD) or increased environmental risk. Discussion with parents for vaccinating patients 16 to 18 years of age is encouraged as an optional recommendation.

Human Papilloma Virus

HSCT recipients are also at risk for HPV complications, including cervical dysplasia. Despite the lack of efficacy studies in the population, recent guidelines recommend using quadrivalent HPV or 9-valent HPV in HSCT recipients because of their high potency in preventing cancers (up to 90% for cervical cancer).[36]

Live Vaccines

Waning antibodies to measles and varicella have been documented after HSCT. However, for both MMR and varicella vaccines, delaying these vaccines for at least 2 years after transplant is recommended, and

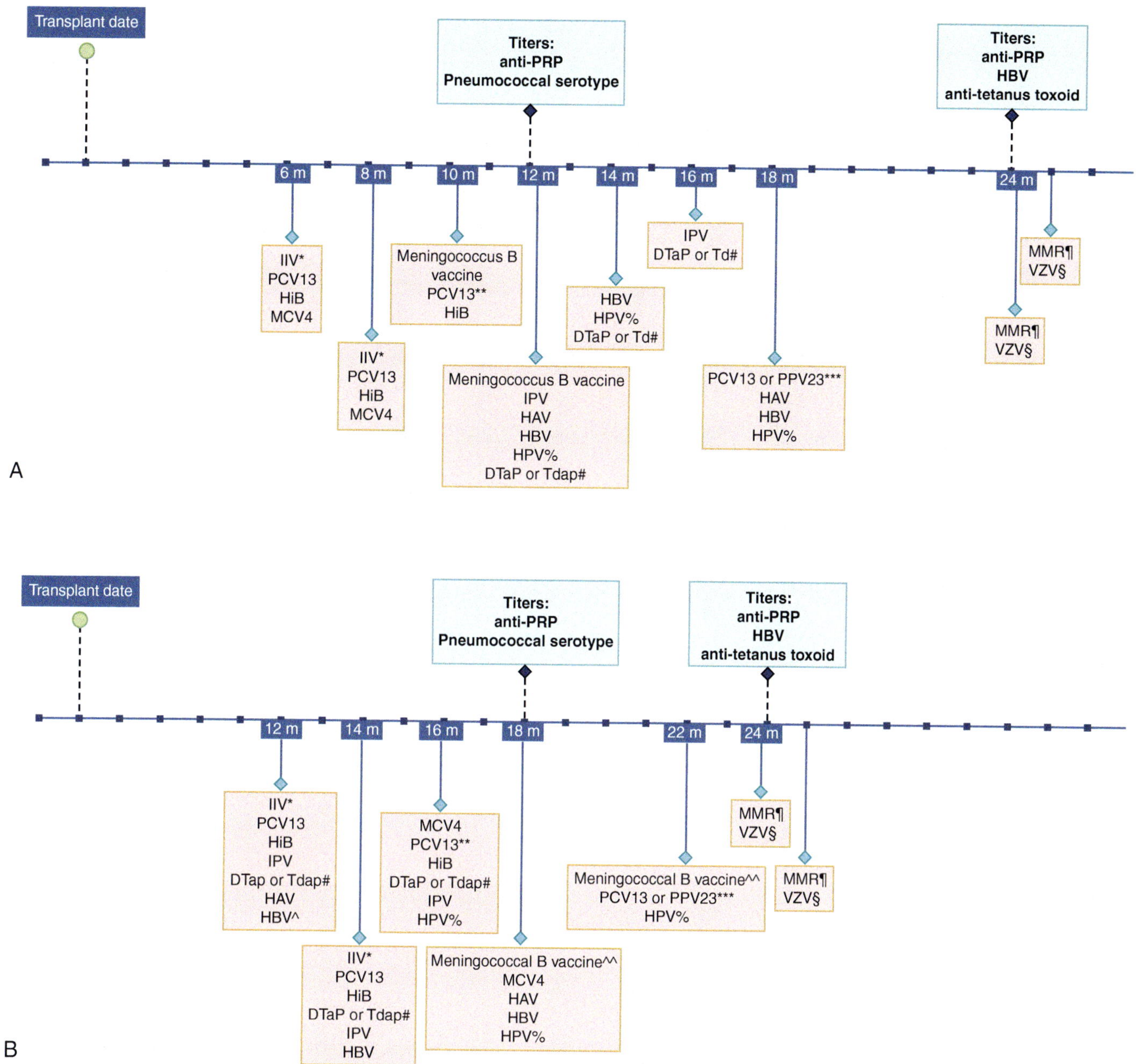

* For IIV vaccine in children <9 years, give a second dose at 8 months
** Check titers at 12 months; if not checked then check at 24 m
*** In patients with chronic GVHD who are unlikely to respond to PPV23 it is preferable to administer a 4th dose of PCV13
^^ In children older than 9 years old
§ Only for vaccination with VZV vaccine seronegative recipients without a history of chickenpox or varicella vaccination, check varicella serology at least 1–2 months after second dose of vaccine to ensure seroconversion. First dose can be given at the same day with MMR
¶ For children <9 years of age, two doses are recommended yearly between transplant and 9 years of age.
\# Go to meningococcal vaccine section in post HSCT
% Either 4vHPV or 9vHPV between the age of 9 years to 26 years

Fig. 9.2 A, Timeline for pediatric vaccination if started before 12 months after hematopoietic transplant. **B,** Timeline for pediatric vaccination if started after 12 months after hematopoietic transplant.

further delay is needed if patients are still receiving active immunosuppression and/or have chronic GVHD.[37]

Vaccines in Special Circumstances

Yellow fever vaccine, rabies vaccine, tick-borne encephalitis vaccine, and Japanese encephalitis vaccine are not routinely administered vaccines, so their use is driven by a disease-specific risk, such as a patient living in a region with a specific risk or patient travels. Traveling patients often do not seek advice before traveling and may become sick abroad.[38] Some general principles should be followed, such as delaying when possible traveling during the first year after transplant, seeking advice in a specialized center from a travel medicine expert with knowledge on immunocompromised hosts, and updating the basic and supplementary vaccines, recommended for the destination. These change yearly and can be found on updated websites from the CDC (www.cdc.gov/travel) or other websites.

CONCLUSION AND FUTURE DIRECTIONS

Although immunization is without a doubt a very important preventive measure in immunocompromised hosts, research should focus on finding ways to increase vaccines' immunogenicity, clinical efficacy, and persistence of immune response in these children. More data should also be gathered on seroresponse and safety of vaccination, especially regarding live-attenuated vaccines, as well as dissecting the differential effects of various immunosuppressive regimes. Until then, providers should focus on vaccinating children before the immunosuppression is started, follow up on vaccination schedules, seroprotection after immunosuppression, and vaccination of health care workers and household members.

10

Microbiome Implications in Transplantation and Oncology

Matthew S. Kelly, MD, MPH and Michael A. Silverman, MD, PhD

At birth, infants become colonized with trillions of commensal microbes that play important roles in health and disease. The majority of these microbes reside in the gastrointestinal tract, reaching densities of 10^{12} bacteria per gram of intestinal content in the colon.[1] Complex microbial communities are also found on all human surfaces, including the skin, oropharynx, vagina, and lung. These microbiomes are highly abundant—bacteria represent an astounding 50% to 90% of the cells within or on our bodies and are accompanied by less well-defined but significant numbers of viruses, fungi, and archaea. Overall, the human microbiome contains thousands of species spanning the microbial phylogenetic tree. Because the majority of these microbes are anaerobic and are not routinely recovered using standard microbial culture techniques, the biological impacts of the human microbiome have historically been underappreciated. However, recent technological advances in high-throughput DNA sequencing provided powerful tools to define and study these microbial communities. The microbiome is now understood to be a complex ecosystem in which there is tremendous cross talk between microbial species and between microbes and their host. This communication and interdependence between potential pathogens and the host is likely especially important in severely immunocompromised hosts, such as transplant recipients and oncology patients.

So how does one understand and study the microbiome and its importance to human health? A first step is to catalog the microbes present in a particular anatomic location. Currently, the most widely used culture-independent approach to identify bacterial and fungal microbes is to amplify and sequence the variable regions of the highly conserved 16S ribosomal RNA (rRNA) gene from bacteria or 18S rRNA gene from fungi. These sequences can then be assigned to specific bacteria or fungi and used to determine the abundances of specific microbes within a sample. This approach is inexpensive and high-throughput but has the disadvantage of identifying only bacterial or fungal members of the community. A second approach, referred to as "shotgun" metagenomics, sequences all of the DNA present in a sample. This approach is more expensive and involves substantially more sophisticated analyses to define the members of the microbial community. However, shotgun sequencing provides information on a broader range of microbes, including viruses and archaea, and yields more detailed information on gene content, which can be used to infer the functional capacity of the microbial community.

Taxonomically, microbes are classified by kingdom, phylum, class, order, family, genus, and species. The gut microbiome consists of bacteria primarily from five phyla (Table 10.1). The neonatal gut microbiome has low diversity (relatively few bacterial species) and is typically composed of bacteria from the genera *Bifidobacterium* and *Lactobacillus* and facultative anaerobes from the family Enterobacteriaceae. During the first 3 years of life, the gut microbiome is fluid and undergoes substantial shifts in composition with the introduction of solid foods, with strict anaerobes from the orders Clostridiales and Bacteroidales replacing the neonatal microbiome.[2] Alteration of this early life gut microbiome can disrupt immune system development and function. This is most evident in germ-free animals that lack commensal microbes and have myriad health consequences, including abnormal development and function of the immune system and increased susceptibility to infections and autoimmunity.[3] Human epidemiologic studies also reported associations between early life microbiome perturbations (e.g., cesarean delivery, antibiotic exposures) and the later development of asthma, atopy, and autoimmune disorders. Taken together, these studies suggest that microbial exposures are important for educating the developing immune system, with a lack of host-microbe interactions predisposing to immune dysregulation. This concept, often referred to as the "hygiene hypothesis," was first proposed to explain the geographic distribution of cases of seasonal allergic rhinitis, but has since been extended to other areas of medicine, including hematopoietic stem cell transplantation, oncology, and solid organ transplantation (SOT).[4,5]

Commensal microbes also prevent infection by providing a barrier to colonization and overgrowth by more virulent bacteria. This concept—referred to as "colonization resistance"—was originally described in 1954 when it was noted that mice treated with the antibiotic streptomycin were susceptible to nontyphoidal *Salmonella* infection at a dose 10,000-fold lower than the typical minimal infectious dose.[6] The mechanisms that account for colonization resistance are becoming increasingly well understood (Fig. 10.1). It is now recognized that commensal gut bacteria can inhibit pathogen colonization through competition for carbohydrates and other micronutrients, secretion of antimicrobial substances (e.g., peptides, short-chain fatty acids), and through interactions with the host immune system. The classic example of an infection that results from a loss of colonization resistance of the gut microbiome is *Clostridium difficile* colitis. A loss of gut microbial diversity and anaerobic commensal bacteria, most frequently after the administration of antibiotics, predisposes to *C. difficile* colonization and infection.[7] Restoration of gut microbial diversity through fecal microbiome transplantation is increasingly being used as a treatment for recurrent *C. difficile* infection and is widely regarded as the most successful microbiome therapeutic in modern medicine.

Several concepts are important to understanding the impact of the microbiome on human health and disease. First, anatomic location is a critical determinant of the microbiome. For example, the skin microbiome is markedly different from the gut microbiome

TABLE 10.1 Taxonomic Classification of Common Gut Bacteria

Phyla	Class	Order	Family	Genus
Actinobacteria	Actinobacteria	Actinomycetales	Corynebacteriaceae	*Corynebacterium*
		Bifidobacteriales	Bifidobacteriaceae	*Bifidobacterium*[a]
Bacteroidetes	Bacteroidia	Bacteroidales[b]	Bacteroidaceae	*Bacteroides*
			Prevotellaceae	*Prevotella*
			Rikenellaceae	*Alistipes*
Firmicutes	Clostridia	Clostridiales[b]	Clostridiaceae	*Clostridium*
				Faecalibacterium
			Eubacteriaceae	*Eubacterium*
			Lachnospiraceae	*Blautia*
			Ruminococcaceae	*Ruminococcus*
	Negativicutes	Veillonellales	Veillonellaceae	*Dialister*
	Bacilli	Lactobacillales	Enterococcaceae	*Enterococcus*[c]
			Lactobacillaceae	*Lactobacillus*[a]
			Streptococcaceae	*Streptococcus*[c]
Proteobacteria	Gamma proteobacteria	Enterobacteriales	Enterobacteriaceae[a]	*Enterobacter*[c]
				Escherichia[c]
				Klebsiella[c]
Verrucomicrobia[b]	Verrucomicrobiae	Verrucomicrobiales	Akkermansiaceae	*Akkermansia*

[a]Bacteria that predominate in infants.
[b]Bacteria that predominate in children and adults.
[c]Endogenous bacteria that commonly cause invasive infection.

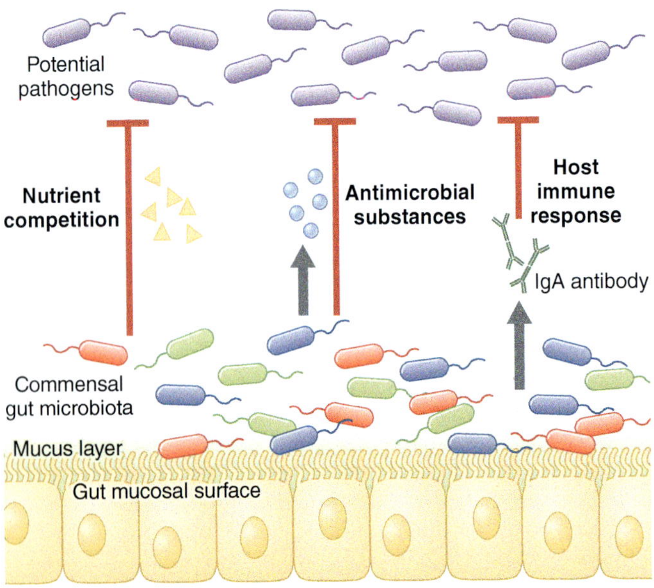

Fig. 10.1 Mechanisms of colonization resistance. *IgA*, immunoglobulin A.

and, within the gut, the microbiome of the small intestine differs substantially from that of the large intestine. This illustrates the importance of local environmental factors, such as nutrient availability, temperature, and pH, in regulating human microbiome composition.[8] Second, the microbiome performs specific functions, such as digesting dietary fiber, secreting metabolites, and modifying bile acids, and microbiomes with varied composition can provide similar functions.[8] In turn, composition cannot be used to accurately predict microbiome function; microbiomes with similar compositions may perform different functions and have different effects on their host.

Third, microbiome alterations observed in the setting of a disease may implicate the microbiome as an important driver of that disease state, or alternatively, may reflect the effect of the disease on the microbiome. Longitudinal studies that include characterization of the microbiome before disease onset are generally needed to establish or refute a causal relationship between the microbiome and a disease state. This is an important distinction to make because it has implications for the potential of microbiome therapeutics to prevent or ameliorate the disease.

In general, microbiomes associated with disease states have lower diversity and high abundances of one or a few potentially pathogenic microbes. This microbiome state is referred to as "dysbiosis" and occurs when the microbiome has a negative impact on the host. A dysbiotic microbiome has disproportionately lost beneficial microbes while microbes that are potentially detrimental to the host have expanded to dominate the microbial community. Such a microbiome may harm the host through loss of microbial metabolic functions that benefit the host. For example, antibiotics that deplete fiber-fermenting anaerobes deprive the host of short-chain fatty acids, which nourish enterocytes and help maintain gut barrier function. Lower abundances of these anaerobes can lead to disruption of the gut mucosal barrier and translocation of intestinal microbes, which can result in bacteremia and sepsis.

In this chapter, we discuss three emerging themes that relate the microbiome to children undergoing hematopoietic stem cell transplantation (HSCT), treatment for cancer, or SOT (Fig. 10.2). First, the microbiome influences risk for infection. Although many infections in immunocompromised patients originate from endogenous microbes, a healthy microbiome also prevents colonization, overgrowth, and invasion by exogenous pathogens. Second, the microbiome influences immune system function in children at risk for graft-versus-host disease (GVHD) and allograft rejection. Third, the microbiome has the potential to be a powerful tool to predict and prevent infections and other complications in immunocompromised children.

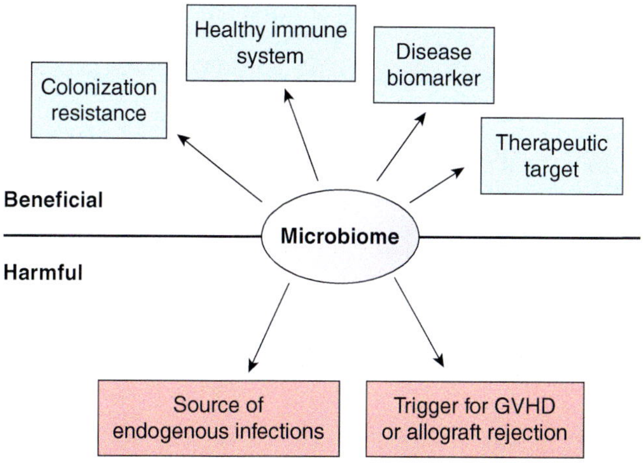

Fig. 10.2 Effects of the microbiome on immunocompromised children. *GVHD*, graft-versus-host disease.

MICROBIOME AND HEMATOPOIETIC STEM CELL TRANSPLANTATION

HSCT is associated with substantial alterations of the gut microbiome. Although the gut of healthy individuals typically contains a diverse microbial community composed of approximately 1000 bacterial species, the gut microbiome of patients early after HSCT is frequently far less diverse and is often dominated by a single bacterial species.[9] These shifts in gut microbial diversity and composition occur rapidly—often over the course of days—and are associated with exposure to antibiotics, chemotherapy-induced gut mucosal injury, and dietary changes. Marked increases in the relative abundances of *Enterococcus* species and Proteobacteria occur frequently after HSCT and are associated with receipt of antibiotics.[10] These shifts are offset by losses of key commensal gut bacteria, including microbes from the genera *Faecalibacterium* and *Ruminococcus*.[11] Changes in nutritional intake and, in particular, a lack of enteral intake early after HSCT also contribute to alterations in the gut microbiome. Enteral feeding via a nasogastric tube has been associated with lower GVHD risk and infectious mortality compared with parenteral nutrition in observational studies of allogeneic HSCT recipients. A randomized controlled trial (the NEPHA study) is currently underway to compare these nutritional approaches.[12]

Several studies suggest that the gut microbiome may be a useful biomarker for the prediction of outcomes after allogeneic HSCT. Most of this research has been conducted in adults and has focused on gut microbial diversity. The diversity of the gut microbiome at the time of engraftment is strongly associated with mortality after allogeneic HSCT. In a study of 80 adults, patients with lower diversity of the gut microbiome had markedly worse survival 3 years after allogeneic HSCT (36% vs. 67%).[13] Gut microbial diversity was most strongly associated with mortality from GVHD and infections, suggesting the importance of the gut microbiome to the pathophysiology of these conditions. The gut microbiome also was associated with the risk of relapse among patients undergoing HSCT as treatment for malignancy. In a study of 541 adult patients with hematologic malignancies, the presence of *Eubacterium limosum* in the gut microbiome predicted a lower risk of relapse at 2 years after allogeneic HSCT.[14]

Graft-Versus-Host Disease

Despite recent advances in histocompatibility matching and donor selection, GVHD remains a leading cause of morbidity and mortality among children after allogeneic HSCT. Our current understanding of the pathogenesis of GVHD suggests that chemotherapy-induced damage to the gut mucosa results in translocation of microorganisms or their products—most notably lipopolysaccharide—triggering an innate immune response that ultimately leads to activation of alloreactive donor T lymphocytes (Fig. 10.3). Research conducted in the 1970s and 1980s established the importance of the gut microbiome to the pathophysiology of GVHD. In these studies, germ-free mice developed GVHD at a far lower rate after allogeneic HSCT than conventionally raised mice.[15,16] These findings spurred numerous efforts to prevent GVHD in patients undergoing allogeneic HSCT through suppression or decontamination of the microbiome. A variety of approaches were attempted, including "sterile" diets, laminar airflow isolation, skin cleansing protocols, and gut decontamination through the administration of high-doses of nonabsorbable oral antibiotics. Unfortunately, these strategies were not consistently effective for GVHD prevention in clinical studies and were thus not widely implemented.

The recent development of high-throughput sequencing technologies led to renewed interest in understanding how the gut microbiome influences the risk of GVHD. Although the diversity of the gut microbiome is a strong predictor of the risk of GVHD, the relative abundances of specific microorganisms also appear to be important. In particular, higher relative abundances of *Enterococcus* have been observed in patients with GVHD, consistent with studies demonstrating that enterococci can impair gut mucosal integrity and stimulate activation of the innate immune system. Other studies suggest that specific gut anaerobes may be protective for GVHD. In particular, higher relative abundances of certain bacteria from the order Clostridiales (e.g., *Blautia*) appear to be associated with a lower risk of GVHD. Limited

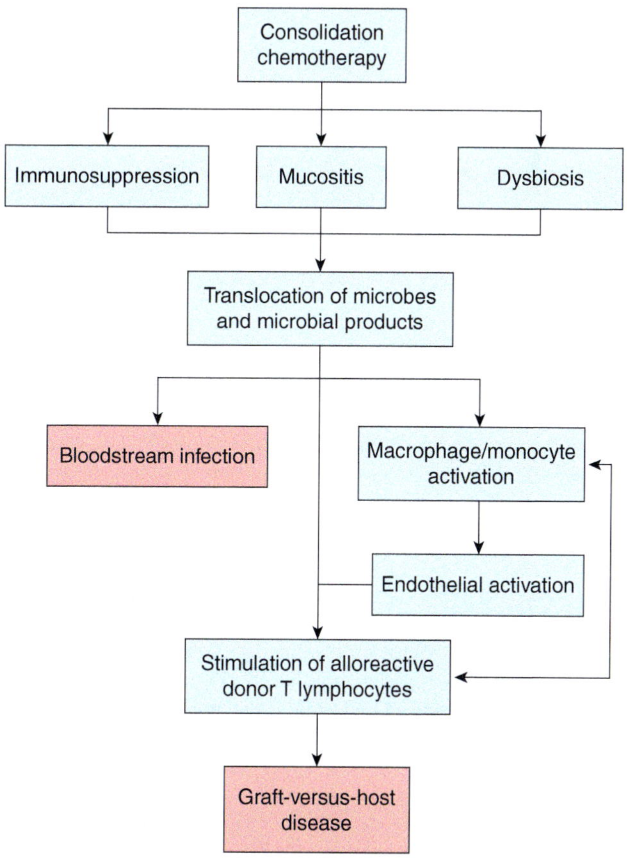

Fig. 10.3 Proposed pathogenesis of bloodstream infection and graft-versus-host disease after hematopoietic stem cell transplantation.

data from clinical studies also suggest that anaerobic bacteria may be protective from the onset of GVHD. In a single-center retrospective study of adult allogeneic HSCT recipients, the use of antibiotics with an anaerobic spectrum of activity during the peritransplant period was associated with higher GVHD mortality.[17] Although the associations identified in these studies are noteworthy, our understanding of the mechanisms by which the gut microbiome influences GVHD risk remains limited. Further research is needed to better delineate the complex interactions that exist between the gut microbiome and the host immune system to inform strategies to prevent GVHD through manipulation of the gut microbiome.

Infections

There has been much interest in investigating whether the gut microbiome modifies the risk of infections in HSCT recipients. Most studies conducted to date focused on bloodstream infections, particularly those caused by enteric bacteria. Overgrowth of the gut microbiome by *Enterococcus* or Proteobacteria is associated with a higher risk of bloodstream infection caused by these organisms among adults after allogeneic HSCT.[10] Moreover, antibiotics appear to be an important precipitating factor for overgrowth of the gut microbiome by these bacteria by decreasing colonization resistance. The administration of metronidazole increases the risk of enterococcal domination, consistent with reports that gut anaerobes provide a barrier to colonization and overgrowth by enterococci, whereas fluoroquinolones reduce the incidence of domination by Proteobacteria.[10] Interestingly, and somewhat unexpectedly, gut bacteria also appear to influence the risk of viral infections, including those arising outside the gastrointestinal tract, which could result from the extensive cross talk that occurs between the gut microbiome and the host immune system. Although our understanding of these complex and bidirectional interactions is limited, the gut microbiome appears to play an important role in establishing and maintaining virus-specific memory T-lymphocyte responses.[18] This finding mirrors those of studies of viral infections in germ-free or antibiotic-treated mice in which the presence of commensal microbes alters susceptibility to some viral infections.[19] In clinical studies, the gut microbiome's influence on viral infections has been most clearly shown for respiratory viruses. Several studies demonstrated associations between antibiotic exposures or the composition of the gut microbiome and the risk and severity of respiratory virus infections among adults after allogeneic HSCT.[20,21]

Microbiome Therapeutics

Given the associations between the gut microbiome and the risk of GVHD and infections after HSCT, the potential exists for microbiome therapeutics to improve outcomes of HSCT recipients. These therapies can broadly be divided into four categories: antibiotics, prebiotics, probiotics, and postbiotics. *Antibiotics* are substances that kill or slow the growth of microorganisms. *Prebiotics* are nondigestible substances that support the growth of specific microorganisms within the host. *Probiotics* are supplements or foods that contain live microorganisms. *Postbiotics* are nonviable microbial products or metabolic by-products that are biologically active within the host.

Antibiotic strategies used in HSCT recipients include antibiotic prophylaxis, de-escalation of antibiotic therapy, and minimizing the duration of antibiotic treatment. Antibiotic prophylaxis is a strategy that is widely used to lower the risk of bacterial infections after HSCT. This practice prevents bloodstream infections and is associated with lower mortality among patients with chemotherapy-induced neutropenia.[22] The most frequent antibiotics used for prophylaxis after HSCT are the fluoroquinolones, most commonly ciprofloxacin. Data from adult HSCT recipients indicate that fluoroquinolone administration prevents overgrowth of Proteobacteria within the gut microbiome, which may provide insight into how these agents reduce bloodstream infection risk.[10] Although antibiotic prophylaxis may be beneficial in HSCT recipients, there is a growing consensus that minimizing disruptions of the gut microbiome after HSCT has the potential to improve patient outcomes. Thus, although patients undergoing HSCT frequently require broad-spectrum antibiotics as empirical therapy for febrile neutropenia, antimicrobial stewardship efforts to limit the duration or spectrum of activity of antibiotics in HSCT recipients should generally be encouraged. As the feasibility of rapidly sampling the microbiome increases in the future, clinicians may be able to serially monitor the gut microbiome to identify patients at high risk of bloodstream infection and to tailor antibiotic therapy to an individual patient's microbiome.

The administration of probiotics to patients after HSCT is currently an active area of investigation, particularly as a strategy for the prevention of GVHD. Most studies conducted to date have focused on *Lactobacillus*-based probiotics because of the safety data available for these products in healthy populations. *Lactobacillus rhamnosus* GG was associated with a lower incidence of GVHD and improved survival when administered to mice after allogeneic HSCT.[23] Moreover, examination of the mesenteric lymph nodes from the mice that received this probiotic demonstrated less translocation of enteric bacteria, suggesting that this treatment improved the integrity of the gut mucosal barrier.[23] Clinical studies of probiotics in HSCT recipients have historically been limited by safety concerns of administering live microorganisms orally in the setting of severe immunosuppression and mucositis. Most notably, there are several well-documented cases of bloodstream infection caused by the microorganisms contained within probiotics among HSCT recipients and other immunocompromised patient populations. However, these complications appear to be rare and there is a growing body of literature to suggest that at least some probiotics may be safe to administer to HSCT recipients. There are currently several clinical trials studying the use of specific probiotics for GVHD prevention in children and adults after allogeneic HSCT. In particular, a double-blind randomized controlled trial of *L. plantarum* is currently being conducted through the Children's Oncology Group. This probiotic formulation was previously shown to be safe and well tolerated in a small group of children and adolescents who underwent allogeneic HSCT.[24]

The use of prebiotics or postbiotics is an appealing strategy for manipulating the gut microbiome of HSCT recipients because these products do not include live microorganisms, and thus do not carry a direct infectious risk. There is currently much interest around the use of prebiotic substances to support the growth of Clostridiales and other bacteria that produce short-chain fatty acids. These short-chain fatty acids induce regulatory T lymphocytes that are important for maintaining gut homeostasis and barrier function that may be protective for GVHD.[25] Use of oral β-lactamases is a postbiotic approach that has been proposed to minimize the effect of antibiotic exposures on the gut microbiome. Various compounds are currently in development and several were shown to prevent alterations of the gut microbiome by antibiotics and preserve the colonization resistance provided by commensal gut bacteria in non-HSCT populations.[26]

Fecal microbiome transplantation (FMT) is an alternative to the targeted approaches to modifying the gut microbiome. FMT involves transfer of an entire gut microbial community, rather than one or only a few live bacterial species, and thus has the potential to profoundly alter the recipient's gut microbiome. Several recent case series reported use of FMT in HSCT recipients. As in other populations, FMT has primarily been used as a treatment for recurrent *C. difficile* infection in patients after HSCT. In a case series of seven HSCT recipients who underwent healthy donor FMT for this indication, including five patients who were still receiving immunosuppressive therapy, no serious adverse events were reported and only one patient experienced a recurrence of *C. difficile*.[27] A clinical trial of autologous FMT, in which a fecal sample collected before HSCT is administered back to an individual after HSCT, is currently underway for the prevention of *C. difficile* infection after allogeneic HSCT. Although the efficacy of this approach remains uncertain, early data from the trial indicate that autologous FMT is effective in restoring microbial diversity to pre-HSCT levels.[28] Finally, based on data implicating the gut microbiome in the pathogenesis of GVHD, healthy donor FMT has occasionally been used with success to treat steroid-refractory or steroid-dependent gut GVHD.[29] However, there is currently little or no experience with the use of FMT during the neutropenic phase that precedes engraftment, and there are concerns that this practice could result in bacterial translocation. Norovirus infection and sepsis have been reported after FMT in other immunocompromised populations, highlighting the need to exercise caution when considering FMT in HSCT recipients.

MICROBIOME AND ONCOLOGY

We normally co-exist in a healthy equilibrium with our approximately 100 trillion commensal microbes. This balance is maintained by three primary mechanisms: colonization resistance against invasion or overgrowth of pathogens, mucosal barriers, and a robust immune system. These protective mechanisms are frequently lost in children with cancer who are receiving chemotherapy, placing these patients at high risk for serious infections from a broad range of microbes, many of which normally reside at mucosal surfaces. As described earlier, the effect of antibiotics on commensal microbes can lead to a loss of colonization resistance. In addition, there is growing evidence that chemotherapeutic agents may have direct and indirect impacts on the microbiome.

The microbiome drives the development of several types of cancer and also affects clinical responses to cancer treatments. Seminal studies in the 1990s of patients colonized with *Helicobacter pylori* demonstrated that this bacteria induces chronic gastritis that can lead to gastric cancer, and more recent studies identified associations between the microbiome and colon cancer.[30] Animal and human studies demonstrate that the commensal microbiome influences the efficacy and toxicity of some chemotherapeutic and immunotherapeutic agents, including cyclophosphamide and immune checkpoint inhibitors.[31-33] The commensal microbiome has also been implicated in the autoimmune complications of immune checkpoint inhibitors; one such case of autoimmune colitis was effectively treated with FMT.[34]

Advances in antimicrobial therapy have improved the outcomes of patients with cancer. In particular, the development of potent antibiotics against *Staphylococcus aureus* and *Pseudomonas aeruginosa* in the 1970s (e.g., methicillin and carbenicillin) provided a means to effectively combat active infection by these organisms during periods of neutropenia. More recent data suggest that use of antibacterial prophylaxis can reduce the incidence of infections from chemotherapy-induced febrile neutropenia. For instance, levofloxacin administered during periods of neutropenia prevents bacteremia and decreases the development of febrile neutropenia among pediatric patients receiving chemotherapy for leukemia.[35] However, antibiotics also have a substantial effect on commensal microbes, and a current challenge in the care of pediatric oncology patients is to effectively use antimicrobial agents to prevent and treat infections while minimizing the deleterious effects on the microbiome. A substantial proportion of serious bacterial infections in oncology patients are caused by endogenous microbes from the oropharynx (e.g., *Streptococcus* species), gastrointestinal tract (e.g., Proteobacteria, enterococci, *Candida* species), and skin (e.g., *Staphylococcus* species).[35] High-throughput sequencing technologies have sparked renewed interest in tracking the abundances of these endogenous microbes in oncology patients with the goal of predicting and preventing infections.

Mucosal barrier integrity is maintained by a protective mucus coat, epithelial cell layer, and the mucosal immune system. These components work in concert to prevent translocation of microbes across mucosal surfaces. Chemotherapy-induced mucositis is a major risk factor for bacteremia caused by endogenous microbes such as viridans group streptococci. Although most studies on the pathogenesis of chemotherapy-induced mucositis have focused on the oral mucosa, the same principles are likely to apply to mucositis occurring in other parts of the gastrointestinal tract. In a model promoted by Sonis, chemotherapy initiates free radical generation, inflammation, and epithelial cell apoptosis, leading to disruption of the oral mucosa and translocation of bacteria into the bloodstream.[36] The resulting infections—referred to as mucosal barrier injury bloodstream infections—are especially frequent in children undergoing treatment for acute myelogenous leukemia and solid tumors. Microbes and microbial components translocating across mucosal barriers lead to local and systemic inflammation. This microbial intrusion triggers an inflammatory cascade that changes the local mucosal environment to favor domination by pathogenic bacteria.[37] The importance of mucosal barrier injury in the pathogenesis of bacterial infections in oncology patients has led to the suggestion that "febrile mucositis" might be a more appropriate term to describe oncology patients with febrile neutropenia.[38]

Commensal microbes may also be important for the development of mucositis. In germ-free and selectively colonized mice, the severity of irinotecan-induced mucositis is influenced by the composition of the gut microbiome.[39] Moreover, among pediatric cancer patients, higher baseline oral microbiome diversity was associated with the development of oral mucositis, and children with mucositis had more substantial alterations in oral microbiome composition than children in whom mucositis did not develop.[40] Recent studies suggest that commensal microbes such as *Bifidobacterium* and *Lactobacillus* may prevent or ameliorate mucositis by decreasing inflammation and improving epithelial integrity.[41] The microbiome may also indirectly affect infection risk through an influence on hematopoiesis. Germ-free mice display reduced proportions and differentiation potential of specific myeloid precursor cells, and colonization of these mice with a complex microbial community corrects these defects in myelopoiesis. This suggests that the microbiome may facilitate reconstitution of the immune system after chemotherapy in pediatric oncology patients.

Recent studies evaluated the extent to which the fecal and oral microbiomes of pediatric and adult patients are influenced by a leukemia diagnosis.[42,43] The largest pediatric study characterized the gut microbiome composition of 199 children receiving treatment for acute lymphoblastic leukemia at St. Jude Children's Research Hospital.[42] Although the precise impact of cancer treatment on the microbiome requires further study, several themes have emerged. First, patients with cancer undergo a loss of diversity of their oral and gut microbiomes, often associated with domination by microbes, including enterococci, streptococci, and Enterobacteriaceae.[42] Proteobacteria such as *Escherichia coli*, which typically are of low abundance in the gut microbiome (<0.1%), can expand up to 1000-fold to dominate the gut microbiome. The gains in these potential pathogens are offset by losses of anaerobic bacteria that are important for colonization resistance. These microbiome alterations may result from a variety of factors, including the cancer itself and the associated immune system defects, treatment with antibiotics and chemotherapeutic agents, and the effects of mucositis. Second, alterations in the composition of the microbiome often precede febrile episodes and may be useful in predicting the risk of febrile neutropenia and invasive infections.[42,44] For instance, higher abundances of Proteobacteria in the gut microbiome are associated with a higher risk of febrile neutropenia among children with acute lymphoblastic leukemia.[42] Further research is needed to explore the ability of the microbiome to serve as a biomarker for the prediction of infection in pediatric oncology patients.

Treatment of children with cancer with chemotherapeutic and antimicrobial agents leads to alterations of the microbiome, a loss of mucosal barrier integrity, and depletion of the immune system that increase the risk for invasive infection. Antibiotic prophylaxis is an effective strategy for infection prevention in these patients, but this strategy can have detrimental effects on the microbiome that facilitate colonization by exogenous pathogens. Thus the judicious use of antibiotics for the prevention and treatment of infections in this patient population is likely to improve infectious outcomes.

MICROBIOME AND SOLID ORGAN TRANSPLANTATION

Long-term survival after SOT requires careful manipulation of the immune system to promote tolerance to the allograft while maintaining immunity to protect from infections. This balance is typically achieved through use of immunosuppressive medications. Recently interest has emerged in determining the extent to which commensal microbes affect outcomes after SOT. One hint that commensal microbes may modify the risk of complications after SOT is the higher rates of poor outcomes in patients receiving allografts from sites colonized by commensal microbes (e.g., intestines, lungs) compared with sterile sites (e.g., kidneys, heart), although these mucosal organs are also rich in immune cells and lymphoid tissue. Experimental evidence from germ-free mice demonstrates that commensal microbes indeed influence skin and cardiac allograft rejection.[45] Recent clinical studies indicate that commensal microbial communities change after SOT, with some data suggesting that dysbiosis affects the risk for infection and allograft rejection.

Relatively few pediatric studies have evaluated changes in the microbiome that occur during SOT, but several important concepts are emerging from studies of adults and children. First, similar to allogeneic HSCT, the microbiome is substantially altered by SOT, often characterized by lower diversity and losses of commensal microbes. For example, in a small study of the oral microbiome in pediatric liver transplantation patients, there were alterations in bacterial and fungal microbes in the first few days after liver transplantation.[46] Similarly, cardiac and renal SOT patients also experience microbial dysbiosis, although the relevant anatomic location to study the microbiome in these setting remains unclear. Second, this dysbiosis is influenced by multiple factors, including antibiotic exposures, immunosuppressive medications, anatomic changes (e.g., placement of an ileostomy in intestinal transplantation), and allograft rejection. Third, the influence of immunosuppressive medications on the microbiome varies by agent, dose, and microbiome site. Finally, targeted manipulation of the microbiome is an attractive therapeutic approach to improving outcomes after SOT, and a more complete understanding of the host-microbiome interactions will support microbiome therapeutics that can be used in clinical practice.

Acute rejection of allografts is also associated with microbial dysbiosis. For example, microbial diversity and composition were altered among patients with acute rejection after intestinal transplantation.[47] The gut microbiomes of these patients had lower abundances of Lactobacillales and higher abundances of Proteobacteria.[47] Some studies indicate that reconstitution of the pretransplant lung microbiome among lung transplant recipients protects from bronchiolitis obliterans syndrome, a form of chronic rejection.[48] Shifts in the microbiome also accompany renal transplantation, characterized by losses of diversity and increases in Bacteroidetes and Proteobacteria.[49,50] Although it remains challenging to predict how a specific patient's microbiome will affect immune system responses such as allograft rejection, there are significant potential therapeutic benefits that require further investigation.

Allograft Rejection

How might commensal microbes influence the risk of allograft rejection? The intestines and, to a lesser extent, the lungs, harbor large numbers of commensal microbes and receive direct signals from these microbial communities. Although the liver is not thought to be colonized with microbes, it receives portal blood rich in intestinal microbial components. Under certain conditions commensal microbes can translocate from the intestine and be recovered from the liver.[51] As such, intestinal, lung, and liver allografts are anatomically positioned to respond to signals from commensal microbes. In addition, commensal microbes may affect allograft tolerance by regulating activation of the innate and adaptive immune systems. Patients with mutations of toll-like receptor 4 have lower rates of bronchiolitis obliterans syndrome and renal allograft rejection, suggesting that innate immune receptor activation influences allograft rejection.[52,53] Finally, in a process referred to as "heterologous immunity," memory T cells generated from prior infections can cross-react with allograft antigens. Because antigen-specific T cells are also generated against commensal microbes, heterologous immunity may include T cells directed against commensal microbes.[54] Mouse models of allograft rejection demonstrate that the commensal microbiome primes antigen-presenting cells to activate alloreactive T cells, which ultimately leads to allograft rejection.[45] Certain microbes also affect the development of specific subsets of effector T cells, which contribute to alloreactivity. Other microbes, most notably *Bacteroides* and *Clostridium* species, promote the development of regulatory T cells that inhibit alloreactivity. Taken together, commensal microbes are critical to the maintenance of balance within the innate and adaptive immune systems, which may in turn influence the risk of allograft rejection.

Microbiome Therapeutics

Modulating communities of commensal microbes has the potential to decrease infection and allograft rejection in SOT. Several studies demonstrate that antibiotic-treated or germ-free mice have improved allograft survival.[45,55] However, the specific microbes that contribute to allograft rejection have not been identified and antibiotics may have differential effects on the microbiomes of individual patients, which make antibiotics a less appealing approach for manipulating the microbiome of SOT recipients. The administration of probiotics with or without prebiotics in the peritranplant period has also been studied in SOT recipients. A meta-analysis found that probiotics and prebiotics resulted in lower rates of urinary tract and intraabdominal infections in liver transplant recipients but had no effect on allograft rejection or all-cause mortality.[56] Although the results of these early studies are promising, more research is needed to determine the differential benefits that may result from different probiotic strains, dosing, and timing of administration in SOT recipients.

KNOWLEDGE LIMITATIONS

Despite the growing consensus regarding the importance of the gut microbiome to the outcomes of immunocompromised children, there are several limitations to current knowledge on this topic. First, much of the existing clinical data come from single-center studies of adult patients that did not account for potential confounders in microbiome data analyses. This is largely because the statistical approaches for analyzing microbiome data have lagged behind the rapid advances in sequencing technologies that have occurred over the past decade. Microbiome data are highly skewed, sparse, and when collected from the same individual over time, correlated. Currently, there are relatively few statistical methods that can take into account these unique data characteristics, adjust for confounders, and identify the microorganisms that are associated with clinical outcomes. In addition, there are a number of inconsistencies in the findings of studies evaluating the importance of the microbiome in immunocompromised patients. These could be related to differences in practice across centers, further highlighting the need for multi-institutional research, or to variation in the collection, processing, and storage of clinical samples. Finally, the majority of microbiome studies in immunocompromised patients have been conducted in adults. Distinct shifts in the gut microbiome occur during infancy and early childhood, and there are substantial differences in the treatment protocols for HSCT, SOT, and malignancies that are used for children and adults. Pediatric studies are urgently needed to more clearly define how the gut microbiome influences the outcomes of immunocompromised children.

FUTURE DIRECTIONS

Our understanding of the importance of the gut microbiome to immunocompromised children advanced rapidly over the past several decades with the development of high-throughput sequencing technologies. However, the overwhelming majority of these microbiome studies have relied on 16S rRNA gene sequencing, which typically does not have the resolution needed to classify sequencing reads to the species level. Moreover, this approach provides information only on the bacteria that are present in a sample, and specifically does not offer insight into the functional activity of these bacteria or the abundances of fungi, viruses, parasites, or archaea. Increasingly, it is apparent that strain-level differences in genetic content or gene expression can profoundly influence how microorganisms interact with the host. In the future, use of sequencing technologies that can identify microorganisms to the species or strain level and provide information on the functional activity of microorganisms promise to improve our understanding of how the microbiome influences the health of immunocompromised children.

A major goal of microbiome research is to develop therapeutics that can improve patient outcomes. To accomplish this objective, associations observed in clinical datasets must be studied in controlled settings (e.g., in vitro cell cultures, animal models) to confirm the findings and gain insight into potential mechanisms. A powerful approach is to transfer human microbes or microbial communities into germ-free animals to develop gnotobiotic model systems capable of isolating the effect of specific microbes on human diseases. Developing gnotobiotic models of the pediatric microbiome will be a powerful tool to define how microbes interact with the pediatric host. Moreover, although studies of currently available probiotics in immunocompromised children are warranted, the complexity of the gut microbial community and its myriad interactions with the host immune system suggest that a consortium of beneficial microorganisms, selected based on observations in preclinical and clinical studies, may be a promising strategy for modifying the gut microbiome of immunocompromised children.

In summary, commensal microbes have a substantial impact on pediatric HSCT, oncology, and SOT patients. The commensal microbiome modifies the risk of developing certain cancers, the response to and complications from chemotherapy and immunotherapy, and most prominently, the risk of infection and immune dysfunction, including GVHD. A deeper understanding of these dynamic interactions between commensal microbes and the immune system may facilitate the development of microbiome therapeutics that improve outcomes of these vulnerable populations of children.

11

Antimicrobial Stewardship in Immunocompromised Hosts

Joshua Wolf, MBBS, PhD, FRACP, Jeffrey S. Gerber, MD, PhD, and Michael J. Smith, MD, MSCE

Antimicrobial stewardship refers to the appropriate selection, dosing, route, and duration of antimicrobial therapy to optimize patient outcomes and minimize toxicity and the development of resistant pathogens.[1] Over the past decade, the number of pediatric antimicrobial stewardship programs (ASPs) has increased. Pediatric ASPs, which typically include dedicated pediatric infectious diseases–trained physicians and pharmacists, have expanded from freestanding children's hospitals to pediatric units within larger hospitals to less traditional settings, such as community hospitals, emergency departments, and outpatient clinics.

Although the prevalence and scope of pediatric ASPs is increasing, the optimal role of ASPs in the management of pediatric immunocompromised patient populations is less defined. Immunocompromised patients represent a small proportion of all pediatric hospitalizations but account for a large proportion of antimicrobial use. We review the goals of antimicrobial stewardship in the transplant population, barriers to its implementation, and offer specific stewardship strategies that may be useful in this population.

GOALS OF STEWARDSHIP IN IMMUNOCOMPROMISED HOSTS

The basic goals of antimicrobial stewardship in immunocompromised hosts are the same as in other children: to maximize therapeutic success by optimizing choice, dose, route, and duration of therapy while limiting unintended consequences such as adverse events and cost. Stewardship can, however, be challenging in immunocompromised hosts, particularly in the transplant population. Because of multiple previous rounds of antimicrobial therapy, which may include prophylaxis, transplant recipients are more likely to be colonized with multidrug-resistant organisms, complicating empiric antibiotic choices. And even when the conditions of these patients improve with empiric therapy, their often profound immune deficiency and comorbid conditions, some of which mimic infection, may make de-escalation difficult as well.

It is crucial that stewardship teams develop expertise in immunocompromised hosts. This requires knowledge not only of the wide array of infectious diseases affecting these patients but also the mechanisms and impact of various immunosuppressive regimens to understand the specific arm(s) of the immune system rendered vulnerable and the opportunistic infectious diseases that exploit these deficiencies. Furthermore, stewardship teams should partner with immunocompromised patient care teams, including oncology, solid organ transplant, and bone marrow transplant services, to develop a working knowledge of protocols and approach to the antimicrobial prescribing by these services. Ideally, stewardship teams should collaborate with immunocompromised patient teams to optimize antimicrobial use in these populations, not dictate unilaterally.

Conducting stewardship requires a complete assessment of the risks and benefits of antimicrobial prescribing. On the one hand, these patients are at high risk of invasive infection and should be treated aggressively. On the other hand, use of broad-spectrum agents will further drive resistance, already present at a higher rate in this population, and may contribute to development of graft-versus-host-disease and *Clostridium difficile* infection (CDI).[2] To further complicate the issue, clinicians may have different thresholds of risk. For example, the primary team may focus on the potential value of aggressive antimicrobial therapy (i.e., broader therapy for a longer duration), whereas the stewardship team may focus more on acute (e.g., organ toxicity, drug-drug interactions) and chronic (e.g., antimicrobial resistance, microbiome disruption) adverse events.

The role of antibacterial prophylaxis is a prime example of the challenges in this population. In adult hematopoietic stem cell (HSCT) recipients, the use of fluoroquinolone prophylaxis is common. The evidence is less clear in children. A recently published randomized placebo-controlled trial of levofloxacin prophylaxis administered during the first 2 cycles of chemotherapy found a significant decrease in the incidence of bacteremia for children with acute myeloid acute and relapsed lymphoblastic leukemia.[3] A smaller, nonsignificant decrease in the incidence of bacteremia was seen in the subgroup of children after HSCT. Therefore implementing prophylaxis in this population depends on how the risks of antibacterial exposure are considered compared with a potential, albeit not statistically significant, decrease in bacteremia.

Although most pediatric stewardship efforts have focused on antibacterial agents, immunocompromised hosts are at high risk for complications from fungal and viral infections. Therefore strategies for antifungal and antiviral stewardship need to be considered in this population. The significant variability in use of these medications across institutions for both prophylaxis and treatment further highlights this need. A review of 2015 data from the Pediatric Health Information System database examined antifungal and antiviral use at 47 freestanding children's hospitals.[4] Although high-risk patients accounted for less than 5% of all hospital discharges, they accounted for nearly half of the antiviral and antifungal use. Specifically, HSCT recipients accounted for 20% of all antifungal use and 24% of all antiviral use. Although this cohort was limited to high-risk patients, there was still significant variation in prescribing, demonstrating the need for stewardship of these agents. Antivirals and antifungals are ideal targets for stewardship interventions because they are often inappropriately prescribed, have narrow therapeutic windows, and are costly. Although the most important strategies for antifungal and antiviral stewardship remain to be elucidated, therapeutic drug monitoring and development of protocols for fungal prophylaxis are examples.

Diagnostic stewardship is another important consideration. In otherwise healthy children, the use of rapid diagnostics has decreased time to optimal therapy, leading to better patient outcomes.[5] Several studies have documented that having a stewardship pharmacist to act on results of these tests is more effective than the mere availability of the results.[6] In addition to helping interpret these test results, stewardship teams can have an active role in determining criteria for laboratory test ordering. Unnecessary testing can lead to increased costs as well as to treatment of organisms that are normal colonizers and not true pathogens.

Other stewardship goals include the reduction of redundant antimicrobial coverage, promotion of the oral route of antibiotics over the intravenous route, and prevention of CDI.

BARRIERS TO ANTIMICROBIAL STEWARDSHIP PROGRAMS IN IMMUNOCOMPROMISED CHILDREN

Understanding barriers and challenges to effective antimicrobial stewardship, especially those that differ between targets and populations, is important to planning, implementing, modifying, and evaluating a stewardship program. Barriers to antimicrobial stewardship in immunocompromised pediatric patients may be similar to those in other populations, but there are some unique aspects.[7-9] Issues particularly challenging to stewardship efforts in the immunocompromised population include the lack of evidence or consensus for optimal prevention and treatment of infection, diagnostic uncertainty, medical complexity and risk of severe or life-threatening infections, and the relatively high risk of antimicrobial-resistant infections.

Paucity of Evidence for Prevention and Management of Infections

Although evidence for management of some infectious syndromes in immunocompromised children exists,[3,10-12] it is the exception rather than the rule. For example, despite intensive research, optimal management of febrile neutropenia in children with cancer remains controversial.[12] The aim of empiric management is to provide immediate, appropriate therapy to prevent progression to sepsis and its associated morbidity and mortality. One issue is stratification of risk for neutropenic children when fever is the presenting symptom, which drives initial antimicrobial therapy decisions. Significant work has attempted to design a system that uses clinical signs, symptoms, and laboratory tests to identify which patients with febrile neutropenia have an underlying serious infection requiring broad-spectrum antibiotic therapy.[13] However, in contrast to effective protocols in adults,[14] many pediatric approaches have performed poorly in validation attempts, and those that have been validated are poorly specific or require collection of relatively large amounts of local data to recalibrate before implementation at each institution.[15] Furthermore, although it seems reasonable that a formal decision support system might be safe and improve antimicrobial use, this has not yet been shown. This lack of evidence can lead to widespread use of unnecessarily broad empiric antimicrobial therapy. Other areas where evidence is lacking include duration of therapy for infections or fever in immunocompromised children,[16] appropriate antibiotic treatment of infectious intraabdominal syndromes such as colitis/typhlitis,[17,18] and the long-term safety or efficacy of antibacterial prophylaxis.[3,19,20]

Diagnostic Uncertainty

There are also difficulties associated with diagnostic tools for infection in immunocompromised hosts. This is problematic because stewardship interventions often rely on identification of a clear clinical syndrome (e.g., by diagnostic imaging) or demonstration of a microbiologic etiology for infection. Most episodes of fever in this population, however, have no etiology identified,[21] and serious infection can exist even without localizing signs or symptoms.[22] One example is lung infection, for which microbiologic diagnostics have low yield for bacterial and fungal etiologies across pediatric populations.[23] However, because the differential diagnosis is broader in immunocompromised patients and the required treatment duration may be longer, the potential impact of diagnostic uncertainty is amplified in this population. Efforts to improve this by early use of bronchoalveolar lavage or biopsy[24,25] have met resistance from clinicians concerned about diagnostic yield, risk-benefit ratio, and cost-effectiveness.[26,27] The phenomenon of poor diagnostic tools in the context of a broad differential diagnosis also applies to a number of other infections, including skin and soft tissue infections, intraabdominal infections, presumed disseminated invasive fungal infections, and persistent fever without source, all of which can be associated with prolonged courses of broad-spectrum antimicrobials without a clear need. This issue is further confounded by the problem of discriminating graft-versus-host-disease and organ rejection from infection in transplant patients.

Contributing to this problem of diagnostic uncertainty is the relative dearth of accurate diagnostic tests for the pediatric immunocompromised population. For example, biomarkers, such as C-reactive protein and procalcitonin, which have been successful in discrimination of patients with bacterial infection from those with viral infection or no infection in some populations, appear to be unreliable in immunocompromised children, possibly because of their altered immune response to infection.[28] Similarly, diagnostic tests that are sensitive and specific for invasive fungal infection in immunocompromised adults, such as (1,3)-β-D-glucan and specific findings on computed tomography scans, perform poorly in children, leading to a high rate of "presumed" fungal infection.[29,30]

Concerns for Polymicrobial or Multiple Infections

Improved diagnostics may not completely solve the problems associated with diagnostic uncertainty. Early data suggesting that use of narrow-spectrum antibiotics for treatment of susceptible infections in profoundly immunocompromised hosts was associated with a high risk of breakthrough infection have contributed to a culture of maintaining broad-spectrum coverage, even when a causative organism is recognized.[12,31] Similarly, improved diagnosis of viral pneumonia in immunocompromised hosts may not lead to reduced antibiotic use because of concerns about undiagnosed polymicrobial infection.[32]

Provider Autonomy and the Stewardship Team

A number of barriers to stewardship have been attributed in the literature to differing approaches between the stewardship team and the primary clinicians caring for immunocompromised patients—for example, transplant physicians, surgeons, and oncologists.[8,9,33,34] It is important to note that many of these factors are subjective and are reported as perceived barriers by stewardship clinicians. The most frequently reported barrier is that, perhaps because of the frequency of serious infections in this population, primary clinicians may be more concerned about rare adverse infection outcomes than about long-term risks or financial costs related to antibiotic use. This may lead to excessive or inappropriate antimicrobial use.[35] Concern about loss of autonomy by allowing external input into routine patient management may also be an issue. ASP clinicians report that their efforts to improve antimicrobial use are hindered by insufficient input into local or protocol-related treatment guidelines. Lastly, it is important to note that despite some positive effects of antimicrobial stewardship interventions in immunocompromised populations, inappropriate prescribing typically persists, albeit at a somewhat lower level.[36-38]

End-of-Life Care

Although the overall chance of long-term survival is high for many immunocompromised pediatric patients, some will enter into palliative care. During the period of palliative care, inappropriate antimicrobial prescribing is common. This can occur because antibiotics are considered harmless or benign, so continuing these can be a way of maintaining treatment even when no therapy is available for the primary disease. This is supported by multiple studies showing that antibiotics are frequently administered at the end of life, often without undertaking appropriate tests and without an infectious disease diagnosis.[39,40]

Antimicrobial Stewardship Programs

Most pediatric antimicrobial stewardship clinicians report that improving antimicrobial use in immunocompromised children is a priority for their program and that they believe that they have sufficient experience in infections in this population.[9] However, because of the issues described earlier, interventions in this population can be extremely time intensive, which can be challenging in environments where only limited stewardship resources are available.[41] Importantly, it seems that not all stewardship providers are equivalent in the immunocompromised setting. In one study, an effective stewardship program became markedly less effective after trainee specialists were substituted for the attending physicians who had originally performed the interventions.[42,43] This suggests that academic or institutional authority may be an important component to stewardship in this population; insufficient power or authority has been previously identified as an issue by ASP clinicians in an international survey.[9] Lastly, it is important to note that building trust with primary clinicians relies on accurate recommendations, and there is evidence that infectious diseases clinicians may underestimate the risk of serious infection related to specific patient presentations, which could lead to inappropriate ASP interventions and erode trust.[35]

STRATEGIES AND TACTICS FOR STEWARDSHIP IN IMMUNOCOMPROMISED HOSTS

Despite these barriers, many centers have developed stewardship initiatives in their immunocompromised populations. Seo and colleagues surveyed 127 adult and pediatric HSCT centers, 107 of which also performed SOT, about their stewardship practices.[44] Responses were received from 71 (56%) centers, of which 62 had active ASPs. Of the centers surveyed, 12 were freestanding children's hospitals, but pediatric-specific results were not reported separately. Survey responses were reported separately for HSCT and SOT, but there were no significant differences in use of specific strategies between these two patient populations.

Formulary restriction and guideline development were the most common interventions and were used by more than 70% of the responding centers. Prospective audit with feedback, education, and dose optimization and prior authorization were also common. Most stewardship strategies were adapted from Infectious Diseases Society of America recommendations for development of stewardship programs in general.[1] Few data exist to determine optimal stewardship strategies in transplant patients, with even fewer data in the pediatric transplant population.

Horikoshi and colleagues report the impact of ASP activities on the hematology/oncology and HSCT units of a metropolitan hospital in Tokyo, Japan.[45] The ASP started with postprescription review of carbapenems, then expanded to include prior authorization for carbapenems and other activities, such as prospective audit with feedback, therapeutic drug monitoring, selective reporting, guidelines for febrile neutropenia, weekly educational series, and implementation of molecular diagnosis for viral infections. Results were not reported separately for oncology and HSCT patients, but the HSCT unit accounted for 36,150 of 49,642 (73%) total patient-days during the study period. Although it is not possible to determine which specific component had the most impact, stewardship bundles led to significant decreases in days of therapy. Notably, there was no difference in infection-related or all-cause mortality associated with this decrease in antibiotic use.

Clinical guideline development is another key stewardship strategy that has been shown to be successful in pediatric transplant patients. Wattier and colleagues reported a decrease in use of second gram-negative antibiotic therapy after creation of a dedicated HSCT fever and neutropenia guideline at a tertiary care children's hospital.[36] Before guideline development, ciprofloxacin and tobramycin were frequently used as double gram-negative coverage. Using time-series analysis, the authors describe a 99% level change decrease for tobramycin and a 95% decrease for ciprofloxacin. Importantly, there was no increase in mortality associated with these reductions in second gram-negative coverage. The protocol for general oncology patients was separate from that for HSCT recipients, highlighting the importance of specific unit and provider group-based guidelines.

Other guidelines commonly used in the transplant population include those for antifungal prophylaxis, treatment for invasive fungal infection, and cytomegalovirus prophylaxis and treatment.[36] De-escalation is another strategy that may benefit from development of a specific guideline. Although challenging in this population, de-escalation may be more likely to be achieved if there is an agreed-upon protocol in place with objective indicators to identify in which patients de-escalation may be safe. Regardless of the specific topic, it is critical to identify key partners on the respective transplant teams to realize the value of stewardship and ensure that the goals of the stewardship and primary teams remained aligned.

Some centers develop individualized treatment plans for patients who are known to be colonized with multidrug-resistant organisms, leading to more appropriate empiric prescribing. Furthermore, by encouraging discussions between the stewardship, infectious diseases and transplant teams before a child becomes ill, this activity in and of itself can help establish a culture of collaboration.

Other strategies less commonly used in the transplant population include the use of automatic stop dates, use of order forms, and antibiotic cycling.[44] Allergy delabeling is another promising stewardship strategy that may be effective in transplant recipients. In the adult oncology population, the presence of β-lactam allergies had been shown to be associated with worse clinical outcomes and increased cost.[46] Although not specifically studied in this population, these findings likely extend to immunocompromised pediatric patients who often require long-term broad-spectrum therapy. It would be beneficial to determine which children have true antibiotic allergies using a combination of patient questionnaires and penicillin skin testing before transplantation to optimize correct antimicrobial use.

STEWARDSHIP METRICS IN THE TRANSPLANT POPULATION

In their survey of transplant centers, Seo and colleagues reported that the rate of CDI was the most common outcome measured by ASPs in the transplant setting, followed by antimicrobial cost.[44] Antimicrobial use was only measured by 34% of HSCT centers and 27% of SOT centers; 23% of centers reported that they did not follow any stewardship outcomes in transplant patients.

Rates of antimicrobial resistance were less commonly measured but should be considered as an important metric. Because of the frequent use and escalating breadth of antimicrobial therapy in the transplant population, patients are likely to become colonized with more resistant pathogens. Some hospitals produce transplant-unit specific antibiograms to capture this information.[44] However, because transplant patients often spend time in and out of the intensive care unit, emergency department, and outpatient clinics, it can be difficult to attribute their pathogens to a specific patient unit. At least one center uses SOT patient-specific compared to unit-specific antibiograms to overcome this issue.[47]

Although some metrics, such as rates of CDI, methicillin-resistant Staphylococcus aureus, vancomycin-resistant enterococci, and antimicrobial cost, are required to be reported, it is important to measure outcomes that are of importance to the transplant teams. This will further serve to build confidence and trust in the stewardship program.

CONCLUSION AND FUTURE RESEARCH

Pediatric HSCT and SOT recipients are important targets for antimicrobial stewardship efforts. There are limited published data to determine the optimal stewardship interventions in this population, but the general strategies outlined in the Infectious Diseases Society of America stewardship guidelines are a reasonable place to start.[1]

Several topics appear well-suited for further study. For example, ongoing pediatric studies of duration of therapy for common infections, such as pneumonia, urinary tract infection, and uncomplicated bacteremia, need to be extended into the immunocompromised host. Additionally, when appropriate, adult transplant initiatives should be extended into the pediatric age group. For example, a recent study of early de-escalation of broad-spectrum antibiotics in adult HSCT recipients with febrile neutropenia and negative culture results found that this strategy did not lead to worse clinical outcomes and successfully decreased days of therapy and the incidence of CDI.[16] Given the relatively small number of pediatric transplants at the national level, multicenter collaborative efforts are needed to answer these important questions.

12

Hospital Infection Prevention for Pediatric Transplant Recipients and Oncology Patients

Ibukunoluwa C. Akinboyo, MD and Dawn Nolt, MD, MPH

GENERAL PRINCIPLES

Children with deficient immune mechanisms, immunologic disorders, or those receiving immunosuppressive therapy (e.g., radiation, cytotoxic chemotherapy, antirejection medication, and steroids) are identified as high-risk patients with the greatest risk of acquiring healthcare-associated infections. Patients in this subset include those who are severely neutropenic for prolonged periods of time (i.e., an absolute neutrophil count ≤500 cells/mL), allogeneic hematopoietic stem cell transplantation (HSCT) patients, and those who have received intensive chemotherapy.[1] Treatment of infection is usually difficult, making prevention strategies paramount.

Handwashing remains the simplest, most effective method of preventing infections, and efforts should be made to optimize proper hand hygiene using soap and water or alcohol-based sanitizers among patients, healthcare workers (HCWs), and visitors, including families. Hands should be washed at hospital room entry and exit. Hand hygiene should also be performed before and after manipulating catheters or performing procedures. Standard precautions, including the use of gloves while handling body fluids, respiratory etiquette, and safe injection practices, should be instituted as part of routine care for hospitalized patients.[2]

Other infection prevention strategies incorporate personal protective equipment (PPE) to minimize modes of pathogen transmission that may vary based on pathogen class. These strategies may be transmission based (i.e., acute clinical syndromes such as diarrhea, meningitis and respiratory tract infections) and should trigger contact and/or droplet isolation precaution that typically includes donning of PPE (i.e., barrier gowns, gloves, and/or masks) when appropriate. The important routes of transmission include contact (i.e., direct transmission from infected person to uninfected person with or without an intermediary object or person, such as contaminated hands of HCWs or contaminated surfaces of hospital equipment) droplet (i.e., a more extensive form of contact transmission that involves exposure to infected respiratory droplets >5 μm in size from expectorated sputum, coughs, or sneezes), and airborne (i.e., transmission of either airborne droplet nuclei or small particles that remain infective over time and distance).[1,2]

Although some pathogens can be transmitted by more than one route, some of the more common examples of organisms transmitted via contact include *Staphylococcus aureus* and *Clostridium difficile,* whereas most respiratory viruses (e.g., influenza) are transmitted via droplet. *Mycobacterium tuberculosis* is a common example of an infection with airborne transmission. Airborne transmission could also occur with environmental pathogens such as fungal spores. Other environmental sources of infection include aerosolized water or ingestion of contaminated water, food, or medications, although standard hospital safety practices should limit these exposures. Numerous guidelines exist to assist with developing appropriate transmission-based precautions and duration of isolation for immunocompromised patients within a healthcare system.[2] Extending the period of isolation for the duration of the hospital stay or until documented clearance of infection may be necessary for respiratory viruses or other transmissible infections owing to prolonged shedding of viruses that can occur in immunocompromised patients. Prevention of vector-borne infections that might spread within a healthcare system or in limited-resource settings is beyond the scope of this chapter.

Close collaboration with a healthcare epidemiologist is important to achieve the shared aims of improving patient safety, performing active monitoring, reporting healthcare-associated infections (HAIs) and promoting strategies that support quality, evidence-based medical care.[3] Within an established culture of safety, the infrastructure for hospital epidemiology should have the capacity for investigation and management of HAIs and should be optimized for rapid outbreak identification.[2,4] Ideal programs incorporate HAI surveillance and antibiotic stewardship.[4] Instituting a culture of safety where all members of the workforce combine efforts to prevent infections, avoid system errors, and adhere to infection prevention practices is pivotal to successfully preventing transmission of healthcare-associated pathogens to immunocompromised patients.

IMPORTANCE OF HEALTHCARE-ASSOCIATED INFECTIONS SURVEILLANCE

The Centers for Disease Control and Prevention (CDC) National Healthcare Safety Network (NHSN) has determined that certain preventable healthcare-associated infections should be actively monitored and reported to federal agencies with a potential to impact reimbursement.[5,6] Surgical site infections and *C. difficile* infections can be consistently determined for hospitalized patients regardless of immune status.

Indwelling catheter use is almost ubiquitous in the oncology and transplant populations owing to their chronic medication administrations and laboratory assessment needs. Stringent adherence to established practices for maintaining central catheters and urinary catheters is advised.[6-8] Nevertheless, central line–associated bloodstream infections (CLABSIs) continue to rank among the most common of HAIs reported to the NHSN. Providers for immunocompromised pediatric patients have often argued that NHSN surveillance definitions may not appropriately characterize the nature of bloodstream infections in immunocompromised hosts, given underlying mucosal and immune defects. To accommodate for some of these concerns, the NHSN adjusted surveillance definitions to incorporate Mucosal Barrier Injury Laboratory-Confirmed Bloodstream Infection.[6] This surveillance definition incorporates risk factors, such as allogeneic hematopoietic stem cell transplant recipients within the past year with high-grade gastrointestinal (GI) graft-versus-host-disease [GI GVHD], recent onset of voluminous (such as ≥1 L stool measured in a 24-hour period), and ongoing neutropenia (defined as at least 2 separate days with absolute neutrophil count and/or white blood cell values less than 500 cells/mm^3 collected within a 7-day period.)[6] These criteria allow infection prevention professionals the ability to determine if bloodstream infections in certain individuals may not be entirely preventable.

Obtaining routinely scheduled surveillance blood cultures is not recommended and may cause more long-term harm if it leads to recovery of skin contaminants and subsequent inappropriate use of antibiotics. Outside NHSN-defined surveillance, medical providers and infection prevention professionals should be aware that there may be atypical clinical presentations of infectious diseases in immunocompromised patients. Each healthcare facility should have a low internal threshold to initiate an investigation if there is an increased number of common infections or unique pathogens within transplant and oncology patients. For example, a single case of *Legionella* pneumonia acquired during a hospitalization or two cases of adenovirus conjunctivitis in immunocompromised hosts within a short period should warrant an immediate investigation to mitigate a possible outbreak.

TABLE 12.1 Summary of Recommendations to Prevent Healthcare-Associated Infections in Pediatric Immunocompromised Patients

Patient Population	Healthcare-Associated Pathogens	Infection Prevention Recommendations
Hematopoietic stem cell transplant	Viruses *Aspergillus* *C. difficile* MDROs	Handwashing Visitor restriction Herd immunization Water quality HEPA filtration Effective environmental cleaning Limitation of aerosolized water, use of carpets, exposure to animals. and live plants Positive-pressure rooms and ≥12 air exchanges/hour
Solid organ transplant	Viruses *Candida* MDROs	Handwashing Herd immunization Effective environmental cleaning
Oncology	Viruses MDROs *C. difficile*	Handwashing Visitor restriction Herd immunization Effective environmental cleaning

C. difficile, *Clostridium difficile*; *HEPA*, high-efficiency particulate air; *MDROs*, multidrug-resistant organisms.

PATHOGEN-SPECIFIC INFECTION PREVENTION STRATEGIES

Infections in immunocompromised patients are often derived from pathogens colonizing the skin, such as *S. aureus* or *Streptococcus* species; colonizing the GI tract, such as *Escherichia coli* and *Pseudomonas aeruginosa*; and from the environment, such as *Aspergillus* species. Although emerging pathogens (e.g., *Candida auris*) or imported highly transmissible pathogens (e.g., viral hemorrhagic fevers) can infect HSCT, oncology, and organ transplant patients, aligning prevention efforts with the institution's infection prevention department should help with preparation for and mitigation of these possible exposures. Efforts to decrease the risk of invasive infections in immunocompromised hosts should focus on areas in which interventions have been shown to decrease exposure or colonization with these microorganisms. Table 12.1 provides a summary of guidelines to prevent HAIs in pediatric immunocompromised patients.

Legionella

This pathogen is the prototypical microbe to highlight transmission of water-borne infections to the immunocompromised host. *Legionella* is a water-borne gram-negative pathogen associated with symptoms that range from a mild febrile illness to pneumonia with respiratory distress. Healthcare-associated transmission of laboratory-confirmed Legionnaires' disease, defined as infection in patients hospitalized for 10 days or longer before confirming diagnosis, has been described among HSCT recipients.[9,10] Transmission occurs through inhalation of aerosolized water particles or exposure to contaminated water. Many published reports note that fountains, showers, water fixtures, and nonaerated faucets have been implicated as the source of outbreaks of water-borne illness. Other organisms with similar transmission routes include *P. aeruginosa, Burkholderia cepacia,* and *Stenotrophomonas maltophilia*. Methods to mitigate risk and curtail outbreaks are detailed in the "Water Quality" section later in the text.

Staphylococcus aureus and Vancomycin-Resistant Enterococci

S. aureus and Enterococci species are ubiquitous in the healthcare environment. The clinical impact of these bacteria includes severe infections in immunocompromised patients, although there remain conflicting data on whether these high-risk populations have increased mortality compared with immunocompetent children.

S. aureus, including methicillin-resistant *S. aureus* (MRSA), is an important cause of morbidity in pediatric immunocompromised patients. Staphylococcal infections in pediatric oncology and HSCT patients are predominately invasive and catheter associated, with a high rate (18%) of complications, not specifically associated with MRSA.[11] In up to 5% of pediatric solid organ transplant (SOT) recipients in whom *S. aureus* infections developed, half of the isolates were identified as MRSA.[11] Despite these reported infections, studies are not entirely supportive of the necessity or timing of MRSA screening and decolonization to reduce infections.

The incidence of infections secondary to vancomycin-resistant *Enterococcus* (VRE) is relatively low among immunocompromised patients and the impact on morbidity and mortality may vary according to the underlying medical or clinical condition. In one registry-based population study, HSCT recipients who experienced VRE bacteremia demonstrated decreased 1-year survival and increased nonrelapsed mortality compared with patients with non-VRE bacteremia, but study findings are limited by the exclusion of known contributing factors, such as GVHD, in the analysis.[12] Among SOT recipients, a meta-analysis reviewing VRE colonization demonstrated that pre- and post-transplant VRE colonization portends a statistically significant risk for VRE infection among transplant recipients.[13]

Accepted infection prevention practices to limit the transmission of multidrug-resistant organisms such as MRSA and VRE include use of PPE (i.e., donning gowns and gloves before caring for a colonized patient).[14] One publication suggests that the routine use of contact isolation to prevent transmission of VRE may not be necessary, although study limitations (exclusion of noninvasive infection, adult population) preclude generalization of these findings to the pediatric population.[15]

S. aureus decolonization, using topical antibiotics to eradicate nasal colonization, is recommended in critically ill patients admitted to the intensive care unit as it decreases the incidence of invasive *S. aureus* infections during their hospitalization.[4,16] There are few studies assessing the utility of screening and routine decolonization of transplant and oncology patients except in the case of preoperative decolonization. Case-by-case decision making for the use of mupirocin for decolonization may be warranted. Although the debate continues on the utility of contact isolation to limit transmission of MRSA and VRE, facilities housing immunocompromised patients should closely monitor for increased incidence of disease if contact isolation for MRSA and VRE is not routinely used.

Clostridium difficile

C. difficile is a bacteria that causes infections in patients with prolonged exposure to antibiotics or exposure to the healthcare system, most of whom are immunocompromised patients. *C. difficile* has been responsible for numerous healthcare-associated outbreaks, even within immunocompetent hosts. The particular strain, toxinotype III, North American pulsed-field type 1, and PCR ribotype 027 (NAP1/027), known to produce large amounts of toxin A and B, has been identified in these outbreaks across the globe.[1] Reduction of antimicrobial use is the predominant modifiable risk factor that decreases the risk for *C. difficile* infection. An infrastructure that supports infection prevention and antibiotic stewardship to reduce HAIs such as *C. difficile* is ideal. In addition, appropriate hand hygiene with soap and water before and after contact with a patient is recommended. Some experts support the use of an alcohol-based hand sanitizer in non-outbreak settings. Contact precautions (i.e., PPE of gown and gloves) should be used by HCWs caring for transplant and oncology patients infected with *C. difficile*.[10,17]

C. difficile spores may persist within the healthcare environment; optimal cleaning of infected patient rooms using a bleach-containing disinfectant (5000 ppm) is advised.[1] During endemic outbreaks or in hospital units with high rates of healthcare-associated *C. difficile*, terminal cleaning with a sporicidal agent and preferential use of soap and water for handwashing are recommended. Other modalities for cleaning and disinfection, such as ultraviolet germicidal irradiation and vaporized hydrogen peroxide, have shown promising results, but data are insufficient at this time to make firm conclusions for use in routine or outbreak settings. Compared to MRSA and VRE isolation, there is little debate and some evidence to support the necessity of contact isolation to decrease transmission of *C. difficile*.[17]

Multidrug-Resistant Gram-Negative Organisms

Microorganisms resistant to one or more classes of commercially available antimicrobial agents are described as multidrug-resistant organisms (MDROs). Gram-negative organisms are emerging as epidemiologically important pathogens owing to the high rate of healthcare-associated transmission, the increasing number of outbreaks, and the increased mortality rates associated with invasive infections in children.[18] Risk factors independently associated with developing a severe infection with an MDRO, specifically carbapenem-resistant *Klebsiella pneumoniae,* include recent organ or stem cell transplantation, prolonged length of hospital stay, and extensive use of antibiotics, all of which are often present in the pediatric immunocompromised population.[19] A carbapenem-resistant Enterobacteriaceae (CRE) infection develops in up to 10% of SOT recipients if they reside in a CRE-endemic area.[20] Preventing the spread of these pathogens has now been listed as an urgent priority by the CDC.[14]

Prevention strategies should incorporate efforts to delay the advent of resistance by promoting judicious broad-spectrum antimicrobial use in highly vulnerable patients. Performing surveillance cultures of the perianal and rectal regions of at-risk patients can identify patients colonized with MDROs and preemptive cohorting or contact isolation may prevent healthcare-associated exposures.[19] Surveillance of CRE or carbapenem-resistant *Klebsiella pneumoniae* and ongoing implementation of bundled infection prevention practices, including hand hygiene, preemptive use of contact precautions for colonized patients, and multidisciplinary teams to monitor adherence to recommendations are part of a comprehensive program to minimize the impact of MDROs.[2,21]

Mycobacteria

Nontuberculous mycobacteria are ubiquitous in the environment and outbreaks have been well described in immunocompromised patients. Transmission may occur through contact with soil or contaminated water. Over a 10-year period, investigators at a U.S.-based cancer treatment institution described clinical risk factors associated with rapidly growing mycobacteria infections, typically within 7 days of culture incubation, in patients with cancer. Although few clinical cases occurred (2.9 per 100,000 patient-days), disease in 59% of patients was diagnosed from respiratory specimen cultures and most infections occurred in SOT patients.[22] Continued assessment of air and water quality (see later text) is needed to decrease the burden of particulates or spores in healthcare areas housing immunocompromised patients. Screening HCWs for *M. tuberculosis* should be based on local prevalence and regulations.[14]

Opportunistic Mold

Opportunistic molds (such as *Aspergillus*) cause significant morbidity and mortality in immunocompromised patients, although mortality rates are highly variable according to the underlying condition of the affected patient population and the advent of antifungal prophylaxis. Opportunistic molds are associated with dusty or moist environmental conditions, such as those found in construction areas. Contribution of the healthcare environment to an invasive fungal infection of a patient is hampered by the unknown incubation period of *Aspergillus* and the threshold spore count necessary for infection. Prevention strategies to protect patients against mold infections should include minimization of dust accumulation and dust disturbance.

Viruses

Pediatric patients are at high risk for transmissible viral infections, especially during seasonal outbreaks. The all-cause mortality among pediatric HSCT recipients who were hospitalized with a respiratory viral infection over a 3-year period was as high as 11%, suggesting significant contribution to outcomes after HSCT.[23] Over a similar period and among more than 1000 pediatric SOT patients hospitalized with respiratory viral infections, intestinal/abdominal transplant recipients (38%) were most often affected; however, case fatality within 3 months of infection was lower (4%) than HSCT recipients.[24] Reverse droplet precautions, where all HCWs wear masks before interactions with neutropenic patients during respiratory viral seasons, are used in various institutions, but no available evidence supports this practice. Early identification of immunocompromised hosts with viral infections and implementation of contact and droplet precautions may attenuate healthcare-associated viral transmission.[25] Limiting exposure to ill HCWs and visitors may help with preventing respiratory viral infections. Routine surveillance for community-acquired respiratory viruses in asymptomatic immunocompromised patients is not advised.

Nonrespiratory viruses also affect the pediatric immunocompromised host. Gastrointestinal (GI) viruses may be acquired from the community (e.g., norovirus) or represent reactivation (e.g., adenovirus, cytomegalovirus). Healthcare-associated transmission of norovirus and adenovirus have been reported in patient populations with oncologic disease and recipients of HSCT and solid organs.[26,27] The presence of GI viruses in immunocompromised patients, regardless of clinical suspicion as to the primary etiology of a diarrheal illness or merely intestinal shedding, should prompt the appropriate isolation precautions to minimize transmission to other vulnerable patients. Although prolonged intestinal shedding is well known to occur in immunocompromised patients, it is unclear whether isolation needs to be extended past resolution of diarrheal symptoms to minimize transmission.

Transmission of viruses, historically known as blood-borne (human immunodeficiency virus, hepatitis B, hepatitis C), have largely been eliminated through national screening programs. Expansion of the screening panel (e.g., inclusion of West Nile Virus) or temporary inclusion of emerging pathogens (Zika virus) further ensures the safety of the blood supply to all patients.

Vaccine-preventable viruses, namely varicella-zoster and measles, can cause virulent infections in immunocompromised patients. Centers with declining community vaccine rates (and likely low herd immunity) may consider restricting incompletely vaccinated children from visiting pediatric transplant units. Sufficient data to support the use of airborne precautions and in tandem N95 masks by vaccinated HCWs to prevent transmission of measles and varicella-zoster viruses do not currently exist. Some have suggested that surgical masks and PPE may be sufficient. However, for consistency among HCWs and to avoid confusion, some facilities may opt to use airborne precautions for all patients being evaluated for or currently being treated for specific viral infections. To comply with airborne precautions and prevent inhalation of infected particles, HCWs should have scheduled fit testing to confirm their ability to use a respirator with N95 or higher filtration.[2]

GOOD PRACTICE RECOMMENDATIONS

Policies Regarding Sick Providers

HCWs with highly transmissible infections, such as GI illnesses, acute influenza-like illness, and exposed skin lesions, should be advised to limit direct patient care for transplant or oncology patients. These syndromes may allow for pathogen spread via contact, droplet, or airborne transmission. HCW restriction should last for the duration of the illness or until clearance is obtained from occupational health or according to national published guidelines.[10]

Vaccinations of Healthcare Workers and Close Contacts

A general principle of infectious diseases and infection prevention is the use of vaccinations as a protective measure. Immunization of selected groups of immunocompromised patients with inactivated/killed vaccines can provide a measure of protection. Herd immunity of HCWs and family members of immunocompromised hosts maintains the protective environment within and outside of the hospital. Recommended vaccinations for family members, close contacts, and HCWs include hepatitis A, influenza, polio, measles-mumps-rubella, *Haemophilus influenzae*, varicella, tetanus, diphtheria, and pertussis.[10]

Visitation Policies

Visitation recommendations may vary among institutions housing immunocompromised patients. Policies regarding visitation should be made in consultation with a multidisciplinary team, including local pediatric infection prevention, nursing, physician, and ancillary staff. At a minimum, policies should restrict ill individuals unless they are critical to the care of the immunocompromised patient. Some facilities restrict visitation based on age, season, or total number of persons allowed in the patient's room at any given time and for a specific duration. These restrictions are based, in part, on concerns that asymptomatic visitors may shed and transmit viruses to patients. Visitor restriction should be balanced with the benefits of the emotional well-being of the patient. Visitor screening could be a useful component to visitation and should assess for immunization status, active symptoms, and recent exposure to possible communicable infections.

Animal Safety

Animals may be encountered in a healthcare setting. Therapy animals serve a beneficial purpose within a healthcare setting, but this benefit should be balanced with risks of transmission of pathogens from the animal's fur, mouth, and paws. These pathogens may originate directly from the animal (such as *Salmonella*, *Pasteurella*, or *Capnocytophaga*) or be acquired as the animal passes through the healthcare facility (such as *S. aureus*). Professionally trained animals should be handled according to institutional policies. It may be prudent to restrict access to therapy animals if patients are immunocompromised, although no formal recommendation addresses this particular situation.[28] A published guidance on animals in healthcare settings showed that up to a third of centers with policies on animal-assisted activities excluded therapy animals from immunocompromised patients, although the definition of those patients may vary (e.g., neutropenia, HSCT pre-engraftment, asplenia).[28] At a minimum, excellent hand hygiene before and after touching/encountering the animal is advised. Animals such as birds and reptiles should be restricted from hospital units owing to the high risk of colonization with infectious organisms. Visitation by an individual's personal pet should be restricted, although end-of-life decisions may be made on a case-by-case basis.

Good Bathing Practices: Showers and Wipes

Personal hygiene is important for prevention of infections from endogenous skin flora. The use of showers has been controversial, as several studies implicate aerosols from showerheads in outbreaks of water-borne pathogens.[29] No formal recommendation against prohibition of showers in immunocompromised patients exist, although shower restrictions may be implemented if there is concern for an outbreak. Experts recommend running showers for up to 10 minutes during routine hospital room cleaning to limit accumulation of stagnant water in showerheads.

Chlorhexidine gluconate (CHG), a commonly used skin antiseptic, is an integral part of catheter insertion and maintenance practices within hospitals. However, data are inconclusive on the use of daily bathing with chlorhexidine-containing products as a means of reducing bloodstream infections in immunocompromised patients. Reported decreases in infections may be largely dependent on decreased blood culture contamination with skin commensals such as coagulase-negative staphylococci, but one multicenter, cluster-randomized study showed statistically significant decreased rates of MDRO (MRSA, VRE) colonization and infection after implementation of CHG bathing with minimal adverse effects in HSCT patients.[30] Despite potential limited utility and reports of mild skin irritation with frequent CHG use and restricted use in premature infants, chlorhexidine remains a safe and effective option for skin cleansing in immunocompromised pediatric patients and could be implemented for critically ill patients or those who are unable to shower.[30,31]

Toys

Toys are commonly colonized with bacteria, and publications regarding outbreaks within pediatric oncology units have implicated toys.[32] There have been no reports of shared toys as an underlying factor in a mold outbreak; however, contaminated bath toys have been implicated in outbreaks of *P. aeruginosa*.[2] Encouraging single-use toys or shared toys with nonporous surfaces that can be easily cleaned or washed is recommended. Manufacturer claims about antimicrobial properties of soft toys or hard toy covers may need to be evaluated further. Guidance is published on appropriate cleaning of toys by the CDC.[33]

Food Safety

Food safety should always be a priority, especially for immunocompromised patients. Food may be a vehicle for bacterial contamination with *E. coli* and *Salmonella*. Immunocompromised patients should avoid raw fruits and vegetables that cannot be effectively washed, peeled, or cooked.[34]

Mask Use in Patients During Ambulation or Transportation Within Hospitals

The issue of whether masks (particularly N95 respirators) should be routinely worn by patients outside hospital or clinic rooms is unresolved.[34,35] Risk factors for inhaling infectious particles include the presence and nature of construction or demolition, the degree of immunocompromised status, and whether patients are receiving antifungal prophylaxis. In areas with active construction, large crowds, or with critically ill patients, N95 or surgical masks may be worn by the pediatric HSCT and oncology patients.[35] There are no existing guidelines or data showing the benefit of masking in SOT patients. No commercially available masks have been systematically evaluated for prevention of spores and mold inhalation. Use of cloth masks or decorated mesh masks is not advised.

Environmental Impact on Medical Care of Immunocompromised Patients

The environment contains a variety of opportunistic pathogens that can be responsible for disease transmission in immunocompromised patients, resulting in significant morbidity and mortality.[1] These reservoirs, such as dust and moisture for mold, may be disturbed during manipulation of the environment. In addition, disruptions of engineering systems for maintaining air and water quality may also promote proliferation of opportunistic infections.[36] Such disruptions increase the pathogen load in the air and water and increase risk of acquisition and severity of infection in the immunocompromised host.

Air Quality

Air quality is absolutely critical to the safety of patients, even in the absence of accompanying construction. Air handling systems (heating, ventilation, air conditioning [HVAC] system) can be ideal environments for microbial growth because pathogens such as opportunistic fungi can proliferate in areas with air, dust, and water.[1] Advance notice of scheduled HVAC maintenance, particularly if it affects areas occupied by high-risk patients, will allow appropriate measures to be taken to minimize dust and moisture intrusion.[36]

The use of high-efficiency particulate absorption (HEPA) filtration may be desired to improve air quality in areas housing high-risk patients. HEPA filters remove at least 99.97% of particles 0.3 μm or smaller in diameter (as a reference, *Aspergillus* spores are 2.5 to 3.0 μm in diameter). Although the purpose of HEPA filtration is to reduce fungal spores from the environment, one meta-analysis showed little survival benefit in immunocompromised patients.[37] Despite this, many existing and new facilities choose to invest in HEPA filtration.

Using a protective environment (PE) during hospitalizations could mitigate the acquisition of environmental fungal infections.[2] PEs combine HEPA filtration, high numbers (≥12) of air changes per hour, and positive pressure. Positive pressure refers to the differential between two adjacent spaces (room and hallway), in which air flows away from the area to keep airborne pathogens from entering the airspace of the room. Patients with anticipated prolonged neutropenia, such as HSCT recipients and patients with leukemia, should have priority placement into PEs. The air pressure gradient of all rooms (especially those designed for PEs and for airborne infections) should be monitored and documented periodically, especially if the rooms are occupied by patients.[1]

Measurements of air quality within a given space may take the form of particle counts (size and total quantity) and/or microbiologic sampling for fungal spores. There are no widely accepted thresholds for air sampling.

Routine air sampling for fungal spores is not recommended for several reasons. There is no clear threshold of spore counts that predicts acquisition of fungal infection and the unknown incubation of *Aspergillus* makes it difficult to attribute fungal infections as healthcare associated, resulting in a lack of standardized protocols for testing (sampling intervals, number of samples per area). In addition, the investment of laboratory resources for microbiologic air testing can be prohibitive. Hence routine microbiologic air sampling is not advised.[34] Individual healthcare facilities may develop their own schedule for airborne particle sampling to assess the performance, maintenance, and cleaning efficiency of airflow systems and dust-control measures.[1,36]

Because air quality is vital to the health of immunocompromised patients, medical providers should have a working understanding of the various mechanisms at their healthcare facility surrounding air handling. The use and placement of HEPA filters (rooms, hallways, central, portable), location of rooms with positive pressure, and priority placement of HSCT recipients and patients with leukemia into PEs should be appreciated. Periodic rounds (at least annually) with infection prevention providers and facility maintenance personnel would provide reciprocal education regarding logistics of air handling and patient safety.

Construction and Renovation

The construction and renovation of healthcare facilities affect air quality control. Clinically significant microorganisms are released into the air when environmental reservoirs (i.e., soil, water, dust, and decaying organic matter) are disturbed and brought into the healthcare environment.[38] Many publications have strongly suggested that construction and renovation activity are independent risk factors for invasive mold infections in heavily immunosuppressed populations.[36,38] The most commonly reported healthcare-associated invasive mold infection is *Aspergillus*,[36] and the primary site of infection is the lower respiratory tract.

Dust control measures during construction can minimize aerosolization of fungal particles. To that end, infection prevention professionals should be notified and involved in hospital projects with anticipated dust disturbance. These projects require completion of an infection control risk assessment (ICRA) that calculates the necessary control measures for dust and moisture containment based on the project type and patient risk groups. These control measures may include (but are not limited to) containment barriers (e.g., rigid, dustproof, airtight seals); close monitoring of air quality with possible use of portable HEPA filters and/or air particulate sampling; and relocating or redirecting high-risk patients away from construction.[39] A multidisciplinary team should discuss and implement appropriate measures as determined by the ICRA. Compliance with recommendations should be monitored with regular visits and feedback by infection prevention professionals.[40]

Surveillance for healthcare-associated mold infection is difficult but crucial to outbreak detection, particularly during periods of construction and renovation. The infection prevention professional should work closely with clinicians to identify and mitigate clusters of possible, probable, or proven cases of fungal infections. Although some facilities may use microbiologic air sampling and particle counts during times of construction, this should not replace or supersede clinical surveillance.[41] There may be a role for microbiologic air sampling or particle counts during outbreak investigation if it becomes necessary to localize an area to determine infection prevention interventions.

Furnishings

To prevent dust accumulation and aerosolization, the use of counters and furniture with smooth, nonporous surfaces that can be adequately scrubbed is advised. Carpeting should not be installed within hospital units as they have been implicated in outbreaks of aspergillosis.[2] Patients should be encouraged to minimize and reduce the clutter that can accumulate over a prolonged hospitalization. This would allow environmental services personnel to easily clean the room, as well as minimize dust accumulation that may serve as a reservoir for mold. One possible strategy for facilities to consider is inpatient room rotations for long-stay patients to allow for optimal deep cleaning of their environments.

Care of Linens and Healthcare Worker Attire

Reports of pulmonary and cutaneous fungal infections have implicated contaminated hospital linen supplies.[42] The linen supply chain, from the laundry facility to the transport of supplies to the hospital, and the storage of linens, should be monitored. Standards for processing of hospital linens are available from the Healthcare Laundry Accreditation Council and should be followed.[43] A single case of healthcare-associated cutaneous fungal infection should prompt investigation of linen care at the laundry facility and in the hospital. The process of soil removal, pathogen removal, and pathogen inactivation will render the laundry free of vegetative organisms, thus becoming hygienically clean. Outside the operative room, it is not necessary to use sterile linens for immunocompromised patients.

Although the attire of HCWs may be contaminated with pathogenic microorganisms,[43] there are no reports directly linking contaminated HCW attire to outbreaks outside the operative arena. There are cost-saving measures in healthcare facilities that have staff launder their own clothing, and no guidance exists for care of nonoperative HCW attire. At a minimum, attire should be clean and free of noticeable dirt and stains.

Plants

Live flowers or plants and their potting materials may harbor large numbers of fungal spores that can easily become aerosolized. Although exposure to plants and flowers has not conclusively been shown to cause invasive mold infections, most experts recommend that plants and dried/fresh flowers should not be allowed in hospital rooms of neutropenic or immunocompromised patients.[34,44]

Water Quality

Outbreaks attributed to contaminated healthcare-associated water supplies have been reported.[29] The most common pathogens associated with outbreaks include *Legionella*, nontuberculous mycobacteria, and *Pseudomonas*, all of which have been identified in municipal drinking water. The infection prevention professional should be knowledgeable of the quality and treatment (filtration, chlorination) of the municipal water before its entry into the hospital water supply.

Water-borne outbreaks occur when pathogen concentrations are increased in the hospital water supply (e.g., introduction of dust or dysregulation of water temperature allowing pathogen growth), or when such water is aerosolized (including open water features such as water walls and decorative water fountains). Measures to reduce bioburden within hospital water systems include scheduled maintenance of faucets and sinks (i.e., cleaning and disinfecting aerators and faucets), insulating recirculation water pipe loops, and evaluating for backflow and cross-connections in high-risk units.[1] Recommendations are to store hot water above 140°F (60°C) and circulate with a minimum return temperature of 124°F (51°C), whereas cold water temperatures should be below 68°F (20°C).[1] Annual inspection of thermostats, water pressurization, and climate control and fire protection systems will ensure that waterways remain adequately functional.

Complete eradication of pathogens and associated biofilms from hospital tap water and the plumbing infrastructure is not realistic given the environmental persistence of many of these microbes. Facilities may add filters to ice machines, showerheads, and/or sinks that are used or in proximity to immunocompromised patients. Ice machines should be dismantled and cleaned according to the manufacturer's recommendation. Various water disinfectant systems are available for use. Flushing chlorinated water through the water system intermittently may be useful; however, there are no standard recommendations for the use of chlorine dioxide, heavy metal ions, such as copper and monochloramine, ozone, or ultraviolet light for water sterilization.[45] It should be noted that use of carbon filters might remove chlorine from water supply and subsequently lead to increased microbial burden. Some centers instruct their immunocompromised patients to consume water only if it is bottled. Many of these measures have little data to support their use outside an outbreak setting and can be costly.

Hospital facilities may elect to monitor their water quality to reduce the risk of invasive infections such as from *Legionella* or nontuberculous mycobacteria infection in their susceptible patients. The optimal strategy (i.e., frequency and number of sites surveyed and determination of a dose-response, bacterial burden necessary for infection) has not been determined.[1] Cost-effectiveness studies are also unavailable.

Water Damage

If not rectified, water damage in structural areas of the hospital can serve as an ideal substrate for the proliferation of mold. Water may gain access through leaking from a broken water pipe or through excessive humidity in the environment (>60%). A number of publications assert that water systems within healthcare facilities may harbor fungal contamination.[46] Policies should outline the response plan to water damage or sustained levels of high humidity. At a minimum, repair and drying of wet materials within 72 hours or the removal of the wet material is recommended.[1] Infection prevention professionals should ensure that appropriate containment measures to minimize dust or mold dissemination are used during repairs of water damage.

Cleaning and Disinfecting Environmental Surfaces Within Hospital Units

Hospital surfaces are frequently contaminated and have been implicated in transmission of HAIs among hospitalized patients.[44,47] Cleaning is defined as the removal of visible soil, stains, dust, and spills. Cleaning should be done as expeditiously as possible in an acute event. Disinfection is defined as the removal of many or all pathogenic micro-organisms, but may not be necessarily sporicidal. Cleaning should be performed prior to disinfection. The Environmental Protection Agency has registered disinfectants that meet safety and disinfection standards for hospital use. Manufacturer instructions for use should be stringently followed. Environmental fogging with chemical disinfectants is not recommended owing to the lack of microbicide efficacy.[45]

To adequately eradicate *C. difficile* spores, disinfectants with sporicidal activity (e.g., hypochlorite-based products) are recommended.[48] There are insufficient studies evaluating ultraviolet germicidal irradiation and other "touchless" disinfection modalities to recommend their use as part of routine *C. difficile* infection prevention bundles. Focal areas of cleaning should include high-touch and high-dust surfaces. Auditing cleaning efficacy with fluorescent markers and black light or an adenosine triphosphate–based system and standard aerobic cultures has been assessed in small studies, with fluorescent systems showing a slight advantage.[49] More research is needed to determine the optimal frequency and tools used for cleaning audits.

INFECTION PREVENTION PRACTICES IN SPECIFIC IMMUNOCOMPROMISED PEDIATRIC POPULATIONS

Hematopoietic Stem Cell Transplantation

Patients undergoing HSCT have prolonged and profound immune deficiencies. Up to four weeks might be needed for neutrophil count recovery, and immune reconstitution may be delayed with use of suppressive medications to treat GVHD. Treatment of active infection in the midst of ongoing immune deficiency is difficult; therefore prevention of infection is paramount in patients with HSCT.

The presence of central venous catheters, which are necessary for supportive medical care, is a well-known risk factor for bacteremia. Increased rates of CLABSIs often highlight a deficiency in catheter insertion and/or maintenance practices. Preemptively, facilities should undertake and maintain a reliable and reproducible workflow for line insertion and maintenance. The development and, most importantly, auditing of central line use should involve nursing leadership, vascular access specialists, infection prevention professionals, quality specialists, and physician leadership of HSCT units. These stakeholders would have a preexisting working relationship to investigate and mitigate increased incidence of CLABSIs if they occur.

Invasive fungal infections are a life-threatening complication in patients undergoing HSCT. As outlined previously, efficient HVAC systems, positive-pressure ventilation, HEPA filtration, and careful risk assessment during construction and renovation projects help to ensure safe air quality. This may mitigate the contribution of the healthcare environment to a patient's risk of invasive fungal infection. Working toward safe air quality within the PE and to prevent invasive fungal infections requires a close and trusting relationship between infection prevention professionals and personnel in facility maintenance and design/construction. A preexisting collaboration can then be easily reassembled to investigate and mitigate possible fungal outbreaks.

The use of PPE for the prevention of HAIs in patients with HSCT may be helpful. Patients undergoing HSCT may wish to use personal N95 respirators or surgical masks to reduce environmental mold exposure while outside PE, particularly before engraftment. There are insufficient data to recommend this routinely, although it may be reassuring to patients.[34]

Solid Organ Transplantation

Common pediatric transplanted organs are kidneys, lungs, and hearts. The numbers of pediatric intestinal transplants are increasing but remain relatively rare in most institutions owing to the nature of the transplants, recurrent exposure to antimicrobials, and the necessity for prolonged immunosuppression. In addition, such patients are often at risk for invasive infections with MDROs. For example, a sizable proportion of patients with CRE bacteremia had received one or more organ transplants and SOT remains an independent risk factor for invasive CRE infections.[20] Screening for MDROs, especially VRE and MRSA, in SOT recipients may be of negligible benefit. However, there has been growing interest in screening organ donors for MDRO, although data on infection prevention and cost analysis are lacking. A focus of the infection prevention professional should be clinical surveillance and mitigation of MDRO outbreaks in SOT recipients.

Infections in transplant recipients may frequently occur at the site of the organ graft (i.e., pneumonia in lung transplant recipients; urinary tract infections in kidney transplant recipients). It is prudent for the infection prevention professional and clinician to use strategies to minimize manipulation into the new organ graft. An infection prevention program may focus efforts to limit medical devices into the graft site (such as expeditiously removing endotracheal tubes and urinary catheters) to decrease the risk of MDRO colonization or biofilm formation.

Viral infections in pediatric SOT recipients may be newly acquired or reactivated after SOT. SOT recipients may be exposed to community-acquired viruses within their homes, within the hospital, or within commonly visited centers such as school or a religious community where they spend considerable amounts of time. These patients are particularly at risk for vaccine-preventable viral infections as live vaccines may be contraindicated and vaccine responses may be attenuated by chronic immunosuppression. In addition, pretransplant vaccination rates in liver and heart transplant recipients have been historically suboptimal.[50] Therefore infection prevention efforts should highlight the importance of appropriate hand hygiene and appropriate vaccination of SOT candidates before receiving transplant, close contacts, HCWs and the local community to reduce viral transmission.

Fungal infections with *Candida* or endemic molds have been rarely reported in pediatric SOT patients except in pediatric small-bowel transplant patients, among whom an invasive *Candida* infection develops shortly after transplant in 20% to 25% of cases .[50]

Donor-derived infections, such as transmission of *Toxoplasma* from infected transplanted cardiac tissue or hepatitis from the donor transplant liver, are also of concern and protocols exist to guide pretransplant risk assessment or testing options to reduce posttransplant infections. Specific guidelines to prevent donor-derived infections are beyond the scope of this chapter.

Oncology

Infection prevention professionals may regard the infection risk of patients with oncologic disease to be minimally less than patients with HSCT. Patients with oncologic disease undergo repeated rounds of chemotherapy but have interval periods of quantitatively normal neutrophils, although neutrophil function may be impaired and thus not protective against invasive bacterial or fungal infections. Preventive measures for central line management and for optimization of air and water quality remain important. Strategies discussed previously should also be applied to oncology patients receiving chemotherapy or those admitted to the hospital.

Future Areas of Research in Standardizing Infection Prevention Practices

Many specific recommendations for infection prevention in immunocompromised patients are based on a common sense approach rather than on precise data.[34] Questions remain regarding the necessity and standardization of microbiologic assessment of air and water quality, how best to minimize development and transmission of resistant pathogens, methods to decrease the burden of MDRO colonization, and the clinical and emotional impact of restricting visitation by asymptomatic individuals. Increasing healthcare costs will also foster interest in whether financial investments, such as central HEPA filtration, will have clinical value. Future studies could target these gaps and optimize care of pediatric immunocompromised patients.

13

Safe Living After Transplantation or Chemotherapy

Blanca E. Gonzalez, MD and Marian G. Michaels, MD, MPH

PREVENTION OF INFECTIONS BY DIRECT CONTACT

Children are particularly prone to infections acquired by direct contact. Frequently, children engage in behaviors that place them at risk, such as placing their hands in their nose or mouth and then touching surfaces, playing in close proximity to others, and coughing or sneezing without observing adequate etiquette. Studies have shown that hand hygiene rates among children and adolescents in schools are low, sometimes not surpassing 50%.[1] However, interventions to improve hygiene in children can be done and have proven to be effective. Increasing handwashing compliance may involve implementation of educational strategies and creativity, especially when educating younger ones who are not knowledgeable or attentive to diseases transmitted through contact. In addition, engagement of people who interact with these children outside the hospital environment is key, especially teachers and day care workers. Social media has become a useful tool for educating children on hand hygiene practices. A myriad of videos geared toward teaching children proper hand hygiene are available online and their use is encouraged.

Many infections, including respiratory viral infections, are transmitted through direct contact. For these microbes, handwashing is the mainstay of infection prevention, particularly in the vulnerable immunocompromised host. There are no pediatric studies that address hand hygiene compliance after transplantation or in immunocompromised patients. An adult survey of lung transplant recipients focusing on safe living strategies after transplant found that the majority of patients surveyed would wash hands before eating or preparing food (87.7%); however, patients younger than 40 years of age were less likely to be compliant with safe living recommendations than older patients.[2]

To prevent infections children should be taught and encouraged to wash hands at the following times:

- Before eating or preparing food
- During and after preparing food
- After coughing, sneezing, or blowing their nose
- After touching animals or handling pet treats
- After playing outside
- After using the toilet
- After touching garbage

Unless dealing with contact with *Clostridiodes difficile* or visibly soiled hands, alcohol rubs are acceptable alternatives to soap and water hand hygiene.

Percutaneous exposures may also lead to infections in children. Walking barefoot is discouraged in children after transplantation as it exposes their feet to a wide variety of hazards that may lead to infection. Organisms such as *Nocardia* and *Alternaria* and other dematiaceous fungi, commonly found in the soil, plants, and decomposing debris, can lead to infections after penetrating injuries. In countries where sanitation is not perfect, parasitic infections such as *Strongyloides* and cutaneous larva migrans may be acquired by walking barefoot. Warts, which may be extensive and difficult to treat in transplant recipients, may also be acquired by ambulating barefoot as the virus is ubiquitous in the environment and can penetrate through small abrasions. If children want to help with gardening chores, using protective gloves is a must to avoid injuries.

Tattoos and piercings are increasingly popular among adolescents and young adults, including immunocompromised patients. Unfortunately, many are performed by unlicensed personnel, increasing the risk of infection acquisition. Tattoos have been associated with infections with organisms such as *Staphylococcus aureus, Aspergillus,* and nontuberculous mycobacteria, among others. Potential transmission of HIV, hepatitis B, and hepatitis C through unsafe tattooing practices is another concern. Piercings, especially tongue piercings, have equally been implicated in the development of severe infections, such as endocarditis, cellulitis, and perichondritis. Even though few reports are available of these infections specifically occurring in transplant or immunocompromised recipients, counseling regarding the potential for infection is critical. Stilley and colleagues noted that the prevalence of tattoos and piercings in adolescent and young adult heart transplant recipients mirrored that of the general adolescent population. Of the 27 patients in their study, 26% had more than two piercings and 33% had tattoos.[3] If body piercing or tattoos are to be obtained, timing should be discussed with the transplant physician and should be avoided until immunosuppression is more stable. In addition, these body modification practices should only be performed by licensed personnel who should be made aware of the immunocompromised status of the patient so they can observe the highest hygiene measures. Home tattoos and piercings should be avoided.

PREVENTION OF RESPIRATORY INFECTIONS

Respiratory tract infections are a significant cause or morbidity and mortality in the immunocompromised hosts. Organisms causing these infections enter the body either through direct contact with contaminated secretions (including fomites) or through inhalation of organisms in the form of aerosols or droplets. Lung transplant and hematopoietic stem cell transplant (HSCT) patients are the most vulnerable because of the high frequency of progression to pneumonia, but all organ transplant recipients are at risk of high severity, especially infants or during times of increased immunosuppression. In an attempt to reduce the transmission and prevent respiratory infections, children should exercise handwashing when in contact with secretions and follow coughing and sneezing etiquette. In periods of high immunosuppression it is prudent to avoid crowded areas. Face masks are frequently used in this population to prevent the acquisition of infections. Several trials have been conducted in community settings evaluating the effectiveness of masks in preventing respiratory infections and are summarized in a comprehensive review by MacIntyre and Chughtai.[4] Most trials had as an endpoint the prevention of influenza in households, and face masks were often combined with hand hygiene strategies. This practice was shown to be useful if wearing the mask was initiated shortly after a case of influenza or other respiratory infection was identified in the household and if patients were compliant.[4] If possible, the immunocompromised host should remain separated from a household contact. In addition, vaccination of patients and their households has been proven to be the best method for influenza prevention.

Molds and endemic fungi may also be acquired via inhalation. Similar to solid organ transplant (SOT) and HSCT patients, those receiving chemotherapy or tumor necrosis factor alpha inhibitors should be counseled about histoplasmosis and coccidioidomycosis. Exposure to caves, chicken coops, bird roosts, and wood piles presents risk for histoplasmosis and should be avoided if possible. For coccidioidomycosis, patients who travel or live in endemic areas should additionally avoid construction and excavation sites and stay inside during dust storms. Extrapolating from infection prevention experience at hospitals where fungal outbreaks have been reported during construction and renovation, it may be prudent to avoid construction and renovation at times of higher levels of immunosuppression.

With the legalization of cannabis in a number of countries and parts of the United States and its increased medical use, adolescents may have easier access to this drug. There are many case reports in the medical literature of HSCT and SOT recipients and cancer patients in whom *Aspergillus* have developed after smoking contaminated marijuana, and therefore its use should be avoided.[5] Information suggests that baked marijuana (at 300°F for 15 minutes) may be safer.[6]

WATER SAFETY/EXPOSURE TO *CRYPTOSPORIDIUM*

Exposure to contaminated drinking and recreational waters is a common source of infections in the general population. Waterborne infections may result from ingestion, inhalation, or direct contact with contaminated water sources. Direct consumption of contaminated drinking water or inadvertent ingestion or contact with contaminated water during activities such as bathing or swimming place immunocompromised patients at risk of acquiring pathogens that cause important morbidity. In the United States, during the period ranging from 2000 to 2014, approximately 500 outbreaks occurred involving contact with treated recreational waters, such as swimming pools, sprinklers, and fountains.[7] Centers for Disease Control and Prevention (CDC) surveillance studies also identified 42 outbreaks in 19 states in 2013 and 2014 related to drinking water; 83% were associated with public community and non-community waters.[8]

Organisms frequently associated with contaminated water include *Escherichia coli, Salmonella* spp., *Giardia lamblia, Ascaris lumbricoides, Pseudomonas* spp., and *Cryptosporidium* spp. *Legionella* can also be transmitted but is less frequently encountered in children. Viral agents such as human noroviruses, which can cause protracted diarrhea in transplant recipients, have been associated with contaminated water sources, including private wells and contaminated drinking water (Table 13.1).

Cryptosporidium infection deserves special attention as it is now considered one of the major etiologies of diarrhea in childhood and has increasingly been identified as a cause of diarrhea in transplant recipients.[9] More than 15 species have been identified, but the majority of human infections are caused by either *Cryptosporidium parvum* or *C. hominis*. The oocysts are chlorine resistant and ingestion of a small inoculum (approximately 50 cysts) can lead to clinically significant infection. Moreover, not all water filters are capable of removing *Cryptosporidium*. The CDC website provides useful information on water

TABLE 13.1 Pathogens Associated With Waterborne Infections

Organism	Most Common Contaminated Water Source Exposure	Common Manifestations
Bacteria		
Aeromonas	Fresh and brackish waters	Pneumonia (near drowning episodes) and skin and soft tissue infections (SSTIs), gastrointestinal manifestations
Edwarsella	Salt water environments	
Vibrio		
Escherichia coli	Recreational waters: lakes, rivers	Diarrhea
Shigella	Well water	
Legionella	Hot tubs/whirlpools Aerosols (i.e. fountains, sprays) Air conditioners Flood waters	Pneumonia, Pontiac fever
Leptospira	Contaminated water especially after floods and natural disasters	Disseminated infections (Weil syndrome), pneumonia
Pseudomonas aeruginosa	Hot tubs/whirlpools recreational waters (swimming pools)	SSTIs Keratitis Pneumonia (near drowning)
Mycobacteria (M. marinum, M. chelonae, other rapid growing mycobacteria)	Fresh and saltwater environments (fish tanks, aquariums)	SSTIs, disseminated infection
Fungi and Algae		
Prototheca	Fresh and stagnant waters, aquariums	SSTIs, disseminated infections

Continued

TABLE 13.1 Pathogens Associated With Waterborne Infections—cont'd

Organism	Most Common Contaminated Water Source Exposure	Common Manifestations
Viral Infections		
Norovirus	Contaminated recreational or drinking water	Diarrhea
Adenovirus		
Hepatitis A, E		Hepatitis
Parasites		
Cryptosporidium	Contaminated recreational and drinking water (lakes, rivers, swimming pools)	Diarrhea
Giardia	Well water	
Free-living amoebas	Warm fresh waters	Meningitis, keratitis, SSTIs

filters. Labels stating an absolute pore size (as opposed to a nominal pore size) of 1 μm or less will filter *Cryptosporidium* oocysts. Similarly, filters that use reverse osmosis protect against *Cryptosporidium*. Manufacturers who have had their filters tested specifically against *Cryptosporidium* label them as National Sanitation Foundation/American National Standards Institute (NSF/ANSI) Standard 53 or 58. Several case reports and series of *Cryptosporidium* infections in pediatric transplant recipients have been published.[9] Exposure to recreational waters was the most common risk factor recognized for those few reports in which a common source was identified. A pediatric cohort study of renal transplant recipients by Bandin and colleagues identified *Cryptosporidium* as the etiologic agent of diarrhea in 18% of the patients studied.[10] Forty-three percent of these children had had a recent exposure to swimming pools and 14% traveled to an area with increased rates of infection. In another pediatric case reported by Hong and colleagues, a 7-year-old kidney transplant recipient with *Cryptosporidium*-related diarrhea had exposure to a swimming pool at a resort in the United States before the onset of symptoms.[11] Data from a nationwide French study of *Cryptosporidium* infections in SOT recipients (the TRANSCRYPTO study) identified 47 SOT recipients with cryptosporidiosis over 4 years. Seven were patients younger than 15 years of age.[12] Environmental risk factors for infections were found in 18 patients, 2 patients drank nonpotable water, 4 used recreational water, and 10 traveled to endemic areas where poor water sanitation is common. The American Society for Transplantation Infectious Disease Community of Practice and the CDC recommendations for water safety in immunocompromised patients are summarized in Table 13.2.[13]

Many transplant centers advocate for the consumption of bottled water. The bottled water industry is regulated by the U.S. Environmental Protection Agency and Food and Drug Administration requiring certain standards to be met. However, bottled water undergoes less scrutiny than tap water. Studies have shown that bacteria will grow in noncarbonated bottled water several days after it has been bottled and stored at room temperature.[14] In a study of the diversity of bacteria in bottled water identified by 16S ribosomal ribonucleic acid sequences, 80% to 98% of the bacteria detected were members of the Betaproteobacteria family (Burkholderiales order).[14] Other studies have identified gram-negative organisms such as *Stenotrophomonas* spp. and *Pseudomonas* spp., bacteria associated with severe infections in immunocompromised hosts.[15] Outbreaks related to contaminated bottled water have also been described. Eckmanns and colleagues reported an outbreak of *Pseudomonas aeruginosa* in six different intensive care units in Germany linked to still bottled water.[16] Pulsed-field gel electrophoresis of the organisms recovered in 15 infected and 4 colonized patients indicated they were identical to each other and matched the environmental sample obtained from an unopened bottled water. The outbreak was terminated by the removal of the remainder of commercial bottled waters existing in the intensive care unit. More recently, an outbreak of norovirus in Spain was also sourced to still bottled water with the detection of high norovirus GI and GII ribonucleic acid levels (10^3 and 10^4 genome copies/L) in the samples obtained.[17]

Although bottled water has not been specifically identified as being contaminated with *Cryptosporidium*, its consumption does not

TABLE 13.2 Water Safety Recommendations

Drinking Water	Recreational Water	Water Safety During Travel
• Boil water for at least 1 minute to completely eliminate risk of *Cryptosporidium* • Pay close attention to "boil water" advisories in the community • When selecting personal filters or bottled water, use only filters with pore size <1 μm or NFS (National Sanitation Foundation) tested or certified • Private or public well water should generally be avoided unless frequently tested for bacterial pathogens • Avoid drinking directly from lakes or rivers. Avoid swallowing water while swimming	• Avoid swimming in bodies of water that are likely to be contaminated by human or animal waste • Pay attention to "do not swim" advisories, especially after rainfalls • Avoid swimming in pools for 2 weeks after diarrhea has resolved for patients with *Cryptosporidium* or other diarrheal illness • Immunocompromised persons should avoid hot tubs • Do not swim with open wounds • Clean wounds that occur while bathing in fresh or ocean water with an uncontaminated water source	• Avoid tap and well water • Avoid fountain drinks • Avoid ice made of tap or well water • Avoid drinks or water ice made from tap or well water • Prefer drinks that are bottled and sealed, keeping in mind that carbonated is better • Follow drinking water and recreational water recommendations

completely eliminate the risk, especially in areas of high prevalence. Sarkar and colleagues conducted a study in a highly endemic area for *Cryptosporidium* with the goal of determining if a protected water source could delay infection transmission.[18] A total of 176 children were enrolled; approximately half were given either bottled water or municipal drinking water. They found that drinking bottled water was not protective against acquisition of the organism, suggesting multiple modes of transmission. The Environmental Protection Agency encourages immunocompromised patients who want to be absolutely safe about bottled water to check the labels or to call the bottling company to inquire about the techniques used to treat the water. Water bottles labeled with any of the following terms "treated with reverse osmosis, distillation, filtration through an absolute 1-μm or smaller filter" are all considered protective against *Cryptosporidium*. In addition, bottled waters that are derived from rivers and lakes tend to be more contaminated than those obtained from protected well or spring water sources.

FOOD SAFETY

According to the CDC, 1 in 6 Americans becomes ill every year due to the ingestion of a contaminated food product.[19] However, the incidence of these infections in SOT recipients or children with cancer is unknown. A study by Boyle and colleagues evaluated the burden of this problem in their HSCT population including children and adults over an 11-year period and found bacterial foodborne events occurred infrequently at a rate of 1/100,000 patient days. However, when contrasted to the number of cases in the general population for the same time periods, the rate in HSCT patients was 10-fold higher than that of the general population, acknowledging that this difference was likely overestimated owing to the lack of reporting in the general population.[20] Younger age and type of transplant may influence the adherence to safer living recommendations. For example, Jain and colleagues found that in lung transplant recipients, younger age was associated with less compliance with hand hygiene and other safer living practices, although in their study almost all patients avoided raw or undercooked meat, poultry, and unpasteurized dairy products.[2] In a small study examining the knowledge and perceptions of food safety in transplant recipients, HSCT patients were more knowledgeable than the SOT patients surveyed and expressed more willingness to adhere to recommendations. In this study, SOT patients viewed themselves as "healthy" more often than HSCT patients after transplantation and found less need to be compliant with safety recommendations.[21]

In addition to transplant recipients (hematopoietic or solid organ) and patients receiving chemotherapy, patients receiving biological agents for the treatment of conditions such as rheumatoid arthritis and Crohn disease are also vulnerable to foodborne pathogens. For example, patients on tumor necrosis factor alpha inhibitors are at increased risk for acquiring infections with foodborne organisms such as *Listeria* spp. and *Salmonella* spp.[22]

Although hepatitis A virus (HAV) has long been recognized as a potential contaminant of foods, other viruses such as norovirus and hepatitis E virus (HEV) have been more recently recognized as potential foodborne infections that can threaten the transplant population. Norovirus has become the leading cause of foodborne illness in the United States, with 58% of cases caused by this organism.[23] This organism has been increasingly reported as a cause of chronic diarrhea in the adult and pediatric transplant population, as previously mentioned.[24] Leafy green vegetables, fresh fruits, and shellfish have been commonly linked to outbreaks, and food service workers are the most common sources of infection. HEV is also transmitted via the fecal-oral route and is suspected to be a zoonosis as strains of this virus are prevalent in wild boars and swine. Kamar and colleagues reported on 14 adult patients from France in whom acute HEV developed several years after transplantation. The infection evolved into chronic hepatitis in 57% of the patients. The testing for this virus was prompted by an increased number of cases in normal hosts in the southwest region of France at the time of presentation.[25] Subsequently, researchers from Canada demonstrated the occurrence of such infection in children after liver transplant. A child in this study who lived in semirural area of Quebec had an HEV infection with serotype 3a, a strain that shares similarities with the swine HEV 3a strain, suggesting that a zoonotic transmission likely occurred in this child.[26] These reports highlight the importance of transplant recipients from abstaining from consuming raw or undercooked meat products. HAV risk is diminished significantly by vaccination, but caution is still needed as outbreaks continue to occur nationally and internationally

Immunocompromised patients should follow basic food safety handling recommendations by the U.S. Department of Agriculture when shopping, preparing, and storing food. The four steps for Food Safe Families are as follows:

- Clean: Wash hands and surfaces frequently.
- Separate: Do not cross-contaminate foods.
- Cook: Always cook to the correct temperature.
- Chill: Refrigerate products promptly.

Eating the following products places patients at risk of a foodborne infection and should be avoided:

1. Unpasteurized milk, fruit, or vegetable juice/cider or cheeses made from unpasteurized milk: *E. coli* O157:H7, *Salmonella* spp., *Brucella*, *Listeria*, *Yersinia enterocolitica*, and *Cryptosporidium*.
2. Raw or undercooked eggs: *Salmonella* spp.
3. Raw dough: Children often are allowed to play with and eat raw dough that is intended to be cooked or to be craft dough. These may be harmful as flour can be contaminated with organisms such as *Salmonella* spp. and *E. coli*.
4. Raw or undercooked meat, poultry or fish: In addition to any bacterial contamination, parasitic infections such as *Taxoplasma gondii* and tapeworms and viruses such as HEV may also be acquired by consuming these raw food products. De novo toxoplasmosis is of particular concern in seronegative transplant recipients, particularly in areas where the disease is endemic.
5. Raw or undercooked seafood (oysters, clams, mussels): *Vibrio* spp., HAV, HEV, *Cryptosporidium* spp., *Campylobacter jejuni*.

Comprehensive recommendations, including a printable resource for transplant recipients, are available at the U.S. Department of Health and Human Services at https://www.fda.gov/food/foodborneillness-contaminants/peopleatrisk/ucm312570.htm.

Probiotics have been increasingly used by the general population and parents often ask about their use in the immunocompromised population. In a recent trial of *Lactobacillus plantarum* given to children and adolescents undergoing HSCT, no cases of bacteremia or other adverse effects were documented. The *Lactobacillus* was administered orally starting at day −7 of transplant and continued to day +14 after transplantation.[27] However, multiple case reports of sepsis, bacteremia, and endocarditis linked to the use of probiotics have been reported. Most of these infections have occurred in immunocompromised patients, patients with intestinal insufficiency syndrome or valvular heart disease, and in patients with central venous catheters. At this time, until further information is available regarding the safety of these products in the immunocompromised population, they should generally be avoided unless participating in a clinical trial.

ANIMAL CONTACT AND PET SAFETY

Many households worldwide own pets, including households where immunocompromised patients reside.[28,29] Pet ownership has been found to be beneficial for children's well-being, but pets are a potential source of infections, especially for the immunocompromised. The rate of zoonotic infections in these patients is not known, but the morbidity and mortality associated with such infections can be high. Companion animals may be the source of more than 70 zoonotic infections and as methods to diagnose infections improve, this number is expected to rise.[28,29] This section is not intended to preclude animal exposure but to educate about the potential risks and offer strategies to minimize risks.

Children may be more vulnerable to acquiring zoonotic infections as they are usually less careful than adults when interacting with pets and their actions could place them at risk of acquiring such infections.[28-30] A survey study from Chile of 70 families of immunocompromised children (defined as children with cancer, HIV, bone marrow and SOT recipients) showed that 55% of families owned pets.[30] Furthermore, a significant number of children engaged in behaviors that would place them at risk of acquiring zoonotic infection, such as kissing or allowing themselves to be licked by their pet (38%), cleaning up animal waste (12%), eating from the pet's plate (7%), and co-sleeping with a pet (2.%).[30] In contrast, adult transplant recipients may be more careful when it comes to pet care after transplantation. A survey study of lung transplant recipients showed that the majority of patients complied with recommendations to avoid infections, such as not cleaning up animal feces, avoiding scratches, thorough handwashing, and a small percentage even gave their pets away before transplantation to avoid the risk altogether.[2] Although this latter action may not be needed for all pets, some pets have higher risk than others for infections and should be discouraged. These include reptiles (lizards, snakes, and turtles), baby chicks or ducklings or any exotic pets, including monkeys. The most common zoonoses affecting transplant and immunocompromised patients are listed in Table 13.3.[26,29,31]

In addition to exposure to animals, certain veterinary live vaccines may pose risk to the immunocompromised host. This is the case with the vaccine against *Bordetella bronchiseptica*, a species related to *Bordetella pertussis* and *Bordetella parapertussis*. This organism causes tracheobronchitis in dogs, also known as "kennel cough." The live vaccine is aerosolized and administered intranasally to dogs and occasionally cats. Anecdotal cases of healthy and immunocompromised patients possibly acquiring this organism after exposure to recently vaccinated pets have been reported.[32] Immunocompromised patients may present with symptoms that range from respiratory symptoms to a severe pneumonia or bacteremia. There is no established treatment or prophylaxis against the organism; therefore it is recommended that immunocompromised patients avoid contact with the nose or face of dogs recently vaccinated with this vaccine or those diagnosed with kennel cough.[32,33] A killed virus version of the vaccine exists and its administration could be discussed with the veterinarian. Finding a temporary accommodation for the pet (1 to 2 weeks after vaccination) may also prevent exposure. In the case of an exposure to this organism, observation of the patient is warranted for the development of symptoms. Some veterinarians use prophylactic doxycycline for 5 days to prevent canine respiratory disease in dog shelters with a high incidence of wild-type disease. However, there are no reports of use of this antimicrobial as prophylaxis in humans who have potentially been exposed.[34]

A thorough discussion of safe pet ownership should take place in the anticipatory guidance of the immunocompromised host. For example, for children listed for SOT, the pretransplant evaluation is a good time to review pet ownership and discuss safer ownership practices. This information should be reviewed again when the patient is ready to be discharged home. Stull and colleagues conducted a study in Canada surveying parents and guardians of children being treated at an oncology and diabetes unit in eastern Ontario regarding their knowledge of pets as sources of disease, concerns regarding pet-derived pathogens, and pet ownership practices. The survey was responded to by 214 households. Interestingly, new pets were acquired by 20% of households after the diagnosis of cancer and in 49% after the diagnosis of diabetes. Moreover, 70% acquired pets that are considered high risk for these patients, such as puppies and kittens younger than 6 months, reptiles, and rodents. Of the respondents, 70% thought that the benefits of owning a pet outweighed any risk associated. Sadly, less than half of the responders recalled having a conversation regarding safe pet ownership practices with their physicians.[28] Another single-center survey of pediatric thoracic organ recipients found 67% had pets before transplant and 68% acquired new pets after transplantation. More than 70% recalled a safe pet ownership discussion specifically during the pretransplant evaluation. One episode of *Bartonella* was documented from a new kitten.[35]

Parents of immunocompromised children should observe the following practices when owning or thinking of acquiring a pet[31,36]:

Pet Consideration. Parents must consider the species and age of the pet they own or plan to acquire. Young pets are more likely to shed zoonotic agents than older animals. Reptiles and amphibians (snakes, iguanas, lizards, and turtles), chicks, and ducklings have a high risk of *Salmonella* infection and should be avoided. Kittens may transmit *Bartonella henselae*, especially through scratches, and cats who go outdoor may transmit *T. gondii*. Young dogs and some cats need live

TABLE 13.3 Infectious Organisms Transmitted From Animals

Pet	Organisms
Dogs and Cats	*Bartonella* spp., *Brucella* spp., *Bordetella bronchiseptica, Campylobacter jejuni, Capnocytophaga canimorsus, Leishmania, Leptospira interrogans, Pasteurella multocida, Salmonella* spp., *Toxocara* spp., *Cryptosporidium* spp., *Giardia lamblia, Ascaris lumbricoides,* hookworm, *Echinococcus,* rabies, *Toxoplasma gondii* (cats), tick-borne infections
Birds	*Cryptococcus neoformans, Chlamydophila psittaci,* Salmonella spp., *Campylobacter jejuni* (migratory water fowl), *Mycobacterium avium, Histoplasma capsulatum*
Reptiles	*Salmonella* spp.
Fish	*Mycobacterium marinum*
Rodents	Lymphocytic choriomeningitis virus, *Leptospira interrogans, Streptobacillus moniliformis, Spirillum minus*
Farm animals (sheep, goats, horses, cows)	*Campylobacter jejuni, Rodococcus equi* (horses), *Cryptosporidium, Salmonella* spp., *Escherichia coli,* hepatitis virus (swine, boar, deer)

vaccinations as previously mentioned, placing owners at some risk; however, there is less risk than if the pet is unvaccinated and develops wild-type disease. Rodents have a risk of transmitting lymphocytic choriomeningitis virus, and exotic pets and stray animals are best avoided altogether. It is recommended that patients who are planning to acquire a new pet do so after the period of heightened immunosuppression has passed (6 to 12 months after transplant).

Petting zoos are very popular among children and have been linked to many outbreaks, including *E. coli* O157-H7, *Salmonella, and Cryptosporidium*. Cases of *Cryptosporidium* in transplant recipients who have had contact with farm and petting animals have been reported.[9] HEV, which can cause chronic hepatitis in children after liver transplantation, has been associated with contact with farm-raised swine.[26] Therefore it is best to avoid petting zoos during periods of intensified immunosuppression, especially those with young animals. Hand hygiene after visiting a petting zoo or farm is also of critical importance.

Pet Care Practices. Pets should be fully vaccinated and have routine checkups with the veterinarian to ensure the animal is and remains healthy. It is important that parents supervise immunocompromised children to avoid scratches and bites, which should be thoroughly cleansed if they occur. Some immunocompromised patients have indwelling lines that need to be kept away from animals. Martin and colleagues reported a case of a 21-year-old undergoing hemodialysis who had *Pasteurella multocida* sepsis after his pet cat bit the catheter.[37] Although the transplant recipient need not be excused from all responsibility associated with having a family pet, it is best for them to avoid being involved with cleaning the cage or tank. This is particularly important during times of higher immunosuppression or neutropenia. If necessary during other times, then attention to hygiene is critical, including wearing gloves and masks if aerosolization is anticipated, as with bird cage cleaning, and strict handwashing afterward. Pets should be fed dry or commercial animal food, avoiding contaminated or spoiled meat. Raw food (i.e., meat, eggs) has been associated with increased *Salmonella* shedding in dogs and therefore should not be fed to pets; outbreaks of *Salmonella* have been reported after ingestion of contaminated dog treats. Keeping a pet indoors is always best, but pets such as dogs need to be taken outside for walks. For this situation, dogs should be kept with a leash to refrain them from eating garbage, feces, or hunting.

Pet Care Hygiene. Good hand hygiene should occur after contact with pets and any animal in general, especially in children younger than 5 years in whom hand hygiene should be supervised by patents. If the pet is ill with a diarrheal illness, children should avoid contact with the animal until it has resolved. Backyard sand boxes should be covered to prevent toxocariasis.

RETURNING TO SCHOOL

Returning to school is a very important component of reestablishing or keeping normalcy during cancer therapy and after transplantation. This may be challenging for the patients in many aspects, including the anxiety and fear of infections. Brauer and colleagues examined the experiences of adolescents and young adults in the return to school process after HCT and found that fear of infections posed a barrier to the return to school process. In their survey study, some transplant recipients expressed concerns and heightened anxiety toward the possibility of being exposed to germs.[38] However, studies have shown that attending school is beneficial and probably safe.[39] Sandberg and colleagues conducted a study to assess whether attending school during the initial cancer treatment was associated with an increased risk of infections. The study, a national cohort study in Sweden, showed that children undergoing cancer treatment were not at a higher risk of starting antibiotic treatment than those without cancer.[39] The appropriate time to return to school is different for every child, but the type of transplant, immune status, and age need to be taken in account. When children return to school, they should continue to observe the same precautions for food, water, and pet safety as discussed previously and exercise good handwashing and cough etiquette. Parents need to partner with teachers to keep children safe during this transition. Unfortunately, with the rise of the antivaccine movement in the United States and other parts of the world, immunocompromised children may be exposed to vaccine-preventable disease for which their immunity may not be strong or may be nonexistent. Therefore the importance of vaccinating the SOT patients as completely as possible before transplant, and for HCT patients systematic reimmunization after transplantation, is pivotal. In some instances when frequent exposures to varicella and measles are expected because of poor vaccination rates in the community, vaccination may be considered in certain SOT recipients if patients meet specific criteria such as stable low level immunosuppression, normal lymphocyte counts, and at least a year after transplantation.[40,41] However, risks and benefits need to be thoroughly discussed with the parents. All members of households of immunocompromised patients also need to have up-to-date immunization. Families can also partner with schools to enforce immunization laws that are applicable in their area. The school should ideally contact the parents of the immunocompromised host if cases of vaccine-preventable diseases occur so that the patient may receive prophylaxis in a timely manner if indicated or be homeschooled during outbreak periods.

RECREATIONAL ACTIVITIES INCLUDING TRAVEL

As survival of children after cancer therapy or transplantation improves with the advances in the respective fields, more children will be leading normal lives and engaging in the same activities as their peers. These may include attendance at camps, travel, sexual activity, and recreational sports, among others. Therefore when children are transitioning from hospital to home and to normal life thereafter, counseling regarding what is and what is not safe for the child to engage in is important for parents and children alike.

Sports

Transplant recipients are at risk of suffering from cardiometabolic conditions and related complications, such as diabetes, hypercholesterolemia, and obesity, among others. Therefore exercise should be a part of the well-being plan of care for the transplant patient, including children. As such, the World Transplant Games serve as motivation for children and adults to engage in healthy lifestyles after transplant. That being said, sport-related infections are not infrequent, the majority of which are transmitted by contact. Skin-to-skin contact during participation in sports like wrestling, martial arts, rugby, and American football render the patient susceptible to infections such as staphylococcal and streptococcal cellulitis, pyoderma and impetigo, viral infections such as molluscum and herpes and fungal infections such as tinea. Swimming in improperly maintained pools and open water also exposes the patient to waterborne infections, as discussed previously. The American Academy of Pediatrics Committee on Infectious Diseases alongside the Council on Sports Medicine and Fitness have published a clinical report with guidance on prevention and outbreak control of infections associated with sports.[42] These recommendations also apply to transplant recipients. Transplant recipients should check with the transplant team before participating in any sport and take the necessary precautions to make the activity safer.

Travel

The importance of adequate travel counseling and preparation before travel cannot be overemphasized. It is evident from studies that immunocompromised patients do engage in travel to areas with low and high risk for infection and that visits to travel clinics before travel are suboptimal in this population.[43,44] A study of travel patterns after HCT found that only 56% sought travel recommendations, and in another study of international travel in SOT recipients, a staggering 96% did not seek pretravel recommendations.[43,44] Pediatric data are not available for the immunocompromised patient, but from the GeoSentinel Surveillance Network noted that children tend to receive pretravel evaluations less often but require hospitalization for travel-related illness more frequently than adults.[45]

Transplant teams should be consulted to approve travel, especially to high-risk destinations. This should be discussed as part of the pretransplant evaluation so that families have time to consider family travel plans well in advance. In general, travel to high-risk areas is discouraged for allogeneic HSCT and SOT patients during the first 6 to 12 months after transplantation or times of heightened immunosuppression. Evaluation by a travel physician is important to review water and food safety precautions and to ensure the patient is up-to-date with vaccines. SOT recipients should avoid live vaccines specific for travel such as bacillus Calmette-Guérin, oral polio (not available in the United States), oral typhoid, and yellow fever vaccine. Non-live vaccines such as inactivated polio vaccine and inactivated typhoid VI capsular polysaccharide vaccine are available. A recent study of the immunogenicity and safety of yellow fever vaccine in HSCT recipients after immunosuppression had been discontinued showed that the vaccine could be safe in this population beyond 2 years of transplant.[46] They looked at 21 allogeneic HCT patients who received the vaccine at an average of 39 months after discontinuation of immunosuppression (and had no evidence of graft-versus-host-disease), finding the vaccine immunogenic and with little side effects; however, more data is needed before widespread use.

In addition to vaccines, water, and food safety recommendations, one of the most important precautions immunocompromised patients should follow during travel is insect precautions. Diseases such as dengue, West Nile virus, chikungunya, Zika virus, yellow fever, malaria, and leishmaniasis, among others, are transmitted by mosquitoes and other vectors. West Nile virus may present as encephalitis or as a flaccid paralysis in pediatric patients, with cases reported in pediatric kidney transplant recipients. Patients should be aware of the peak time and places for exposure to mosquitoes, wear appropriate clothing, and use mosquito nets and repellents containing at least 20% DEET (*N,N*-diethyl-*m*-toluami). During hikes, wearing long sleeves and long pants is recommended as well as tick checks.

Sexual Activity

As part of this process of feeling "normal," adolescent transplant recipients tend to engage in risky activities, including use of alcohol, street drugs, and high-risk sexual activities.[3,47] In a study by Ashoor and colleagues, the burden of sexually transmitted infections among pediatric kidney transplant recipients was high; 30% of the sexually active adolescents had diagnoses with at least one sexually transmitted infection (STI). Girls in the study were more sexually active than boys (58% vs. 15%) and the prevalence of STIs was also higher in girls (37.5% vs. 20%). These infections included gonorrhea, chlamydia, HIV, human papillomavirus (HPV), and herpes simplex virus, among others.[47] It is paramount to discuss sexual activity with adolescent transplant patients as part of routine follow-up and to counsel them regarding pregnancy and STI prevention. Patients should always use latex condoms for sexual intercourse to prevent STIs and should avoid contact with feces during sexual activity. Cytomegalovirus and Epstein Barr virus are also transmitted through secretions associated with intimate contact, but they are not always considered during counseling of adolescents who received their transplants at a younger age and therefore are more likely than older recipients to be seronegative.

HPV reactivation is common in HCT survivors and is a risk for the development of vulvar or cervical cancer.[48] In SOT recipients, HPV accounts for 2% to 3% of cancers that involve the anogenital region.[49] These findings highlight the importance of immunizing children before sexual activity. Attention should be given to administering HPV immunizations to adolescents and teenagers on SOT transplant lists before transplant as the immunogenicity of the vaccine may be inferior when administered after transplant.[50]

14

Multidrug-Resistant Gram-Negative Infections in Transplant and Oncology Patients

Mehreen Arshad, MBBS, Andrew Nowalk, MD, PhD, and Pranita D. Tamma, MD, MHS

COMMON MECHANISMS OF GRAM-NEGATIVE RESISTANCE

Gram-negative organisms are divided into the Enterobacteriaceae (e.g., *Escherichia coli, Klebsiella* species, *Enterobacter cloacae*) and the glucose nonfermenting gram-negative organisms (*Pseudomonas aeruginosa, Acinetobacter baumannii, Stenotrophomonas maltophilia*). Drug resistance in Enterobacteriaceae is often due to the production of β-lactamases. Common β-lactamases include extended-spectrum β-lactamases (ESBLs), AmpC β-lactamases, and carbapenemases. ESBLs and carbapenemases are generally plasmid mediated, whereas Amp C β-lactamases can either be plasmid mediated or chromosomally mediated.

Common ESBL genes include bla_{TEM}, $bla_{CTX\text{-}M\text{-}type}$, and bla_{SHV}, and the associated enzymes result in the hydrolysis of penicillins, cephalosporins, and aztreonam. SHV and the widely spread TEM enzyme were among the first to be recognized from this group; however, CTX-M enzymes are now rapidly becoming a common mechanism of bacterial resistance in many parts of the world.[1] Mechanisms of AmpC β-lactamase resistance in Enterobacteriaceae are divided into three categories: (1) inducible resistance by chromosomally encoded *ampC* genes (e.g., *E. cloacae, Citrobacter freundii, Serratia marcescens*), (2) noninducible chromosomal resistance owing to promoter and/or attenuator mutations (e.g.; *E. coli, Shigella* spp.); or (3) plasmid-mediated resistance (e.g., *E. coli, Klebsiella pneumoniae, Salmonella* spp.). Common carbapenemase genes include bla_{KPC}, bla_{NDM}, and $bla_{OXA\text{-}48\text{-}like}$. Plasmids that carry ESBL and carbapenemase genes also frequently encode fluoroquinolone resistance, trimethoprim-sulfamethoxazole resistance, and aminoglycoside resistance.[2]

Resistance mechanisms common to *P. aeruginosa* include OprD porins, hyperproduction of AmpC β-lactamases, upregulation of efflux pumps, and mutations in penicillin-binding proteins, with the minority producing carbapenemases. Drug resistance in *Actinobacter baumannii* is generally the result of the production of carbapenemases such as OXA-23-like, OXA-40-like, OXA-58-like, and OXA-143-like carbapenemases.

EPIDEMIOLOGY AND RISK FACTORS

Hematopoietic Stem Cell Transplant Recipients. Patients undergoing allogenic hematopoietic stem cell transplant (HSCT) are at particular risk for invasive infections with gram-negative enteric pathogens. This may be related to conditioning therapy, intestinal graft-versus-host disease, or a prolonged need for parenteral nutrition, all of which can damage the gut epithelium and allow greater translocation of enteric pathogens, resulting in bloodstream infections (BSIs).

A multicenter observational study evaluated the risk factors associated with 848 episodes of multidrug-resistant gram-negative (MDRGN) BSIs in children after HSCT in the United States between 2004 and 2008 and 2011 and 2014.[3] All positive blood culture results between days −10 and +365 surrounding allogenic HSCT were included. Approximately 53% of patients had at least one episode of a gram-negative rod (GNR) BSI; the most frequent pathogens implicated were *Klebsiella* spp. (26%), *Enterobacter* spp. (17%), *Pseudomonas* spp. (16%), *E. coli* (13%), *Stenotrophomonas* spp. (7%), and *Citrobacter* spp. (2%). Approximately 15% of GNR BSIs were caused by organisms resistant to three or more classes of antibiotics. Age older than 16 years and more than one BSI event were risk factors for infection with a resistant organism.

A large study from 65 institutions across 25 countries in Europe, Asia, and Australia was conducted by the European Bone Marrow Transplantation Group to study antibiotic resistance among patients of all ages undergoing autologous or allogenic HSCT.[4] The study results showed that 13% percent of the study participants were 18 years of age or younger. Enterobacteriaceae were significantly more resistant to fluoroquinolones compared with non-Enterobacteriaceae (57% vs. 31%), whereas carbapenem resistance (51% vs. 8%), and multidrug-resistance (47% vs. 32%) was more common in non–lactose-fermenting GNRs, which include *P. aeruginosa* and *A. baumannii.* Rates of resistance against all classes of antibiotics were significantly higher in allogenic versus autologous HSCT recipients. In general, GNR resistance in children mirrored proportions in adults, except for fluoroquinolones and antipseudomonal β-lactam/β-lactamase inhibitor combination drugs, for which resistance was higher in adults.

Heart and Lung Transplant Recipients

Infections are a leading cause of death in pediatric heart transplant patients, especially in the first year after transplant, with more than half of infections caused by bacterial pathogens. The Pediatric Heart Transplant Study, a prospectively maintained multiinstitutional research database in the United States, studied bacterial infections in children younger than 18 years less than 1 month, 1 to 6 months and more than 6 months after transplant.[5] Among the GNRs, *P. aeruginosa* was the most common cause of infection at all time points and was especially more likely to occur in patients with cardiac devices or nosocomial infections. Other important GNRs, regardless of the time point, included *Enterobacter* spp. (5%), *Klebsiella* spp. (5%), and *E. coli* (5%). Data regarding antibiotic resistance were not collected; however, the investigators noted that 2% to 5% of the infections in the first month after transplant were due to organisms commonly resistant to first-line antibiotic agents (e.g., *Serratia* spp., *Citrobacter* spp., *Stenotrophomonas* spp., and *Acinetobacter* spp.).

Data from a study in adults receiving a solid organ transplant (SOT) showed a steady increase in MDRGN infections (5% in 2007-2008 to 39% in 2014-2015).[6] This was largely driven by an increase in ESBL Enterobacteriaceae. A study in Italy showed that *Klebsiella* spp., *A. baumannii*, and *P. aeruginosa* (49%, 44%, and 31%, respectively) caused the majority of carbapenem-resistant infections.[7] Infection with carbapenem-resistant organisms was more common in patients with a history of lung or heart transplant.

Data are limited in the pediatric lung transplant population to estimate determinants of MDRGN infections. Data from adult lung transplant recipients without underlying cystic fibrosis indicated that *P. aeruginosa* and *Enterobacter* spp. were the most common MDRGNs (20% and 19%%, respectively).[8] Any previous exposure to broad-spectrum antibiotics, the presence of a tracheostomy, and an intensive care unit (ICU) stay longer than 14 days were associated with MDRGN bacterial acquisition. Prior colonization with MDRGN bacteria in donors or recipients was not associated with MDRGN infections or worse survival after transplant. Similar results were observed in a cohort of adult cystic fibrosis lung transplant recipients colonized with pan-resistant bacteria, including *P. aeruginosa, S. maltophilia*, and *Burkholderia cepacian*.[9]

Liver and Intestinal Transplant Recipients

Children undergoing liver transplants are at high risk of MDGN infections. However, limited data exist regarding the epidemiology of multidrug resistance in this population. In a single-center study of U.S. adults between 2010 and 2014 who received a liver transplant, 53% of bacterial infections were found to be MDR.[10] Among the Enterobacteriaceae, 55% were found to be MDR and 82% were resistant to antibiotics that were used for bacterial prophylaxis.

Among children undergoing intestinal transplants, a U.S. single-center study of BSIs within the first year after transplant showed that almost 24% of the *Klebsiella* spp. were MDR.[11] Similarly, another U.S.-based study including both adults and children showed that despite use of prophylactic therapy based on individual bacterial resistance patterns, 45% of subsequent infectious episodes were due to MDR organisms.[12] A Spanish study of both children and adults who received an intestinal transplant showed that the most common GNRs isolated were *P. aeruginosa, E. coli*, and *A. baumanni*, with 65%, 50% and 100% of respective isolates being MDR.[13]

Renal Transplant Recipients

A systematic review including both pediatric and adult studies showed that 10% of renal transplant recipients develop urinary tract infections (UTIs) with ESBL-producing *Enterobacteriaceae*.[14] In a Canadian study enrolling adult renal transplant patients, most UTIs were caused by antibiotic-resistant *E. coli* or *K. pneumoniae*; 5% of isolates were ESBL-producing. Furthermore, resistance to trimethoprim-sulfamethoxazole or fluoroquinolones occurred in 52% and 21%, respectively, of isolated microorganisms. Another study in adult renal transplant recipients showed that although infection with carbapenem-resistant Enterobacteriaceae (CRE) occurred in only 1% of patients, it was associated with higher mortality (30% vs. 10%) and a higher rate of recurrence (50% vs. 22%) compared with patients with more susceptible isolates.[15]

Oncology Patients

Approximately one-third of all BSIs in pediatric oncology patients are caused by gram-negative bacteria.[16] A large multicenter study that included both pediatric and adult hospitals in Europe reported that at individual institutions, ESBL-producing bacteria represented 15% to 24% of infections, and carbapenem-resistant *P. aeruginosa* caused 5% to 14% of infections.[17] Pediatric data from the United States are lacking, but a case-control study in adults was conducted in two New York oncology hospitals to determine the risk factors associated with carbapenem-resistant CRE between 2008 and 2012.[18] Overall, 2% of all BSIs and 5% of all GNR BSIs were caused by CRE. The majority (68%) of CRE organism were *K. pneumoniae*.

CLINICAL MANIFESTATIONS OF MDRGN INFECTION

Although MDRGN infections in immunocompromised patients occur frequently, clinical manifestations and sites of infection vary widely.[19] Previously noted risk factors for MDRGN infection are shared across all patients, including long hospital stays, ICU admission and ventilation, indwelling catheters and drains, and frequent antibiotic exposure. Prior colonization with MDRGN is also common. Specific sites of infection and clinical disease are often dependent on the method of immune suppression and modifying medical and surgical factors. Although pediatric data are often limited, general lessons drawn from adult literature can be applied to these patients as well.

Solid Organ Transplant Patients

Recipients of SOTs vary in their typical sites of infection by graft type.[19] Many of the pediatric conditions that lead to transplant—intestinal insufficiency, hepatic failure, congenital heart disease, cystic fibrosis—require intensive inpatient care, which can lead to a significant risk for infection before receipt of the graft. The complex postsurgical care needs often involve catheter placement and risk for catheter-related infection and associated bacteremia, whereas mechanical ventilation puts many recipients at risk of ventilator-associated pneumonia. Specific graft types also lead to increased incidence of specific clinical syndromes. In renal transplant recipients, both UTIs and surgical site infections with MDRGN develop. For kidney transplant recipients, ESBL-producing *E. coli* accounts for up to 12% of infection, especially in high-risk adult patients.[20] Approximately 70% of the complications caused by ESBL-producing GNR are UTIs. In contrast, liver transplantation requires extensive abdominal surgical procedures and post-transplant infections reflect this. A 2008 survey of pediatric liver transplant recipients noted that 38% of patients have bacterial infection in the first year after transplant, composed of central line (39%), intraabdominal (35%), wound (14%), and biliary infections (7%).[21] Gram-negative infections predominate in all these sites, and the overall prevalence of MDRGN among these infections was recently estimated at 7%, although for bacterial infection, respiratory tree syndromes predominate. A recent survey of pediatric lung transplantation noted a 22% rate of postoperative infection.[22] Whereas bacteremia predominated in the first month postoperatively, respiratory tract infection with MDRGN was seen more commonly after that period. In this study, prior history of MDRGN, especially in the setting of cystic fibrosis, led to elevated overall risk of infection. Infections in pediatric heart transplant are dominated by bacteremia, pneumonia, and surgical site infections. Recent data show that although BSIs (25%) are more common than pneumonia (21%), MDRGN infections are more commonly associated with respiratory infection.[5]

Oncology and Hematopoietic Stem Cell Transplant Patients

Regardless of type of malignancy or HSCT, oncology patients all share the risks for MDRGN infection similar to other chronically hospitalized patients. The presence of indwelling catheters, exposure to immune suppression and mucositis risk, and colonization with prior pathogens all increase this risk. Patients in a large prior survey of infections in children with cancer found that bloodstream (29%), pulmonary (18%), and skin and soft tissue (15%) are the most common sites in pediatric patients.[23] Among these, bacteremia associated with mucositis and catheter infections is the most common MDRGN infection found in oncology patients.

Disease Prophylaxis and Prevention

Decolonization practices and benefits for MDRGN disease are less well established than for gram-positive pathogens. Decontamination of the respiratory and digestive trees is based on presumed reduction of infection risk by altering the biome to reduce the burden of MDRGN in these sites. Methods include oropharyngeal decontamination with antiseptic agents and selective digestive tract decontamination with nonabsorbable antibiotics. Prior studies have indicated that selective oral and digestive tract decontamination reduces rates of bacteremia and mortality in ICU patients, although the overall benefit appears modest and conflicting data exist.[24] Use in U.S. hospitals has been limited by concerns for induction or worsening of antibiotic-resistant pathogens, as initial studies in the European centers were conducted in hospitals with low rates of antibiotic resistance.[24] These differences in incidence limit the generalizability of findings for areas more endemic for MDRGN resistance. Oral decontamination regimens typically use chlorhexidine (CHG) gluconate, an antiseptic with broad-spectrum bacterial activity, including MDRGN. Daily CHG bathing has been shown to decrease CRE skin colonization, and large-scale studies have shown benefit of CHG bathing in reducing the risk of hospital-acquired BSIs. Although studies specifically focusing on the role of CHG bathing in preventing MDRGN transmission have not been conducted, various bundles that have been successful in reducing MDR GNR transmission have included daily 2% CHG bathing. Concerns of gram-negative microorganisms developing resistance to CHG have tempered some of the enthusiasm for it, although some recent data suggest this may not be a drawback.[25]

Screening for colonization of SOT recipients with MDRGN is generally recommended in the pretransplant period.[26] As noted previously, risk factors for MDRGN infection include colonization in the pretransplant period, which has been linked to infection after graft placement. Despite the strong connection between colonization and infectious complications, no clear data exist regarding the effectiveness of perioperative prophylactic regimens in children. Screening of potential donors specifically for MDRGN colonization is not recommended by any major society, although targeted therapy to treat donor-derived infections is considered on a case-by-case basis. American Society for Transplantation guidelines for recipients who are ESBL carriers are limited to specific prophylaxis not exceeding 48 hours of duration, with the exception of lung transplant recipients for whom longer courses are acceptable.[19] Specific recommendations for other MDRGN do not exist except for standard surgical prophylaxis.

Oncology patients and bone marrow transplant recipients are at high risk for MDRGN infections. One series documented that isolation of MDRGN from any site in the prior 12 months increased the risk for MDRGN bacteremia almost 9-fold.[27] However, no consensus guidelines beyond those noted in the aforementioned recommendations exist for pretransplant screening or ongoing screening of recipients for MDRGN colonization at specific sites. Although routine use of levofloxacin prophylaxis in high-risk patients undergoing chemotherapy and bone marrow transplant has increased in frequency, some data suggest an increase in development of resistant GNR in response to this approach.[28] Modification of levofloxacin prophylaxis in selected oncology patients with a prior history of MDRGN has not been extensively studied and thus no definitive recommendations exist for this clinical scenario in either pediatric or adult patients.

Diagnosis

With limited options for the treatment of MDRGN infections, it is essential to adequately differentiate true invasive infection from colonization. Bacterial cultures from endotracheal aspirates and urine in the absence of appropriate signs and symptoms suggestive of infection may lead to the unnecessary overuse of antibiotics and associated downstream consequences.[29] Fig. 14.1 provides an overview of clinical signs and symptoms to assist with determining if a bacterial isolate is likely a pathogen or a contaminant when isolated from nonsterile sites.

Treatment

The selection of appropriate antibiotic therapy for critically ill transplant and oncology patients can be challenging. In general, antipseudomonal regimens such as cefepime or piperacillin-tazobactam are recommended as first-line agents. Avoiding universal empiric carbapenem therapy for this population is prudent, unless the child had previous colonization or infection with an organism resistant to other commonly used antipseudomonal β-lactams, is critically ill, or became ill while receiving or recently completing other antipseudomonal β-lactams. Although additional β-lactam agents with coverage broader than carbapenems are available (e.g., ceftazidime-avibactam, ceftolozane-tazbobactam, meropenem-vaborbactam imipenem/cilastatin-relebactam (herein, referred to as imipenem-relebactam), to preserve the efficacy of these agents, their use drugs should be limited to when in vitro activity has been confirmed and no other β-lactams present viable treatment options (Table 14.1).

Extended-Spectrum β-Lactamase-Producing Enterobacteriaceae. The continued rise in infections caused by ESBL-producing pathogens is one of the most pressing concerns facing the health care community. Previously, use of non–carbapenem β-lactams, most notably piperacillin-tazobactam, for the treatment of ESBL infections yielded conflicting results.[30] However, with the publication of the MERINO study, a randomized trial demonstrating the superiority of carbapenem therapy over piperacillin-tazobactam for the treatment of invasive ESBL infections, this question appears to be settled and carbapenem therapy is considered the first-line therapy for invasive ESBL infections.[31] If in vitro activity is confirmed, agents such as fluoroquinolones or trimethoprim-sulfamethoxazole can be considered for step-down therapy or for milder infections.

Carbapenem-Resistant Enterobacteriaceae. Optimal treatment regimens for CRE have not been definitely established. In general, treatment approaches do not differ based on underlying medical conditions (e.g., transplant vs. nontransplant patients) or by age (e.g., children vs. adults). Data evaluating the comparative effectiveness of various regimens, alone or in combination, for CRE infections are largely limited to observational studies. CRE are defined by resistance

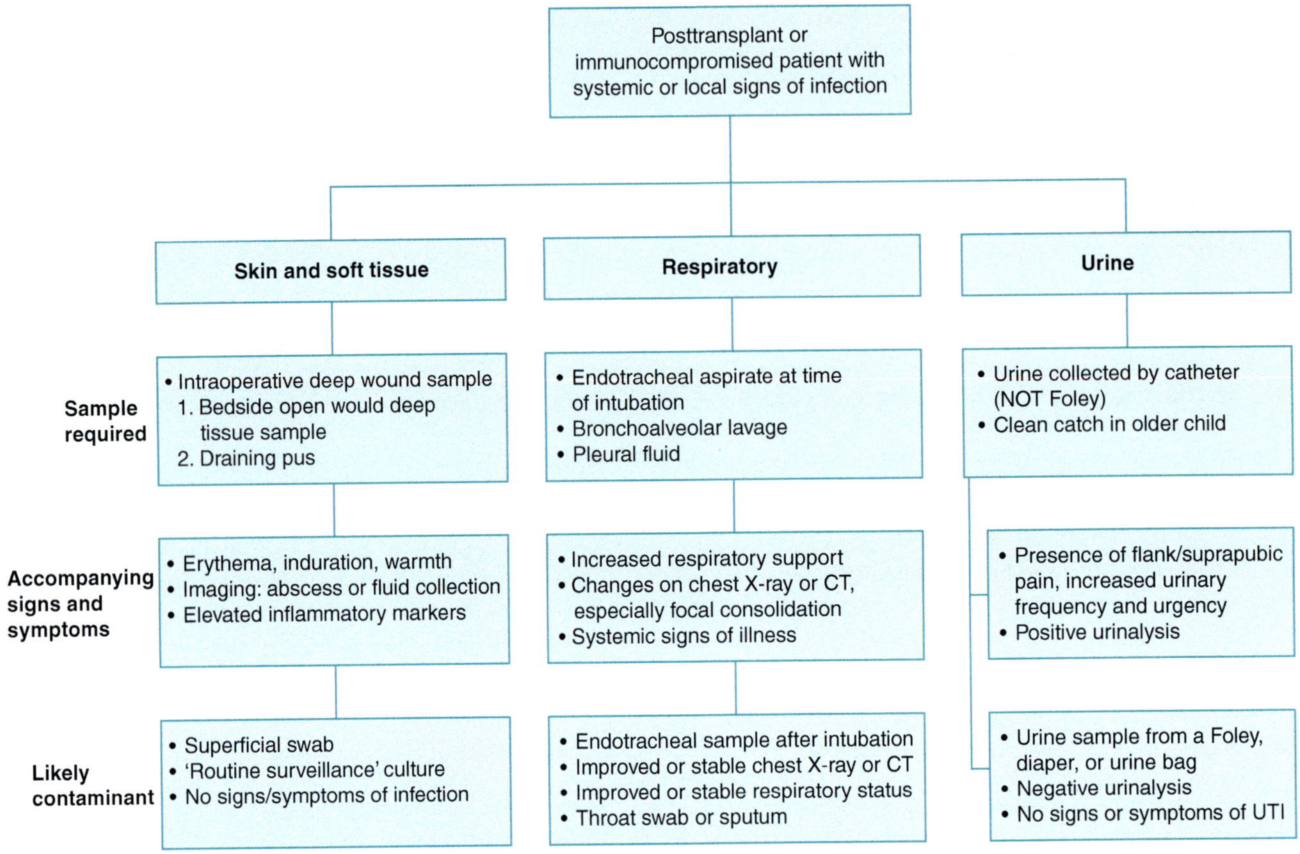

Fig. 14.1 Schematic diagram to determine pathogen versus contaminant from common patient samples. *CT*, computed tomography; *UTI*, urinary tract infection.

TABLE 14.1 Suggested Treatment Regimens for Carbapenem-Resistant Enterobacteriaceae

Considerations	Agents	Notes
Meropenem or imipenem-cilastatin MIC 1 μg/mL	Meropenem or imipenem-cilastatin as standard infusion	• As CRE implies resistance to at least one carbapenem agent, not infrequently, resistance to ertapenem may be observed, but susceptibility to other carbapenems may be present
Meropenem or imipenem-cilastatin MIC 2 μg/mL	Extended-infusion meropenem (or imipenem-cilastatin) ± a second agent	• Extended-infusion meropenem preferred over imipenem-cilastatin due to prolonged stability at room temperature • Second agent should be considered when a carbapenem is being administered serious infections, at least until an appropriate clinical response is observed • Determine second agent based on in vitro susceptibilities and source of infection. In order of preference: aminoglycosides > fluoroquinolones > trimethoprim-sulfamethoxazole > polymixins = tetracyclines (minocycline, tigecycline, eravacycline)
Meropenem or imipenem-cilastatin MIC ≥4 μg/mL	Ceftazidime-avibactam, meropenem-vaborbactam, or imipenem/cilastatin-relebactam	• Always perform in vitro susceptibility testing prior to prescribing ceftazidime/avibactam or, meropenem/vaborbactam or imipenem/cilastatin-relebactam

CRE, carbapenem-resistant Enterobacteriaceae; *MIC*, minimum inhibitory concentration.

to at least one carbapenem, yet frequently resistance to ertapenem is observed, and susceptibility to meropenem or imipenem-cilastatin (e.g., minimum inhibitory concentration [MIC] ≤1 μg/mL) is retained. In these scenarios, treatment with a susceptible carbapenem agent (e.g., meropenem or imipenem-cilastatin) as monotherapy is generally sufficient.

For carbapenem MICs of 2 μg/mL, combination therapy can be considered (see Table 14.1). For carbapenem MICs of 4 mcg/mL or above, agents such as ceftazidime-avibactam, meropenem-vaborbactam, or imipenem-relebactam should be considered as first-line agents. Although these agents can also be considered for CRE infections with MICs below 4 μg/mL, consideration of severity of illness and likely bacterial burden should be weighed against the risk of the development of resistance to these newer agents, precluding them as future treatment options for critically ill immunocompromised patients.

The possible benefit of combination antibiotic therapy (e.g., carbapenem plus colistin) for CRE infections has been explored in several observational studies. Although some of these studies have suggested improved outcomes with combination therapy, and more specifically, carbapenem-containing combination therapy, these studies have significant methodologic limitations, including relatively small sample sizes, differences in combination regimens, heterogeneity in patient population and source of infection, varied definitions of carbapenem resistance, limited consideration of confounding factors, and varying outcome evaluations. One of the largest observational studies (343 patients with monomicrobial carbapenemase-producing CRE BSIs) demonstrated a benefit of combination therapy only in the subgroup of patients at higher risk of mortality (e.g., severe sepsis, source other than urine of biliary tract).[32] A single randomized trial evaluated the impact of combination therapy on mortality among patients with infections caused by CRE, but this study primarily enrolled patients with *A. baumannii* infections.[33] Although this trial demonstrated no difference in outcomes when colistin monotherapy was prescribed compared to colistin plus meropenem, only 18% of patients were infected with CRE, making it unclear whether the results can be applied to patients infected with CRE. The available data support a potential role for combination therapy for treatment of CRE in high-risk patients but suggest that monotherapy may be effective for lower risk patients, with consideration given to illness severity, site of infection, source control, and the carbapenem MIC in stratifying patients as high or low risk. With the novel beta-lactam-beta-lactamase inhibitors, however, available data do not suggest a benefit with combination antibiotic therapy.

When a carbapenem is being considered for CRE treatment, extended-infusion strategies are generally recommended to increase the likelihood of appropriate time of the carbapenem above the MIC of the organism (e.g., meropenem infused over 3 hours).[34] Intermittent dosing (e.g., meropenem infused over 30 minutes) can lead to precipitous drops in serum drug concentrations as meropenem may be rapidly cleared through the kidneys. If a second agent is added to the extended-infusion carbapenem, potential options for combination therapy include aminoglycosides, fluoroquinolones, trimethoprim-sulfamethoxazole, polymixins, or tetracyclines (e.g., minocycline, tigecycline, eravacycline). The second agent should be selected based on in vitro activity. In general, aminoglycosides are preferred,[34] in large part because of a nuanced understanding of their pharmacokinetics and pharmacodynamics. If gentamicin, tobramycin, or amikacin do not provide activity against the CRE in question, plazomicin can be considered. As plazomicin is able to withstand modification by most aminoglycoside-modifying enzymes that inactiviate other aminoglycosides, it could provide a valuable role as combination therapy for CRE infections.[35]

Polymyxin antibiotics, which include colistin and polymyxin B, achieve bactericidal killing by binding to the negatively charged lipopolysaccharide layer of the cell membrane, disrupting the cell membrane and resulting in cell death.[35] Several clinical studies have demonstrated poor clinical outcomes with colistin monotherapy.[35] Complex pharmacokinetics, controversy surrounding the appropriate breakpoint and in vitro testing methodology, challenges with optimal dosing, and associated toxicities represent additional challenges.

Tigecycline is an injectable agent designed to be a poor substrate for tetracycline-specific efflux pumps. It generally has excellent in vitro activity against CRE isolates.[35] Tigecycline use as monotherapy is concerning given its unfavorable pharmacokinetics as serum concentrations peak at less than 1 μg/mL and promptly decline because of rapid tissue distribution, making it an unfavorable choice for BSIs.[35] However, use of tigecycline as part of a combination regimen for other sites of infection may prove valuable. Eravacycline is a newer tetracycline derivative with a similar mechanism of action as tigecycline; however, it is two- to fourfold more potent than tigecycline against Enterobacteriaceae.[36]

With carbapenem MICs of 4 μg/mL or greater ceftazidime-avibactam, meropenem-vaborbactam, or imipenem-relebactam should be considered.[37] Available data suggest these agents can generally be used as monotherapy. Ceftazidime-avibactam has in vitro activity against common CRE, including *K. pneumoniae* carbapenemase (KPC)-producers, OXA-48-like producers, and non–carbapenemase-producing CRE (e.g., ESBL producers in the setting of porin mutations or efflux pumps).[37] Several postmarketing observational studies have highlighted the potential for development of ceftazidime-avibactam resistance after even a limited duration of therapy. These findings underscore the importance of vigilance for emerging resistance on therapy.

Meropenem-vaborbactam has excellent in vitro activity against KPC-producing Enterobacteriaceae but is limited to no activity against other mechanisms of carbapenem resistance found in Enterobacteriaceae.[37] Randomized controlled trial data indicate it has superior outcomes to the best available therapy for these infections.

Imipenem-relebactam is highly active against KPC-producing isolates, but not MBL-producing isolates. More data are needed for its activity against OXA-48-like producing isolates. In vitro data suggest that relebactam can significantly lower the imipenem MIC for isolates with imipenem MICs of >64 μg/mL, as would be expected given the structural similarities to avibactam.[38] Randomized controlled trial data indicate that this agent improves clinical outcomes and is associated with less acute kidney injury compared to the combination of imipenem/cilastatin and colistin.

Carbapenem-Resistant *Pseudomonas aeruginosa*. Carbapenem-resistant *P. aeruginosa* generally evolve because of an interplay of multiple complex mechanisms, making the selection of effective agents more challenging than with CRE. In general, although conclusive trial data are lacking, combination therapy is generally preferred for the treatment of carbapenem-resistant *P. aeruginosa*. As with CRE, extended-infusion meropenem or imipenem-cilastatin is preferred. Tigecycline and eravacycline do not provide coverage against *P. aeruginosa*; all other agents described as options for CRE can be considered as second agents to combine with extended-infusion carbapenem therapy. Plazomicin has similar activity as amikacin against carbapenem-resistant *P. aeruginosa* and does not afford enhanced coverage over amikacin as it does with CRE. Meropenem-vaborbactam is highly unlikely to provide enhanced coverage against carbapenem-resistant *P. aeruginosa*.[37] Ceftazidime-avibactam has been shown to be active against 67% to 88% of meropenem-nonsusceptible *P. aeruginosa* isolates.[37] Ceftolozane-tazobactam and imipenem-relebactam offer broad coverage against carbapenem-resistant *P. aeruginosa*.[38]

Ceftolozane-tazobactam was 93% active against extensively drug-resistant *P. aeruginosa* isolates in the United States.[40] In a separate cohort of 42 carbapenem-resistant *P. aeruginosa* isolates, ceftolozane-tazobactam remained active against 95% of isolates; whereas ceftazidime-avibactam retained activity against 71% of the same isolates.[41] Therefore when carbapenem-resistant *P. aeruginosa* organisms are isolated, it is prudent to test ceftolozane-tazobactam and/or imipenem-relebactam as a potential treatment option.

Infection Prevention and Anticipatory Guidance

Infection Prevention. Prevention efforts for MDRGN infection reflect recent comprehensive recommendations regarding the management and prevention of MDRGN in health care facilities. The 2007 Healthcare Infection Control Practices Advisory Committee guidelines established isolation precautions to prevent transmission of MDRGN and other pathogens in hospital settings where solid organ and bone marrow transplant recipients receive care.[42] These publications provide guidance with regard to the following:

1. Education of health care workers
2. Surveillance for targeted multidrug-resistant organisms
3. Application of infection control precautions during patient care
4. Environmental cleaning and disinfection measures
5. Decolonization practices
6. Judicious use of antibiotics

The CDC also issued a 2015 update to their "Guidance for Control of CRE," which recommends core measures for acute and long-term care facilities to decrease the transmission of CRE.[43] The CDC document recommends core interventions, including hand hygiene, contact precautions, patient cohorting, and active surveillance. The CDC recommends preemptive contact precautions pending the results of screening cultures and that all patients colonized or infected with CRE have contact precautions in place. The duration of contact precautions remains unknown, and no controlled data informing this decision for MDRGN are available. In 2014, the European Society of Clinical Microbiology and Infectious Diseases published guidelines for infection control measures to reduce transmission of MDRGN.[44] These evidence-based guidelines were developed after review of published literature on infection prevention strategies aimed at reducing the transmission of MDRGN and include standard recommendations for all acute care facilities and enhanced recommendations for ongoing transmission of MDRGN.

Anticipatory Guidance. Invasive infections with MDRGN often require treatment for several weeks, increasing the risk of drug toxicities. Treatment with broad-spectrum antibiotics, is necessary with MDRGN infections, also increases the risk of antibiotic-associated diarrhea, particular those due to *C. difficile*. Therefore testing for this pathogen is recommended in a patient with diarrhea receiving prolonged broad-spectrum therapy. β-lactams such as cephalosporins and carbapenems have rarely been associated with hypersensitivity reactions, drug fevers, and bone marrow suppression after prolonged use. Carbapenems, especially imipenem, can decrease the seizure threshold in some patients. Colistin can cause nephrotoxicity, and patients' urine output and creatinine should be closely monitored.

15

Bartonella, Legionella, Mycoplasma, and *Ureaplasma*

Daniel Dulek, MD and Victoria A. Statler, MD, MSc

BARTONELLA

Epidemiology and Risk Factors

Bartonella species are fastidious, slow-growing, gram-negative bacilli. There are 45 different species that can cause disease in zoonotic hosts, with *Bartonella henselae* and *Bartonella quintana* causing most *Bartonella*-related disease in human hosts in the United States.[1] *B. henselae* has been reported to cause infection in pediatric and adult heart, liver, and renal transplant recipients and in adult lung transplant recipients. There have been rare reports of *B. quintana* causing disease in adult solid organ transplant (SOT) recipients. Both species have been reported to cause infection in pediatric patients undergoing chemotherapy for hematologic malignancies.

Cat-scratch disease (CSD), a syndrome of regional lymphadenopathy or granulomatous disease in the liver and spleen, is the most widely recognized illness attributed to *B. henselae*. The highest incidence of CSD in the United States is reported in people who live in the Southeast and among children 5 to 9 years of age.[2] Granulomatous disease/CSD is the most common presentation of *B. henselae* in SOT recipients and is found in 19 of 32 (59%) reported cases.[3] *B henselae* infection disproportionately affects children. Moulin and colleagues reported that 25% of the cases of *Bartonella* infection in transplant recipients occurred in children younger than 18 years, despite pediatric patients representing only 3% to 4% of the overall transplant population.[4]

Bacillary angiomatosis (BA) and bacillary peliosis (BP) are vasoproliferative manifestations of both *B. henselae* and *B. quintana* in immunocompromised hosts. They are most commonly described in adults with very low $CD4^+$ lymphocyte counts caused by human immunodeficiency virus (HIV). Cases have been described in pediatric and adult SOT recipients and those with hematologic malignancies. All patients reported with BA associated with cancer have had full resolution of their disease with treatment. Interestingly, in SOT recipients, BA tends to develop on average 1.9 years after transplantation, whereas granulomatous disease/CSD develops 5.2 years after transplantation. The reason for this is unknown but may be explained by greater immunosuppression close to the time of transplant, predisposing patients to vasoproliferative manifestations.[5]

B. henselae causes bacteremia in cats, its natural reservoir. The seroprevalence of *B. henselae* is 13% to 90% in domestic and stray cats in the United States.[6] Other animals, including dogs, can become infected and have been associated with human disease. Kittens and stray or sheltered cats are more likely to have bacteremia, which can last for weeks to months. Despite this, cats are usually asymptomatic. Transmission between cats occurs through the cat flea, whereas transmission to humans occurs through the lick, bite, or scratch of a bacteremic cat; the claws of the cat are thought to be contaminated by the feces of *Bartonella*-infected fleas. The incubation period from scratch to the appearance of a cutaneous lesion is 7 to 12 days. Lymphadenopathy usually occurs 5 to 50 days, with a median of 12 days, after the scratch.[6]

There have been no cases of person-to-person *B. henselae* transmission.[6] One case of possible donor-derived transmission has been reported in an asymptomatic liver transplant recipient with granulomatous hepatic lesions appearing 2 months after transplant. Subsequent 16S PCR of DNA from the lesion was positive for *B. henselae*. This patient had no reported contact with cats, raising the possibility of donor-derived infection.[7]

B. quintana is closely related to *B. henselae* and is more commonly associated with louse-borne trench fever. Risk factors for infection with *B. quintana* include homelessness, chronic alcoholism, and body lice.

Clinical Manifestations

In general, *Bartonella*-mediated disease in transplant recipients can be divided into two distinct groups: cat-scratch disease (typical and disseminated) and BA and BP.

Cat-scratch disease commonly occurs in immunocompetent children as a self-limited febrile illness characterized by a cutaneous papule at the site of a cat scratch and accompanied by regional lymphadenopathy. Cases of this "typical" regional presentation of CSD have also been reported in pediatric SOT recipients.[8,9] Lymph nodes are generally tender and can have central necrosis and suppuration. Nodes may regress spontaneously within 2 to 4 months in immunocompetent hosts, but usually respond promptly to antimicrobial therapy in SOT patients. Systemic symptoms are mild in immunocompetent hosts, whereas transplant recipients can present with fever, fatigue, myalgias, joint pain, and night sweats. Importantly, although fever is the most common symptom present in any manifestation of *Bartonella* disease in SOT recipients,[3] the absence of fever does not rule out this infection. At least two cases of *B. henselae* infection without fever have been reported in children,[7,10] with another two cases reported in adults,[3] one of whom died from infective endocarditis.[4]

Lymphadenopathy can also be accompanied by hepatosplenic lesions, concerning for disseminated disease in SOT recipients. Children often present with prolonged fever, abdominal pain, joint pain, headache, weight loss, and chills. Immunocompromised patients may have splenic or hepatic enlargement or both, and abdominal imaging usually identifies hypodense lesions in either or both organs.[9] Transaminase levels often remain normal. In almost all cases, cat, kitten, or flea exposure is given in the history. Recurrence has been reported, with one case of recurrent cat-scratch lymphadenitis described in a pediatric kidney transplant recipient.[9] More unusual manifestations of CSD in immunocompetent hosts include endocarditis, osteomyelitis, encephalopathy, retinitis, optic neuritis, and Parinaud oculoglandular syndrome. A case of posterior uveitis and one case of pulmonary nodules caused by *B. henselae* have been described in pediatric kidney transplant recipients.[10] Acute rejection of the renal allograft has been reported in conjunction with *Bartonella* infection in two children.[8] Reports in adult renal transplant recipients have described a patient with sternal abscess and one with septic shock, encephalopathy and seizures, and bacteremia has been described in a hematopoietic stem cell transplant (HSCT) recipient.[5]

BA and BP vasculoproliferative cutaneous or subcutaneous lesions are due to either *B. henselae* or *B. quintana*. Lesions of BA are most commonly seen on the skin but may involve subdermal structures, bones, and mucous membranes of the mouth, conjunctivae, and the gastrointestinal tract. BP lesions may appear as hemorrhagic parenchymous and cystic lesions usually seen in the liver or spleen. *B. henselae* is almost exclusively associated with lesions in the lymph nodes and the liver, whereas bone lesions are more associated with *B. quintana*.[11] Children may be systemically asymptomatic, or more commonly, present similarly to those with CSD with systemic symptoms of fever, abdominal pain, anorexia, myalgias, nausea, vomiting, weight loss, night sweats, and weakness. Liver and spleen lesions, lymphadenopathy, and hepatomegaly have also been reported.[4,10] Vasculoproliferative cutaneous lesions can be papular, nodular, or vascular; are usually red or violaceous in color; and may be hemorrhagic, ulcerating, or have a collarette of scale. They can be solitary or multiple and may grossly resemble Kaposi sarcoma. Recurrence of BA is seen in HIV-positive patients and has been described in a pediatric renal transplant recipient despite prolonged therapy for the first episode.[4,5]

Providers should also have a low index of suspicion for secondary hemophagocytic lymphohistiocytosis in transplant recipients with *Bartonella* infection, as it has been described in both children and adults.[4,12] Pancytopenias, elevated transaminase levels, low fibrinogen level, and a very elevated ferritin level should prompt the clinician to consider this diagnosis. Treatment of the underlying cause is prudent, but patients may also require corticosteroid therapy. Consultation with a hematologist may be warranted.

Disease Prophylaxis/Prevention

Because cats and kittens carry *B. henselae* and because cat fleas play a major role in cat-to-cat transmission, it is prudent to discuss pet ownership with transplant recipients and their families. They should be educated about obtaining and caring for pets, particularly cats and kittens. All pets should be seen regularly by a veterinarian and before introduction of the pet into the home. Flea control is essential. New pets should not be introduced during times of heightened immunosuppression (immediate posttransplant period or during treatment for rejection). Immunocompromised hosts should avoid all contact with cats younger than 1 year, stray cats, cats with fleas, or cats that bite or scratch. Although declawing of cats is not routinely recommended, patients should not engage in behavior that would cause a scratch or bite. If a scratch or bite should occur, it should be cleaned immediately and thoroughly. Testing cats for *Bartonella* infection is not recommended because cats can be transiently bacteremic. Good hand hygiene is always encouraged, especially after petting or caring for cats or kittens.

Diagnosis

The differential diagnosis of cat scratch disease includes other causes of lymphadenopathy and systemic symptoms in transplant recipients: cytomegalovirus, Epstein-Barr virus, and posttransplant lymphoproliferative disease, lymphoma, fungal or mycobacterial infections, and pyogenic abscesses. BA may mimic Kaposi sarcoma, pyogenic granuloma, or angiosarcoma. *Bartonella* infection should be considered in any transplant recipient with cat or cat flea exposure who presents with unexplained fever, culture-negative endocarditis, granulomatous or necrotic regional or disseminated lymphadenopathy, BA or BP, new hepatomegaly, new splenomegaly, or hepatosplenic lesions.

Confirmatory diagnosis can be challenging in immunosuppressed patients. The indirect immunofluorescent antibody assay for detection of serum antibodies to antigens of *Bartonella* species is available at many commercial laboratories and through the Centers for Disease Control and Prevention. Immunoglobulin (Ig) M production is brief and may easily be missed. Immunofluorescent antibody IgG titer greater than 1:256 is consistent with acute infection, although lower titers (>1:64) have been used for diagnosis. Documentation of a fourfold increase in IgG titers can also be suggestive of recent infection. In one review of the literature, of 23 SOT patients with *Bartonella* infection who had serologic testing performed, all were at least IgG or IgM positive initially or had evidence of a fourfold increase in titers on follow-up testing.[5] The sensitivity of the indirect fluorescence antibody test in immunocompromised patients is lower than in immunocompetent hosts (75% vs. 82-95%).[11] Furthermore, serologic test results can be negative early in the course and may take 2 to 4 weeks to develop.[8,10] In some cases, patients may never mount a response, even when serology is obtained later in the course.[4] It is important to note that cross-reactions between the different *Bartonella* species exist, as well as with other zoonoses such as *Rickettsiae*.[6]

Histologic examination of lymph nodes from affected patients can reveal lymphocytes with epithelioid granulomas, which may later in the course have central zones of necrosis or appear suppurative; some may contain stellate microabscesses. Warthin-Starry or Steiner silver stain demonstrates aggregates of small coccobacilli. This test, however, is not specific for *B. henselae*. Immunohistochemistry of lymph node tissue with *B. henselae*–specific antibodies may also reveal evidence of infection.

On biopsy, BA of lymph nodes or skin contains a dense vascular proliferation with plump endothelial cells that protrude into the vascular lumina. There is often a mixed inflammatory infiltrate of both lymphocytes and neutrophils. Biopsies of BP lesions differ from those in BA. Lesions often demonstrate dilated capillaries and cystic blood-filled spaces scattered throughout the hepatic or splenic parenchyma. As do biopsies of lymph nodes in typical CSD, both BA and BP demonstrate clusters of bacilli seen on Warthin-Starry or Steiner silver stain.

Identification of *Bartonella* in cultures is difficult due to its fastidious growth and culture techniques that are not sensitive. Culturing of *Bartonella* can require 1 to 4 weeks of incubation on blood agar plates under specific conditions. If culture is performed, specialized laboratories with experience in isolating *Bartonella* organisms are recommended for processing of cultures.

Polymerase chain reaction (PCR) of DNA extracted from tissue may confirm species identity.[5] PCR assays are available commercially and in research settings for testing of tissue or body fluids, including blood. PCR of tissue has been used to determine the etiology from lymph nodes, hepatosplenic lesions, and lung nodules in immunocompromised hosts.[11] This technique is both sensitive and specific.

Treatment

The need for treatment of CSD in the immuocompetent host is not well established. In the only prospective, randomized trial of treatment of typical CSD in immunocompetent children, there was no clinical difference except in lymph node size at 30 days between those treated with azithromycin versus placebo.[13]

Because severe, progressive, disseminated disease can occur in immunocompromised patients, treatment for *Bartonella*-associated infections is always recommended in this population. There are no established treatment guidelines for *Bartonella* infection in transplant recipients. Unlike in immunocompetent hosts, response to treatment is usually prompt in the immunocompromised patient. Pediatric transplant recipients with granulomatous or suppurative disease, including hepatosplenic lesions, have been successfully treated with single agents or combinations of agents: aminoglycosides (gentamicin, amikacin), macrolides (azithromycin, erythromycin), tetracyclines (doxycycline), fluoroquinolones (ciprofloxacin), and trimethoprim-sulfamethoxazole.[7-10] Durations of therapy have ranged from 2 weeks to 6 months. In most cases, therapy was discontinued when all lymphadenopathy and/or hepatosplenic lesions had resolved. Shorter therapy has been associated with at least one reported recurrence of lymphadenitis in a pediatric kidney transplant recipient.[9]

Azithromycin, doxycycline, and ciprofloxacin have been used successfully in pediatric transplant recipients with BA treated with a 3- to 4- month duration of therapy. In adult SOT recipients, reported length of therapy has ranged from 4 weeks to 6 months, which is similar to reported guidelines for HIV-infected patients with BA.[10] In presumed disseminated CSD and BA or BP, prolonged therapy is generally administered (for at least 3 months and until lesions resolve) with a macrolide antibiotic or tetracycline, either alone or in combination with another efficacious antimicrobial, such as rifampin, an aminoglycoside, or ciprofloxacin. It is important to note, however, that children younger than 8 years in whom a macrolide may be given, doxycycline is not recommended for more than 21 days.[6] Clinicians should also be aware that a Jarisch-Herxheimer reaction may develop after the first few doses of treatment of BA.[10]

Drug-drug interactions must be considered in SOT recipients. Macrolides can increase the serum concentration of some calcineurin inhibitors like tacrolimus, and rifampin is a potent hepatic enzyme inducer and interacts with many drugs.

In addition to antimicrobial therapy, a decrease in immunosuppression is recommended if possible.

Infection Prevention and Anticipatory Guidance

Standard precautions are recommended for children with *Bartonella* infections.

LEGIONELLA

Epidemiology and Risk Factors

The term "Legionnaires' disease" (LD) was first used to describe an outbreak of pneumonia that occurred among members of an American Legion convention in Philadelphia in 1976. Eventually, *Legionella pneumophila* was identified as the etiologic agent responsible for the outbreak, and LD became the name given to pneumonia acquired by susceptible people through inhalation of aerosols that contain *Legionella* species.

Legionella is a fastidious gram-negative bacillus, of which there are at least 60 different species. There were 6141 cases of legionellosis reported in the United States in 2016, more than a fourfold increase in reported cases since 2000.[14] The most common species that cause disease in the United States is *L. pneumophila* serogroup 1. Other serogroups and species are also pathogenic and have been reported to cause disease in children, including *L. micdadei*, *L. dumoffii*, and *L. bozemannii*. *L. longbeachae* has been described in patients in the western United States who have had exposure to potting soil. It is the second most common cause of legionellosis in Australia and has been reported in adult transplant recipients.[15]

Legionellosis is a rare cause of both community-acquired and nosocomial-acquired pneumonia in children. Between 2000 and 2009, 1% of cases reported in the United States were in children 19 years and younger.[16] The incidence of legionellosis in immunocompromised children is unknown, but there have been numerous cases reported sporadically and in health care–associated outbreaks.

Risk factors for disease fall into two broad categories: those that increase exposure to contaminated water sources (well water and water in large buildings such as hotels or hospitals) and those with impaired pulmonary or immune defense mechanisms, especially transplant recipients, children with hematologic malignancies, and those who use glucocorticoids.[17] Both are identified as risk factors in the cases reported in the pediatric population. There have been no reports of transmission between patients and health care providers or between patients and other patients, although there has been one report of possible transmission between a son and his mother who cared for him in a nonventilated residential room for several hours.[18] Incubation periods have ranged from 2 to 19 days, most commonly 2 to 10 days.[19]

Clinical Manifestations

Legionellosis often manifests as a severe pneumonia in immunocompromised children.[20-22] Symptom onset is often abrupt. Children tend to have fever, which may be the only initial symptom, but respiratory symptoms eventually become more prominent. Cough is the most frequent symptom and can be accompanied by dyspnea, tachypnea, and pleuritic chest pain. Hemoptysis is infrequently reported. Legionellosis in immunosuppressed patients may rapidly progress to respiratory failure. Hypoxia and abnormal finding on lung examination are the most common signs. Chills, abdominal pain, nausea and vomiting, headache, malaise, anorexia, and/or fatigue may occur. Diarrhea is a common extrapulmonary finding in adults but is infrequently reported in children.[22,23] There have also been case reports in adults of pericarditis, myocarditis, endocarditis, arthritis, and central nervous system manifestations.[17]

Without appropriate antibiotic therapy, immunocompromised hosts often progress to severe respiratory compromise, multiorgan failure, and eventual death with a reported mortality rate in immunosuppressed children of 42%.[22] In fact, delay in diagnosis has been considered a risk factor for increased morbidity and mortality in adults.[24] Empyema or cavitation can occur. Extrapulmonary manifestations rarely occur in children, including *Legionella*-associated transverse myelitis and liver abscesses.

Unlike the interstitial pneumonias caused by other "atypical bacteria," radiographic findings of LD are more often lobar consolidations with or without pleural effusion. Bilateral and/or nodular infiltrates may occur, mimicking invasive fungal infection, mycobacterial infection, or *Nocardia*. When nodules are present, patients may be asymptomatic.[25] Cavitation can occur for up to 14 days after presentation, despite appropriate antibiotic therapy. Abscess can also occur. Chest computed tomography often reveals a mixture of ground-glass opacities and consolidation. Later in the course, an organizing pneumonia pattern may also be seen.

Nonspecific abnormal laboratory results are common and may not help in the diagnosis. Leukocytosis, leukopenia, lymphopenia, and thrombocytosis can be seen. Elevated transaminase levels and renal dysfunction are common. Recurrence can occur and has been noted in children after HSCT.[21]

Disease Prophylaxis/Prevention

Minimizing *Legionella* growth in large buildings and hospital water systems, including potable water, showers, hot tubs, decorative fountains, and cooling towers, is key to prevention of this infection. A word of caution should be given to transplant recipients who travel or who will be around fountains or other manmade water sources that may aerosolize water droplets.

Diagnosis

Pneumonia is common in children and it may be difficult to distinguish between pneumonia caused by *Legionella* and pneumonia caused by other etiologies. Lobar consolidation may easily be confused with other bacterial causes of pneumonia, whereas those with nodular infiltrates or cavitation may be difficult to distinguish from fungal or mycobacterial infection. *Mycoplasma*, psittacosis, and Q fever may be suspected but tend to have an interstitial pattern on chest radiographs. If the respiratory symptoms are accompanied by systemic symptoms, viral causes such as influenza may also be considered.

Laboratory diagnosis can be challenging, and clinicians must have a high index of suspicion to ensure appropriate testing. Most assays and culture methods must be requested because they are not considered routine at many institutions. Culture of *Legionella* from sputum and other lower respiratory tract specimens remains the gold standard and allows for the diagnosis of all *Legionella* species, outbreak investigations, and antimicrobial susceptibility testing. However, culture requires special media (buffered charcoal yeast extract supplemented with α-ketoglutaric acid) and is not time efficient (it may take up to 7 days to grow). Sensitivity also varies widely (20% to 80%) and depends on the type of sample.[17] Blood and pleural fluid cultures have very low yield. Urinary antigen detection allows for the most rapid method of diagnosis, but this test detects only *L. pneumophila* serogroup 1, and therefore results may be negative in disease caused by other species or other serogroups. It does have a high specificity and sensitivity for legionellosis caused by serogroup 1 and should be performed in any transplant recipient with pneumonia for which an underlying etiology is not readily apparent.

Detection of *L. pneumophila* antigen from lung tissue or sputum by immunofluorescence can be performed within 1 to 2 hours and is highly specific (99%) but may be insensitive (25% to 75%).[26] Appropriate diagnosis requires expertise and training of laboratory personnel and many laboratoriess do not perform this test.

Detection of *Legionella* DNA in respiratory tract specimens and urine can be done by PCR and may detect other serogroups and species. Sensitivity and specificity are excellent, but different laboratory assays vary. Additionally, no commercial laboratories in the United States offer PCR testing for specific *Legionella* species.[26]

Serologic diagnosis is not helpful in immunocompromised patients. The average time to seroconversion in immunocompetent patients is 2 weeks. Measuring convalescent serum is delayed and therefore is not efficient for acute case diagnosis and initiation of therapy. Finally, seroconversion may not occur at all in the immunosuppressed patient.

Treatment

Adequately sized prospective clinical studies of antimicrobial therapy for legionellosis are lacking. Newer macrolides such as azithromycin can be considered for therapy in immunocompromised children. A dosage of 10 mg/kg once daily (maximum dose 500 mg) for 5 to 10 days is recommended. Azithromycin is available in intravenous and oral forms and approved by the U.S. Food and Drug Administration for the treatment of legionellosis in adults. Macrolides often interact with immunosuppressive therapies such as tacrolimus, and their use may prove challenging in the transplant population. Fluoroquinolones also have efficacy in vitro and in vivo, and levofloxacin is the drug of choice for *Legionella* pneumonia in adult transplant recipients. It is approved by the Food and Drug Administration for the treatment of LD in adults. Length of therapy should be 14 to 21 days with a quinolone because of the shorter half-life compared with azithromycin. Improvement in most patients occurs within a few days to a week after starting therapy.

One observational study of non-immunocompromised adults with legionellosis compared those who received levofloxacin with those who received erythromycin or clarithromycin therapy. The levofloxacin group had a significantly shorter time to defervescence and a shorter length of hospital stay.[27] Although combination antibiotic therapy has been reported, there is no clear benefit to this beyond what is achieved with use of a fluoroquinolone or a macrolide alone.

Infection Prevention and Anticipatory Guidance

Standard precautions are recommended for children with legionellosis. Multiple nosocomial and community outbreaks of legionellosis have been reported. Reservoirs include potable water distribution systems, air conditioning cooling towers, hot tubs, decorative fountains, and others. Hospital water systems should maintain hot water at the highest temperature allowable, usually stored at a minimum of 60°C (140°F) and with a minimum returned temperature of 51°C (124°F). If even a single case of legionellosis is detected, an epidemiologic and environmental investigation is warranted.[19]

Hospitals with transplantation programs should maintain a high index of suspicion for legionellosis. Using sterile water for nebulization equipment is recommended. Periodic culturing of the hospital's potable water system should also be considered, particularly after construction has been done or hospital additions built. Outbreaks have been halted by emergency superheating of water to 70°C to 80°C. Measures for long-term prevention include the use of water management systems and decontamination using copper-silver ionization, hyperchlorination, and ultraviolet light.

Legionellosis is a nationally notifiable disease in the United States.

MYCOPLASMA AND *UREAPLASMA*

Mycoplasmas and ureaplasmas are small, fastidious organisms that lack a cell wall and cause an array of clinical symptoms in both immunocompetent and immunocompromised patients.[28,29] Species that cause human disease include *Mycoplasma pneumoniae, M. hominis, M. genitalium, Ureaplasma urealyticum*, and *U. parvum*. Disease processes caused by these pathogens are numerous and include lower respiratory tract infection, necrotizing pneumonia, meningoencephalitis, genitourinary infections, bone and joint infections, and intraabdominal infections as well as parainfectious and postinfectious syndromes, including erythema multiforme and Stevens-Johnson syndrome (SJS).

Epidemiology and Risk Factors

The epidemiology of *Mycoplasma* and *Ureaplasma* infections is highly species dependent. *M. pneumoniae* causes upper and lower respiratory tract infections in both endemic and epidemic patterns.[28] Classically, *M. pneumoniae* causes a significant proportion of community-acquired pneumonia in otherwise healthy school-age and adolescent children. In a recent Centers for Disease Control and Prevention–sponsored multicenter pneumonia epidemiology study of pneumonia causing hospitalization in children younger than 18 years, *Mycoplasma* accounted for 8% of pneumonia overall and 19% in children 5 to 18 years.[30] The epidemiology of *M. pneumoniae* is not well defined in pediatric SOT, HSCT, or oncology patients with only case reports and case series defining the occurrence of infection in these populations (see later text). In one prospective active surveillance study of upper or lower respiratory tract infection in children with cancer, *M. pneumoniae* respiratory infection occurred in 4 of 253 (1.6%) children over a one-year period.[31]

Urogenital colonization by *M. hominis* and *M. genitalium* is well documented in sexually active adults.[32] Despite this predilection, nongenitourinary infections are described, although they occur often in adolescents (see "Clinical Manifestations" later). Donor-derived acquisition of *M. hominis* is reported in an adult lung transplant recipient in whom bilateral pneumonia, pleural effusion, and multijoint arthritis developed early after transplant.[33]

Ureasplasma species colonize the male and female genital tracts with infants becoming colonized during passage through the birth canal.[29] Before the onset of sexual activity, detection of *Ureaplasma* species from the genital tract of prepubertal children is infrequent. Similar to *M. hominis*, donor-derived transmission of *Ureaplasma* is documented.[34] Additionally, hypogammaglobulinemia may be a risk factor for severe or disseminated *Ureaplasma* infection.[35-37]

Clinical Manifestations

An array of clinical manifestations are associated with *Mycoplasma* and *Ureaplasma* spp. infections. It is important to note that disease manifestations are highly dependent on the species of infecting organism. Although literature reports of *Mycoplasma* and *Ureaplasma* infections in pediatric transplant or oncology patients are limited to case reports and case series, several patterns emerge from the literature, including occurrence of a greater variety of species causing disease, the occurrence of atypical locations and manifestations of infection, chronicity, and pyogenicity.

Pneumonia can occur as a consequence of infection with both *Mycoplasma*. and *Ureaplasma* spp. *M. pneumoniae* is a frequent cause of pneumonia in children; numerous studies have defined the typical age of occurrence ranging from young school-age (4 to 5 years) to the early teenage years (10 to 14 years).[28-30] Of note, many of the early studies used culture and serologic assays, which likely underestimate the contribution of *M. pneumoniae* to pneumonia incidence compared with current molecular assays.[38]

In immunocompetent children, respiratory *Mycoplasma spp.* infections are typically limited to *M. pneumoniae* and cause acute onset of pulmonary manifestations. A variety of radiographic patterns are reported in the literature, including scattered interstitial infiltrates, consolidative lobar pneumonia, pleural effusions, and occurrence of clinically severe and extensive pulmonary disease. In immunocompromised subjects, subacute to chronic presentations and purulent infections are also described. Chronic, recurrent focal consolidative pneumonia caused by to *M. pneumoniae* was diagnosed in a 4-year-old child who presented with persistent fevers and weight loss 3 years after kidney transplantation.[39] Empyema caused by *M. hominis* was reported in an 18-year-old lung transplant recipient.[40] In adult transplant patients, *M. hominis* pulmonary infection has been accompanied by surgical site infections.[41] *U. urealyticum* was detected in the lower airways by culture in three pediatric cancer patients (2-year-old boy and 16-year-old girl each with HSCT, and a 16-year-old girl with rhabdomyosarcoma) with radiographic findings of lower respiratory tract infection; two of these three patients had diffuse bilateral pneumonitis.[42] Thus lower respiratory tract infections caused by *Mycoplasma* and *Ureaplasma spp.* can present as either focal and purulent/pyogenic or diffuse, bilateral infection.

Nonrespiratory sites of infection are reported primarily as those caused by *M. hominis* and *Ureaplasma* spp., with infection sites including urogenital, intraabdominal, bone/joint, and central nervous system. In a series of 10 adult kidney transplant patients with pyuria and detection of *U. urealyticum* and/or *M. hominis*, five patients were asymptomatic and three patients had pyelonephritis that responded to directed therapy.[43] Intraabdominal abscesses caused by *M. hominis* and *U. urealyticum* have been reported in adult kidney transplant recipients.[44] Septic arthritis of the hip caused by *M. hominis* was diagnosed in a 15-year-old woman in whom leukopenia and right hip weakness and pain developed 6 weeks after kidney transplantation.[45] Septic polyarthritis caused by *U. urealyticum* was reported in an 18-year-old acute lymphocytic leukemia patient and a 28-year-old HSCT patient.[36,46] Meningitis caused by *U. urealyticum* has also been reported in SOT patients.

In addition to direct infections, parainfectious and postinfectious complications such as SJS and toxic epidermal necrolysis after *Mycoplasma* infection may occur.[47] Attribution of causality of these events to *Mycoplama* is difficult given that immunocompromised pediatric patients are often receiving multiple medications that may cause SJS or toxic epidermal necrolysis.

The occurrence of severe and fatal hyperammonemia syndrome as the result of disseminated *U. urealyticum* infection has not been reported in children. However, potential exists for rare but severe occurrence in this population. Therefore understanding of the pathophysiology and features of this syndrome is critical for practitioners caring for immunocompromised pediatric patients. Primarily reported in lung transplant recipients, hyperammonemia syndrome occurs with a gradual elevation in serum ammonia concentration that ultimately results in severe neurologic dysfunction and progresses to cerebral edema and death. In 2015, the development of hyperammonemia syndrome in a cohort of adult lung transplant recipients was linked to disseminated *Ureaplasma* infection.[48] The initial correlation with *Ureaplasma* infection was made in four patients who had died of neurologic sequelae of hyperammonemia syndrome. Identification of *U. parvum* and timely treatment in two subsequent patients resulted in resolution of hyperammonemia and excellent outcomes.[48] Detection and treatment of *U. parvum* infection in a 21-year-old patient 2 weeks after matched unrelated HSCT led to resolution of hyperammonemia and associated neurologic abnormalities.[49] Idiopathic hyperammonemia has been reported as a rare complication of HSCT and has not yet been associated with *Ureaplasma* infection. Practitioners caring for children undergoing transplantation should have a high index of suspicion for *Ureaplasma* infection in the setting of acute neurologic changes and/or altered mental status, especially when accompanied by hyperammonemia.

Disease Prophylaxis/Prevention

Prophylaxis against *Mycoplasma* and *Ureaplasma* spp. infections is not typically performed. Importantly, levofloxacin prophylaxis used in the setting of certain oncologic or HSCT therapeutic plans would theoretically provide prophylaxis against these infections (see "Treatment" section), although this has not been formally studied.

Diagnosis

Diagnosis of *Mycoplasma* and *Ureaplasma* spp. can be achieved by serologic, PCR, or culture-based methods.[28] Serologic assays to detect both *M. pneumoniae*–specific IgG and IgM are readily available. As the currently available serologic assays have low specificity in otherwise healthy children, concern exists regarding both the sensitivity and specificity of these assays in immunocompromised children. Clinically available serologic assays for other *Mycoplasma* spp., such as *M. hominis* and *M. genitalium* and for *Ureaplasma* spp., are not available.

Detection of *M. pneumoniae* by PCR has been reported and is clinically available from a variety of specimens, including sputum throat, nasopharynx, cerebrospinal fluid, urine, synovial fluid, and tissue. Detection of *M. pneumonia* by PCR has greater sensitivity than serologic assays though may also detect asymptomatic colonization.[38] More recently, *M. pneumoniae* detection has been included on several multiplex PCR platforms for evaluation of respiratory infections. PCR detection of other *Mycoplasma* and *Ureaplasma* spp. is also readily available through commercial laboratories.

Culture-based diagnosis of *Mycoplasma* and *Ureaplasma* spp. is challenging given the generally slow-growing and fastidious nature of these pathogens and may require up to 6 weeks of incubation to confirm negative results.[28] Further, species-level identification requires either biochemical tests or PCR-based identification from subculture.

Treatment

Because all *Mycoplasma* sand *Ureaplasma* spp. lack a cell wall, these organisms are intrinsically resistant to β-lactams and glycopeptides. Treatment options for these infections include macrolides, such as azithromycin and clarithromycin, tetracyclines including doxycycline, and "respiratory" fluroquinolones such as levofloxacin.[28] In the case of *M. pneumoniae*, macrolides and levofloxacin have the lowest MICs and are bactericidal.[50] Importantly, macrolide resistance in *M. pneumoniae* develops after point mutations in the 23S rRNA target of these antibiotics. Because of their high mutation rate and small genomes, mutations can occur rapidly during therapy. The frequency of resistance varies geographically with resistance as high as 90% in areas of Japan and China, as low as 1% to 2% in some European countries, and approximately 10% to 13% in the United States.[50] Although the clinical significance of macrolide resistance in *M. pneumoniae* is not well defined, macrolide resistance is of importance to immunocompromised pediatric patients given their increased reliance on antimicrobial activity in the clearance of infection. Resistance to tetracyclines and fluoroquinolones has not been detected in clinical isolates of *M. pneumoniae*.

Treatment options for other *Mycoplasma* and *Ureaplasma* spp. are highly dependent on the infecting species. *M. hominis* is always resistant to macrolides but is susceptible to clindamycin.[40] Variable susceptibility to doxycycline and rare resistance to fluoroquinolones exist in *M. hominis* isolates. In contract, *U. urealyticum* remains susceptible to macrolides, tetracyclines, and fluoroquinolones but is not susceptible to clindamycin.[29] *M. genitalium* is frequently resistant to macrolides and nonresponsive to tetracycline-based therapy, although fluroquinolones maintain susceptibility.[32]

Infection Prevention and Anticipatory Guidance

M. pneumoniae is transmitted from symptomatic persons via respiratory droplets, and transmission to household contacts as well as outbreaks has been reported.[28] When hospitalized, patients with suspected respiratory illness caused *M. pneumoniae* should have droplet precautions. Immunocompromised children exposed to a household contact with atypical pneumonia or documented *Mycoplasma* infection should be counseled regarding the potential for transmission and advised to contact their primary and appropriate subspecialty providers if symptoms of fever or respiratory illness develop.

16

Nontuberculous and Tuberculous *Mycobacterium*

Flor M. Munoz, MD, MSc and Philana Ling Lin, MD, MSc

MYCOBACTERIUM TUBERCULOSIS INFECTION

Epidemiology, Risk Factors, and Pathogenesis

Mycobacterium tuberculosis (MTB) is among the most successful respiratory pathogens worldwide as the majority of those infected are asymptomatic and will live their lifetime without clinical manifestations. Latent infection is defined as having asymptomatic MTB infection, as the immune system can control but not eradicate the pathogen. In low-incidence areas, latent infection is treated to reduce the risk of reactivation occurring later in life. Those with active tuberculosis (TB) disease (either as primary infection or reactivation) are typically symptomatic or have microbiologic (including sputum or other sterile site) or radiographic evidence of disease. Immunosuppressed hosts can have minimal symptoms or symptoms that are difficult to discern from their underlying disease, so a heightened level of clinical suspicion and knowledge of disease in these high-risk patients are necessary.

The risk of TB among adult solid organ transplant (SOT) recipients is approximately 4 to 74 times greater than the general population.[1,2] Risk should always be referenced with local TB incidence as rates can vary substantially by geographic location. For example, TB prevalence rates among SOT patients are reported between 0.4% and 6.6% in populations with low TB risk (e.g., United States and Western Europe) compared with rates as high as 15.2% in areas with high TB rates.[2-5] The TB-associated mortality among SOT recipients ranges from 6% to 29%[3,6] compared with the less than 5% mortality attributed to TB in the United States. Mortality rates are higher in renal transplant recipients and especially those with graft rejection, miliary TB, and those receiving T-cell–depleting immune suppression.[6] Although there are only limited data, the estimated mortality in pediatric SOT TB cases was more than 30% in a small series.[7]

Risk factors associated with TB among SOT recipients are multifactorial. Lung transplant recipients appear to have the highest incidence of TB among organ transplant types, followed by liver and then kidney transplant recipients.[6] Other risks include a history of prior TB, the use of T-cell–depleting antibody as well as immune modulators that impair T-cell function (e.g., basiliximab, alemtuzumab), chronic renal insufficiency, graft rejection, augmented immune suppression, diabetes mellitus, hepatitis C, chronic liver disease, increased recipient age, and presence of other co-infections (e.g., cytomegalovirus, *Pneumocystis jiroveci* pneumonia).[1,6,8,9] Among renal transplant recipients, the incidence of TB was associated mammalian target of rapamycin (mTOR) inhibitors or azathioprine use.[1] Higher rates of TB are observed in those who are older at the time of transplant, as older patients are more likely to have latent infection due to having lived in an era where TB was more prevalent.[9,10] Recognized behavioral risk factors include increased cumulative time residing in high–TB-endemic countries and exposure within prisons or homeless populations.[11] Independent risk factors of mortality among SOT recipients with TB include the presence of acute cellular rejection after the diagnosis of MTB infection, use of three or more TB drugs (likely reflecting active TB), and disseminated MTB.[12]

Four different mechanism of pathogenesis exist in SOT recipients:

1. Reactivation TB, in which the recipient has preexisting latent infection before SOT is believed to be the most common etiology in non–TB-endemic areas like the United States.[1] This is more common in adults compared with children, as adults are more likely to have latent MTB.
2. Donor-derived transmission either from a donor who had unrecognized active TB or latent infection. The reported risk of TB transmission is estimated at 30% when a donor has active TB.[11] Although lung transplants are recognized to have the greatest risk of donor-derived TB transmission, given that the lung is the most common organ to harbor MTB, all SOT types have been associated with donor MTB transmission.[3] In the United States, donor-derived TB accounts for less than 5% of TB cases after transplant[3,13] and estimates are likely higher in countries with more TB-endemic rates.
3. Active TB in a recipient who is either unrecognized or recognized (undergoing treatment but requires emergent transplant).
4. Primary infection that occurs after the time of transplantation.

The overall contribution of each listed category of TB transmission is not well characterized and it remains unclear what the actual risk of TB disease is associated with each potential transmission modality. Thus the overall TB risk is likely cumulative based on the contribution of both the recipient and donor risk factors as well as the endemic TB rates inherent to the geographic area, behavioral risk, and degree of immune suppression.

Very few data are available for pediatric SOT populations as significantly fewer children undergo transplant compared with adults. In general, the risk of developing active TB is greatest among those younger than 5 years and then during adolescence/early adult ages.[7] The incidence of TB after pediatric SOT has been reported as high as 2.4% in nonendemic areas to 9.7% in high–TB-endemic areas.[14-16] Within the same geographic area, the rates among adult SOT recipients are higher than in children after SOT[15] and are likely due to the fact that transmission in children is more likely from primary infection (recent exposure) and less likely from reactivation and other transmission modes discussed previously.

Hematopoietic stem cell transplant (HSCT) is an independent risk factor for TB, and it is estimated that HSCT recipients have a 10 to 40 times greater risk than the general population.[17,18] The incidence of TB varies based on geographic area with rates estimated at 0.1% to 5.5% in low-endemic areas but 16% in high endemic areas.[17,19] For example, in India, a high endemic area, nearly 2% of all infections after HSCT are due to TB.[20] Risk factors include allogeneic transplantation with unrelated donors or mismatched donor, graft-versus-host-disease (GVHD), use of total body irradiation, busulfan, cyclophosphamide, corticosteroid treatment, T-cell–targeted immune modulators, or prior history of TB.[18,19] Although there are no direct comparisons, it is generally accepted that HSCT recipients are at less risk of TB than SOT recipients. Despite HSCT recipients being more severely immune suppressed before and during HSCT compared with SOT recipients, the duration of immune suppression is only transient until engraftment ensues. This contrasts with SOT recipients, who require more prolonged (in many cases a lifetime of) immune suppression to prevent graft rejection.[21] Moreover, donor-derived transmission of MTB is rare; the primary mode of pathogenesis is either reactivation from underlying latent infection or primary infection immediately before or during HSCT. Mortality from TB ranges from 0 to 50%.[19] Like adults, children who have undergone HSCT are believed to be at higher risk of TB than the general population, although data are not well defined. While data are limited in pediatrics, some have reported that the risk of TB is lower in HSCT than SOT recipients.[22] Up to 25% of pediatric TB patients do not have an obvious risk factors for TB, and there are no universal screening practices in pediatric HSCT candidates as most hematology/oncology physicians believe that the tuberculin skin tests (TSTs)/interferon-gamma release assays (IGRAs) do not work in HSCT candidates receiving immune suppression.[20] More efforts are needed to better characterize TB in both adult and pediatric HSCT recipients.

Clinical Manifestations

Variable presentations and delays in diagnosis likely contribute to the higher TB mortality rates observed in SOT. Most cases of posttransplant TB occurred within the first 6 months of transplant (reported medians of 4 to 9 months) with the exception of renal transplant recipients, in whom TB occurred later.[6,7,16] The interval of time between SOT to clinical presentation of TB appears to be associated with transmission modality as earlier onset of disease is associated with reactivation or donor derived, whereas later onset of disease likely occurs from primary infection.[6] In pediatric SOT cases of TB, the reported time intervals between transplant and diagnosis was 8 months to 8 years and were presumed to be predominantly from primary infection after transplant.[14,22] Presenting symptoms of TB may be nonspecific and associated with site of involvement (~24% of cases).[12] Although pulmonary TB is the dominant manifestation in the general population, extrapulmonary disease is more prominent in SOT patients (79% to 84%). Miliary disease was reported in 44% to 63% of SOT TB cases, pulmonary disease in 12.2% to 36%, and genitourinary disease in 4% of cases.[13,23] Other reports showed extrapulmonary disease or disseminated (35% to 67%) as the most common manifestation of TB in SOT recipients and included involvement in the liver, gastrointestinal tract, lymph nodes, pericardium, bone, orbital, central nervous system, and genitourinary sites.[6,12,13,24] Fever was reported in 64% of cases with localized disease and 94% of disseminated cases[6] in addition to weight loss and night sweats. Many have suggested that TB should be considered in any SOT recipient with prolonged fever, especially in the first 3 months after transplant.[13] Renal transplant recipients often present with increased creatinine as the first sign of MTB, which can progress to disseminated disease.[1] Some have suggested that donor-derived disease more commonly presents as sepsis and organ dysfunction when a nonpulmonary organ is involved.[5] Thus a high index of clinical suspicion is important as most patients may have atypical clinical presentations. Clinical manifestations in children were also highly variable as more than 50% of reported cases had extrapulmonary disease.[7] In a series of seven cases of TB among children after renal transplant, almost all presented with fever, cough, and most had weight loss.[14] In another series, four of six children presented with fever of unknown origin (with cervical lymphadenopathy or deafness/meningitis).[22]

Unlike SOT recipients, clinical manifestations of TB in HSCT recipients are primarily pulmonary (87%),[17] including a spectrum of symptoms that can be indolent or overt with fever, cough, dyspnea, and hypoxia. Similar to the workup for SOT recipients, a wide range of symptoms can occur with TB and a high clinical suspicion is necessary for evaluation and workup. The median time to diagnosis from HSCT was 1.22 years (range between 22 days and 4.63 years).[17]

Diagnosis

Currently, there are no universal screening/evaluation guidelines for TB among SOT candidates and recipients, although most organizational bodies include a thorough history (including an individualized risk assessment for TB), physical examination, and IGRA or TST at a minimum.[8,25] Some experts also recommend a chest radiograph within 3 to 6 months of transplant and review of any prior chest imaging to be more thorough (Fig. 16.1). The experience from TB-endemic areas has suggested that the most accurate screening for active TB should not only include not IGRA/TST, sputum, careful evaluation of patient symptoms, and history but also the patient's prior TB contact history and chest imaging.[1] Chest radiography within 3 to 6 months before transplant is recommended regardless of TST/IGRA results in such cases. Recent exposure to a TB contact and chest radiographic evidence of prior TB were both factors that increased the risk of posttransplant TB. Pretransplant chest computed tomography (CT) evidence of "healed" or prior TB was more predictive of posttransplant TB than chest radiographs (which in some cases were interpreted as normal). For this reason, chest CT should be considered in patients for whom there is a high clinical suspicion despite negative test results.[1] That said, imaging modalities are not diagnostic and must be considered in the context of other TB-specific testing. Above all, it is important to understand that the current existing assays for MTB are limited and no assay has 100% negative predictive value. When appropriate, a high level of suspicion is required during the evaluation.

TSTs and IGRAs are currently the mainstay of diagnostic assays but are only able to detect MTB infection without distinguishing active TB or latent infection. TST is inexpensive and there has been long-standing experience with this test for decades in all age groups; however, it has many disadvantages. The TST requires a return visit at 48 to 72 hours to measure induration, which can be subjective and false-positives can occur as a result of cross-reactivity with non-tuberculous *Mycobacterium* and BCG bacilli Calmette-Guérin (BCG) vaccine. The IGRA (either in the form of QuantiFERON (QFT [Qiagen]) or T-Spot.TB (Oxford Immunotec) measures the production of interferon-gamma in response to MTB-specific antigens and therefore has less cross-reactivity with nontuberculous *Mycobacterium* and BCG vaccination. These assays require only a single visit with an objective result (i.e., positive, negative, or indeterminant) with improved specificity over the TST. However, the IGRA is more expensive and requires a laboratory infrastructure to perform the assay. Both the IGRA and TST assays are dependent on immune-specific responses against MTB and are therefore not optimal in patients with underlying immune suppression, the population at most risk for TB disease. Even among immunocompetent hosts, these assays have limited diagnostic yield, in each, in part, owing to the lack of gold standard and the inherent testing bias in each population tested. In general, the pooled sensitivity of TST, QFT, and T-Spot.TB assays is estimated at 77%, 84% and 88%, respectively. The pooled specificity of TST, QFT and T-Spot.TB assays is estimated at 97%, 98%, and 93%, respectively, although reports vary based on risk of TB in study cohort, state of infection studied, and so on.[26] The sensitivity and specificity of these tests

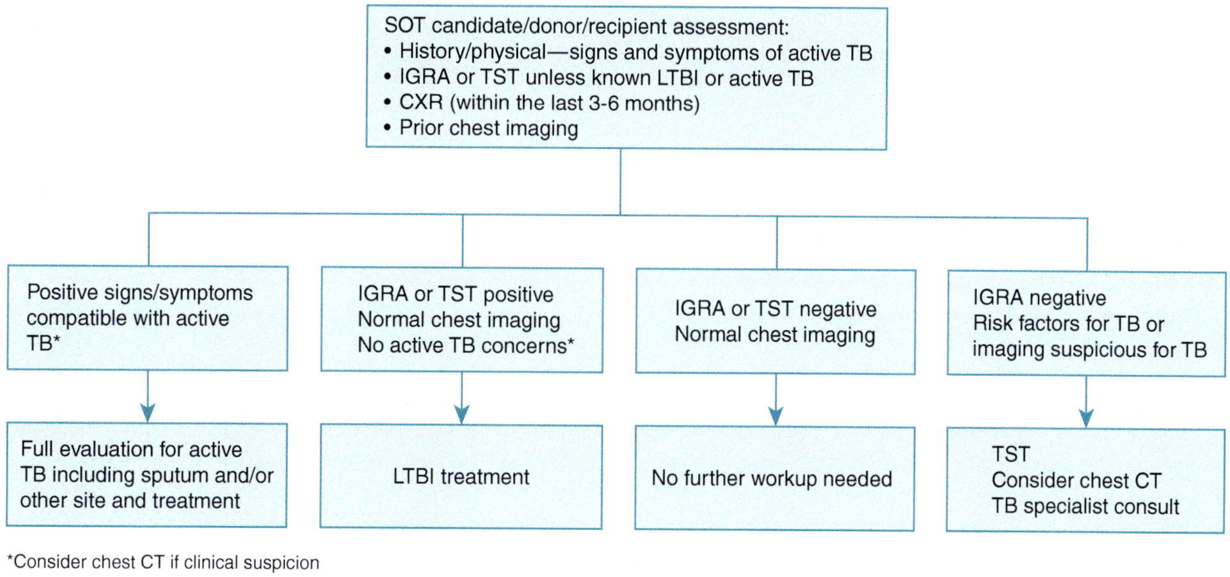

Fig. 16.1 Algorithm for tuberculosis screening/evaluation in solid organ transplant candidate/ donor/ recipient. *CT*, computed tomography, *CXR*, chest x-ray; *IGRA*, interferon-gamma release assay; *LTBI*, latent tuberculosis infection; *SOT*, solid organ transplant; *TB*, tuberculosis; *TST*, tuberculin skin test. (Modified from Epstein DJ, Subramanian AK. Prevention and management of tuberculosis in solid organ transplant recipients. *Infect Dis Clin North Am.* 2018;32(3):703-718.)

have not been thoroughly tested in SOT candidates and recipients. Patients with end-stage liver disease are known to have false-negative TST results owing to cutaneous anergy[27] and high rates of indeterminant results by IGRA.[28] Concordance between IGRA and TST assays was compared among 1500 SOT adult recipients; fewer positive TST results were observed among SOT recipients compared with IGRA results but this did not reach statistical significance.[29] Although limited, studies thus far have shown that a negative IGRA result before SOT was associated with a low risk of active TB after SOT.[30] Thus many experts have preferred IGRAs over the TST as they may be more sensitive (especially in cases of end-stage liver or renal disease). Even less is understood regarding the interpretation and predictive value of the IGRAs and TST in HSCT recipients as there are little published data. One report suggested that the IGRA may be more sensitive than the TST with a high degree of discordance found between the two assays.[31] Regardless, a negative IGRA result does not rule out the diagnosis of active TB as numerous case reports have described patients with culture-proven TB despite a negative IGRA test result.[30] Unfortunately, more recent host biomarker diagnostics in TB, focused on biomarkers/host-dependent signatures (i.e., host gene expression profiles from blood, serum proteins, or metabolites), are still in development but are likely to be prioritized for healthy adults or those with human immunodeficiency virus (HIV) and not targeted for SOT or HSCT recipients.[32]

Among immunocompetent children with active TB, the pooled sensitivity of the TST, QFT, and T-SPOT.TB tests was estimated to be 80%, 83%, and 84%, respectively. Similarly, the pooled specificity of the TST, QFT, and T-SPOT.TB tests were from 95%, 91%, and 94%, respectively.[26] Some smaller studies have shown that a positive IGRA result was a more accurate predictor of active TB after recent infection.[33] In a report of 30 pediatric SOT candidates with end-stage renal disease (all of whom were vaccinated with BCG at birth, median age 8 years), results of TST and IGRA testing were concordant in all but 1 case.[34] The TST result was positive in all six pediatric TB SOT cases in a small series; IGRA was performed in only two and both had indeterminant results.[22] Some experts suggest that both IGRA and TST be performed in children with high-risk families,[22] and a positive test result from either assay should warrant further evaluation. It is worth mentioning that these reports were conducted when IGRAs were approved for children 5 years and older. The assay was recently approved for children younger than 2 years and a newer version of the QFT (i.e., QFT-plus) is being marketed. As assays continue to advance and upgrade, the sensitivity, specificity, and hopefully, predictive value will also improve. Regardless, more data are needed to assess the value of TST and IGRA in the pediatric SOT and HSCT populations, as there are currently no compelling data to suggest that one assay is better than the other.

Because of the prominence of both pulmonary and extrapulmonary manifestations in SOT patients, diagnostic imaging is critical as well as the consideration of the type of organ transplanted. In one report of TB among liver transplant recipients, the chest radiographic pattern was identified as the most important risk factor for TB.[27] In another review of SOT-associated TB cases, all pulmonary cases were observed in lung transplant recipients,[13] in whom as many as 75% of all cases reported had some radiographic abnormality.[13] Chest radiographic findings in TB SOT cases can vary widely, including focal infiltrate, miliary pattern, nodules, cavitary disease, pleural effusion, or diffuse interstitial infiltrate.[6,7] CT is a more sensitive measure of disease. Patterns reported in SOT-associated TB cases include pulmonary findings of ground-glass opacity, consolidation, cavitation, tree-in-bud pattern, mediastinal lymph node enlargement, and miliary pattern.[35] Extrapulmonary disease may have variable yield as only 30% of renal transplant recipients with TB had pulmonary findings and only 30% had lymph node enlargement.[35]

HSCT recipients with active TB are most likely to have pulmonary manifestations. Chest radiographic patterns are similar to those as the general population, such as airspace consolidation or nodules, although unusual patterns such as diffuse alveolar hemorrhage has been reported.[19] Chest CT findings such as consolidation, nodules, tree-in-bud, ground-glass appearance, cavitary formation, and lymphadenopathy have been described and are common. Although pulmonary involvement is common, some authors have reported higher rates of extrapulmonary disease (as high as 46%) compared with the general population.[36]

A high level of clinical suspicion and low threshold for microbiologic testing/confirmation (either by sputum or biopsy) should be maintained when evaluating for TB in a SOT recipient. Acid-fast smear and culture (with susceptibility testing) from sputum or sterile sites suspected for MTB involvement are considered the standard microbiologic methods. The limited sensitivity and slow growth of MTB by standard culture methods suggest that early investigation and empiric treatment may be required for optimal management. To date, standard clinical laboratory–based nucleic acid amplification methods are reliable only when performed on acid-fast bacillus smear–positive samples for which a high bacterial burden is present. The advent of the GeneXpert assay (Cepheid Inc.) (and now new version, Xpert MTB/RIF Ultra) as a rapid method of MTB detection (cartridge-based, nucleic acid amplification) and isoniazid (INH)- or rifampin (RIF)-resistance testing on sputum samples has markedly improved TB diagnosis and treatment strategies worldwide. This assay has been endorsed in by the World Health Organization (WHO) for use in HIV-positive patients, and testing is currently being expanded to other biologic specimens (e.g., cerebrospinal fluid).[32] These assays have evolved as the primary diagnostic method in areas where standard acid-fast bacillus smear and culture testing are not available. The yield in pediatric samples (pooled sensitivity of only 66%) is less optimal given the paucibacillary nature of TB disease in children compared with adults,[37] and studies exploring the use of the GeneXpert test in other samples, such as bronchoalveolar lavage samples, pleural fluid, and other areas, have not been encouraging. Other non–culture-based assays are under development. For example, the Alere Determined TB LAM Ag assay (Abbott) is a non–culture-based assay that detects urinary lipoarabinomannan, an antigen of MTB, and has been endorsed by the WHO for HIV-infected patients with CD4 T-cells counts below 100 cells/μL in whom pulmonary or extrapulmonary TB is suspected as the bacterial burden and degree of dissemination is presumed to be high.[32] The utility of these newer diagnostic assays has not been assessed in SOT or HSCT recipients to date.

Treatment

Active pulmonary TB should be treated with the standard regimen of INH, RIF, ethambutol (ETH), and pyrazinamide (PZA) for 2 months followed by 4 months of INH/RIF for drug-susceptible disease (with pyridoxine). Prolonged treatment may be necessary if clinical or microbiologic response is suboptimal or if central nervous system involvement or other circumstances occur. Unfortunately, this regimen (specifically the rifamycins) interacts with many of the immunsuppressive drugs used to prevent graft rejection, including calcineurin inhibitors (cyclosporine, tacrolimus), mTOR inhibitors (sirolimus, everolimus), and steroids. The inadvertent reduction in immunosuppressive drugs increases the risk of rejection, a recognized event during TB treatment among SOT recipients,[7] although other reports have cited similar rates of rejection regardless of RIF use.[24] Direct liver toxicity from INH, RIF, and/or PZA can occur and close monitoring of liver function test results is recommended. SOT recipients are at further risk of drug-induced toxicity; ETH, PZA, and INH require renal clearance and renal insufficiency is a common comorbidity in these patients.[7,11] In a meta-analysis review, 30 of 88 liver transplant recipients with TB had to stop or change medications because of adverse drug effects. The mean time to occurrence was 3.1 months from initiation of TB treatment. The majority of those cases (73%) were due to hepatotoxicity, whereas the remaining were due to drug interactions with immunosuppression.[12] Those with rejection were more likely to have hepatoxicity. To prevent the risk of rejection, close monitoring of immunosuppressant drugs (e.g., cyclosporine, tacrolimus) is required as well as empirically increasing steroid levels by 50% until a period of stability is observed. RIF induction of cytochrome P450 reduces the drug levels as early as a few hours after RIF administration with maximal effect in 1 to 2 weeks. It is not unusual for the drugs such as cyclosporine or tacrolimus or mTOR inhibitors to increase two- to fivefold while RIF is used. The effects of RIF slowly decline over 2 weeks after it has been stopped.[11] Similar issues arise among HSCT recipients who require treatment for active or latent infection as RIF will decrease levels of immunosuppressant agents and can lead to worsening GVHD.[19] It is not uncommon to taper the cyclosporine and add corticosteroids during this period among HSCT recipients being treated for TB. Despite rifabutin having less cytochrome P450 induction, immunosuppressant medications can still be difficult to maintain. It is important to keep in mind that RIF, INH, and PZA are critical backbones in the shortened TB regimen of 6 months. Although the RIF-sparing regimens may seem more attractive, they are less effective, requiring longer treatment durations (e.g., 12 months).[1] Similarly, PZA can be replaced with a quinolone but requires longer treatment durations.[1] Thus standard TB treatment regimens should be encouraged as much as possible in SOT recipients with constant vigilance toward drug interactions and toxicity. Lastly, some experts have suggested that IGRA conversion results from positive to negative could be used as a surrogate for monitoring treatment response. However, although most studies show a reduction in the IGRA response to MTB antigens during treatment, the responses were variable and therefore not useful for drug treatment monitoring, especially in immunocompromised SOT recipients.[38]

There are a number of different first-line treatment regimens for latent MTB infection that include 9 months of INH, 4 months of RIF, and 12 weeks of INH and rifapentine.[1] In a randomized trial among adults, 4 months of RIF was associated with lower rates of hepatotoxicity compared with 9 months of INH (0 vs 8%). Alternative regimens include 6 months of INH, 4 months of rifabutin, or 3 to 4 months of INH/RIF but these regimens have not been well studied.[1] Pyridoxine should be given in any regimen when INH is used. The use of levofloxacin with ETH was compared to INH in SOT recipients with latent infection but the trial was stopped early because of high rates of adverse events in the levofloxacin group.[11] Although INH has higher rates of hepatoxicity, fewer drug interactions may make it more attractive than RIF despite the longer treatment duration. Timing of when to start treatment may also depend on the stability of the patient's condition, liver function, and immunosuppressed status as drug interactions will likely cause some fluctuation. Unlike the treatment of active TB, for which treatment should begin immediately, many experts have deferred treatment of latent infection.[1] Decisions on treatment regimens must be individualized based on baseline liver function, potential drug-related interactions, toxicity risk, compliance, and so on. Some have recommended monitoring liver function testing with prothrombin time every 2 to 4 weeks during INH treatment and then monthly once laboratory findings and clinical status are stable. Treatment with RIF should include monitoring of a complete blood count.[1]

The treatment regimens are the same in children with the same concerns regarding drug interactions and toxicity. Although the incidence of drug-induced hepatotoxicity is generally less common in healthy children compared with healthy adults, the incidence in pediatric SOT patients is not well described and monitoring as described earlier would be reasonable. In a report of six cases of pediatric SOT TB, half used RIF treatment (all had INH and PZA in their treatment regimen). Hyperuricemia developed in two patients related to PZA; transaminases increased 2 to 7 times higher than baseline presumably from INH in four of six cases.[22] More data are needed to assess the true risk of TB treatment in pediatric SOT recipients.

Prevention and Screening Practices

Screening practices among SOT candidates and donors can be difficult and vary based on epidemiologic risk and duration of exposure time in both the donor and recipient. For example, donors may be divided into low, moderate, and high risk for TB based on social history (e.g., homelessness, prison, alcohol use, low body mass index, known TB contact) and prior exposure or residence in other countries.[5] The risk of TB can vary based on the type of SOT, choice of immunosuppression, and genetic predisposition of the recipient. Thus the guidelines discussed later vary based on endemic epidemiologic risks, experience, and practices of each institution within a given region.

As discussed earlier, screening of SOT candidates plays a key role in preventing reactivation TB after organ transplant (Fig. 16.1). In a meta-analysis of liver transplant–associated TB, 35% of TB cases a prior positive TST result but were not treated.[12] All candidates should be screened either with TST or IGRA (especially those with prior BCG vaccination), risk assessment of possible exposure (e.g., homeless, recent exposure to active TB), and chest raidography.[28] Some experts have suggested the use of IGRAs only in low-incidence areas to prevent false-positive results, whereas others have argued that both tests should be used to maximize the sensitivity of both screening modalities.[11] Similar to the evaluation of SOT candidates and recipients, some have suggested both TST and IGRA can be used if there is high pretest probability for latent infection[7] and any positive IGRA or TST result should be further evaluated (Fig. 16.1). Chest CT has been used to detect MTB-suspicious lesions in the lung, especially in high TB-endemic areas.[3] The Tuberculosis Network European Trials (BNET) Consensus Committee (largely European experts) developed broad-based guidelines based on local endemic TB rates that include empiric treatment for latent infection without screening in areas with high TB-endemic rates (>100 per 100,000).[7] As for HSCT candidate screening, both the IGRA and TST have reduced sensitivity in the setting of a person undergoing evaluation for HSCT who is already receiving chemotherapy.[21]

Although the experience and data are limited, the guidelines for pediatric SOT candidates are essentially the same as the earlier adult guidelines with some caveats. As IGRA assays are not approved for children younger than 2 years, TST remains the primary diagnostic in very young children. Results of the TST should be interpreted regardless of BCG vaccination as it is not possible to disprove the positive test results. Unlike adults, whose prior experience and travel contribute to the risk of MTB exposure specific to the patient's risk, a thorough assessment of risk factors among the parents and other household contacts is important as they are most likely to transmit MTB to the child. Close contacts or family members were the source of MTB infection in 66% to 80% of pediatric TB or latent SOT cases.[7,16] Similarly, children whose parents were born outside the United States had a higher risk of SOT-related TB.[11]

Treatment of latent infection in a SOT candidate is important but can be delayed. In two large cohorts of liver transplant patients, treatment of latent infection was associated with fewer cases of active TB among those treated compared with those not treated.[12] The advantage of treated latent infection before SOT includes a higher efficacy in the absence of immunosuppression with fewer drug interactions, lower medication burden, and better tolerance. However, there may not be adequate time for treatment before transplant, drug-induced liver disease may be difficult to distinguish from underlying liver disease, and drug-induced injury could prompt fatal injury or require emergent liver transplant.[3] Many institutions wait to treat latent infection soon after SOT during the period at greatest risk for reactivation (discussed earlier). The disadvantages to this practice include the difficulty in discerning drug-induced liver toxicity from graft rejection (in the case of liver transplant), jeopardizing injury to a new liver graft, high pill burden, managing drug interactions, and the theoretically less effective treatment during immunpsuppression.[12] Among the first-line latent infection regimens mentioned earlier, RIF or rifapentine/INH use is likely a better option before transplant given the shortened duration and is less attractive after transplant owing to the increased incidence of drug-drug interactions with immunosuppressive medications, respectively.[11] The INH regimen is more likely to be a better option after transplant as it has fewer drug-drug interactions. Any decision not to treat latent infection should be discussed with the patient and medical team weighing all risks and benefits.

TB screening among donors plays a key role in prevention of SOT-related TB given that donor-derived transplanted allografts result in both pulmonary (e.g., lung donor) and extrapulmonary (non–lung donor) TB. For obvious reasons, only limited information regarding TB risk is available in deceased donors. Although some committees have endorsed the use of IGRA or TST (if time permits) when a potential donor is identified,[25] to date there is insufficient evidence on the sensitivity and specificity of these tests on dying or deceased donors. That said, a positive result should prompt further workup for active TB, as such a donor should be excluded for transplant. Some have suggested that chest radiography or CT may play a role in identifying patterns consistent with TB.[3] A thorough review of donor risk factors (perhaps from family members) should be performed and considered, including homelessness or recent incarceration, travel or residence in a high TB-endemic area, history of TB, alcoholism, history of recurrent pneumonia, and so on.[5,13] For donors with probable latent infection, most experts suggest that the recipient should be treated for latent infection as the lungs carry the highest risk of donor-derived TB.[7]

Living donors should be tested in a fashion similar to SOT candidates/recipients, especially as the diagnosis of active TB is a contraindication for organ donation. In the United States, all living donors have a routine chest radiograph and those with a risk for TB also have testing with either IGRA or TST. Symptoms consistent with TB or concerning chest radiographic findings should prompt a workup for active TB.[25] In a European survey of transplant centers, 48% of centers used TST, 30% used IGRA alone, and 16% used both,[11] demonstrating the variety of approaches. More rigorous screening recommendations have also been endorsed that include a careful epidemiologic and personal medical history, physical examination and chest radiography (regardless of TST/IGRA results), both IGRA and TST testing (with TST booster if no recent testing has been performed and IGRA especially in BCG-vaccinated patients), bronchoscopic testing for mycobacterial growth before lung donation, and urinalysis with microscopy or genitourinary testing for donors living in intermediate- or high-risk countries before kidney transplant donation.[5] For donors with latent infection, treatment should be offered to the donor. The risks of delaying transplant if no other donor is available and the benefits of treatment (and risk of drug interactions) should be individualized as treatment need not be completed before transplant.[5] As many as 30% to 40% of organ donors in TB-endemic countries are recognized to have latent infection and require treatment before transplant would significantly reduce the donor pool.[25] Some institutions with high TB-endemic rates treat the recipient with INH without donor screening, assuming that this regimen after transplant will prevent reactivation, donor transmission, and de novo infection during the time of maximal immunosuppression.[5]

There are some distinctions between TB evaluation among HSCT candidates. For example, there are no formal recommendations to screen HSCT donors, as the risk of transmission is rare.[7,21] Donors with active TB should undergo treatment and avoid donation. However, most experts believe that transplanting HSCT from an untreated, latently infected donor poses no risk to the recipient.[21] There is no consensus regarding screening practices for HSCT candidates.[19] A survey of HSCT centers in Europe reported that only 10% of centers systematically screen for TB and only 51% would screen once clinical suspicion arose.[19] Some guidelines recommend that candidates be assessed by history for TB risk factors and the extent of the evaluation after that is somewhat controversial.[39] Certain guidelines dissuade the use of TST, suggesting that IGRA may be more useful.[39] Anyone with TB risk factors (e.g., prior TB exposure, history of active TB, or positive TST/IGRA) should undergo evaluation for active TB or latent infection (Fig. 16.2). Active TB disease should warrant treatment with delay of HSCT. The timing of when to start the HSCT after initiating anti-TB drugs should be individualized to the patient and involve discussion with the patient, infectious disease consultant, and primary HSCT team. Latent infection does not require delay in HSCT but should be treated based on a positive TST/IGRA result or recent exposure to someone with high-risk active TB (e.g., smear-positive sputum with pulmonary or laryngeal TB) regardless of the TST/IGRA result.[21] Interestingly, two large studies in Korea, a high TB-endemic country, demonstrated that INH treatment for latent infection before HSCT (defined by IGRA positive result) did not reduce the incidence of TB, although this may have been due to TB cases that occurred from reinfection after HSCT.[36] Although there is no question that TB in HSCT recipients is an important infectious complication, the role of TB screening and its benefits are less defined.

Despite well-intentioned guidelines, the limited nature of the current diagnostic assays, variable risk of transmission and disease, and complex treatment regimens require both individualized and evidence-based methods of management. It is important for HSCT and SOT transplant teams to work with transplant infectious disease specialists to help guide practice and optimize preventive, diagnostic, and treatment issues to critically analyze and maximize the benefits while minimizing patient risks. For example, given the unpredictable nature of organ transplant, the timing of how long a patient with active TB must receive treatment before transplant can be performed should be individualized based on donor availability, MTB load, and duration of anti-TB treatment. Given that organ procurement and donor organ distribution can span a large region, systems have been put in place such that all donor-derived diseases are reported to the Organ Procurement and Transplantation Network, which then promptly distributes the information to other donor sites,[3] where decisions regarding risk and management can be considered. Lastly, a high index of suspicion for TB is critical to prompt full evaluation in the hopes that improved diagnostic assays will be developed and become available for this high-risk patient population.

NONTUBERCULOUS *MYCOBACTERIUM* INFECTION

Epidemiology, Risk Factors, and Pathogenesis

Nontuberculous mycobacteria (NTM) are ubiquitous in the environment, present in soil, water, animals, and food. Although more than 140 species have been described, only a few cause infection in

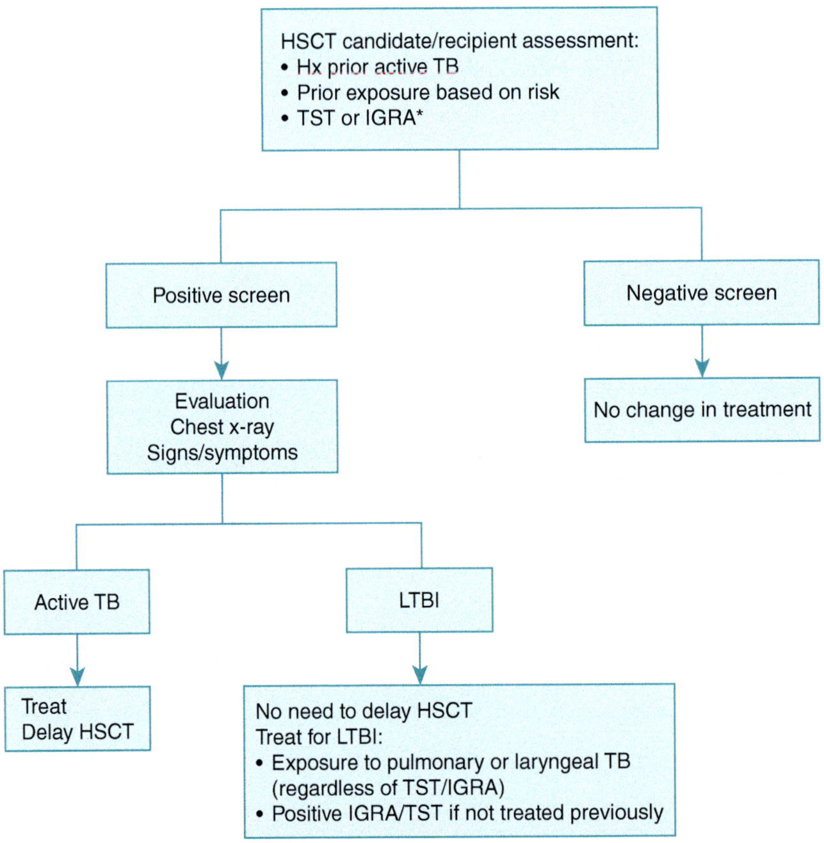

Fig. 16.2 Algorithm for tuberculosis screening for hematopoietic stem cell transplant candidate/recipient. *HSCT*, hematopoietic stem cell transplant; *HX*, history; *IGRA*, interferon-gamma release assay; *LTBI*, latent tuberculosis infection; *TB*, tuberculosis, *TST*, tuberculin skin test. (Data from Tomblyn M, Chiller T, Einsele H, et al. Guidelines for preventing infectious complications among hematopoietic cell transplantation recipients: a global perspective. *Biol Blood Marrow Transplant.* 2009;15(10):1143-1238.)

humans. NTMs are classified based on their growth rate in culture. Several species form visible colonies on solid media within 3 to 7 days, which allows for prompt identification; these are referred to as rapid growers, whereas most NTM take several weeks to show sufficient growth to allow identification and are therefore known as slow growers. Numerous NTM species have been reported to cause infection in transplant recipients, some more frequent and pathogenic than others (Table 16.1)

NTM are an uncommon but important causes of pulmonary and extrapulmonary infection and disease after SOT. The incidence of infection has been reported in a few, mostly single-center studies in adults and is higher in thoracic (0.2% to 2.8%) than in abdominal (<0.5%) transplant recipients, with the majority of disease occurring after lung transplantation (0.46 to 8%).[40,41] Lung transplant candidates are more likely to have infection with NTM, resulting in increased risk for morbidity and mortality after transplant and potential contraindications for transplantation.[42] Chronic lung disease in general, but particularly cystic fibrosis (CF), is a risk factor for NTM colonization and infection before transplant. At least one of every five patients with CF and advanced lung disease have positive sputum cultures for NTM.[43] *M. abscessus* and *M. avium* complex (MAC) are the most common and challenging pathogens. The incidence of NTM infections in HSCT recipients in adults has been reported to range from 0.4% to 4.9%, with higher rates reported in more recent studies, and a related mortality rate of 7.5%.[41,44] The most common type of infection in HSCT is pulmonary, and the most common species is MAC. Identified risk factors for NTM infection in allogeneic HSCT recipients include the presence of chronic GVHD and cytomegalovirus viremia.[44] Person-to-person transmission of NTM does not occur; however, concern for indirect person-to-person transmission in settings where high-risk CF patients congregate has been recently raised.[43] Contaminated water in the community (tap water) and within the health care system (respiratory and hemodialysis equipment, and so on) is a common source of infection. Other sources of infection include organic material, penetrating trauma, skin abrasions, surgical and puncture sites, and the oropharynx.

TABLE 16.1 Pathogenic Nontuberculous Mycobacteria in Transplant Patients Classified According to Growth Characteristics.

Rapid-Growing Nontuberculous Mycobacteria	Slow-Growing Nontuberculous Mycobacteria
M. abscessus[a]	*M. asiaticum*
M. boletti	*M. avium-intracellulare complex*[a]
M. chelonae[a]	*M. celatum*
M. fortuitum[a]	*M. genavense*
M. mageritense	*M. haemophilum*[a]
M. massiliense	*M. gastri*
M. mucogenicum	*M. gordonae*
M. neoaurum	*M. kansasii*[a]
M. smegmatis	*M. malmoense*
	M. marinum[a]
	M. scofulaceum
	M. simiae
	M. szulgai[a]
	M. terrae
	M. thermoresistible
	M. triplex
	M. xenopi

*Most commonly a cause of human disease.

Clinical Manifestations

Clinical manifestations of disease caused by NTM are diverse, depending on the site of infection. Pulmonary disease is most common in SOT, with variable and often nonspecific manifestations, including pulmonary infiltrates, solitary pulmonary nodules, abscesses, and cavitary lesions, with symptoms including chronic cough with or without sputum production, dyspnea, and hemoptysis. These symptoms may be associated with fever, fatigue, and weight loss. In thoracic SOT recipients, NTM infection can involve anastomotic sites, resulting in potentially life-threatening complications in the early postoperative period, such as hemorrhage, mediastinitis and extension into adjacent organs and the thoracic cavity. Cutaneous infection, surgical site infection, lymphadenitis, catheter-related infections, and disseminated disease also occur more frequently in these immunocompromised hosts.

HSCT recipients also have pulmonary disease as the predominant clinical manifestation of NTM infection, but they are also are more likely to present with extrapulmonary NTM disease, including catheter-related bloodstream infection, lymphadenitis, bone and joint involvement, and disseminated disease. Manifestations of disseminated NTM infection include fever, night sweats, weight loss or poor weight gain, fatigue, abdominal pain, diarrhea, and musculoskeletal pain.

M. abscessus infection in lung transplant candidates, such as patients with CF, is a particularly difficult challenge because of its ability to cause aggressive and persistent disease and limited options for treatment when multidrug resistance develops.[43,45] Infection with *M. abscessus* may be considered a contraindication for lung transplantation when patients have progression of disease despite optimal therapy, and when treatment options are not available owing to multidrug resistance or intolerance, according to the International Society for Heart and Lung Transplantation.[46] Although successful lung transplantation has been reported in patients chronically infected with *M. abscessus* and it is therefore not an absolute contraindication, the decision to proceed with transplant is typically determined on a case-by-case basis and based on the expertise of the transplant center.[47]

Diagnosis

A high index of suspicion and consideration of risk factors are necessary to diagnose NTM infection in transplant candidates and recipients. Definitive diagnosis requires isolation of the organism from a relevant specimen source. Given that NTM are often present in the environment, it is important to work with the microbiology laboratory to ensure that culture specimens are properly handled and to determine whether a positive culture result represents a true infection or contamination, particularly when obtained from a nonsterile site. Identification of NTM isolates to the species level and routine susceptibility testing are recommended. Isolation of NTM from sterile sites, such as blood, bone marrow, cerebrospinal fluid, pleural fluid, tissue biopsy samples or surgically excised tissue, is likely to represent true infection. Isolation of NTM from infected wounds and draining sinus tracts is also usually clinically significant. However, respiratory samples, including sputum and lower respiratory tract samples obtained by aspiration or bronchoscopy, may or may not represent true infection. In patients who have more than one positive respiratory culture result for NTM, the challenge is to ascertain whether these represent a chronic colonization or disease in order to decide on the need for antimicrobial treatment. In transplant candidates with CF, a sudden or rapid decline in lung function, as measured by standard pulmonary function tests, is associated with disease when NTM has been isolated from respiratory sample cultures. Positive smears in sputum samples and abnormal imaging studies that show progressive disease are also more likely to represent NTM disease. Suggestive findings of NTM disease in chest radiographs and CT imaging studies include nodular pneumonia with a tree-in-bud appearance, lymphadenopathy, and cavitation. Diagnostic criteria for NTM lung disease in adults published by the American Thoracic Society and the Infectious Diseases Society of America include the identification of NTM in two or more separate sputum samples or one bronchial alveolar lavage specimen, or a transbronchial or other lung biopsy specimen with mycobacterial histopathologic features (granulomatous inflammation or acid-fast bacilli) and positive culture results, in patients with characteristic clinical symptoms and radiographic findings in whom other etiologies of disease have been excluded.[48] However, these guidelines are difficult to apply in certain populations, including CF, children, and transplant patients, in whom they have not been validated. An approach for the evaluation and diagnosis of pulmonary NTM disease in SOT and HSCT candidates based on American Thoracic Society/ Infectious Diseases Society of America guidelines is shown in Fig. 16.3.

Treatment

Diagnosing NTM infection does not imply that antimicrobial therapy should be started. The decision to treat includes consideration of the type and extent of the disease, the expected benefit, and potential risks of the therapy. This is particularly challenging in making decisions about the adequacy of a transplant candidate before transplantation. There are no established guidelines for management of these patients, particularly patients with chronic infection requiring lung transplantation. Consultation with an infectious diseases expert in the management of NTM is recommended. For some NTM species, treatment to reduce disease burden and achieve disease control before transplantation may improve outcomes. Many practitioners would initiate antimicrobial therapy as soon as lung transplantation is considered for those with *M. abscessus* infection, but case-by-case assessment is recommended. Successful treatment requires documentation of consistent smear and culture negativity by collecting serial samples during treatment to demonstrate that the infection is being controlled and assurance that the patient can tolerate the selected antimicrobial regimen without experiencing significant/limiting toxicities.

Treatment of NTM consists of a multiple-drug combination tailored to the species and susceptibility testing results. Antimicrobial susceptibility testing depends on the species. Clarithromycin susceptibility testing is recommended for MAC isolates, whereas *M. kansasii* isolates should be tested for RIF susceptibility. *M. abscessus, M. fortuitim,* and *M. cheloneae* organisms tend to be multidrug resistant; accordingly, susceptibility testing to various agents, including amikacin, imipenem (*M. fortuitum*), doxycycline, quinolones, trimethoprim-sulfamethoxazole, cefoxitin, clarithromycin, linezolid, and tobramycin (for *M. chelonae*), is needed. The presence of intrinsic antimicrobial resistance, development of resistance on therapy, poor drug tolerability, and the potential for drug-drug interactions pose particular challenges in transplant recipients.

Treatment of *M. abscessus* pulmonary disease is the most challenging, given that there are no standardized or proven effective drug regimens. Multiple-drug combinations are used based on in vitro susceptibility testing, most including a macrolide and intravenous agents such as amikacin and either cefoxitin, imipenem, or tigecycline, for a prolonged duration. Aerosolized amikacin has been used as an adjunct to multidrug regimens, and in patients in whom combination

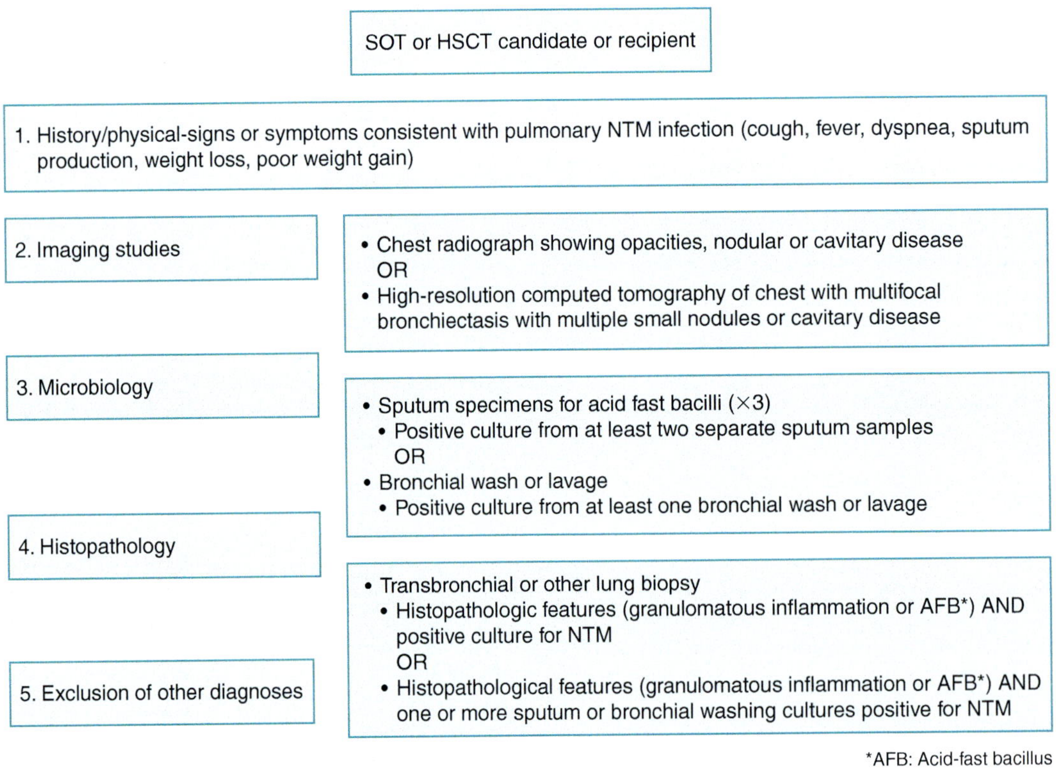

Fig. 16.3 Algorithm for evaluation and diagnosis of nontuberculous mycobacterial lung infection in solid organ and hematopoietic stem cell transplant candidates and recipients. *HSCT*, hematopoietic stem cell transplant; *NTM*, nontuberculous Mycobacterium; *SOT*, solid organ transplant. (Data from Griffith DE, Aksamit T, Brown-Elliott BA, et al. An official ATS/IDSA statement: diagnosis, treatment, and prevention of nontuberculous mycobacterial diseases. *Am J Respir Crit Care Med.* 2007;175(4):367-416.)

SOT or HSCT candidate or recipient with NTM infection

Rapid growing NTM

Pathogen	First line	Second line
M. abscessus	Azithromycin Amikacin Imipenem or Cefoxitin	Clarithromycin Linezolid Tigecycline Clofazemine
M. chelonae	Azithromycin Amikacin or Tobramycin Linezolid Tigecyline or Imipenem	
M. fortuitum	Amikacin Quinolone Sulfonamide	Sulfonamides Doxycycline or minocycline Imipenem Tigecycline

Slow growing NTM

Pathogen	First line	Second line
MAC	Azithromycin Ethambutol Rifabutin	Clarithromycin Rifampin Amikacin or Streptomycin Clofazemine
M. kansasii	Rifabutin Ethambutol Isoniazid	Rifampin Clarithromycin or Azithromycin Sulfamethoxazole Moxifloxacin
M. marinum	Azithromycin Ethambutol Rifabutin	Rifampin Clarithromycin or Azithromycin Sulfonamides Doxycycline or Minocycline
M. Haemophilum	Azithromycin Rifabutin Ciprofloxacin	Clarithromycin or Azithromycin Sulfonamides Doxycycline

Fig. 16.4 Algorithm for treatment of non-tuberculous mycobacterial infection in solid organ and hematopoietic stem cell transplant candidates and recipients. *HSCT*, hematopoietic stem cell transplant; *MAC*, Mycobacterium avium complex; *SOT*, solid organ transplant. (Data from Rao M, Silveira FP. Non-tuberculous mycobacterial infections in thoracic transplant candidates and recipients. *Curr Infect Dis Rep.* 2018;20(6):14; Beswick J, Shin E, Michelis FV, et al. Incidence and risk factors for nontuberculous mycobacterial infection after allogeneic hematopoietic cell transplantation. *Biol Blood Marrow Transplant.* 2018;24(2):366-372; and Griffith DE, Aksamit T, Brown-Elliott BA, et al. An official ATS/IDSA statement: diagnosis, treatment, and prevention of nontuberculous mycobacterial diseases. *Am J Respir Crit Care Med.* 2007;175(4):367-416.)

oral drug therapy failed.[49,50] Even if treatment is started before transplant, treatment during and after transplant are often necessary to reduce the risk of recurrent disease, which can be more difficult to control and have risk for dissemination after transplantation. Similar regimens are used for extrapulmonary disease. When pertinent, surgical debridement/debulking of disease can improve treatment success. Treatment of MAC pulmonary disease requires a combination regimen of a combination regimen of a macrolide, RIF, and ETH, which can be administered 3 times weekly.

Patients with MAC cavitary disease or severe nodular/bronchiectatic disease are treated with a daily combination of a macrolide, RIF or rifabutin, and ETH , to which intravenous amikacin or streptomycin could be added. Prolonged treatment is necessary for at least 1 year after the first negative respiratory or tissue sample culture results. Patients with disseminated MAC after HSCT can be treated with a combination of a macrolide and ETH, with or without rifabutin, until resolution of symptoms and reconstitution of cell-mediated immunity. Treatment for these and other relevant NTM species is summarized in Fig. 16.4.

Disease Prophylaxis and Infection Prevention

Screening for NTM is recommended for patients with CF undergoing evaluation for lung transplantation, but not for other SOT or HSCT candidates. Measures to decrease intraoperative contamination in patients known to be previously infected include paying close attention to surgical technique to avoid contamination, irrigation of the chest cavity with antimicrobial agents to which the isolate is susceptible, and continuation of the antimicrobial regimen both perioperatively and postoperatively. It is also important to closely monitor the surgical wound and any other catheter sites and areas of skin breakdown for evidence of NTM infection. In addition, prevention of NTM infections in the health care setting among SOT and HSCT recipients relies on the prevention of exposure of surgical wounds, injection sites, and intravenous and other indwelling catheters to potentially contaminated water and other fluids. This includes the proper sterilization of instruments such as endoscopes. Prophylaxis for NTM is not routinely used in SOT or HSCT patients. Macrolide or rifabutin prophylaxis in patients with low $CD4^+$ T-lymphocyte counts is effective in preventing susceptible NTM.[48]

17

Cytomegalovirus

Lara A. Danziger-Isakov, MD, MPH and Tanvi Sharma, MD, MPH

Viral infections represent a significant cause of morbidity and mortality among children who have undergone either solid organ (SOT) or hematopoietic stem cell transplantation (HSCT), as well as in children undergoing therapy for malignancies. Herpesviruses, which possess a unique ability in their life cycle to establish latent infection, are especially significant within these patient populations because of their capacity to reactivate in the setting of immunosuppression. Cytomegalovirus (CMV) is the most common herpesvirus causing disease among adult transplant recipients and represents an especially important pathogen among pediatric immunocompromised patients.

CMV is a β-herpesvirus that shares many of the characteristics of other herpesviruses. It has a large, double-stranded DNA genome with a viral capsid and envelope, and core of proteins that are conserved within all of the herpesviruses.[1] The pathogenesis of CMV in otherwise healthy individuals is directed by viral transcripts that interfere with viral antigen presentation on the cell surface and lead to lytic viral replication. Symptoms that occur with viral replication are primarily associated with the immune response to the infection rather than direct viral destruction; therefore symptoms may be blunted in immunocompromised hosts with an ineffective immune response.[1] Most healthy hosts are asymptomatic with CMV infection but shed virus in saliva and other mucous membranes, leading to transmission between hosts.

CMV infects epithelial cells, lymphocytes, and monocytes and ultimately establishes latency within these cells as well as in macrophages through a balance of viral immune evasion mechanisms and host immune control. The innate immune response through Toll-like receptor (TLR) inflammatory pathways, as well as memory natural killer (NK) cells and γδ T cells, is important for initial control of CMV replication and disease. This primary immune response is sufficiently restricted, however, to allow the virus to establish latency rather than be eradicated.[2,3] Adaptive immunity mediated through $CD4^+$ and $CD8^+$ T-cell responses is necessary for immune surveillance to prevent viral reactivation and proliferation of virus-infected cells. Humoral immune responses mediated by B cells are also needed for immune memory, but viral reactivation can occur despite adequate antibody responses in infected individuals. In transplant recipients, the disruption of effector T cells through immunosuppressive therapies leads to the potential for viral reactivation, replication, and associated CMV disease. Similarly, in oncology patients, chemotherapeutic agents as well as lymphoid malignancies that impair T-cell function promote CMV replication and may lead to disease. An unusual feature of herpesviruses, especially CMV, is the ability to precipitate graft rejection, graft-versus-host-disease (GVHD), autoimmunity, malignancies, and lead to a heightened risk of other opportunistic infections.[4-6] This concept is known as heterologous immunity and is characterized by alteration of the immune response to new pathogens or to the transplanted graft by memory immune responses to the previously encountered viral pathogen.[1,7-9] These varied interactions of CMV with the immune system and the balance between disease owing to viral replication versus graft rejection present challenges for effective management of infection in immunosuppressed transplant recipients.

EPIDEMIOLOGY AND RISK FACTORS

Seroprevalence rates of CMV in the general population have been reported to range from 30% to 97%; therefore it is likely that many children will develop CMV infection during their lifetime.[10] CMV is ubiquitous, and transmission occurs horizontally through person-to-person contact with virus-containing secretions from infected individuals (saliva, urine, genital secretions), vertically from mother to infant (in utero, during delivery, or postnatally through breastfeeding), through transfusions of blood products from infected donors, and through SOT or HSCT from infected donors.[11] Among children in day care settings, transmission through urine and saliva is frequent and represents a common scenario for primary CMV acquisition. Transmission among household contacts also occurs frequently. Children with primary CMV acquisition often shed virus for prolonged periods, leading to the potential for ongoing transmission to other children and caregivers. Sexual transmission among adolescents and adults also occurs.

In the setting of SOT, individuals who are CMV seronegative before transplantation and receive an organ from a seropositive donor ([D]-positive/recipient [R]-negative: D^+/R^-) are at high risk of primary CMV infection at the time of organ transplantation and ultimate development of CMV disease.[4] Children are more likely to be CMV seronegative at the time of transplantation than adults and are at risk for newly acquiring CMV from their organ donor, particularly if the donor is an older child or adult. Before the routine use of antiviral prophylaxis, the incidence of symptomatic CMV infection among liver transplant recipients had been reported to be 20% to 60% within the first 30 to 90 days after SOT.[12] Simultaneous receipt of induction immunosuppression may potentiate the risk of CMV disease among SOT recipients with donor and recipient seropositivity mismatch. SOT recipients who are previously CMV infected before transplantation (R^+) are at risk of CMV reactivation after initiation of immunosuppression after SOT. The risk of CMV disease among SOT recipients also varies depending on the transplanted organ, owing to variation in immunosuppressive strategies to prevent organ rejection. Lung and small intestine transplant recipients have a higher risk of developing CMV disease, even in the setting of recipient seropositivity before transplant, whereas liver, heart, and kidney recipients have a lower risk of reactivation.[4]

TABLE 17.1 Risk Assessment in SOT: Cytomegalovirus Reactivation and Disease

Organ	Donor CMV Serostatus	Recipient CMV Serostatus	Risk Assessment
Kidney, liver, heart	Negative	Negative	Low
	Positive or negative	Positive	Intermediate
	Positive	Negative	High
Lung, intestine	Negative	Negative	Low
	Positive or negative	Positive	High[4]
	Positive	Negative	High

CMV, cytomegalovirus; *SOT*, solid organ transplant.
From Martin JM, Danziger-Isakov LA. Cytomegalovirus risk, prevention, and management in pediatric solid organ transplantation. *Pediatr Transplant.* 2011;15:229-236.

TABLE 17.2 Serologic Risk Assessment in HSCT: Cytomegalovirus Reactivation and Disease

Recipient CMV Serostatus	DONOR CMV SEROSTATUS: Negative	DONOR CMV SEROSTATUS: Positive
Negative	Low risk	Intermediate risk
Positive	High risk	Intermediate risk

CMV, cytomegalovirus; *HSCT*, hematopoietic stem cell transplantation.
From Styczynski J. Who is the patient at risk of CMV recurrence: a review of the current scientific evidence with a focus on hematopoietic stem cell transplantation. *Infect Dis Ther.* 2018;7(1):1-16.

Risk assessment of SOT recipients based on donor and recipient serostatus is summarized in Table 17.1.

Recipients of allogeneic HSCT who are CMV seropositive but receive cells from a CMV- seronegative donor or from cord blood (D^-/R^+) are similarly at risk of primary CMV infection and heightened potential for CMV disease.[13] Risk assessment of HSCT recipients is summarized in Table 17.2. T-cell lymphopenia and prophylaxis against GVHD also contribute to the risk for CMV disease. CMV-infected HSCT recipients who undergo unrelated donor or mismatched donor transplants have higher rates of CMV reactivation or disease compared with those who undergo matched, related transplantation. HSCT recipients who require increased immunosuppression for treatment of GVHD also have higher rates of CMV reactivation and disease,[13] although autologous HSCT recipients generally have low rates of CMV reactivation and disease. In other immunocompromised hosts, such as patients with hematologic malignancies receiving chemotherapy, primary CMV acquisition through person-to-person contact or infected blood products or reactivation of previous CMV infection can create a risk for CMV disease given the effects of both the tumor and treatment on the immune system. Children with primary immunodeficiencies in whom HSCT is pursued as a curative treatment may have had CMV infection and disease before HSCT. In these patients, if T-cell immune dysfunction is significant, control of CMV before HSCT may be difficult and leads to greater risk of CMV reactivation after HSCT. Lymphoid malignancies are associated with a greater risk of CMV reactivation compared with myeloid malignancies, and certain therapies such as alemtuzumab, fludarabine, and rituximab are also associated with higher risk.[13]

CLINICAL MANIFESTATIONS

Primary CMV infection in immunocompetent individuals is often asymptomatic but may manifest as a self-limited febrile illness or mononucleosis-like syndrome before establishing life-long latency.[11] Among immunocompromised hosts, clinical manifestations may vary widely from asymptomatic replication to CMV-associated end-organ disease. Updated definitions to describe the various categories of CMV infection and disease have recently been published to standardize reporting of CMV-associated outcomes among transplant recipients, taking into consideration advanced diagnostic testing techniques.[14] Additional definitions are also used to describe CMV characteristics in patients with hematologic malignancies or those undergoing HSCT.[15] The terminology used throughout this chapter aligns with definitions from the American Society of Transplantation as well as the CMV Drug Development Forum recommendations for definitions used in clinical trials[14-16]:

- *Latent CMV:* CMV seropositivity without infection/replication.
- *CMV infection:* Virus isolation or detection of viral antigens or nucleic acid in any body fluid sample or tissue. CMV replication is evidence of viral multiplication and may be used instead of CMV infection.
- *Primary CMV infection:* First detection of CMV infection in an individual with no evidence of prior CMV exposure before transplantation or other immunosuppression.
- *Recurrent CMV infection:* New CMV infection in an individual with previous evidence of CMV infection in whom the virus has not been detected for at least 4 weeks during active surveillance. Recurrent infection may result from reactivation of latent virus (endogenous) or reinfection (exogenous).
- *CMV syndrome:* Detection of CMV in blood in the setting of a constellation of symptoms that may include fever, fatigue, leukopenia or neutropenia, or elevation of liver enzyme levels in an immunocompromised host.
- *CMV disease:* The combination of CMV detection or CMV syndrome plus end-organ disease. CMV disease often involves the transplanted organ in an SOT recipient but may affect many other organ systems as well. Table 17.3 summarizes the clinical manifestations and criteria required for proven CMV disease at various sites.

Primary CMV infection from a graft, CMV reactivation, and CMV disease were traditionally most likely to occur within the first 3 months after OT or within the first 100 days after HSCT.[10,13] CMV reactivation in HSCT recipients during this period could also manifest as delayed engraftment. Implementation of prophylaxis strategies with antiviral agents during this early stage after SOT or after HSCT has shifted the timeline for reactivation and disease to periods after prophylaxis has been discontinued. Immunocompromised children who acquire primary CMV infection through community exposures are at risk for prolonged CMV replication and disease, particularly SOT recipients who remain to take lifelong immunosuppression, compared with immunocompetent children with community acquisition. Primary CMV infection or reactivation in the setting of immune dysfunction as the result of immunosuppression may also precipitate indirect effects of CMV infection, including organ rejection, GVHD, and disease due to opportunistic pathogens.

TABLE 17.3 Definitions of Cytomegalovirus Disease

Site of Disease	Clinical and Diagnostic Criteria
CMV syndrome	CMV detection[a] in blood plus two or more of the following symptoms: fever, malaise, leukopenia, neutropenia, thrombocytopenia, elevation of liver enzymes, elevation of % atypical lymphocytes.
CMV pneumonia	CMV detection in lung tissue or in bronchoalveolar lavage fluid plus clinical symptoms and/or signs of pneumonia such as new infiltrates on imaging, tachypnea, hypoxia. CMV detection by bronchoalveolar lavage suggests probable disease, not proven disease.
CMV gastrointestinal disease (e.g., colitis, esophagitis)	CMV detection in biopsy tissue with macroscopic mucosal lesions and upper and/or lower gastrointestinal tract symptoms and/or signs. In HSCT recipients, information regarding the presence of absence of graft-versus-host-disease on histopathology should also be included.
CMV hepatitis	CMV detection in liver biopsy tissue plus presence of abnormal liver enzymes.
CMV ventriculitis/encephalitis	CMV detection in tissue plus clinical symptoms and/or signs of central nervous system infection. CMV detection in cerebrospinal fluid suggests probable disease, not proven.
CMV nephritis	CMV detection in renal allograft tissue in the setting of renal dysfunction and histologic features of CMV infection. Detection of CMV in urine is not sufficient for diagnosis, as asymptomatic viral shedding in urine is common.
CMV cystitis	CMV detection in bladder biopsy in a patient with clinical symptoms and/or signs of cystitis. Detection of CMV in urine is not sufficient for diagnosis, as asymptomatic viral shedding in urine is common.
CMV myocarditis	CMV detection in heart biopsy specimen in a patient with clinical symptoms and/or signs of myocarditis.
CMV retinitis	Typical ophthalmologic signs identified by an ophthalmologist experienced with CMV retinitis. Although CMV detection in vitreous fluid is recommended, it is not required for this diagnosis.
Other organ involvement	CMV detection in tissue of ot her organs and compatible clinical symptoms and/or signs of specific organ involvement.

[a]CMV detection methods in biopsy or other samples include virus isolation, rapid culture, immunohistochemical analysis, in situ hybridization, nucleic acid testing, and quantitative polymerase chain assay.

CMV, cytomegalovirus.

From Ljungman P, Boeckh M, Hirsch H, et al. Definitions of cytomegalovirus infection and disease in transplant patients for use in clinical trials. *Clin Infect Dis.* 2017;64(1):87-91.

DISEASE PROPHYLAXIS AND PREVENTION

Table 17.4 summarizes the antiviral agents that may be used for CMV prophylaxis and treatment. Identification and prevention of CMV disease in immunocompromised pediatric patients, including HSCT, SOT, and those receiving cancer chemotherapy, is paramount to decreasing morbidity and mortality in these populations. Methods to prevent CMV disease can be classified as prophylaxis or preemptive. Prophylaxis occurs when antiviral therapy is provided to all (universal) or at-risk (targeted) patients for a predetermined period of time after transplantation. Preemptive therapy is the initiation of antiviral therapy with the identification of CMV replication, usually by quantitative polymerase chain reaction (PCR) during scheduled screenings at predetermined intervals, with or without evidence of symptoms of CMV. A mixed model of short-term prophylaxis followed by surveillance at scheduled intervals, currently referred to as "surveillance after prophylaxis", can also be used. The advantages and risks of each prevention method must be assessed, including the risk for side effects, costs, and potential emergence of resistance with prophylaxis and the risk of indirect CMV effects, missed surveillance blood samplings, or delay in intervention with the preemptive approach. In general, prophylaxis is more commonly used in SOT and preemptive therapy is more common in HSCT.

Solid Organ Transplant–Specific Strategies

As discussed previously, the risk for CMV in SOT is based on both the organ type, with small intestine and lung transplant recipients at higher risk, and the donor/recipient serostatus, with D^+/R^- mismatches at higher risk. These two factors have primarily driven recommendations around the choice of preventative strategy and duration of intervention. Based on extensive literature review, the Transplantation Society International CMV Consensus Group recommends a spectrum of prevention strategies based on both organ type and D/R serostatus (Table 17.5). Additional considerations in the determination of prevention include the use of T-cell–depleting induction therapy and the planned chronic suppressive immunosuppression regimen. Overall, either prophylaxis for a predetermined duration, usually 3 to 12 months depending or organ transplanted, or surveillance after prophylaxis is recommended.[16-21] Exceptions to prophylaxis recommendation include monitoring for symptoms in non–small intestine low-risk (D^-/R^-) patients, and preemptive therapy in intermediate-risk (R^+) kidney transplant recipients,[19] intermediate-risk liver transplant recipients,[22] and low-risk (D^-/R^-) small intestine transplant recipients. In adult heart transplant recipients with hypogammglobulinemia, the addition of CMV-enhanced immunoglobulin (CMV Ig) decreased the risk of CMV infection.[23] Additionally, both CMV Ig and antiviral prophylaxis have been associated with decreased mortality in pediatric heart transplant recipients.[24] Support for the use of CMV Ig independent of other antiviral prophylaxis is lacking; however, CMV Ig administration can be considered in addition to antiviral prophylaxis specifically in thoracic transplantation based on the available literature.[24-26] As more data emerge regarding the risk for CMV disease and impact of various prevention strategies and emerging therapeutics, the landscape of CMV prevention in pediatric SOT will certainly require recommendation modification.

TABLE 17.4 Antiviral Agents for Prevention and Treatment of Cytomegalovirus

Agent	Route of Administration	Pediatric Dosing: Prevention	Pediatric Dosing: Treatment	Toxicity Monitoring
Ganciclovir	IV	5 mg/kg q24h[a] (after 5-7 days of twice daily induction in HSCT)	5 mg/kg q12h[a]	Leukopenia, renal dysfunction
Valganciclovir	Oral	7xBSAxCrCl q24h[a]	7xBSAxCrCl q12h[a]	Leukopenia, renal dysfunction; should be used with caution in patients with malabsorption such as recent small intestine transplant recipients
Foscarnet	IV	60 mg/kg per dose q12h for 7 days, followed by 90-120 mg/kg per dose once daily until day 100 after HSCT[a]	60 mg/kg/dose q12h for 7-14 days, followed by 90-120 mg/kg per dose once daily until CMV indicator is negative[a]	Renal dysfunction, electrolyte disturbances
Cidofovir	IV	Variable: 3-5 mg/kg weekly[a] ± probenicid	Variable: 3-5 mg/kg weekly[a] ± probenicid	Renal dysfunction
Letermovir	Oral	Only approved in adults; pediatric studies in development	Not approved for treatment	Interaction with tacrolimus, limited activity against other herpesviruses
CMV immune globulin	IV	Variable: 100-150 mg/kg per dose	Variable: 100-150 mg/kg per dose	

[a]Dose adjust for renal dysfunction.
BSA, body surface area; *CrCl*, creatinine clearance; *h*, hour; *q*, every.

TABLE 17.5 Recommendations for Cytomegalovirus Prevention in Pediatric SOT

Organ	Risk Category	Primary Prevention Strategy
Kidney	Intermediate (R+)	3-6 months of VGCV *OR* preemptive therapy
	High (D+/R−)	3-6 months of VGCV
Liver	Intermediate to High (any D+ or R+)	2-4 weeks of GCV/VGCV with SAP *OR* 3-4 months of VGCV *OR* preeemptive therapy
Heart	Intermediate (R+)	2-4 weeks of GCV/VGCV with SAP *OR* 3 months of GCV/VGCV
	High (D+/R−)	4 weeks of GCV/VGCV with SAP *OR* 3 months of GCV/VGCV
Lung	High (any D+ or R+)	6-12 months of GCV/VGCV
Small intestine	Low (D+/R+)	Preemptive therapy *OR* 2 weeks of GCV with SAP
	High (R+)	2 weeks of GCV with SAP *OR* 3-12 months of GCV/VGCV
	High (D+/R+)	3-12 months of GCV/VGCV

D, donor; *GCV*, ganciclovir; *R*, recipient; *SAP*, surveillance after prophylaxis; SOT, solid organ transplant; *VGCV*, valganciclovir.
Adapted from Kotton CN, Kumar D, Caliendo AM, et al. The Third International Consensus Guidelines on the Management of Cytomegalovirus in Solid-organ Transplantation. *Transplantation.* 2018;102(6):900-931.

HSCT-Specific Strategies

HSCT-specific strategies for the prevention of CMV rely on the understanding of both risk and the potential impact of antiviral therapies on engraftment. As discussed earlier, HSCT CMV seropositive recipients from CMV seronegative donors (D−/R+) and patients with pre-HSCT CMV DNAemia are at the highest risk for CMV infection and disease.[13] Furthermore, the type of transplant indicates that matched related donors have a decreased risk of CMV after transplant compared with both matched unrelated donors and human leukocyte antigen–haploidentical donors.[27] Concomitant therapy may also affect the decisions regarding preventative strategies with reports of increased risk of CMV infection in patients who did not receive intravenous IG supplementation after HSCT.[28] The risk of CMV must be balanced with the potential impact of antiviral therapy.[29] Ganciclovir and valganciclovir are marrow suppressive, and there is concern for delayed engraftment with routine prophylaxis. Additionally, foscarnet has renal toxicity that may limit its use. Although approved for CMV prophylaxis in adult HSCT recipients, letermovir has not yet been evaluated in pediatric patients. Pediatric data are lacking to support the use of CMV IG as a component of prevention therapies. Additional consideration in HSCT should be given to the potential indirect effects of CMV as well. CMV DNAemia has been associated with improved immune reconstitution[30] and decreased risk of post-HSCT relapse of acute lymphocytic leukemia (ALL),[31] but this must be balanced by an increased risk of nonrelapse morbidity. As with SOT, either preemptive therapy or prophylaxis can be considered in most HSCT.

Oncology-Specific Strategies

Based on limited studies, the risk for CMV disease in oncology patients is less acute than for SOT or HSCT. In one recent study,[32] although nearly 39% of ALL patients in whom CMV developed had at least one positive CMV viral detection during therapy, only those with persistent DNAemia and symptoms received intervention. Persistence of infection has been associated with younger age of diagnosis, high-risk ALL, and relapsed ALL.[32,33] Therefore serial screening by viral load and symptoms for high-risk oncology patients can be considered, although transient detection of CMV in the blood does not always require immediate intervention. CMV incidence and prevention strategies in pediatric patients with solid tumors require additional study as the literature is substantively limited in this area.

Emerging Prevention Therapies and Strategies

In addition to screening, prophylaxis, and preemptive therapy, additional medications and cellular therapies are under investigation for the prevention of CMV infection and disease. Letermovir, a novel agent that blocks viral replication by interacting with the viral pUL56 subunit without inhibiting the synthesis of progeny CMV DNA or viral proteins, has been approved for prophylaxis to prevent CMV in adult HSCT recipients and has less bone marrow toxicity and nephrotoxicity than other antivirals. Pediatric studies are currently in development and an adult study evaluating letermovir in SOT is ongoing. Brincidofovir, an oral prodrug of cidofovir, has activity against CMV; however, a randomized double-blind, placebo-controlled study in adult HSCT did not show a decrease in CMV infections and patinets in the brincidofovir arm had increased risk for adverse events including GVHD.[34] Brincidofovir is currently not approved or under investigation for CMV prevention in pediatrics SOT or HSCT populations. Cellular therapy with CMV-specific cytotoxic T cells has been used in the treatment of CMV in HSCT and SOT recipients (see later text). Evaluation of preemptive administration of these cells with CMV detection is under investigation in pediatric HSCT recipients. Additionally, CMV vaccines remain under investigation, although a candidate for adequate prevention has not yet emerged.

DIAGNOSIS

Diagnosis of CMV infection has evolved substantially with improved reliability, sensitivity, and specificity as new methodologies emerge. Testing modalities for CMV are summarized in Table 17.6. CMV serology (IgG) in both the donor and recipient for HSCT and SOT assists in the determination of risk for posttransplant CMV; however, serology should not be used to diagnosis CMV infection or disease in the posttransplant period as it is a marker of prior exposure and not active CMV replication. CMV viral culture is an outdated method as it requires several weeks for the virus to grow, missing the window of opportunity for intervention. Shell vial culture, a more rapid method providing results in approximately 48 hours, relies on centrifuge inoculation of a cellular monolayer and incubation followed by CMV-specific antibody staining for viral detection, but it remains too insensitive for routine blood monitoring.[29] Detection of CMV pp65 antigen in peripheral blood leukocytes, known as antigenemia testing, is a rapid semiquantitative test used in some centers, but it suffers from technical difficulties and poor interrater reliability. Therefore quantitative CMV PCR has become the most sensitive and reliable methodology for diagnosing CMV in the transplant and oncology populations. As assay results can be affected by sample type (serum, plasma, or whole blood), assay primers, and extraction methods, consistency in these parameters should be paramount and appropriate comparisons performed with any modification of testing methods. The introduction of WHO standardization has enhanced the reproducibility of testing across laboratories and assays,[35] and all results currently should be reported in international units/mL (IU/mL) to identify that the assay has been calibrated to the WHO standard. A definitive threshold value indicating risk for significant infection or disease has not been

TABLE 17.6 Cytomegalovirus Testing Modalities

	SENSITIVITY				
Test Name	**Prior CMV Infection**	**Active CMV Infection and Disease**	**Specimen Type**	**Useful for Monitoring Disease/Treatment?**	**When to Test**
CMV antibody (IgG)	High	Low	Blood	No	Before transplant to determine serostatus; infants <18 mo should also have a urine or saliva shell vial culture or qualitative PCR if seropositive.
Quantitative PCR	Low	High	Blood	Yes	Surveillance, monitoring for progression of disease, monitoring of response to treatment.
Qualitative PCR	Low	High	Urine, saliva, BAL	No	Detection of viral shedding; many centers are using this test in place of shell vial culture for screening of infants. Interpretation of positive result in BAL is difficult and does not directly correlate with disease.
Shell vial culture	High (age <18 mo)	Low	Urine, saliva, BAL	No	Infants <18 mo should be screened for CMV before transplant using urine or saliva in addition to serology.
Histopathologic examination with in situ hybridization	Moderate to high	Moderate	Tissue	No	Biopsy samples, done by pathology demonstrating viral inclusions and cytopathic effect are suggestive; CMV-specific staining should be performed.
Tests No Longer Routinely Used					
Conventional viral culture	Low to moderate	Low	Blood, tissue, urine, BAL	No	Prolonged turnaround time.
pp65 Antigenemia test	Low	High	Blood	Yes	More difficult to interpret treatment response, no longer widely available; not reliable in neutropenic patients.

BAL, bronchoalveolar lavage; *CMV*, cytomegalovirus; *IgG*, immunoglobulin G; *PCR*, polymerase chain reaction.

universally determined, but clinicians should consider both the absolute value above a lower limit of quantitation as well as the rate of change in determining the timing of intervention. In addition, quantitative PCR from bronchoalveolar lavage fluid has been evaluated as a potential biomarker for CMV pneumonia, but specific thresholds have not been reliably determined.[36]

Tissue-based testing modalities, including histopathologic examination for viral cytopathic effects. can be used to document invasive CMV disease. Additional testing with in situ CMV-specific antigen staining provides more specificity that the histopathologic changes are resulting from CMV rather than other viral infections.

Testing for Antiviral Resistance

SOT and HSCT recipients with prolonged exposure to antiviral agents for prophylaxis or treatment of CMV are at risk for development of antiviral resistance over time.[37,38] In SOT, resistance is most likely to develop in CMV D^+/R^- children, whereas in HSCT resistance is most likely in R^+ children. Significant T-cell depletion, high viral loads, and suboptimal antiviral concentrations may all contribute to development of resistance. In children, dose optimization with weight gain and changes in renal function is critical to ensuring adequate antiviral drug levels and avoiding resistance. The most practical assessment of antiviral resistance is currently a genotypic assay to sequence the genes in which antiviral resistance mutations are known to occur.[16] Resistance mutations to ganciclovir have thus far only been identified in two genes, the UL97 phosphotransferase gene and the UL54 viral polymerase gene. Mutations identified in the UL97 gene typically confer resistance to ganciclovir/valganciclovir but not to foscarnet or cidofovir. Mutations in the UL54 gene may confer resistance to all three antiviral agents. In additional, evaluation for mutations in the UL56 gene that may confer resistance to letermovir can be performed. Laboratory identification of mutations in these genes does have limitations. Although mutations may be detected in the UL97, UL 54, or UL56 genes, involvement of certain codons is more likely than others to result in true resistance to the antiviral agent, whereas involvement of other codons may be less suspicious. Therefore familiarity with interpreting genotypic testing and an understanding of the likelihood of resistance arising from mutations in particular codons becomes important for clinical use of such tests.[37] In addition, genotypic tests are qualitative and do not provide quantitative data regarding the percentage of a viral population that may be affected by a mutation. Antiviral resistance testing provides valuable information by helping to clarify whether rising CMV viral loads are due to an ineffective antiviral agent owing to resistance compared with other factors, such as worsening immune function or medication nonadherence. Fig. 17.1 provides an algorithm for evaluation and management of suspected antiviral resistance as recommended by The Transplantation Society International CMV Consensus Group in the Third International Consensus Guidelines on the Management of Cytomegalovirus in Solid-organ Transplantation.[16]

Cellular Assays to Document CMV-Specific Immunity

Cellular assays to assess CMV-specific immunity in immunocompromised patients that can be used to assess risk for infection are developing. Several assays assess exist that measure T-cell responses to CMV antigens, providing a quantitative evaluation of CMV-specific immunity. A preliminary report in a small population of pediatric HSCT recipients indicates that the development of CMV-specific cellular immunity is associated with a decreased risk of CMV infection and relapse similar to adult HSCT studies.[39] Although several studies have evaluated the utility of these assays to determine duration of antiviral prophylaxis, risk of infection, and CMV recurrence in adult SOT, pediatric studies evaluating these cellular immunity assays in pediatric SOT have not been published to date. The optimal use of these assays remains to be determined in pediatric HSCT and SOT, especially as results may be different in infants and pediatric patients with developing immune systems.

TREATMENT

Treatment of symptomatic CMV infection and disease currently relies on several strategies that depend on the relative immune status of the patient. Options include reduction of immunosuppression, antiviral therapy, and cellular therapy including CMV-specific cytotoxic T cells. Immunosuppression reduction can be used if feasible, especially in HSCT patients as therapy for GVHD and SOT recipients. Modification of immunosuppressive regimens by reducing mycophenolate administration or substitution with mammalian target of rapamycin inhibitors have been associated with improved CMV infection profiles and may be considered.[40]

For all patients administration of antiviral therapy can be implemented (see Table 17.4). Generally, intravenous therapy is suggested for patients with severe disease or those who have significant concerns with absorption of oral agents. For SOT, first-line therapy is ganciclovir for severe disease. Based on data from preemptive strategies documenting clearance of CMV DNAemia, valganciclovir is now recommended for treatment of mild disease in pediatric SOT.[16] Other antiviral agents, including foscarnet and cidofovir, are second-line therapies because of their hematologic toxicity and nephrotoxicity. In HSCT, first-line therapy is variable, depending on the status of immune reconstitution related to either engraftment or treatment for GVHD. As noted earlier, concerns exist for marrow suppression with ganciclovir/valganciclovir before engraftment; in these circumstances, alternate agents, such as foscarnet and less commonly cidofovir, have been used. CMV Ig is not routinely recommended for therapy of CMV disease in pediatric SOT.[16] Although there are limited studies describing the use of CMV Ig as an adjunctive treatment with antiviral therapy in adult HSCT recipients with CMV-associated pneumonia, pediatric data are lacking and the use of this agent is not routinely recommended.[41,42]

For patients with concern for antiviral resistance based on clinical suspicion, especially in those with persistent or recurrent CMV DNAemia during prolonged antiviral exposure with at least 2 weeks of full-dose antiviral therapy, antiviral therapy can be empirically modified (Fig. 17.1). For patients receiving ganciclovir therapy, options include increased doses of ganciclovir and addition or transition to foscarnet while genetic resistance test results are pending. Results of resistance testing and specific clinical scenarios including risks for antiviral toxicity should be considered in the development of individualized antiviral treatment plans. Maribavir, another oral antiviral agent that previously failed in a clinical trial assessing its use for CMV prevention in SOT,[43] is currently under investigation for the treatment of refractory and resistant CMV disease in both the SOT and HSCT populations including patients as young as 12 years (clinical trial identifier NCT02931539). Letermovir has not been studied for treatment of CMV disease, although case reports do exist. However, the development of rapid resistance from in vitro studies has dampened the enthusiasm for the potential of letermovir to treat CMV disease with high viral burdens.[44] Brincidofovir additionally has potential for treatment of CMV infection and disease; however, there are no ongoing studies aimed to assess its efficacy for CMV in the pediatric transplant populations.

Emerging Cellular Treatment Strategies

In addition to antiviral therapy, adoptive cellular therapy with CMV-specific cytotoxic T cells (viral-specific T-cells [VSTs]) for

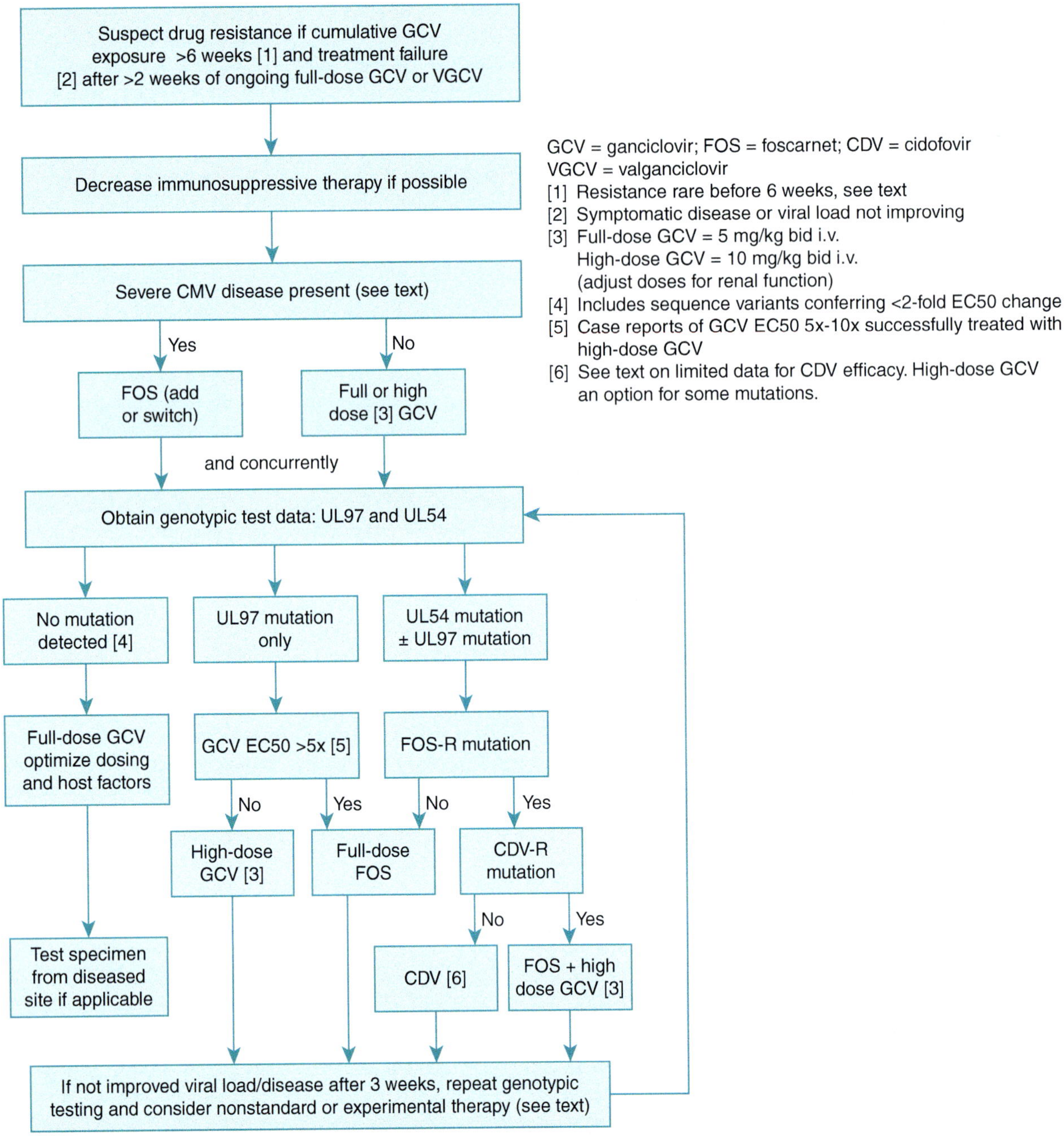

Fig. 17.1 Suggested algorithm for evaluation and management of suspected cytomegalovirus resistance in transplant recipients. (From Kotton CN, Kumar D, Caliendo AM, et al. The Third International Consensus Guidelines on the Management of Cytomegalovirus in Solid-organ Transplantation. *Transplantation*. 2018; 102(6):900-931.)

the treatment of CMV infection and disease is emerging. Primarily reported in HSCT, CMV VSTs are predominantly derived from either the donor or a third party, although generation from naïve T cells from umbilical cord donors has been performed. Administration of CMV VSTs has resulted in CMV clearance and recovery from refractory and resistant disease in HSCT recipients.[45-47] The development of GVHD as the result of incomplete human leukocyte antigen matching—a theoretical concern for third-party VSTs—has not been reported, although it may decrease the efficacy of the therapy.[48] The use of CMV VSTs in SOT is sparse, but administration in adult lung and kidney transplantation described in case reports has been successful.[49,50] The type of CMV VSTs, timing, dosing, and duration of therapy require additional investigation including evaluation for unanticipated side effects.

INFECTION PREVENTION AND ANTICIPATORY GUIDANCE

Although CMV infection and disease are most often considered in the context of donor-derived acquisition or reactivation of latent infection in transplant recipients or oncology patients, immunocompromised children who are CMV negative are also at risk of acquiring primary CMV from community exposures, as are their otherwise healthy, immunocompetent counterparts. Primary CMV infection in immunocompromised children may be more likely to lead to symptomatic disease and may be associated with graft rejection in transplant recipients.[6] Education of patients and families regarding CMV exposure and prevention practices for children who are CMV negative is an integral part of routine peritransplant counseling regarding protection against infections and safer living post-transplantation.

Immunocompromised children in day care settings may acquire CMV through exposure to saliva or other secretions from other children. Shared toys and sharing eating utensils or exposure to nasal secretions are common ways in which toddlers become exposed to the virus in group play settings. Educating children and caregivers to practice frequent handwashing and use alcohol-based hand sanitizers can help to minimize transmission of virus in such settings.

Adolescents and young adults may also acquire CMV through saliva or other secretions from close contacts, similar to younger children, but are also at risk for CMV acquisition through sexual contact. Immunosuppression associated with transplantation or chemotherapy creates a greater risk of CMV disease with primary infection in these settings. Sexually active adolescent and young adult women who acquire primary CMV and become pregnant have a higher risk of transmitting virus to their infant. Offering guidance regarding safer sexual practices is an important part of posttransplant infection prevention counseling.

Transplant recipients, oncology patients, and other children with immunocompromising conditions should receive CMV-negative or leukoreduced blood products to avoid transmission of CMV, particularly in patients who are not previously CMV infected.

Mothers who are breastfeeding have the potential to transmit CMV through breast milk to their infants. Otherwise healthy infants are typically asymptomatic in the setting of such postnatal acquisition of CMV and may not be identified as being CMV infected. Although young infants with congenital cardiac disease, biliary atresia, and other diagnoses may be listed for SOT in early infancy and there may be concern regarding breast milk–associated CMV acquisition in these infants in the setting of possible immunosuppression, there are currently no data to support avoiding breastfeeding in such infants. Transplant centers may restrict breastfeeding of infants with primary immunodeficiencies for whom HSCT is being considered, but no such restrictions are typically implemented for infants undergoing evaluation and listing for SOT.

CONCLUSIONS

CMV and other herpesviruses are important pathogens in immunocompromised children, especially those undergoing SOT or HSCT. Although many advances have been made in diagnostic methods, treatment of CMV disease, and strategies for screening and prevention, there are unique challenges for children who are often vulnerable to primary CMV acquisition while immunosuppressed. Novel antiviral therapies for prophylaxis and treatment, immunomodulatory strategies, and development of vaccines will ultimately be needed to curtail the burden of CMV infection and disease in immunocompromised pediatric populations. Expansion of research efforts to investigate the utility of new approaches to CMV management remains a significant need in the pediatric setting.

18

Epstein-Barr Virus and Posttransplant Lymphoproliferative Disorder

Michael D. Green, MD, MPH, Thomas Gross, Jr., MD, PhD, and Upton D. Allen, MBBS

Epstein-Barr virus (EBV) is a human γ-herpesvirus that is associated with important syndromes in both the immunocompetent and immunocompromised host. It is a ubiquitous virus, as it is found worldwide. In community settings, EBV is primarily transmitted by exposure to human saliva since humans are the only known host of the virus. Peaks of primary infection occur in early childhood and young adulthood, with the highest rates in persons 10 to 25 years of age. In nonindustrialized countries, 90% of children are infected before age 5, where infection is typically asymptomatic. In industrialized countries, this level of seropositivity is not attained until the fourth decade of life.[1] Although many episodes of EBV infection may be asymptomatic or associated with mild, nonspecific respiratory symptoms, it classically presents with the mononucleosis syndrome with rare progression to more severe disease (e.g., EBV-driven hemophagocytic lymphohistiocytosis [HLH]) in the immunocompetent individual. In contrast, the spectrum of EBV-driven disease broadens to include lymphoproliferative syndromes, including malignancies among individuals with congenital or acquired immune deficiencies, particularly those associated with impairment of cell-mediated immunity. In this chapter, we discuss EBV infection and its complications in children undergoing solid organ transplantation (SOT), hematopoietic stem cell transplantation (HSCT), and those being treated for cancer. EBV-driven primary cancers (e.g., Burkitt lymphoma) are not discussed.

EPIDEMIOLOGY AND RISK FACTORS

Epstein-Barr Virus in Solid Organ Transplant Recipients

In the SOT setting, donor-transmitted EBV infection is extremely common in EBV-mismatched (donor-seropositive/recipient-seronegative [D^+/R^-]) patients. Transmission is also possible when non-leukoreduced blood products are used. The EBV genome is found in the majority (>90%) of B-cell posttransplant lymphoproliferative disorders (PTLDs) occurring within the first year after SOT. However, PTLD occurring later after transplant is frequently EBV-negative.[2] The highest rate of PTLDs in the SOT setting is seen in the first year after transplant, typically among individuals who are EBV-seronegative recipients of seropositive donor organs.

Primary EBV infection is a major risk factor for PTLD in SOT recipients; therefore pediatric populations are at much a higher risk of developing PTLD than their adult counterparts.[3] Individuals who are R^+ are not devoid of PTLD risk and account for up to 25% of PTLD cases in children.[4] This may be due to reactivation of latent EBV in the recipient or acquisition of a new strain of EBV. Beyond the specific role of EBV serostatus, the incidence of PTLD varies according to several factors including the type of organ transplanted. Risk related to the latter may reflect immunosuppressive regimens, lymphoid load in the allograft and chronic antigenic stimulation resulting from direct communication and exposure to environmental antigens, or chronic allograft dysfunction including antibody-mediated rejection.[2] Small intestine transplant recipients are at the highest risk for development of PTLD (up to 32%), whereas recipients of pancreas, heart, lung, and liver transplants are at moderate risk (3% to 12%). Renal transplant recipients are at relatively low risk (1% to 2%). Although PTLD lesions in SOT recipients are most often of recipient origin (as this relates to the source of the proliferating cells), lesions that are limited to the graft occurring early after transplant are predominantly donor in origin.[5]

Antilymphocyte globulins that result in selective T-cell depletion, particularly when used in high-dose or repetitive courses, have historically been associated with increased PTLD risk. Among the newer biologic agents, high rates of PTLD presenting predominantly as primary central nervous system (CNS) lymphoma were observed in renal transplant patients who received belatacept and were EBV seronegative before transplant.[6] Beyond these specific scenarios, it is likely that with other immunosuppressants, the risk of PTLD reflects the net state of immunosuppression in specific patients. Indeed, the duration of immunosuppression is a risk factor for late PTLD development.

Studies among pediatric SOT recipients suggest that children receiving heart transplants who are chronic high-EBV load carriers may be at significantly increased risk of late-onset EBV-positive PTLD.[7] This level of risk might not apply to other organ recipients.[8,9] Data from prospective studies would clarify the pathogenesis and natural history of chronic viral load carriage in relationship to subsequent PTLD risk in specific allografts.

Cytomegalovirus (CMV) infection may inconsistently contribute to the net state of immunosuppression and is a known PTLD risk factor. However, more contradictory evidence exists for the role of the following as risk factors for primary disease: tacrolimus in pediatric recipients; specific human leukocyte antigen (HLA) epitopes; HLA matching; certain cytokine gene polymorphisms; preexisting chronic immune stimulation; hepatitis c infection; viral strain virulence (EBV-1 vs. EBV-2 and viral gene mutations).

Although PTLD rates increased after the calcineurin inhibitor tacrolimus became the backbone of most immunosuppressive regimens in the 1990s, it is likely that the net state of immunosuppression, an entity that is difficult to measure, is a major risk factor. Attempts to quantify the risk associated with specific immunosuppressive agents used for induction or maintenance therapy have often led to inconsistent results, which highlights the need for studies to optimize minimization of long-term immunosuppression in individual patients.

Epstein-Barr Virus in Hematopoietic Stem Cell Transplantation

The epidemiology of EBV and PTLD after HSCT differs somewhat from that after SOT in that both the source of EBV and the infected

B cells in PTLD after HSCT are of donor origin in the majority of cases. This is explained in part by the fact that the intense conditioning regimens used in HSCT usually eradicate host EBV latently infected B cells. The period of risk for PTLD after HSCT is also more limited compared with SOT recipients. Although EBV loads may initially become positive 3 to 4 weeks after transplant, PTLD rarely occurs in the first 30 days after HSCT, and the majority of cases occur within 6 months, with the peak incidence in the third month after transplant.[10,11]

The incidence of PTLD after HSCT ranges from less than 1% to approximately 25% depending on the presence of risk factors.[10,11] In HSCT, unlike SOT, EBV status of the recipient is not a strong risk factor for PTLD; however, increasing donor age is a risk factor. Donor source of stem cells has been associated with risk and seems to relate to duration of lymphopenia, and hence recovery of functional T-cell immunity after transplant. PTLD is very rare after autologous bone marrow transplant.[10] The incidence of PTLD is higher with unrelated donors than with matched related donors and increases with degree of HLA mismatching.[10,11] Because cord blood does not contain EBV-infected B cells, it was first believed that PTLD would not occur with this source of stem cells. However, the incidence of PTLD after cord blood transplant is similar to matched related donors. The time to PTLD after cord blood transplant is usually longer, likely owing to prolonged lymphocyte recovery and the need to acquire EBV from a source other than the stem cell graft. T-cell depletion (TCD) is a strong risk factor for PTLD, but it depends on the methodology of TCD.[10,11] Methods that specifically remove T cells confer a higher risk of PTLD compared with methods that deplete all lymphocyte types, including posttransplant cyclophosphamide. It is believed that in the latter approach, depletion of EBV-infected B cells in addition to T cells from the donor lowers the risk for PTLD compared with those that deplete only T cells. Development of graft-versus-host disease (GVHD) has not consistently been demonstrated to be a risk factor for PTLD, although the agents used to prevent and/or treat GVHD, such as anti–T-cell antibodies, do increase the risk of PTLD.[10,11]

Epstein-Barr Virus in Cancer

Complications of chemotherapy resulting from EBV infections are very rare. However, there are anecdotal reports of EBV lymphoproliferative disease, usually associated with prolonged immunosuppressive therapy, such as maintenance therapy for acute lymphoblastic leukemia.[12] Reducing or withholding chemotherapy allowing anti-EBV T-cell immunity to recover is often sufficient to resolve these complications. HLH can be triggered by EBV infection and can be the predominant symptom of some EBV-associated malignancies, particularly mature T/natural killer (NK) cell non-Hodgkin lymphomas (NHLs), or HLH can develop as a complication of EBV infection in patients receiving chemotherapy. In either scenario, aggressive therapy is required.[13]

Clinical Manifestations

Clinical manifestations of EBV infection range from asymptomatic illness to clinically significant and potentially life-threatening disease in children who have undergone SOT or HSCT. As noted earlier, although EBV disease is much less frequently reported in children undergoing treatment for cancer, an increased rate of primary infection compared with children without cancer has been reported to occur,[14] and cancer therapy–associated lymphoproliferative disorders have been reported, though rarely, in the pediatric population.[15] At least some evidence supports that EBV may be a cause of fever alone in transplant recipients and cancer patients with active EBV infection.

EBV infection can either be primary (new infection occurring in an immunologically naïve patient) or as the result of reactivation of latent EBV in the immunocompromised child. Additionally, reinfection with a new EBV strain may occur. For SOT recipients, primary infection is associated with more clinically significant disease, whereas reactivation or reinfection tends to be mild or even asymptomatic. The spectrum of clinical disease in SOT recipients includes a nonspecific febrile illness that can resemble the CMV syndrome, typical mononucleosis, and PTLD, including EBV-associated malignant lymphoma (e.g., Burkitt lymphoma [BL]). In addition, organ-specific manifestations such as enteritis and hepatitis in the absence of PTLD can also be seen. Rarely EBV has been associated with posttransplant smooth muscle tumors in SOT recipients as well, and EBV-positive T-cell PTLDs are also rare occurrences and are associated with a very poor prognosis.

The clinical presentations of the spectrum of EBV disease including PTLD frequently overlap and may affect a large number of sites within the body (Table 18.1). Each of these syndromes can present with prolonged episodes of fever. Adenopathy and hepatosplenomegaly are frequently but not always seen. Gastrointestinal disease occurs frequently and is particularly common in recipients of intestinal transplantation. The presence of diarrhea associated with microscopic or gross blood warrants investigation for EBV. Hematologic changes, including leukopenia, neutropenia, and thrombocytopenia, all frequently occur. Of note, some children with EBV-associated PTLD may be asymptomatic with mass lesions involving nodes or organs found on examination or imaging. In general, variation in severity and extent of disease is believed to be related to the degree of immunosuppression and adequacy of the host immune response in the pediatric organ transplant recipient. For SOT recipients, onset of viral syndrome, mononucleosis, and polymorphic PTLD occur primarily within the first year, whereas monomorphic PTLD and lymphoma tend to occur later.

In contrast to the variability and spectrum of disease in pediatric SOT recipients, the development of EBV infection before immune reconstitution places all EBV-infected pediatric HSCT recipients at risk for progression to PTLD. Clinical symptoms most frequently include fever but manifest the range of symptoms seen in SOT recipients; EBV-negative PTLD or non–B-cell disease is extraordinarily rare. Finally, there are only limited data describing the clinical presentation of EBV disease in children undergoing treatment for cancer. Although it is clear that development of lymphoproliferative disorder after primary infection is rare, data describing clinical presentation in the absence of this have not been generally reported.

TABLE 18.1 Presenting Symptoms and Signs in Patients With Epstein-Barr Virus Disease Including Lymphoproliferative Disorder

Symptoms/Complaints	Signs
Swollen lymph glands	Lymphadenopathy
Weight loss	Hepatosplenomegaly
Fever or night sweats	Subcutaneous nodules
Sore throat	Tonsillar enlargement
Malaise and lethargy	Tonsillar inflammation
Chronic sinus congestion and discomfort	Signs of bowel perforation
Abdominal pain	Mucocutaneous ulceration
Anorexia, nausea, and vomiting	Mass lesions
Gastrointestinal bleeding	Focal neurologic signs
Symptoms of bowel perforation	

PREVENTION OF EPSTEIN-BARR VIRUS INFECTION AND PTLD

The impact of EBV disease including PTLD in children undergoing SOT and HSCT has prompted interest in the prevention of EBV infection and its complication in these populations. Accordingly, evidence assessing the potential efficacy and impact of preventive strategies against EBV have been published, although with few exceptions, prospective randomized comparative trials are generally lacking. Potential prevention strategies against EBV can be categorized as immunoprophylaxis, chemoprophylaxis, and preemptive therapy. In addition to these strategies, the use of leukocyte-reduced blood products also serves as an important barrier to the spread of EBV because the virus is typically carried in B lymphocytes, which are eliminated through the process of leukoreduction. Because of the relatively low frequency of recognized EBV disease in children undergoing treatment for cancer, evidence assessing the efficacy and impact of preventive strategies against EBV in this population is not available and will not be discussed.

IMMUNOPROPHYLAXIS

Immunoprophylaxis can be categorized as active or passive. Active immunoprophylaxis would be accomplished through use of an EBV vaccine but none is available for clinical use. Passive immunoprophylaxis can be accomplished by providing anti-EBV antibody through the infusion of intravenous immunoglobulin (IVIG) or through infusion of EBV-specific cytotoxic T lymphocytes (CTLs). Published data demonstrated a protective effect of IVIG on the development of EBV disease in a SCID mouse model.[16] The potential role of IVIG was further supported by a large retrospective analysis that found that SOT recipients receiving anti-CMV immunoglobulins for CMV prophylaxis did not develop PTLD during the first year (during the time of prophylaxis).[17] However, several prospective studies failed to confirm this finding. A randomized controlled trial using anti-CMV immunoglobulins prophylaxis versus placebo in pediatric liver transplant recipients did not identify significant evidence of prevention of either EBV disease or EBV-associated PTLD, although a trend toward less EBV disease and PTLD was observed in patients receiving immunoglobulins.[18] Similarly, no impact on time free from any EBV viral load, mean viral load, time free from achieving a "high" EBV viral load, or development of EBV-associated PTLD was observed in a prospective study of IVIG versus placebo in EBV-mismatched (donor EBV-seropositive/recipient EBV-seronegative) organ recipients (adult and pediatric), all of whom received 12 months of antiviral therapy consisting of intravenous ganciclovir followed by oral antivirals (acyclovir or ganciclovir).[19] Evidence on the protective effect of IVIG in HSCT recipients against EBV is lacking.

The use of EBV-specific CTLs as adoptive immunotherapy has been proven to be efficacious in stem cell transplant recipients,[20] although the limited availability of access to CTL therapy affects the extent of its use. For HSCT recipients, the EBV-positive donor is often the source of the EBV-specific T cells, though third-party donors have been successfully used. Rates of prevention approaching 100% have been reported by centers with access to EBV-specific T-cell therapy. In contrast to the successful use of this approach in HSCT recipients, efforts to translate these benefits to the prevention of EBV/PTLD in SOT recipients have been limited and have not succeeded as of this time.

Chemoprophylaxis

Chemoprophylaxis using antiviral agents, such as acyclovir and ganciclovir, represents another possible approach to preventing EBV/PTLD. Unfortunately, this has not been the subject of randomized trials. Ganciclovir, or its prodrug valganciclovir, may be the preferred drug for EBV prophylaxis because of its higher in vitro antiviral activity. Nevertheless, these drugs are only effective against the lytic forms of EBV. This might translate into inefficiency in preventing latently driven disease, providing a potential explanation for the lack of clear evidence of benefit of the use of antivirals to prevent EBV. Initial support for the potential role of antiviral therapy in the prevention of EBV infection was derived from several single-center retrospective studies that, although encouraging, suffered from methodologic concerns, including lack of appropriate controls or concomitant changes in clinical practice that could have affected the development of EBV and PTLD. Although a U.S. case-controlled study suggested a potential role of ganciclovir given for CMV prophylaxis in the reduction of PTLD incidence in kidney transplant recipients,[21] other studies have not confirmed the efficacy of ganciclovir, valganciclovir, or acyclovir against EBV/PTLD in SOT recipients.[17] A randomized prospective trial of 2 weeks of ganciclovir compared with 2 weeks of ganciclovir followed by 50 weeks of oral acyclovir in EBV- seronegative pediatric liver transplant patients did not establish any benefit to extended use of antiviral therapy to prevent EBV disease.[22] A 2016 meta-analysis showed that the use of antiviral drugs (ganciclovir, valganciclovir, acyclovir, and valacyclovir) in mismatched EBV transplant recipients (D^+/R^-) had no effect on PTLD incidence in children and adults undergoing SOT.[23] No significant differences were seen across all types of SOTs, age groups, or antiviral use as prophylaxis or preemptive strategy. Despite the results of the meta-analysis, definitive conclusions on the presence or absence of clinical benefits of the use of ganciclovir and related antiviral agents to prevent EBV and it complications likely require prospective multicenter randomized trials.

Because transmission of EBV from the donor to the EBV-naïve recipient is a major risk factor for EBV disease and PTLD, the role of antiviral chemoprophylaxis given to the donor to limit transmission has also been explored. Two pilot studies in the setting of adult kidney recipients of living donors provide encouraging preliminary results that treatment of the donor or recipient before transplant might affect EBV transmission and potentially PTLD. The first study was a randomized treatment of the donors with 2 weeks of valganciclovir.[24] Although the second study used a single dose of rituximab, as opposed to an antiviral, it highlights the principle of potentially interrupting viral replication before transplantation.[25]

Viral Load Monitoring and Preemptive Prevention Strategies

Among pediatric SOT recipients, surveillance monitoring of EBV loads to inform preemptive reductions in immunosuppression has resulted in a decreased incidence of EBV/PTLD compared with historical controls. McDiarmid and colleagues reported a decreased incidence of PTLD from 10% to 5% using EBV viral load monitoring to guide the combined use of reduced immunosuppression and intravenous ganciclovir in pediatric liver transplant recipients with rising EBV loads.[26] Other studies demonstrated decreased incidences of PTLD using decreased immunosuppression alone without ganciclovir in response to elevated EBV loads.[27] One limitation of this approach is that the development of a detectable load does not necessarily predict progression to EBV disease, and additional risk factors that reliably add specificity to the predictive value of an elevated load beyond developing primary EBV infection after SOT have not been identified. Accordingly, reductions in immunosuppression were carried out based on elevated load alone. Owing to the risk of rejection, these reductions have been conducted carefully with ongoing attention for the presence of findings suggestive of early rejection.

Some centers have considered the preemptive use of the anti-CD20 monoclonal antibody rituximab for pediatric SOT patients with elevated EBV viral load, although little published data are available. Martin and colleagues reported encouraging results using EBV load monitoring to inform the preemptive use of rituximab in EBV D^+/R^- adult kidney transplant recipients.[28] However, the majority of treated patients actually had clinical evidence of EBV disease at the time of treatment. Accordingly, these data relate more to the use of rituximab for early treatment and not prevention of EBV disease. Additional experience is needed to confirm the efficacy and long-term safety of rituximab in a prevention/preemption model against EBV in the SOT setting.

Rituximab is more often used among HSCT recipients than among SOT recipients. Because such recipients, who are at high risk for PTLD, often develop EBV infection before reestablishment of adequate cell-mediated immunity, reduction of immune suppression is frequently not an option. As the period of risk is much more predictable and relative early after HSCT, monitoring with EBV viral load polymerase chain reaction (PCR) and preemptive therapy with rituximab appears to reduce the incidence of PTLD.[29] Although no randomized trials have been published to date, this approach of serially monitoring high-risk patients (e.g., patients who receive TCD) by weekly EBV blood PCR and giving rituximab for patients with elevated EBV DNA levels or persistently increasing levels has become standard of care at many institutions, especially for centers without access to adoptive immunotherapy against EBV (see earlier text).

In summary, it appears that the strategy of using EBV load monitoring in SOT to inform preemptive reduction in immunosuppression to prevent EBV/PTLD in SOT recipients is the optimal currently available preventive strategy, although more data evaluating the comparative safety and efficacy of rituximab with reduced immunosuppression alone in response to rising or elevated EBV loads are needed. For HSCT recipients, preemptive use of rituximab in addition to the use of prophylactic or preemptive EBV-specific T cells are current optimal preventive strategies.

DIAGNOSIS

Diagnosis of EBV disease can be difficult in the setting of chemotherapy or transplantation, as it may present as anything in a spectrum of clinical manifestations from primary infection, reactivation, EBV-associated disease, or PTLD. Serologic findings can be difficult to interpret in this population with false-negative results (owing to immunosuppressive therapy), false-positive results (from receipt of blood products including immunoglobulin), or changes in titers as the result of immune dysregulation. PCR detection of virus in blood or plasma is quite sensitive but can lack specificity. Imaging, such as computed tomography scan, magnetic resonance imaging, or metabolic imaging (e.g., positron emission tomography scan), is sensitive in detection of PTLD and is useful for determining extent of disease, but specificity is poor, limiting diagnostic value. The most reliable method of diagnosis of EBV disease is tissue biopsy, and this should be done whenever it is safe to perform. When biopsy is not safe to perform, a presumed diagnosis can sometimes be made based on rising EBV viral loads and characteristic findings on imaging. An algorithm highlighting the approach to the diagnosis of EBV associated PTLD is shown in Fig. 18.1.

Classification of PTLD is difficult, as it refers to a heterogeneous group of lymphoproliferative diseases. The most widely used classification system is the World Health Organization classification, which is

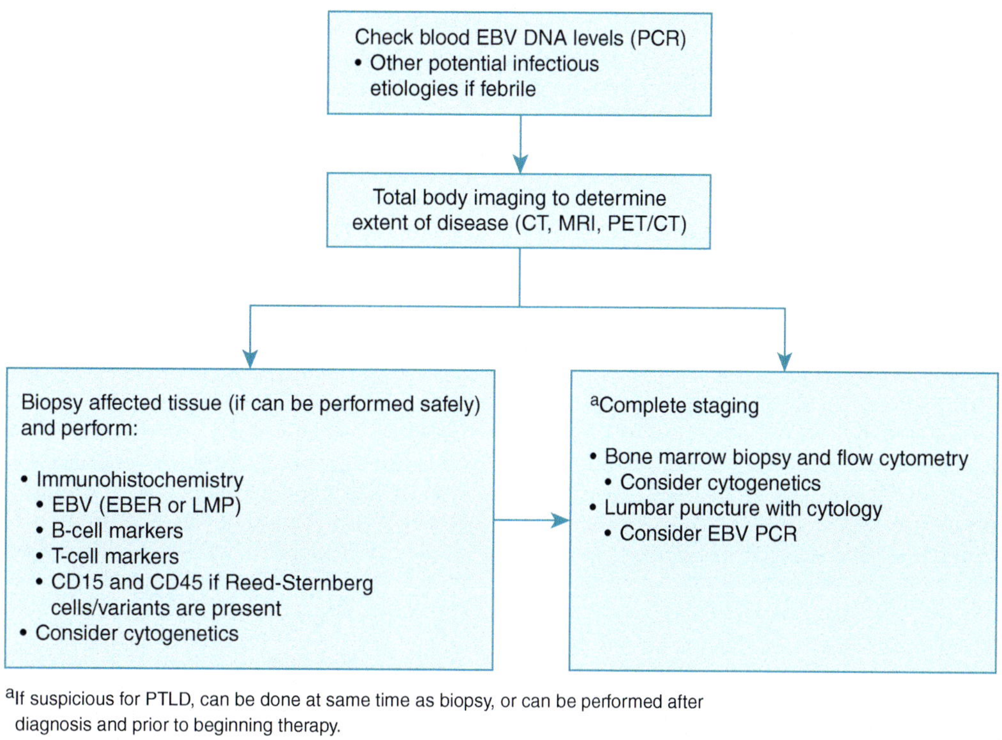

Fig. 18.1 Algorithm for Epstein-Barr virus disease diagnosis. *CT*, computerized tomography; *EBER*, EBV early RNA; *EBV*, Epstein Barr virus; *LMP*, latent membrane protein; *MRI*, magnetic resonate imaging; *PCR*, polymerase chain reaction; *PET*, positron emission tomography; *PTLD*, posttransplant lymphoproliferative disorders.

TABLE 18.2 Modified WHO Classification of EBV-Associated Lymphoproliferations in Immunodeficiency

Classification	Histologic Characteristics	EBV	Clonality	Comments
B-cell hyperplasia • Follicular • IM-like • Plasmacytic	Nondestructive	Rarely EBV-negative	Polyclonal; occasionally small clones can be found	IM-like; can mimic cHL
Polymorphic PTLD or B-LPD	Destructive	Usually EBV-positive	Polyclonal or monoclonal	Can mimic cHL
Monomorphic PTLD or LPD • B-cell lymphoma • Diffuse large B-cell • Marginal zone B-cell • Burkitt • T/NK cell lymphoma • cHL	Destructive	Usually EBV-positive (B-, T/NK, cHL)	Monoclonal Rarely polyclonal Chromosomal aberrations may be detected	

B-LPD, B-cell lymphoproliferative disorder; *cHL*, classical Hodgkin lymphoma; *EBV*, Epstein-Barr virus; *IM*, infectious mononucleosis; *LPD*, lymphoproliferative disorder; *PTLD*, posttransplant lymphoproliferative disorder; *T/NK*, T-cell/natural killer cell.

Data from Swerdlow H, Campo E, Pileri SA, et al. The 2016 revision of the World Health Organization classification of lymphoid neoplasms. *Blood.* 2016;127:2375-2390; Natkunam Y, Gratzinger D, Chadburn A, et al. Immunodeficiency-assciated lymphoproliferative disorders: time for reappraisal? *Blood.* 2018;132:1871-1878.

based on histology; the latest revision was in 2016 (Table 18.2).[30] This classification has also been applied to EBV lymphoproliferations associated with other immunodeficiency states (HIV infection, primary immunodeficiencies, and non–transplant therapy-related immunodeficiencies [e.g., rheumatologic diseases]).[31] The 2016 classification includes an expansion of the "early lesions" category, defined as lesions that, despite cellular proliferation retain their normal histologic architecture. Such lesions now include plasmacytic hyperplasia PTLD, infectious mononucleosis PTLD, and florid follicular hyperplasia PTLD. These are rarely monoclonal but often EBV positive, usually determined by immunohistochemical staining for EBV early ribonucleic acids (Epstein-Barr virus–encoded small RNA [EBER]) or latent antigen membrane expression, although plasmacytic hyperplasia can be EBV negative. Next is polymorphic PTLD, defined by disruption of normal architecture, but containing a heterogeneous admixture of cells. Polymorphic PTLD is often monoclonal and EBV positive. Monomorphic PTLD is defined as PTLD that is histologically identical to NHL—that is, diffuse large B-cell lymphoma (DLBCL), BL, plasma cell PTLD (myeloma-like or plasmacytoma-like), or mature NK/T-cell lymphoma. Monomorphic PTLD is almost always monoclonal. Both B-cell and T-cell PTLD are often EBV positive, but plasma cell PTLD is usually EBV negative. Finally, there is classical Hodgkin lymphoma (cHL)-like PTLD. This has the same immunophenotype as cHL (i.e., $CD45^-$, $CD15^+$ Reed-Sternberg cells or variants). Some polymorphic PTLD can have Reed-Sternberg–like cells, but the immunophenotype is $CD45^+$ and $CD15^-$ and should be verified before making the diagnosis of cHL-like PTLD.

This classification does present some challenges. Sampling bias can lead to false-negative results, and as opposed to most cancers, a biopsy from a single lesion can have a mix of histologies and there can be a discordance in histology between different lesions in the same patient.[32] Also, for disease primarily affecting non-nodal tissue, the criteria of disruption of normal nodal architecture can be problematic. This leads to confusion about classification of EBV disease (e.g., EBV enteritis or pneumonitis) versus PTLD. The clinical importance of this classification has also been questioned, particularly outside the setting of SOT. In general, early lesions and polymorphic PTLD tend to respond to less aggressive therapy (i.e., reduction of immunosuppression),[33] but it has been a challenge to correlate histology with outcome.[32]

THERAPY FOR POSTTRANSPLANT LYMPHOPROLIFERATIVE DISORDERS

An approach to the treatment of EBV disease including PTLD in SOT and HSCT recipients is shown in Figs. 18.2 and 18.3. Treatment strategies for PTLD often require tailoring to the individual patient taking into consideration multiple factors, including disease presentation, pathology, patient comorbidities and performance, risk of organ rejection or GVHD, organ graft function, and immunosuppressive regimen. Clinical decision making is optimized with multidisciplinary team input (e.g., pathology, oncology, transplant speciality, and infectious disease). Also, there remains a challenge in interpreting results in the literature because of (1) mixture of SOT and HSCT recipients in studies, (2) heterogeneous populations (e.g., age of patients, allograft types, histologies, and EBV status of disease), and (3) lack of large randomized trials. Often, the best evidence is from smaller, prospective phase II trials, with inherent selection bias, or from larger retrospective registry data with less control of data quality and completeness. It has been equally challenging to determine prognostic or predictive factors for all the aforementioned reasons. These issues need to be kept in mind when assessing treatment strategies for individual patients. However, there appears to be some consensus that EBV-negative, fulminant disease, late onset, and CNS disease are poor prognostic factors.[33-38] Although there is no universally accepted standard treatment for PTLD, both a risk-adapted and response-adapted approach are increasingly being used.

PTLD Treatment in Solid Organ Transplant Recipients

Reduction of Immunosuppression. The initial approach to managing patients with PTLD after SOT is still reduction of immunosuppression (RI), whenever the graft function allows. The goal with this approach is to restore sufficient EBV-reactive CTL function to control the proliferative process. One challenge is that there is no standard

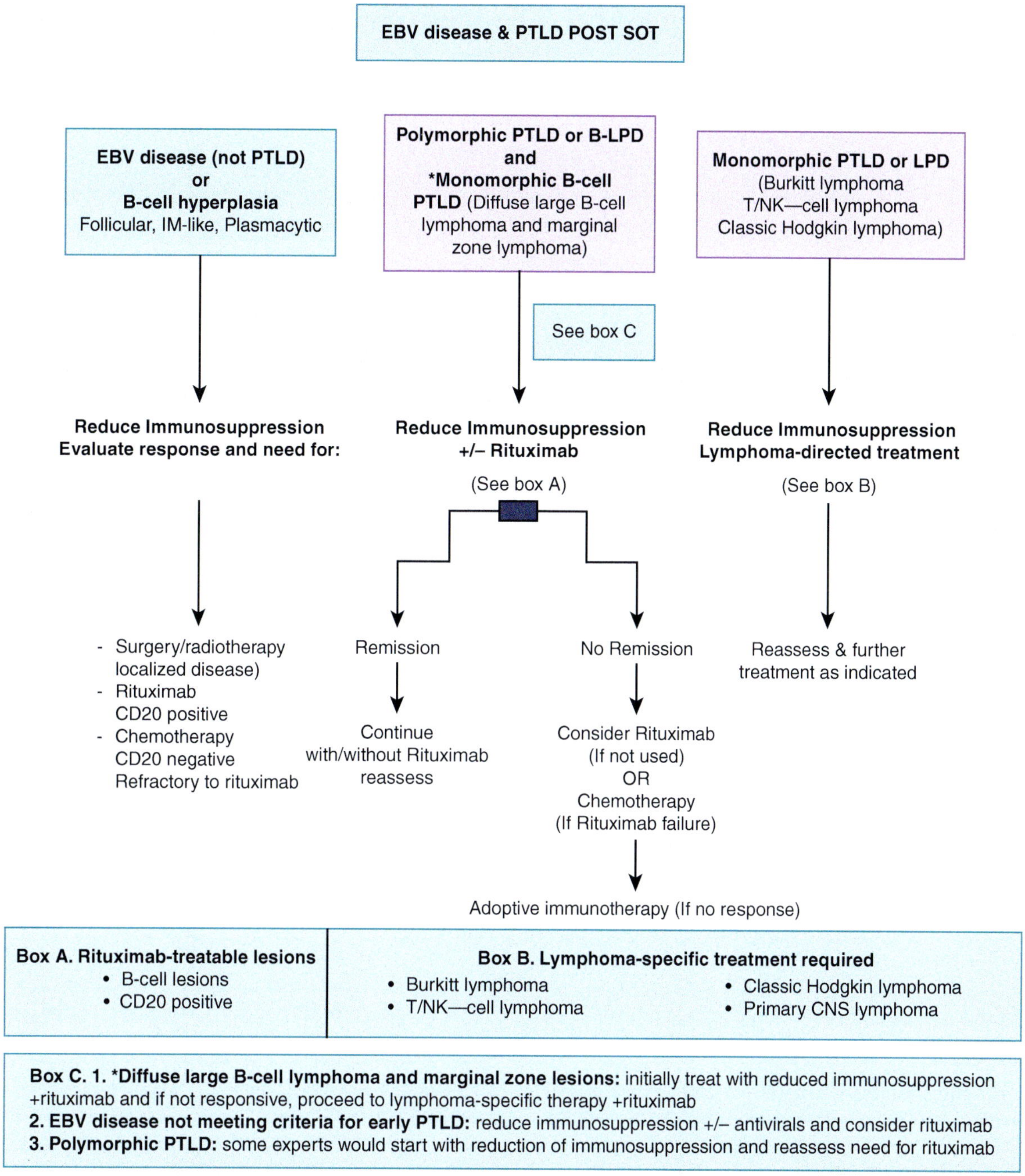

Fig. 18.2 Algorithm for Epstein-Barr virus disease and posttransplant lymphoproliferative disorders in solid organ transplant treatment. *B-LPD*, B-lymphocyte lymphoproliferative disorder; *CNS*, central nervous system; *EBV*, Epstein-Barr virus; *IM*, infectious mononucleosis; *LPD*, lymphoproliferative disorder; *PTLD*, posttransplant lymphoproliferative disorder; *SOT*, solid organ transplant; *T/NK*, T-cell/natural killer cell.

definition of RI—that is, how much and which agents to reduce or discontinue—and these decisions must take into account the type of allograft, time from transplant, and previous history of rejection. Generally, the recommendation is to first reduce immunosuppression by 25% to 50%. Early lesions, polymorphic disease, and patients with PTLD diagnosed early after transplantation appear to respond more often to RI; however, success with monomorphic PTLD has been described.[33,34] Reported response rates for RI vary greatly, ranging from 20% to 89%.[33,34] Switching to a different class of immunosuppression (e.g., mammalian target of rapamycin inhibitors) has been suggested to be beneficial but more studies are required to determine if this is effective.

Local Disease Control. Complete resection of a solitary lesion may be curative but is usually combined with RI.[3] PTLD is usually radiation sensitive, but this is usually reserved for disease that requires rapid local responses (e.g., airway compression) and in inoperable, local disease (e.g., CNS PTLD.

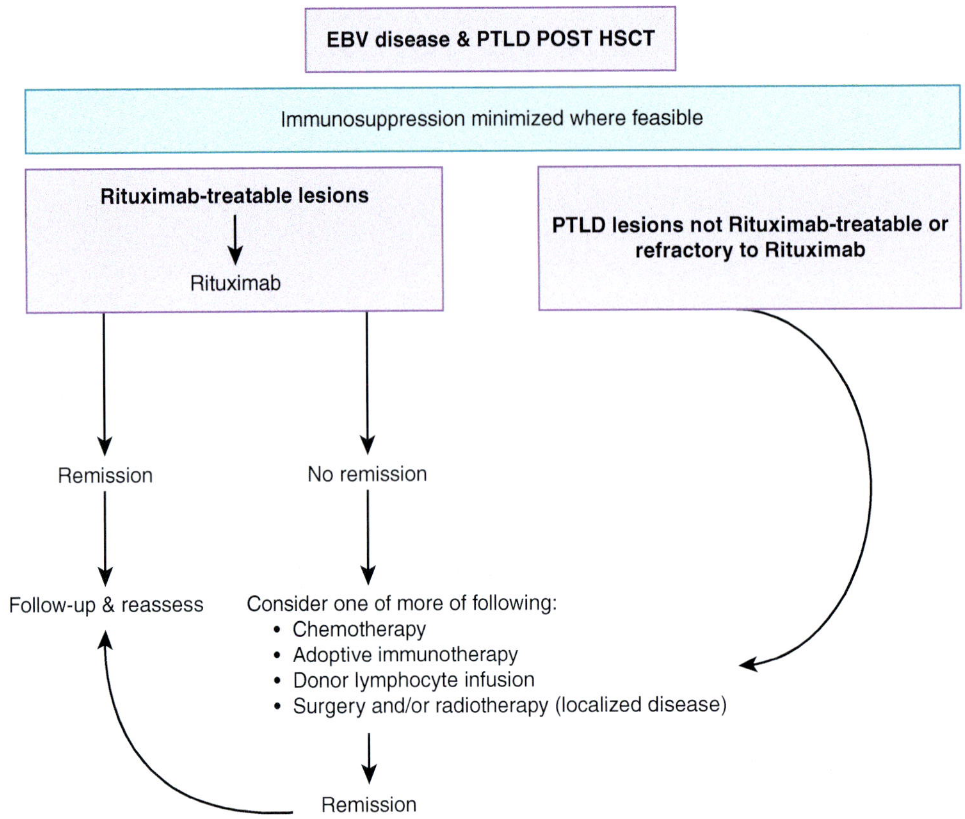

Fig. 18.3 Algorithm for Epstein-Barr virus disease and posttransplant lymphoproliferative disorders in hematopoietic stem cell transplantation treatment. *EBV*, Epstein-Barr virus; *HSCT*, hematopoietic stem cell transplantation; *PTLD*, posttransplant lymphoproliferative disorder.

Systemic Therapy

Chemotherapy. Historically, conventional lymphoma treatment protocols to treat PTLD have resulted in poor outcome because of high treatment-related toxicity, such as infections and multiorgan failure, resulting in high mortality rates. Therefore low dose-chemotherapy regimens were studied with the hypothesis that these regimens would be effective by simultaneously controlling the lymphoproliferative process, preventing allograft rejection, and minimizing treatment-related mortality. A multicenter, phase II study using-low dose cyclophosphamide and prednisone every 3 weeks for 6 cycles in PTLD patients with failed RI achieved an overall survival (OS) rate of 75%.[36]

Anti-CD20 monoclonal antibody. Because the majority of PTLDs express CD20, rituximab is an attractive option as it is less toxic than chemotherapy. Using rituximab (usually weekly for 6 doses) OS has been 60% to 75% in pediatric SOT recipients with PTLD.[39,40] In a phase II study, rituximab was added to the low-dose chemotherapy regimen and an 85% OS was achieved with fewer relapses than with chemotherapy alone.[32] An interesting observation was that 75% of patients with radiographic-evidence of persistent disease at completion of therapy achieved a complete remission at 1 year without any further therapy, suggesting a delayed immunologic effect of the rituximab and/or CTL recovery. Building on these results, a phase II study was conducted using the response to three doses of rituximab to stratify patients. Good responders (two-thirds of patients) received another three doses of rituximab, whereas poor responders received low-dose chemotherapy and a 85% OS was still achieved for the entre cohort, saving two-thirds of children from exposure to chemotherapy.[41] There are no studies directly comparing low-dose chemotherapy versus rituximab, the anti-CD20 monoclonal antibody currently used in clinical practice.

Adoptive immunotherapy. EBV cytotoxic T-cell therapy (EBV-CTL) targets cells expressing EBV viral antigens, usually latent membrane proteins, and are produced in vitro. EBV-CTL therapy for PTLD in SOT recipients is more problematic than in HSCT. Although they have been shown to be safe, the prolonged duration of immunosuppressive drugs limit the ability of EBV-CTLs to expand and persist in vivo.[42,43] To date, the cost and availability of EBV-CTLs have limited the use as first-line treatment, although this may be changing as third-party donor pools become more available. There is an ongoing multicenter study of the feasibility of using third-party EBV-CTLs for patients with incomplete response to 3 cycles of rituximab.

PTLD of "True" Lymphoma

Although monomorphic PTLDs appear like NHLs, most will respond to less aggressive therapy. However, there are situations when the general consensus is to treat with more conventional lymphoma front-line therapy. Burkitt histology is one such case, especially if evidence of a *c-MYC* translocation is present. Another situation is monomorphic disease with any cytogenetic abnormality found, suggesting a true malignant clonal transformation has occurred requiring more aggressive therapy. These patients tend to have a worse prognosis, as one must balance enough therapy to achieve control versus treatment-related toxicity/mortality. Another case is Hodgkin-like PTLD. As stated previously, some polymorphic PTLDs can closely resemble Hodgkin lymphoma, so classic immunohistochemical confirmation of Hodgkin lymphoma is required. As opposed to PTLD presenting as true NHL, Hodgkin-PTLD has a more favorable outcome with a conventional regimen to treat Hodgkin lymphoma.[44]

PTLD Therapy in HSCT

For HSCT recipients in whom PTLD develops, including those despite the use of preventive strategies, rituximab is recommended first-line therapy for biopsy-proven PTLD. However, adoptive T-cell therapy with EBV-specific T-cell has also been effective where available.[20] Unmanipulated lymphocyte infusions are more readily available than EBV-CTL (viral-specific T-cell) in many centers, and this can lead to disease regression; however, it was also associated with significant GVHD caused by alloreactive T cells.[20] Studies have shown complete remission rates between 68% and 85% with persistence of the EBV-CTLs in vivo up to 10 years, and minimal toxicity, including no significant GVHD.[20] The drawback of this approach is the time required to wait while donor-specific CTLs are generated, which is not always an option in this patient population. Thus "off-the-shelf" third-party EBV-CTLs closely matched by HLAs are being manufactured and studied because these could be readily available for patients. There are a few small, single-center reports describing efficacy in HSCT recipients. Better response rates are noted with closer HLA matches, and no immediate or delayed toxicity using third party EBV-CTLs has been described.[42]

Exceptional Clinical Situations

CNS-PTLD after SOT or HSCT is rare. Most pediatric prospective studies have excluded patients with CNS involvement. PTLD with CNS involvement has been described as having a very poor prognosis, although localized CNS PTLD may have a better prognosis compared with multifocal disease.[37] Although tissue biopsy is recommended for diagnosis, the EBV-DNA load in the CSF may be sufficient for diagnosis and monitoring disease response.[45] Anecdotes of RI alone resulting in complete remissions exist, but typically other modalities are required. Retrospective studies have described radiation, systemic chemotherapy, most often high-dose methotrexate and/or intrathecal chemotherapy, and all have been reported to be successful in some patients.[20,37] The concentration of rituximab achieved in the cerebral spinal fluid is only a fraction of the intravenous concentration, but complete responses have been reported with intravenous rituximab, although RI has also been used. There are also some anecdotal reports of patients achieving response with intrathecal rituximab, often combined with systemic chemotherapy. EBV-CTLs have also been shown to be efficacious and safe in a few patients with CNS PTLD.

Other Treatment Modalities

The antiviral agents acyclovir and ganciclovir are sometimes used with or without the use of immunoglobulin. The rationale for antiviral use is that although latent viral infection predominates in PTLD lesions, lytic virus gene and protein expression are also seen in some cases. This notwithstanding, there is no evidence to support the use of antiviral agents (with or without immunoglobulin) in the absence of interventions such as decreasing immunosuppression or anti-CD20 therapy. Future research might examine the role of agents that induce the lytic cycle of EBV in combination with antiviral agents. For example, arginine butyrate, a histone deacetylase inhibitor, induces the lytic cycle of EBV, making EBV-infected cells sensitive to ganciclovir. In addition, the proteosome inhibitor bortezomib induces lytic virus replication in EBV-infected cells and is being evaluated in clinic trials of γ-herpesvirus–associated malignancies, including PTLD.[46]

Historically positive responses have been reported in small numbers of PTLD patients using interferon-alfa and anti–interleukin 6 therapy; however, these agents are no longer commonly used in the treatment of PTLD. The potential for disease response to programmed death ligand 1 blockade using immune checkpoint inhibitors (pembrolizumab, nivolumab) has been proposed in situations when there is refractory disease positive for these markers. However, there is a concern regarding precipitating rejection and/or exacerbating autoimmune diseases.

Prognostic Indicators of Treatment Outcomes

In recent years, the outcomes for patients with $CD20^+$ PTLDs have improved as evidenced by recent adult[13-14,47] and pediatric phase II clinical trials.[35] A clear difference in outcomes has not been demonstrated among EBV-negative compared with EBV-positive PTLDs.[47,48] Outcomes are generally poorer for patients with T-cell PTLD and primary CNS lymphoma compared with other PTLD patients. Outcomes might also be influenced by the sites of initial PTLD, involvement with better outcomes documented for patients with tonsillar/adenoidal PTLD compared with other sites of involvement.[49]

Infection Prevention and Anticipatory Guidance

Preventing EBV primary infection and/or boosting EBV immunity to prevent EBV disease using active immunization would be particularly useful in SOT, but no vaccine is currently available. Vaccine development is still in progress and has largely targeted the EBV glycoprotein 350, which contains major neutralizing epitopes.

The use of leukoreduced blood products may reduce the risk of transfusion-transmitted EBV in a manner similar to cytomegalovirus in individuals who are EBV D^-/R^-. In community settings, seronegative transplant patients are at risk of acquiring primary EBV through contact with oropharyngeal secretions. This is notable among teenage patients, who represent a group known to be at increased risk of primary EBV infection, which among immunocompetent patients would be infectious mononucleosis or kissing disease.

In the post-transplant setting, the identification of patients who are also at risk of primary EBV infection or those receiving antithymocyte globulin therapy would identify a vulnerable subgroup of recipients who are at increased risk of PTLD. This would allow for such patients to be monitored closely for clinical and laboratory evidence of PTLD.

19

Herpes Simplex and Varicella-Zoster Viruses

William J. Muller, MD, PhD and Betsy C. Herold, MD

Herpes simplex virus (HSV) types 1 and 2 (HSV-1 and -2) and varicella-zoster virus (VZV) comprise the human α-herpesviruses, a subfamily of enveloped, double-stranded DNA viruses defined in part by the ability to be transmitted and replicate in mucoepithelial surfaces and to establish latent infection in sensory ganglia of the nervous system. Infection with HSV is common, with serologic evidence of HSV-1 infection in about 48% and HSV-2 infection in about 12% of 14- to 49-year-old people living in the United States.[1] The incidence of infection with either serotype has declined in the United States in the past decade. However, globally the prevalence is quite high with an estimated 3.7 billion people infected with HSV-1 and 0.4 billion with HSV-2.[2] VZV causes the formerly common childhood disease known as chickenpox. A live-attenuated vaccine protecting against VZV disease has been available in the United States since 1995, with a Centers for Disease Control and Prevention recommendation for 2 doses since 2006.[3] This has led to dramatic decreases in VZV cases.[3]

Both HSV and VZV uniformly establish latency in neuronal cells and periodically reactivate to cause cutaneous, or less commonly, neurologic or disseminated disease. Clinically silent HSV reactivation is far more common than previously recognized and the long-term consequences of this are not yet fully understood.[4] Clinical recurrences typical manifest as painful eruptions of grouped vesicles. These are generally self-limited but may be associated with variable levels of viral DNA detected in the blood using quantitative polymerase chain reaction (PCR) assays (referred to as DNAemia).[5] VZV reactivation, which occurs less frequently than HSV reactivation, presents clinically as zoster or shingles and manifests as a painful, dermatomal vesicular rash. Zoster is most common in adults older than 60 years or in immunocompromised patients, including transplant recipients. Zoster-associated pain can persist well beyond the duration of the rash and may occur in the absence of rash. Transmission of VZV is less common with zoster than with primary varicella, reflecting lower viral loads, but may contribute to an increasing proportion of varicella cases in the postvaccine era.[6] Both wild-type and the vaccine strain (vOka) of virus may reactivate, although reactivation occurs far more frequently with wild-type viral strains. Moreover, a new subunit protein vaccine (Shingrix, GlaxoSmithKline) provided 97% protection against zoster and was approved by the U.S. Food and Drug Administration at the end of 2017 for adults older than 50 years.[7] Thus the overall incidence of shingles, which has already decreased with the implementation of the live vOka vaccine for primary varicella and zoster, will undoubtedly continue to decline with the introduction of this new and highly effective subunit protein zoster vaccine.

HERPES SIMPLEX VIRUS IN TRANSPLANT AND ONCOLOGY

Epidemiology and Risk Factors

There are limited data on the epidemiology of HSV infection in pediatric oncology or transplant patients. In the general population, the most recent large-scale U.S studies indicate a prevalence of approximately 27% for HSV-1 and less than 1% for HSV-2 among 14- to 19-year-olds.[1] Rates of HSV-1 infection are likely higher in developing countries.[2] HSV clinical disease is more common in stem cell transplant (SCT) patients than in cancer and solid organ transplant (SOT) patients, reflecting the greater net state of immunosuppression.[8] HSV disease may develop in up to 80% of HSV-seropositive SCT patients without prophylactic antiviral treatment.[8] In contrast to other herpesviruses such as CMV or Epstein-Barr virus, in which the donor is often the source of infection, HSV disease almost always reflects reactivation of latent virus in the recipient and/or primary community-acquired infection. Donor-derived HSV infection is rare[9] because the virus, which is latent in sensory neuronal cells, is rarely transferred, except in unusual instances in which a donor has significant DNAemia and/or disseminated HSV disease. Reactivation of latent HSV may occur in HSV-seropositive SOT recipients who are not receiving antivirals for CMV prophylaxis.[10]

Specific triggers for HSV reactivation independent of immune status include stress, ultraviolet light exposure, and disruption of the epithelial barrier. A quantitative or functional reduction in cellular, humoral, or innate (natural killer cells) immune responses also increases the risk of HSV reactivation.[11] Notably, neutropenia alone has not been recognized as a trigger.

Clinical Manifestations

HSV manifests clinically as oropharyngeal, nasolabial, ocular, esophageal, pulmonary, genital, and less commonly, meningoencephalitis or disseminated disease. Oncology patients and transplant recipients are at risk for more severe and prolonged symptoms with each of these diseases and are at greater risk for viral dissemination compared with immunocompetent hosts.[10] The duration and severity of disease and likelihood of clinical recurrences are affected by the net state of immunosuppression.[10,12]

The most common clinical syndrome associated with primary or recurrent HSV is gingivostomatitis.[10,13] HSV is readily detected in oral secretions during episodes of stomatitis, but it may also be detected in absence of symptoms, complicating the interpretation of causality.[12] An important, but relatively uncommon, complication of herpes stomatitis is Stevens-Johnson syndrome.[14] Local dissemination of primary oral

HSV or reactivation of virus from the trigeminal ganglia may lead to ocular disease, including keratitis or uveitis, with potentially devastating outcomes.[10]

HSV-associated esophagitis may occur in the setting of mucositis, a common sequela of chemotherapy, radiation therapy, and/or graft-versus-host disease (GVHD). Nasogastric tubes may also disrupt the epithelial barrier and promote viral spread to the esophagus. Esophagitis may be polymicrobial with HSV, CMV and *Candida* species being detected. Early endoscopic findings include vesicles, which may progress to diffuse mucosal necrosis.[12]

Pulmonary infection has been recognized more frequently in the past decade, reflecting the advent of molecular testing. In a study of 45 adult SOT patients with pneumonia, 19 (42.2%) had positive results for HSV-1 PCR in bronchoalveolar lavage (BAL) samples and 11 (24.4%) of these were diagnosed with HSV-1 pneumonia; a definitive case was defined as one in which HSV was the only pathogen identified in the BAL and consistent pathology was present. The HSV viral loads in the cases ranged between 10^3 and 10^7 copies/mL.[15] CT findings of HSV-1 pneumonia are relatively nonspecific and may include bilateral ground-glass attenuation or airspace consolidation.

Disseminated disease, which is uncommon outside the neonatal period, may occur in transplant patients. Typical sites of dissemination include the liver, lungs, adrenal glands, or central nervous system and may manifest as pneumonitis, hepatitis, or meningoencephalitis.[8] Primary HSV has also been identified as a rare trigger for hemophagocytic lymphohistiocytosis in immunocompromised hosts, including oncology patients.

Diagnosis

Detection of HSV-specific antibodies by serology identifies whether a patient is infected and at risk for viral reactivation. However, seropositivity does not preclude superinfection with a related viral strain or different serotype. Screening for HSV serotype-specific immunoglobulin (Ig) G is universally recommended for HSCT but is performed more selectively for oncology patients or as part of the SOT pretransplant evaluation. There is no role for IgM testing as it may be elevated in response to viral reactivation and thus does not accurately identify primary infection. The persistence of maternal antibodies in younger infants can complicate interpretation of serologic test results.

Detection of HSV DNA by PCR has emerged as the diagnostic test of choice for disease and has replaced viral culture or antigen detection methods at most centers. However, the detection of HSV DNA in secretions does not differentiate shedding from disease and must be interpreted carefully. This is particularly important when assessing for HSV pneumonia with oropharyngeal swabs or BAL. Higher viral load in the setting of a compatible clinical presentation supports causality, but the gold standard for invasive disease requires tissue for pathology.

More recently, commercially available assays to detect HSV DNA in the blood (DNAemia) have been recommended for the diagnosis of neonatal HSV disease.[16] The frequency and clinical significance of DNAemia in other clinical settings, including primary or recurrent disease or asymptomatic viral reactivation in either immunocompetent or immunosuppressed hosts, has not been defined. Several studies explored the utility of routine screening for HSV DNA in the blood in SCT patients with variable results. In one study of adult allogeneic SCT recipients who were receiving acyclovir prophylaxis, HSV DNA was detected in weekly obtained blood samples during the first 100 days after transplant in more than 20% of patients, even in the absence of symptomatic disease.[17] However, a retrospective study of more than 500 pediatric SCT patients found that routine PCR screening for HSV or VZV DNA in the blood rarely detected either virus.[18] The authors concluded that targeted testing in patients with mucocutaneous lesions, neurologic symptoms, unexplained fever, or elevated liver enzyme levels may be more appropriate than routine surveillance testing, but no controlled studies have evaluated whether DNAemia warrants antiviral therapy.

Culture-based and immunofluorescent methods of detecting HSV may still have a role for diagnosis of disease in certain settings. Many clinical laboratories continue to use direct detection of HSV with fluorescent antibodies and microscopic analysis to diagnose skin infections, though the availability of PCR-based analyses of samples from skin lesions is increasing. HSV is readily recovered in cell culture from many sites except for cerebrospinal fluid and blood,[13] although culture may take up to 5 days for the virus to grow.

Viral culture, rather than PCR diagnostics, is also important for antiviral resistance testing. Clinically significant infections with acyclovir-resistant HSV strains are more commonly described in immunocompromised patients.[19] Numerous mutations in the thymidine kinase (*TK*) gene or, less commonly, DNA polymerase, are associated with resistance to acyclovir, rendering it difficult to diagnose resistance using sequencing-based methods. Phenotypic resistance testing using a culture-based plaque-reduction assay is the current gold-standard[19] but can take several weeks to obtain a result. A high index of suspicion for development of resistance and empiric changes in antivirals is clinically recommended while resistance test results are pending.

Suppressive Therapy and Treatment

Suppressive Therapy. Suppressive therapy, designed to limit replication of reactivating virus, with the nucleoside analog acyclovir or its prodrug, valacyclovir, is recommended by many experts for select transplant and oncology patients who are not receiving ganciclovir or valganciclovir for CMV prophylaxis and are at risk for severe HSV disease (Table 19.1).[20] HSV phosphorylates acyclovir or ganciclovir to the monophosphate, which is further phosphorylated by host cellular kinases to generate acyclovir or ganciclovir triphosphate. The latter are incorporated into replicating viral DNA, leading to premature chain termination. Notably, CMV kinases do not efficiently phosphorylate acyclovir; thus acyclovir is relatively specific for HSV and VZV.[20]

Rates of HSV disease in oncology patients may be reduced with suppressive therapy during periods of intense chemotherapy[13]; however, there have been surprisingly few randomized clinical trials to evaluate the efficacy of suppressive therapy in this population. In a study conducted in the early 1980s, 29 HSV-seropositive adults with acute leukemia receiving chemotherapy participated in a randomized, double-blind, placebo-controlled trial of acyclovir starting 4 days after their initial chemotherapy.[21] Culture-positive HSV disease developed in 11 of 15 patients who received placebo compared with none of the 14 patients who received acyclovir ($P < .001$). Based on these data, suppressive therapy is often recommended, particularly among patients with higher-than-usual risks, including treatment with alemtuzumab (Campath), a monoclonal antibody that binds CD52 on the surface of mature lymphocytes, or other therapies associated with significant suppression of T-cell immunity.[22] B-cell suppression alone with therapies such as rituximab has not been associated with an increased risk of HSV.[22] Some guidelines also support the use of acyclovir in patients at risk for mucositis, although there are limited supporting data.[13]

The risk of HSV disease after SCT is greater than in patients with cancer, leading to universal recommendations for serologic screening and suppressive therapy in seropositive SCT recipients from the start of conditioning through at least neutrophil engraftment and/or until the $CD4^+$ T-cell count is more than 200 cells/μL.[13,23] Acyclovir or valacyclovir is also considered during treatment for GVHD, but there are more limited data to support these recommendations. The recommended

TABLE 19.1 **Antiviral Prophylaxis Regimens for Herpes Simplex in Patients at Risk of Severe Disease[a]**

Population	Drug	Dose[b]	Duration	References
Oncology Patients				
HSV-seronegative		No prophylaxis recommended		Styczynski et al.[13]
HSV-seropositive	Acyclovir[c]	250 mg/m^2 or 5 mg/kg IV q12 h *OR* Up to 200 mg PO tid to 800 mg PO bid	3-5 weeks after start of chemotherapy	Styczynski et al.[13]
	Valacyclovir	Up to 500 mg PO bid	3-5 weeks after start of chemotherapy	Styczynski et al.[13]
	Famciclovir	Up to 500 mg PO bid	3-5 weeks after start of chemotherapy	Styczynski et al.[13]
HSV-seropositive leukemia patients undergoing induction or reinduction treatment	Acyclovir	250 mg/m^2 IV q8 h	Up to 30 days after start of chemotherapy	Saral et al.,[21] Freifeld et al.[23]
Stem Cell Transplantation Patients				
HSV-seropositive recipient	Acyclovir[c]	750 mg/m^2 IV daily	At least until engraftment, longer if ongoing GVHD treatment	Styczynski et al.[13]
	Valacyclovir	Up to 500 mg PO bid		Styczynski et al.[13]
	Famciclovir	Up to 500 mg PO bid		Styczynski et al.[13]
HSV-seropositive, allogenic or autologous SCT recipient	Acyclovir	250 mg/m^2 IV q8 h	D–3 through D+18	Freifeld et al.[23]
Solid Organ Transplantation Patients				
HSV-seropositive recipient not receiving CMV antiviral prophylaxis	Acyclovir[c]	30-80 mg/kg PO divided tid *OR* 5 mg/kg IV q8	At least to D+30, longer if clinical recurrences or if immunosuppression escalated for treating rejection	Wilck et al.,[10] *Red Book*[16]
	Valacyclovir	15-30 mg/kg PO tid		Wilck et al.[10]

[a]Transplant patients not receiving CMV antiviral prophylaxis and highly suppressed oncology patients.
[b]Dose should be decreased in patients with renal impairment.
[c]Oral acyclovir has lower bioavailability than valacyclovir; valacyclovir is generally preferred if oral drug is given.
bid, twice a day; *CMV,* cytomegalovirus; *D,* day; *GVHD,* graft-versus-host disease; *h,* hours; *HSV,* herpes simplex virus; *IV,* intravenous; *PO,* oral; *q,* every; *tid,* three times a day.

duration of antiviral treatment in SCT patients depends on the duration and intensity of immunosuppression. There is also some controversy regarding dosing. Lower doses may be effective and are less likely to cause or exacerbate neutropenia or anemia, although concerns about lower acyclovir dosing contributing to resistance have been raised.[24] The renal toxicity attributed to intravenous (IV) acyclovir results from crystallization of drug in the kidneys and can be prevented by IV hydration and slower infusion rates.

Concerns about development of acyclovir resistance during suppressive therapy have not been supported by the limited number of randomized controlled clinical studies. For example, a retrospective study comparing 30 days versus 1 year or longer of antiviral suppressive therapy found that prolonged antiviral therapy was associated with lower rates of viral resistance and significantly decreased rates of HSV disease.[24] As noted earlier, most resistance maps to the gene for thymidine kinase, the viral protein responsible for acyclovir phosphorylation, but mutations in viral DNA polymerase have also been described.

HSV is generally less of a concern in SOT than SCT, and experts vary on recommendations for routine donor or recipient screening and on whether seropositive recipients should receive suppressive therapy. One exception is the rare scenario when a donor has documented HSV at the time organs are harvested. There are few studies on acyclovir suppressive therapy in SOT recipients. One recent Swiss study of 2781 SOT recipients assessed the impact of CMV prophylaxis on rates of HSV or VZV infections. Overall, 1264 (45%) patients received antiviral prophylaxis, primarily ganciclovir or valganciclovir. The incidence of HSV 1 year after transplant was 3.0% (95% confidence 2.2 to 4) in patients receiving antiviral prophylaxis versus 9.8% (95% confidence interval 8.4 to 11.4), in patients without prophylaxis.[25]

Treatment. IV acyclovir or oral (PO) valacyclovir are the primary drugs for treatment of HSV disease and the choice of IV versus PO depends largely on severity of disease and the ability to tolerate oral therapy. PO acyclovir has relatively poor bioavailability, requiring more frequent dosing, and is less commonly recommended (Table 19.2). Valacyclovir, which is rapidly absorbed, is converted to acyclovir by a hepatic hydrolase. Approximately 55% of an orally administered dose of valacyclovir is available as acyclovir. Pharmacokinetics may be affected by liver disease. Maintaining a high suspicion for HSV disease in the correct clinical context is important, as earlier initiation of treatment can improve outcomes.[26] As with CMV and Epstein-Barr virus, a reduction in immune suppression, if feasible, is also recommended as part of HSV treatment.[10] Steroids have been administered to patients with HSV encephalitis or severe corneal disease as an adjunctive antiinflammatory therapy, but randomized clinical trials to establish benefit have not been completed.

Resistant HSV may be more common in pediatrics than in adults, with one study reporting frequencies as high as 14 to 30% in allogeneic bone marrow transplant recipients.[27] As noted above, most resistance maps to

TABLE 19.2 Treatment of Herpes Simplex Virus Disease in Oncology and Transplant Patients

Population	Drug	Dose[a]	Duration	References
Oncology or SCT Patients				
Severe mucocutaneous or visceral disease	Acyclovir	250 mg/m^2 or 5 mg/kg IV q8h		Styczynski et al.[13]
Pneumonia, meningitis, or encephalitis	Acyclovir	500 mg/m^2 or 10 mg/kg IV q8h	14-21 days	Styczynski et al.[13]
Milder disease	Acyclovir[b]	200-400 mg PO 5 times daily	10 days	Styczynski et al.[13]
	Valacyclovir	500 mg PO bid	10 days	Styczynski et al.[13]
	Famciclovir	500 mg PO bid	10 days	Styczynski et al.[13]
Acyclovir-resistant virus				
	Foscarnet	60 mg/kg IV q12h *OR* 40 mg/kg IV q8h	7-21 days or until complete healing	Styczynski et al.[13]
Acyclovir-resistant and foscarnet-resistant virus				
	Cidofovir	5 mg/kg IV once weekly for 2 weeks, then once every 2 weeks, combined with probenecid and IV hydration		Styczynski et al.[13]
Optional topical treatment for accessible cutaneous lesions	Trifluridine 5% ophthalmic solution	q8h		Styczynski et al.[13]
	Cidofovir gel 0.3 or 1%	Once daily		
Solid Organ Transplantation				
Disseminated, visceral, extensive mucocutaneous disease, or encephalitis/meningitis	Acyclovir	10-20 mg/kg IV q8h	14-21 days	Wilck et al.[10]
Milder mucocutaneous disease	Acyclovir	5-10 mg/kg IV q8h	5-7 days or until complete healing of the lesions (can transition to PO when improving)	Wilck et al.[10]
	Acyclovir[b]	80 mg/kg PO divided 3-5 times daily, up to 1000 mg/day	5-7 days or until complete healing of the lesions	Wilck et al.[10]
	Valacyclovir	20 mg/kg per dose PO twice daily, up to 1000 mg/dose		Wilck et al.[10]
	Famciclovir	500 mg PO bid (adult dose)		Wilck et al.[10]
Acyclovir-resistant virus	Same recommendations as for oncology and SCT patients			Wilck et al.[10]

[a]Dose should be decreased in patients with renal impairment.
[b]Oral acyclovir has lower bioavailability than valacyclovir; valacyclovir is generally preferred if oral drug is given.
bid, twice a day; *h,* hour; *IV,* intravenous, *PO,* oral; *q,* every.

the *TK* gene, resulting in cross-resistance to other drugs that require virally mediated phosphorylation, such as ganciclovir. Continuous infusion of high-dose acyclovir has been successful in some patients, but most infectious disease physicians recommend alternative drugs. First-line drugs for resistant HSV infection include foscarnet or cidofovir (see Table 19.2). Foscarnet, a pyrophosphate, acts by inhibiting viral DNA polymerase, but unlike the nucleoside antivirals used to treat HSV, does not require phosphorylation. It is available only in IV formulations and is nephrotoxic. Cidofovir is an acyclic nucleoside phosphonate that is converted to cidofovir diphosphate by cellular kinases, bypassing the requirement for viral TK. Cidofovir diphosphate competitively inhibits viral DNA polymerase, is also nephrotoxic and is routinely administered with probenecid and with IV hydration. The orally bioavailable prodrug brincidofovir may be less nephrotoxic and may be an alternative treatment for resistant HSV, but there are no controlled studies. A new class of anti-HSV drugs, helicase-primase inhibitors, is represented by pritelivir. Preclinical studies support efficacy for pritelivir, and a phase II clinical trial showed that the drug was more effective than valacyclovir in suppressing HSV genital recurrences.[28] However, the FDA put a hold on further clinical development because of skin and blood abnormalities shown in a macaque study.

Infection Prevention

Contact precautions (gown and gloves) are generally recommended for any inpatients, including immunocompromised patients, with severe mucocutaneous or disseminated HSV infection until lesions are dry and crusted.[16] Patients should be counseled to avoid close contact with individuals who have active lesions, and sexually active patients should be counseled to use latex condoms during sexual contact outside long-term monogamous relationships to reduce exposure to HSV and other sexually transmitted infections.

Household contacts of oncology and transplant patients should be instructed about the importance of careful hand hygiene before and after caring for their children. Those with recurrent HSV lesions should minimize contact with immunocompromised children until the lesions have crusted, and if the lesions are oral or perioral, they should not kiss or nuzzle the patient until lesions have cleared. Lesions on other skin sites should be covered.

Active or Passive Immunization

There have been substantial efforts to develop prophylactic or therapeutic vaccines to prevent primary or recurrent HSV, respectively, but clinical trial results have been uniformly disappointing. Most of these efforts were focused on subunit vaccines designed to elicit high-titer neutralizing antibodies that target the immunodominant viral envelope glycoprotein D. New approaches, including live single-cycle viral vaccines, have shown promise in more stringent animal models.[29] Any vaccines that progress to human trials are unlikely to be tested in oncology and transplant patients until substantial safety and efficacy data are available in immunocompetent individuals. Immunotherapy with anti-HSV specific antibodies may play a role in the future in treating patients with severe disease, but currently there are no commercially available specific products. Pooled IV immunoglobulin has been administered in select cases, but there are no controlled studies documenting utility.

VARICELLA-ZOSTER VIRUS IN TRANSPLANT AND ONCOLOGY

Epidemiology and Risk Factors

In the prevaccine era, both primary (chickenpox) and reactivating (shingles or zoster) disease from VZV were common in children with cancer and those undergoing hematopoietic stem cell transplantation.[30,31] Significant morbidity and mortality was documented among children receiving chemotherapy, with VZV dissemination leading to pneumonitis or hepatitis in severe cases.[30] Severity of disease in patients with acute lymphoblastic leukemia was associated with intensity of chemotherapy or recent steroid treatment.[32]

The morbidity and mortality associated with varicella in pediatric cancer patients drove the development of a live-attenuated varicella vaccine in Japan in 1974. Since the implementation of a vaccine program in the United States in 1995, there has been a significant decline in primary VZV disease in pediatric populations.[3] The overall effect of the vaccine on zoster incidence is more complex because exposure to primary chickenpox and/or zoster is presumed to play an important role in boosting immunologic memory. Thus there was a concern that the incidence of zoster might increase early in the postvaccine era in the absence of boosting from exposure to primary chickenpox in the community. This notion was supported by one study demonstrating an increased incidence of zoster among children in the years 2000 to 2006.[33] However, other studies have demonstrated a decrease in zoster rates in children,[34] and because the vaccine strain is less likely than wild-type virus to establish latency, it is projected that zoster will continue to decline as more of the population is immunized early in childhood. Moreover, as noted earlier, a new highly effective subunit protein vaccine (Shingrix), recently approved for adults to prevent zoster, should lead to an even greater reduction in incidence.

Currently, the overall incidence of zoster in both pediatric and adult SCT recipients remains at approximately 20% and continues to be associated with dissemination and persistent pain (postherpetic neuralgia).[35] Chronic GVHD is an additional risk factor for zoster after SCT.[13] Varicella-zoster after SOT is overall less common than among oncology and SCT patients, but rates remain significant, ranging in one study from approximately 5% in liver transplant recipients to 17% in heart transplant recipients.[36] Use of mycophenolate mofetil as part of the immunosuppressive regimen may confer increased risk for zoster disease.[36] It is thought that the increased rates of zoster among recipients of lung and/or heart transplants relative to other organs are related to the higher immunosuppression requirements in those patients.[26] Donor-derived infection is rare but has been described.

Clinical Manifestations

Primary varicella infection in immunocompetent pediatric patients is well described. After a 2- to 3-week incubation period, progressive pruritic skin lesions develop, beginning as flat erythematous macules, that subsequently evolve into papules, vesicles, and pustules before forming crusted scabs.[16] Rash often begins on the face and spreads inferiorly across the trunk and may spare the palms and soles. It is accompanied by fever, and mucosal lesions involving the mouth or conjunctivae are not uncommon. New lesions appear for approximately 1 to 7 days after the initial rash, with worse disease in children who acquire infection from household exposure or in older children.[37]

Varicella-zoster typically manifests as vesicular skin lesions grouped within one to three sensory dermatomes, which may be accompanied by localized pain and/or pruritis.[16] Other complications of zoster may include keratitis or other eye involvement, neurogenic bladder, ileus, and transverse myelitis.[37] Postherpetic neuralgia as a complication of zoster is less common in immunocompetent and immunocompromised children compared with adults.[38]

The clinical presentation of primary varicella and zoster in pediatric cancer patients and transplant recipients is similar to that described in the general pediatric population. However, severe disease with dissemination to liver and lungs and visceral dissemination in the absence of skin findings is more common in immunocompromised hosts.[13] Notably, atypical skin manifestations of primary or reactivating VZV such as the presence of hemorrhagic lesions may also be observed in immunocompromised populations, requiring a high index of suspicion in the appropriate clinical setting. Zoster may disseminate and mimic primary varicella in highly immunosuppressed patients.

Diagnosis

In healthy hosts, the diagnosis of varicella or zoster is typically clinical with little indication for viral culture, PCR, or serologic testing. However, because of the risk for clinical complications, the need to treat, and the potential infection control issues, virologic confirmation is indicated in oncology patients and transplant recipients. A high degree of suspicion in the right clinical context, along with characteristic cutaneous findings, increases the pretest probability of diagnostic testing for either primary varicella or varicella-zoster. Similar testing methodologies are available for detection of VZV as for HSV,[26] with most centers relying on PCR detection of viral DNA from samples collected from skin scrapings or a skin biopsy. Viral DNA may also be detected in blood or CSF. Direct fluorescent antibody staining for viral antigens in skin scrapings may be used but is less sensitive and less specific than PCR. Culture-based methods are generally not available and rarely used for diagnosis of VZV.[37]

Treatment, Prophylaxis, and Prevention

Treatment. Although antiviral therapy is not routinely recommended in immunocompetent hosts, acyclovir or valacyclovir is recommended for pediatric oncology patients and transplant recipients with either varicella or zoster, because the duration of viral replication is presumably longer (Table 19.3).[16] Ideally, therapy should be initiated within

TABLE 19.3 **Treatment of Varicella-Zoster Virus Disease in Oncology and Transplant Patients**

Population	Drug	Dose[a]	Duration	References
Oncology or SCT patients				
Primary varicella or varicella-zoster	Acyclovir	10 mg/kg IV q8h (<2 years) 500 mg/m^2 IV or 10 mg/kg IV q8h (≥2 years)	Until all lesions are crusted, then switch to oral	Styczynski et al.,[13] *Red Book*[16]
	Acyclovir	20 mg/kg PO 4 times daily	To complete a minimum 7 day total course after IV treatment, until at least 2 days after all lesions crusted. May be used for mild varicella-zoster in some cases.	Styczynski et al.[13]
Acyclovir-resistant disease	Foscarnet	60 mg/kg IV q12h	To complete a minimum 7 day total course, until at least 2 days after all lesions crusted	Styczynski et al.[13]
	Cidofovir	5 mg/kg IV once weekly for 2 weeks, then once every 2 weeks if still needed, combined with probenecid and IV hydration	To complete a minimum 7 day total course, until at least 2 days after all lesions crusted	Styczynski et al.[13]
Solid Organ Transplantation				
Primary varicella or varicella-zoster	Acyclovir	10 mg/kg IV q8h	To complete a minimum 7 day total course, until at least all lesions crusted. Can change to oral after significant improvement.	Zuckerman et al.[26]
Acyclovir-resistant disease	Foscarnet	80-120 mg/kg per day IV in 2-3 divided doses	To complete a minimum 7 day total course, until at least all lesions crusted	Zuckerman et al.[26]
	Cidofovir	5 mg/kg IV once weekly for 2 weeks, then once every 2 weeks if still needed, combined with probenecid and IV hydration	To complete a minimum 7 day total course, until at least all lesions crusted	Zuckerman et al.[26]

[a]Dose should be decreased in patients with renal impairment.
h, hour; *IV,* intravenous, *PO,* oral; *q,* every.

24 hours of onset of rash. The decision whether to use IV acyclovir or oral valacyclovir depends on the patient's net state of immune suppression and ability to tolerate oral therapy. Moreover, IV acyclovir therapy is typically preferred for disease involving the face, owing to concern for extension of disease to the eye or complications involving the facial nerve (Ramsay-Hunt syndrome or weakness of facial muscles and unilateral hearing loss).[26] IV immunoglobulin or varicella immunoglobulin (Varizig, Saol Therapeutics) provides no additional treatment benefit, but as described later, may prevent or modulate disease if administered shortly after exposure. Salicylates should be avoided in the setting of varicella or zoster because of a historic link to Reye syndrome.

Acyclovir-resistant disease is much less common for VZV compared with HSV and may be treated with foscarnet or cidofovir. Brincidofovir may be an orally available alternative for acyclovir-resistant disseminated varicella.

Prophylaxis. Oral valacyclovir prophylaxis against VZV reactivation is generally recommended for seropositive HSCT recipients.[20] A 1-year regimen has been shown to have excellent efficacy and is well tolerated,[39] and most recommendations are to continue prophylaxis in patients being treated with systemic immunosuppressive regimens for chronic GVHD or other reasons.[20] Drugs prescribed for CMV prophylaxis have efficacy against both HSV and VZV, and no additional antiviral therapy is needed for patients receiving CMV prophylaxis.[26] However, the recommendation for VZV prophylaxis is supported primarily by studies in adults and will likely need to be readdressed with increasing implementation of both varicella and zoster vaccines. There are no specific recommendations for antiviral prophylaxis against zoster in seropositive SOT recipients and, similar to HSV, varicella is rarely if ever transmitted from a donor to recipient.

Infection Prevention

Airborne and contact precautions are recommended for hospitalized patients with either primary varicella or zoster because the virus can be transmitted via respiratory droplets and skin.[16,26] Standard precautions and covering of lesions are recommended for immunocompetent patients with localized zoster. Susceptible individuals (i.e., no history of primary disease or vaccination or known to be seronegative) should not enter the room of a patient with primary varicella or zoster.[16,26] Isolation should continue until all lesions are crusted, and localized lesions should be covered, if possible, to decrease transmission risk.[26]

Exposure Avoidance and Immunization of Contacts. VZV serostatus should be determined for children diagnosed with cancer and those who are candidates for SCT or SOT. Family members and close contacts of oncology patients, and SCT or SOT recipients should be counseled to have up-to-date immunizations, including against VZV.[40] Seronegative patients should avoid exposure to people with primary varicella or varicella-zoster and should avoid contact with any vaccine recipients experiencing a rash after vaccination.[13,20] Although rare, there is at least one report of transmission of vaccine strain VZV from a vaccine recipient with varicella lesions to susceptible household contacts.[41] Primary disease in a previously immunized patient receiving chemotherapy has also been reported,[42] suggesting it would be prudent to generally recommend that immunosuppressed patients minimize exposure to individuals with primary infection or zoster.

The optimal prophylaxis for varicella exposure is administration of the live-attenuated viral vaccine within 3 days but up to 5 days after exposure. However, this option is not available for pediatric oncology patients receiving chemotherapy or transplant recipients. Antiviral therapy and/or immunoglobulin is recommended for stem cell transplant recipients and for seronegative, unknown, or incompletely vaccinated oncology patients or SOT recipients. If initiated, preemptive oral valacyclovir should be prescribed starting 7 to 10 days after exposure and continued for 7 days.[16] Varicella-zoster immunoglobulin (Varizig) should be administered ideally within 96 hours of exposure, although it may still provide benefit if administered within 10 days of exposure.[16] If Varizig is not available, IVIG dosed at 400 mg/kg is recommended as an alternative, although the effectiveness of pooled IVIG is not known and the titer of varicella antibodies in pooled IVIG has declined after the advent of universal immunization.[16] Patients receiving monthly high-dose IVIG (400 mg/kg or greater) may still benefit from Varizig but do not require additional IVIG if their last dose was within 3 weeks of exposure.

Vaccination

Pretransplant Vaccination. The CDC Advisory Committee on Immunization Practices recommends a 2-dose regimen of the live-attenuated varicella Oka strain vaccine with the first dose administered between 12 and 15 months of age and a second dose between 4 and 6 years of age in healthy children.[16] Thus depending on the age at presentation, pediatric oncology and transplant candidates may have been fully, partially (one dose), or never vaccinated before presentation for cancer treatment or transplantation. Because routine vaccination has made wild-type varicella less common, fewer children have preexisting immunity from natural disease.

Immunization is recommended for SOT candidates if the transplant is not expected to occur within the next 4 weeks. The first dose of VZV vaccine, administered as the single-component VZV vaccine, may be given as early as 9 months of age, with the second dose as soon as 4 weeks later. Either the single-component VZV vaccine or the combination vaccine with measles, mumps, rubella, and varicella (MMRV) may be administered to SOT candidates older than 1 year.[43] SOT candidates who have previously completed the 2-dose series should be screened for varicella seroconversion and reimmunized if seronegative. As for other live vaccines, receipt of blood products (particularly IVIG) can interfere with host responses, and a delay of 3 months is recommended. If this delay is not possible (i.e., transplant likely to occur 4 to 12 weeks from the time of pretransplant evaluation), then the vaccine may be administered, recognizing that the response may be suboptimal. Also, if the single-component VZV vaccine is given separately from the MMR vaccine, they should be given at the same time or separated by 4 weeks to avoid compromising responses.

If transplant is expected to occur within 4 weeks, current recommendations are to not administer live virus vaccines (MMR and VZV).[26,43] Although the literature lacks reports of outcomes in patients who may have received live virus vaccines within 4 weeks before transplantation, cases of severe disease from vaccine-strain varicella in children immunized just before immunosuppressive chemotherapy[44] raise concern that suppression of cellular immunity after SOT could lead to varicella replication and disease. If a patient inadvertently receives live viral vaccines shortly before transplantation, antiviral prophylaxis and/or IVIG or varicella immunoglobulin could potentially prevent vaccine-related disease, but there are no data to support such a recommendation.

Vaccination After Chemotherapy or Transplant. Because of the high morbidity associated with primary varicella in pediatric cancer patients, the initial varicella vaccine studies were conducted in varicella-susceptible pediatric leukemia patients in remission.[45] A 2-dose vaccine regimen was safe and immunogenic. The vaccine was associated with rash in 149 (40%) of recipients, which was treated with acyclovir in 16 patients. Based on these and other studies, a 2-dose varicella vaccine regimen is currently recommended for cancer patients in remission after at least 3 months since chemotherapy and who have evidence of restored immunocompetence.[40] A delay of 6 months is recommended after treatment with B-cell-depleting antibodies.[40] However, there are no standardized approaches to assess immunocompetence. Some centers recommend quantifying T-cell numbers and function using a mitogen proliferation assay. Vaccination boosting is also recommended after chemotherapy in children who had been previously seropositive because a significant number lose preexisting humoral immunity to VZV (as well as MMR) after completion of chemotherapy.[46]

More recently, researchers have begun to assess whether VZV vaccine can be safely administered to pediatric oncology patients without chemotherapy interruption. In a small single-center study, 31 patients were vaccinated early during their course of chemotherapy.[47] The vaccine was safe and after one dose, the majority had VZV-specific $CD4^+$ T-cell responses with seroconversion occurring in half by antibody assay.

Initial concerns about safety of a live-attenuated vaccine in HSCT recipients have been addressed by studies demonstrating safety and immunogenicity after immune reconstitution. For example, a retrospective study of 46 varicella-seronegative patients younger than 20 years who achieved a $CD4^+$ T-cell count of 200/μL or higher and were vaccinated at a median of 4 years after transplant found seroconversion in 64% after one dose.[48] A self-limited varicella-like rash developed in 3 patients within 2.5 weeks of immunization and shingles did not develop in any patient. Currently, a 2-dose series beginning 24 months after transplant is recommended in SCT recipients, provided they are not being treated with immunosuppressive therapy for GVHD or other reasons, and it has been 8 to 11 months since they last received IVIG.[40] Again, some centers assess immune cell number and function before reintroducing any vaccines. Some centers prefer to document immune response to subunit vaccines (e.g., hepatitis B or pneumococcal vaccines) before administering the varicella vaccine. However, there are no data indicating that the response to subunit vaccines predicts an effective immune response to a live viral vaccine and the mechanisms of generating immune responses are distinct.

Unfortunately, few controlled studies have been conducted for SOT recipients and varicella vaccines are not routinely recommended for them. However, based on the experience with HSCT patients, many centers have adopted policies to introduce varicella vaccine in kidney or liver transplant patients receiving minimal or no immunosuppressive agents.[40,49] Many experts continue to recommend caution in applying these policies.[26,43]

Vaccines for Zoster. There have also been studies to assess the role of vaccines to prevent zoster in adult HSCT recipients. A recent randomized, double-blind, placebo-controlled phase III trial was completed in patients 18 years or older who received 4 doses of inactivated varicella virus vaccine or placebo within the first 5 to 60 days before autologous HSCT and then 30, 60, or 90 days after transplantation. The vaccine was safe and effective, with zoster developing in 42 of 538 (8%) vaccine recipients, compared with 113 of 535 (21%) of placebo recipients during a mean follow-up of 2.4 years.[50]

More recently, a liposome-based subunit glycoprotein E vaccine (Shingrix) combined with adjuvants to stimulate strong $CD4^+$ T-cell responses (AS01B, the Toll-like receptor agonist monophosphoryl lipid A combined with saponin QS-21) was evaluated for prevention of zoster. Phase III placebo-controlled trials in healthy adults demonstrated 97% protection against zoster compared with the 51% efficacy observed in response to the live-attenuated shingles vaccine Zostavax (Merck).[7] Shingrix was approved by the FDA at the end of 2017. Studies are ongoing in adult transplantation recipients and may include pediatric patients in the future. Notably, this vaccine was developed to prevent zoster and not primary varicella, and there are no data regarding immunogenicity in seronegative individuals.

SUMMARY AND FUTURE DIRECTIONS

The human α-herpesviruses HSV and VZV remain pathogens of concern in pediatric oncology and transplant recipients because of their ability to uniformly establish latency and to periodically reactivate throughout the life of an individual. Reactivation, which occurs more often than previously appreciated, is typically controlled by an intact cellular and humoral immune system. Immunosuppressive therapy to prevent graft rejection and as part of chemotherapy regimens results in more frequent and more severe disease in these vulnerable pediatric patients. The epidemiology of disease continues to change with the introduction of protective vaccines, the development of safer and more effective antiviral agents, and changes in immunotherapies for cancer and transplantation. For example, clinically significant primary or recurrent VZV has declined with the introduction of universal vaccination and, hopefully, future effective HSV vaccines will have a similar beneficial impact. New immunotherapies for cancer and transplantation, including checkpoint inhibitors, chimeric antigen receptor T-cell and specific monoclonal antibodies, also affect the risk of HSV or VZV reactivation. The development of more rapid and sensitive molecular diagnostics coupled with safer orally bioavailable antivirals has contributed to improved clinical outcomes. However, physicians must maintain clinical suspicion and intervene with prompt diagnostic testing and treatment to prevent morbidity associated with these viruses.

20

Human Herpesvirus 6, 7, and 8

Debra J. Lugo, MD and Danielle M. Zerr, MD, MPH

Over the past several decades, three novel human herpesviruses (HHVs) have been identified and designated HHV-6, HHV-7, and HHV-8. HHV-6 has since been designated as two distinct species, HHV-6A and HHV-6B. HHV-6 was first isolated from the white blood cells of patients with human immunodeficiency syndrome and lymphoproliferative disease in the 1980s. The virus was initially designated as human B-lymphotropic virus, but the name was changed to HHV-6 once it was identified to preferentially infect CD4 T-lymphocytes[1] rather than B cells. While pursuing additional strains of HHV6, HHV-7 was identified,[2] a virus closely genetically related to HHV-6. HHV-8, also referred to as Kaposi sarcoma (KS)–associated herpesvirus, was identified while researchers were searching for the etiology of KS. HHVs 6, 7, and 8, like the other members of the HHV family, are double-stranded DNA viruses that establish a latent, persistent infection after primary infection. All three viruses can manifest active infection and, in some cases, disease in immunocompromised patients, either owing to reactivation of latent infection or transmission of infection from donors.

HHV-6A and HHV-6B are members of the β subfamily of the HHV, along with cytomegalovirus (CMV). HHV-6A and HHV-6B are closely related but have distinct biologic, epidemiologic, and clinical features. Although the natural history of HHV-6A is unknown, HHV-6B infects most people before the age of 3 years. Primary infection is characterized by a febrile illness often accompanied by respiratory symptoms, diarrhea, and rash. In a large proportion of immunocompromised patients, HHV-6B reactivates, and reactivation has been associated with fever, rash, bone marrow suppression, pneumonitis, acute graft-versus-host disease (GVHD), and graft rejection. In allogeneic hematopoietic stem cell transplant (HSCT) recipients, HHV-6B is the most common cause of encephalitis.

HHV-7 is also a member of the β subfamily of HHVs. In the majority of the population, HHV-7 antibody becomes detectable during childhood, where it has been implicated as an alternative cause of roseola, pityriasis rosea, and nonspecific febrile illness. HHV-7 infection is common after solid organ transplantation (SOT) but is transient and usually not associated with any clinical symptoms.[3] There are few studies that have investigated HHV-7–associated disease, but viremia has been associated with febrile syndromes, thrombocytopenia, acute myelitis, and liver allograft rejection in a small number of studies and case reports. More frequently HHV-7 has been detected as a co-infection with CMV, but further studies are needed to determine if HHV-7 infection affects CMV disease.

HHV-8, or KS-associated herpesvirus, is a γ-herpesvirus along with Epstein-Barr virus (EBV), and like EBV, it is an oncogenic virus. HHV-8 contains a large number of genes that are transduced from the host cellular genome, a process known as molecular piracy. These genes can induce angiogenesis and cell growth while avoiding immune detection.[4] Infection with HHV-8 is less common than HHV-6 and HHV-7, but in endemic areas typically occurs in childhood. Owing to immunosuppression of CD8$^+$ response and lack of humoral immunity, uncontrolled HHV8 replication can lead to neoplastic disease, including KS.[3] HHV-8 is also a rare trigger of hemophagocytic lymphohistiocytosis (HLH), a disorder of immune regulation.[5]

EPIDEMIOLOGY AND RISK FACTORS

Human Herpesvirus 6

The natural history of HHV-6A is unknown. In contrast, HHV-6B infects most children before the age of 3 years and is characterized by fever, respiratory symptoms, diarrhea, and rash. In 25% of patients it causes roseola, an acute febrile illness defined by a maculopapular rash appearing as the fever declines. HHV-6B primary infection is also associated with febrile seizures and possibly epilepsy. Most HHV-6B transmission events are thought to occur via shared saliva early in life. Congenital infection had been estimated to occur in approximately 1% of births,[6] although this is now recognized to be mostly the result of inherited chromosomally integrated HHV-6.

After primary infection, HHV-6B can establish latency in mononuclear cells and serve as a reservoir for endogenous viral reactivation. HHV-6B reactivates in approximately 40% of SOT recipients, typically within 2 to 6 weeks after transplantation or after episodes of rejection when they are receiving increased immunosuppression. HSCT recipients are at greatest risk of reactivation during the peri-engraftment period and after diagnosis of GVHD due to treatment with immunomodulatory medications. Patients receiving cord blood transplant are at an especially increased risk of HHV-6B reactivation, with rates as high as 80% to 90%. HHV-6B has been associated with a number of important outcomes, particularly in allogeneic HSCT recipients, including encephalitis, bone marrow suppression, pneumonitis, GVHD, and mortality. The evidence supports a causal association between HHV-6B and encephalitis, an outcome that is rarely reported in non-HSCT recipients.[7,8] A more specific entity, HHV-6B posttransplant acute limbic encephalopathy, has been estimated to occur in 0.7% of adult donor HSCT recipients and 9.9% of cord blood transplant recipients in the United States.[9]

Reactivation of HHV-6B has been reported in up to 52% of adults receiving cytotoxic chemotherapy,[10] although the clinical significance remains poorly understood. In pediatric patients, one study found that the incidence of HHV-6 DNA detected in blood rose from 17% at time of diagnosis to 37% during chemotherapy and was associated with fever.[11]

The preferential target cell for HHV-6 is CD4$^+$ lymphocytes; however, cellular host cells include CD8$^+$ T lymphocytes, natural killer (NK) cells, macrophages, megakaryocytes, glial cells, and epithelial cells. HHV-6A and -6B establish latency by integrating into the telomere regions of the host chromosomes.[12] When this occurs in a germ cell, it can result in chromosomally integrated HHV-6 (ciHHV-6), which can occur in an estimated 1% of the population. Affected individuals have the HHV-6 genome present in every cell of their body. As a result, affected individuals have persistently detectable HHV-6 viral DNA in tissues, blood, and cerebrospinal fluid (CSF). In addition, viral transcripts and antigens have been demonstrated in immunocompetent and immunocompromised patients with inherited ciHHV-6.[7,13] More recently, the majority of congenital infections have been shown to be due to ciHHV-6.[14]

When ciHHV-6 is not recognized, it can lead to inappropriate treatment of patients. It is important to note that detection of viral DNA does not correlate with symptoms or signs of disease in patients with ciHHV-6. However, there is some evidence that ciHHV-6 can lead to active viral infection and symptomatic disease in severely immunocompromised patients. [7]

Human Herpesvirus 7

Most people become seropositive for HHV-7 at a slightly later age than HHV-6B, typically by 5 years of age. Transmission of HHV-7 is similar to other HHVs, typically through shared saliva. HHV-7 exhibits selective tropism for $CD4^+$ cells, using the CD4 cell receptor for entry. HHV-7 has been described as slower to replicate than HHV-6 and less lytic, with the cytopathic effects similar to HHV-6 but less pronounced.[15] Salivary glands are the major identified site of persistence and replication.

Similar to HHV-6B, HHV-7 may reactivate in SOT recipients. HHV-7–seropositive pediatric patients have been shown to have a 20% to 60% incidence of HHV-7 DNA detection 2 to 6 weeks after transplant.[16] Most reactivation is brief with minimal viremia. Specific risk factors for reactivation have not been clearly defined. Primary infection can also occur in SOT recipients who were seronegative before transplantation. HHV-7 infections are rarely symptomatic in SOT recipients, but rare cases of tissue-invasive disease have been reported and are often associated with other viral infections, including CMV or EBV.

Human Herpesvirus 8

HHV-8 has a broad cellular tropism, including infection of B cells, endothelial cells, macrophages, and epithelial cells. Similar to HHV-6 and HHV-7, primary infection is most often through saliva and can be transmitted from caregivers to children through premastication. It can also be spread through infusion of contaminated blood products. HHV-8 seropositivity rises throughout adolescence and varies geographically. HHV-8 seropositivity is lower in North America compared with countries where it is considered endemic.[17] In Israel, 9% of children and up to 18% of adults are seropositive[18] compared with less than 5% of human immunodeficiency syndrome–negative adults in the United States.[17] HHV-8 seropositivity occurs more often in children whose parents are seropositive, with maternal seropositivity being the most important risk factor.[19]

KS has only rarely been reported in HSCT recipients.[20] KS lesions in transplant recipients can develop as the result of reactivation of latent virus or via transmission of the virus or KS lesions from the allograft. In SOT recipients, most KS (80%) appears to result from reactivation of latent virus.[21] The incidence of KS varies geographically and is dependent on local seroprevalence of HHV-8. KS affects less than 1% of transplant recipients in the United States and has been reported as low as 0.1% in central Europe.[22] In areas of high seroprevalence, KS can account for the majority of posttransplant malignancies. In posttransplant recipients who were previously positive for HHV8, increased immunosuppression can lead to of development of lesions and progression of disease, but no specific regimen is associated with increased risk. The risk of disease decreases with time after transplant.[23] In addition to KS, HHV-8 has also been associated with other malignancies, including primary effusion lymphoma and multicentric Castleman disease, a B-cell lymphoproliferative disease. HHV-8 can also be a trigger for HLH.[5]

CLINICAL MANIFESTATIONS

HHVs can have direct and indirect sequelae. Indirect sequelae have been described as immunomodulatory effects that may increase risk of co-infections with other viruses, specifically CMV, and/or potentially lead to outcomes such as GVHD and organ rejection. HHV-6B infection has been identified in several studies as a significant risk factor for symptomatic CMV disease in both liver and kidney transplant recipients.[24] In the following text we discuss the clinical manifestations for HSCT recipients, SOT recipients, and oncology patients specifically.

Hematopoietic Stem Cell Transplant

The majority of HHV-6B reactivation episodes in HSCT recipients are asymptomatic, transient, do not impact overall survival, and do not require antiviral treatment. HHV-6 has been commonly associated with fever and rash after transplantation, and common hematologic effects associated with HHV-6B infection include delayed platelet engraftment and leukopenia.[25] HHV-6 has also been associated with pneumonitis and hepatitis. There is strong evidence that HHV-6B causes encephalitis, particularly after allogeneic HSCT. In most reports and studies of HHV-6B encephalitis, it is defined as encephalopathy without another cause identified. HHV-6B encephalitis in HSCT recipients presents with symptoms that commonly include confusion and altered consciousness. Other symptoms may also include seizures, amnesia, and syndrome of inappropriate antidiuretic hormone secretion. Laboratory findings may include mild CSF pleocytosis and elevated protein. Distinct imaging findings are medial temporal lobe changes on brain magnetic resonance imaging (MRI). HHV-6B–associated posttransplant acute limbic encephalitis is defined by anterograde amnesia, syndrome of inappropriate antidiuretic hormone, mild CSF pleocytosis, temporal electroencephalogram abnormalities, and MRI hyperintensities in the limbic system.[26]

HHV-7 reactivation is rarely associated with clinical symptoms, although it has been suggested that HHV-7 also can be associated with higher CMV viral loads and delayed clearance of viremia.[27]

HHV-8 reactivation or primary infection after HSCT has rarely been reported in the absence of malignant disease. Studies of the natural history of viral reactivation after HSCT are lacking; other than malignancy, the frequency and outcome of viral reactivation has not been well described. Clinical symptoms described include fever, rash, hepatitis, and bone marrow failure.[28] HHV-8 has rarely been reported to cause KS in HSCT recipients. Symptoms of KS in HCT recipients can include graft failure and pancytopenia in addition to skin lesions. The median time of onset has been reported as 8.5 months after HSCT,[29] and diffuse disease developed in 50% of these patients, with mortality rates reported up to 70%.

Solid Organ Transplant

The most common clinical syndrome of HHV-6B infection in SOT recipients is a nonspecific febrile illness occasionally associated with rash. HHV-6B infection can also have marrow-suppressive effects, including chronic myelosuppression, but this is more frequently seen in HSCT recipients, as described earlier.

HHV-6B has also been associated with significantly higher mortality after liver transplant and has been linked to a higher risk of invasive fungal infections after transplant, likely owing to immunomodulatory effects.[30] HHV-6B has been associated with increased severity of hepatitis C recurrence in positive recipients but is not clearly an independent risk factor for recurrence.[31] This may be clinically relevant as hepatitis C mismatch transplants are increasing.

HHV-7 viremia has been detected after transplant and has been considered as a possible cofactor in CMV disease after SOT. In one study, renal transplant recipients in whom both CMV and HHV-7 were detected had more severe CMV disease.[32] HHV-7 has also been reported in association with pneumonia and bronchiolitis obliterans in a lung transplant recipient.[33]

HHV-8 can lead to KS in SOT recipients, and the disease can be rapidly fatal if not identified in a timely fashion. HHV-8 can also be inciting factor for development of HLH. In addition, nonneoplastic lesions have been associated with HHV-8, including cytopenias and hepatitis.

Oncology

Owing to multimodal treatment with chemotherapy, risk of reactivation persists throughout treatment, peaking during times of intense immunosuppression. Similar to HSCT recipients, reactivation often occurs as a co-infection with CMV and EBV. Most HHV6 and EBV reactivations in the first 100 days of chemotherapy are subclinical.[10] Severe HHV-6 disease is rare, but detection of HHV-6 DNA is more commonly associated with fever, lymphopenia, rash, and hepatic dysfunction.[11]

More studies are needed to determine the frequency of reactivation of HHV-7 in patients with oncologic malignancies and receiving chemotherapy and the clinical impact. Severe disease is rarely reported.

HHV-8 has been linked to several lymphoproliferative diseases, including KS and multicentric Castleman disease, plasmablastic lymphoma, and primary effusion lymphoma in oncology patients. Patients with chronic blood disorders or underlying immune dysfunction have been described at greater risk of developing malignancy from this virus, and HHV-8 is considered a predisposing factor for several malignancies.[34]

Disease Prophylaxis/Prevention

Small studies exploring the utility of antiviral prophylaxis or preemptive therapy with ganciclovir or foscarnet for HHV-6B have been performed in SOT and HSCT recipients with variable results.[35-40] Although these antiviral agents may reduce the rate or delay HHV-6B reactivation, evidence is lacking to support prophylaxis or preemptive monitoring and treatment aimed at preventing HHV-6B–associated disease.

Preemptive testing for HHV-7 and HHV-8 viremia is not routinely recommended after transplant. Antiviral prophylaxis does not appear to alter the appearance of HHV-7.[36,41]

Primary infection with herpesviruses can be acquired through sexual activity, contaminated blood products, or close nonsexual contact owing to active shedding in saliva. Patients at risk should be encouraged to limit any high-risk behaviors, including practicing safe sex and avoidance of premastication.

DIAGNOSIS

Human Herpesvirus 6

Direct viral detection is the preferred method for identifying HHV-6B after transplantation. Viral serologic test results are not helpful given the high prevalence of latent infection, limitations in the available assays, and the immunocompromised state of the targeted patient population. Detection of viral nucleic acids also allows differentiation between HHV-6A and HHV-6B.[42]

Detection of viral DNA by PCR may reflect active or latent infection, depending on the specimen tested. Quantitative viral DNA PCR obtained on noncellular samples such as serum, plasma, or CSF has been shown to correlate with active viral replication[43] and is the most studied and widely available method available. Quantitative assays also allow for the potential of risk assessment as higher viral loads have been more predictive of encephalitis in some studies. Quantitative assays may also help determine trends over time. If whole blood samples are used, it is important to have established thresholds for significance levels owing to the presence of latent virus in peripheral blood mononuclear cells. Reverse transcriptase PCR on whole blood might be the best indicator for active viral replication. However, this test is not commercially available and has also not been studied to determine its ability to predict clinical outcomes.

Detection of HHV-6B in CSF in a patient with acute encephalopathy is generally considered diagnostic of HHV-6B encephalitis in the absence of another etiology of encephalopathy. In a small percentage of patients, HHV-6 has been detected in the CSF in the absence of symptoms.[44] Patients with acute encephalopathy without a clear etiology should have serum or plasma and CSF tested for HHV-6B, and empiric antiviral therapy should be initiated while results are pending. It is important to note that detection of virus in blood or CSF may underestimate tissue-level disease. Despite clearance from CSF or blood, virus may persist in tissue for a prolonged time. CSF findings and results from brain imaging can help in the diagnosis of HHV-6B encephalitis. CSF studies in patients with HHV-6 encephalitis generally demonstrate mild pleocytosis and elevated protein levels. Brain MRI findings consistent with HHV-6B encephalitis include medial temporal lobe changes, typically described as well-circumscribed, hyperintense, nonenhancing lesions involving the medial and temporal lobes, especially the hippocampus.

Persistent high levels of HHV-6 in blood, with or without treatment, should raise suspicion for ci-HHV6.[45] Diagnosis of ci-HHV6 can be confirmed with fluorescence in situ hybridization analysis demonstrating the virus integrated in the chromosome, or alternatively, by testing tissues that would not normally have detectable HHV-6, such as hair follicles. However, these methods are not widely available. More recently, digital droplet PCR methods have been developed for detection of ciHHV-6. In this case, the ratio of viral to human genomes at 1:1 is highly suggestive for the presence of ci-HHV6.[46]

HHV-6 quantitative PCR (serum or plasma) should be performed for the following groups of patients:

1. Posttransplant or severely immunocompromised patients with encephalopathy or encephalomyelitis. CSF should also be obtained for HHV-6 testing (Fig. 20.1).
2. Post-HSCT patients with delayed engraftment (>28 days) or other signs of end-organ disease: hepatitis or interstitial pneumonia without another identified explanation (Fig. 20.2).

Human Herpesvirus 7

Routine testing for HHV-7 is not recommended as clinical relevance has not been established. However, if testing is to be pursued for HHV-7, quantitative PCR on serum or plasma is preferred.

Human Herpesvirus 8

HHV-8, serology may be sent before transplant to determine risk for reactivation. After transplantation, clinical suspicion for HHV-8–associated disease should be heightened when patients present with skin lesions, including nodules or maculopapular lesions, lymphadenopathy, and unexplained pleural or peritoneal effusions. Unexplained febrile illness, respiratory distress, or blood dyscrasias can also be signs of HHV–8-related disease. Diagnosis of KS disease is made on the basis

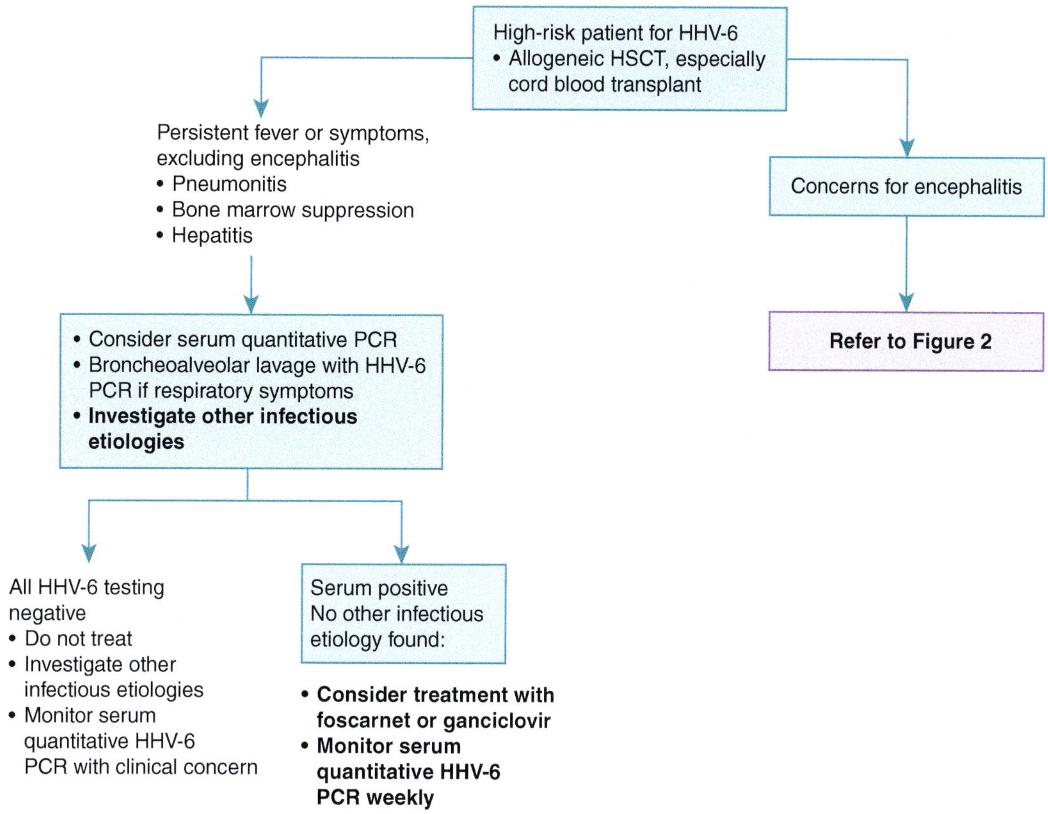

Fig. 20.1 Diagnosis of human herpesvirus 6. *HHV,* human herpesvirus; *HSCT,* hematopoietic stem cell transplant; *PCR,* polymerase chain reaction.

of clinical presentation, histopathologic features of skin lesions, and detection of virus on tissue biopsy. Histopathology demonstrates spindle cells, which can stain positive for endothelial cell markers but also express proteins to other cell types. HHV-8 quantitative PCR of serum can be used for screening for infectious causes. However, biopsy should be used to confirm disease when malignancy is suspected (Fig. 20.3).

TREATMENT

For all symptomatic disease with HHV-6, HHV-7, and HHV-8, withdrawal or reduction of immunosuppression is the best initial approach to treatment. However, this is often not possible in HSCT or oncology patients.

Human Herpesvirus 6

There is no U.S. Food and Drug Administration–approved antiviral for treatment of HHV-6B. Foscarnet, ganciclovir, and cidofovir have been shown to have variable in vitro activity against HHV-6A and HHV-6B. Although limited clinical data suggest that the antiviral agents can affect viral levels, randomized controlled trials that show clinical benefit are lacking.

In a retrospective observational study that included 145 allogeneic HCT recipients with HHV-6B encephalitis, differences between response rates of neurologic symptoms were not significant in the 123 patients treated with foscarnet monotherapy versus ganciclovir monotherapy.[47] However, full-dose ganciclovir or foscarnet was associated with lower incidences of sequelae or death caused by HHV-6B encephalitis compared with lower-dose therapy. In that study, full-dose foscarnet was associated with 93% success versus 74% success with low-dose foscarnet therapy, and full-dose ganciclovir was associated with 84% success compared with 58% success with lower-dose therapy. The rate of death from any cause within 30 days after the development of HHV-6 encephalitis was lower in patients who received foscarnet. Further research is needed to determine if one antiviral is more effective.

Given the existing evidence, we recommend the use of foscarnet and/or ganciclovir for treatment of encephalitis. Full induction dosing of foscarnet (180 mg/kg per day divided every 8 or 12 hours) or ganciclovir (10 mg/kg per day divided every 12 hours) should be initiated immediately while waiting for laboratory and radiology results. Adequate hydration should be maintained and appropriate adjustments to dosing should be made for patients with decreased renal function. Although the optimal duration is unknown, it may be reasonable to extrapolate from recommendations for HSV encephalitis and consider at least 3 weeks of therapy with resolution of viral detection in the blood and CSF.

Treatment is not recommended for asymptomatic patients with isolated viremia. However, treatment for HHV-6B may be considered in patients with viremia and HHV-6B–associated end-organ disease, such as pneumonitis or hepatitis. Treatment courses have not been defined, but it may be reasonable to consider 2 weeks pending clinical improvement. In practice, this course can be shortened if viremia resolves and there is clinical improvement of end-organ disease.

Human Herpesvirus 7

HHV-7 reactivation does not typically require treatment in HSCT, SOT, or oncology patients owing to low risk of disease. However, if treatment is desired, it should be noted that acyclovir is only minimally active, whereas ganciclovir, foscarnet, and cidofovir have increased in vitro activity.

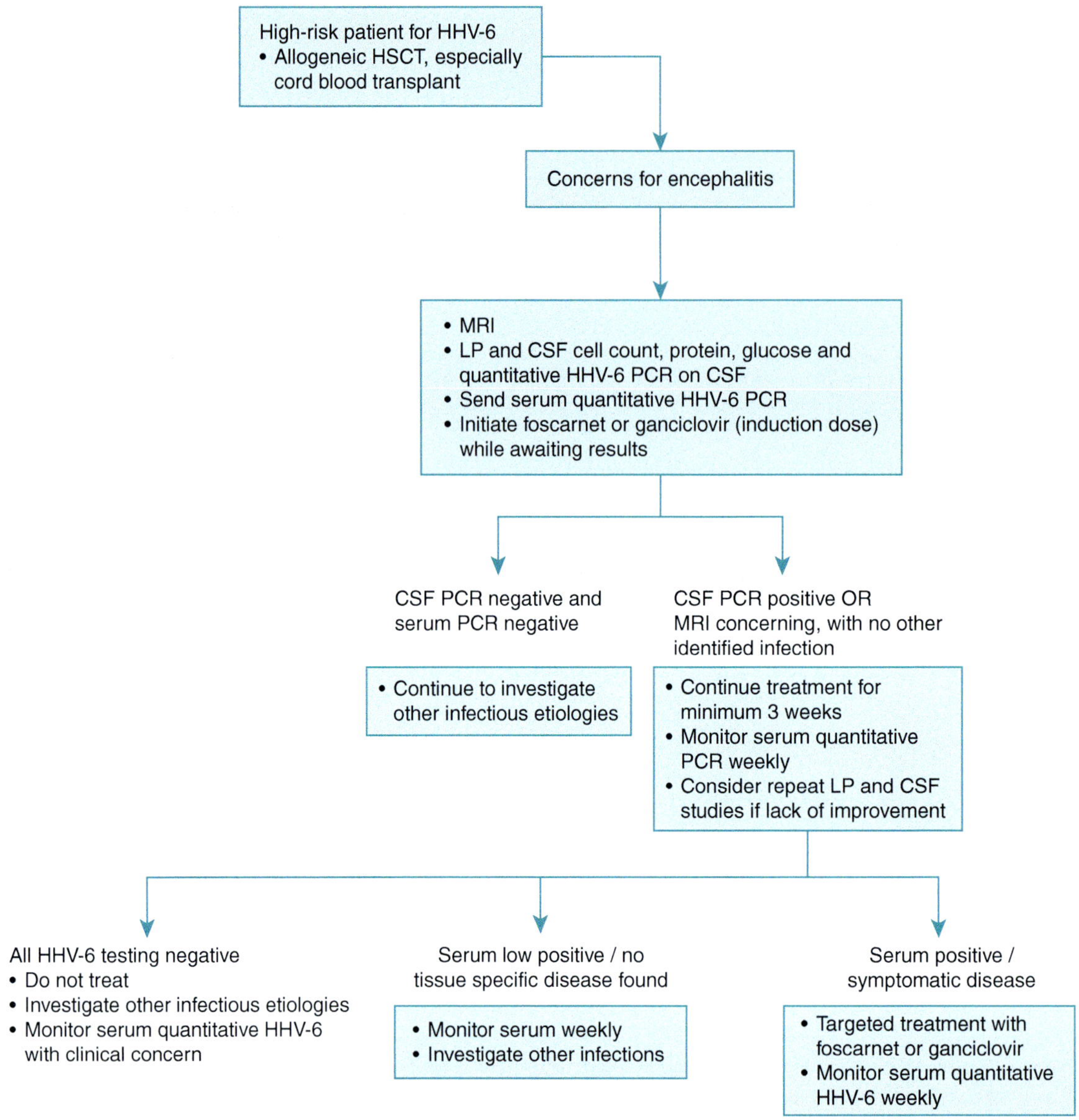

Fig. 20.2 Diagnosis of human herpesvirus 6 encephalitis. *CSF,* cerebrospinal fluid; *HHV,* human herpesvirus; *HSCT,* hematopoietic stem cell transplant; *LP,* lumbar puncture; *MRI,* magnetic resonance imaging; *PCR,* polymerase chain reaction.

Human Herpesvirus 8

Treatment for HHV-8 viremia is limited as ganciclovir, foscarnet, and cidofovir have not been effective clinically despite having in vitro activity. Fortunately, malignant disease does not develop in most patients who are positive for HHV-8. However, if lesions develop, treatment should be based on staging and disease burden. Treatment approaches for lymphoproliferative diseases caused by HHV-8 can involve a combination of antiviral therapy, immunomodulation, and chemotherapy, depending on the severity of disease. Initial treatment of KS focuses on reduction of immunosuppression, which can lead to rapid regression of disease. Alternatives include changing to mammalian target of rapamycin inhibitors with cessation of calcineurin inhibitors. In severe or disseminated disease, chemotherapeutics may be used. Antiviral therapies are not clinically effective in KS disease, as it is due to latent infection of the virus. Current antiviral therapies available require active viral replication to be effective (Table 20.1).

INFECTION PREVENTION AND ANTICIPATORY GUIDANCE

With all herpesviruses, after primary infection a latent infection is established and patients remain at risk for reactivation during periods of immunosuppression. In SOT recipients, this risk is ongoing because of persistent immunosuppression.

Posttransplant patients with HHV-6 encephalitis may experience significant morbidity and mortality despite antiviral therapy.[48] Up to 25% of patients with HHV-6B encephalitis may experience progressive encephalitis and death, and persistent neurocognitive deficits may be present in up to 40% of survivors.[26,49,50] Routine neurocognitive follow-up should be scheduled after encephalitis to monitor progression, as well as speech, occupational, and physical therapy as indicated.

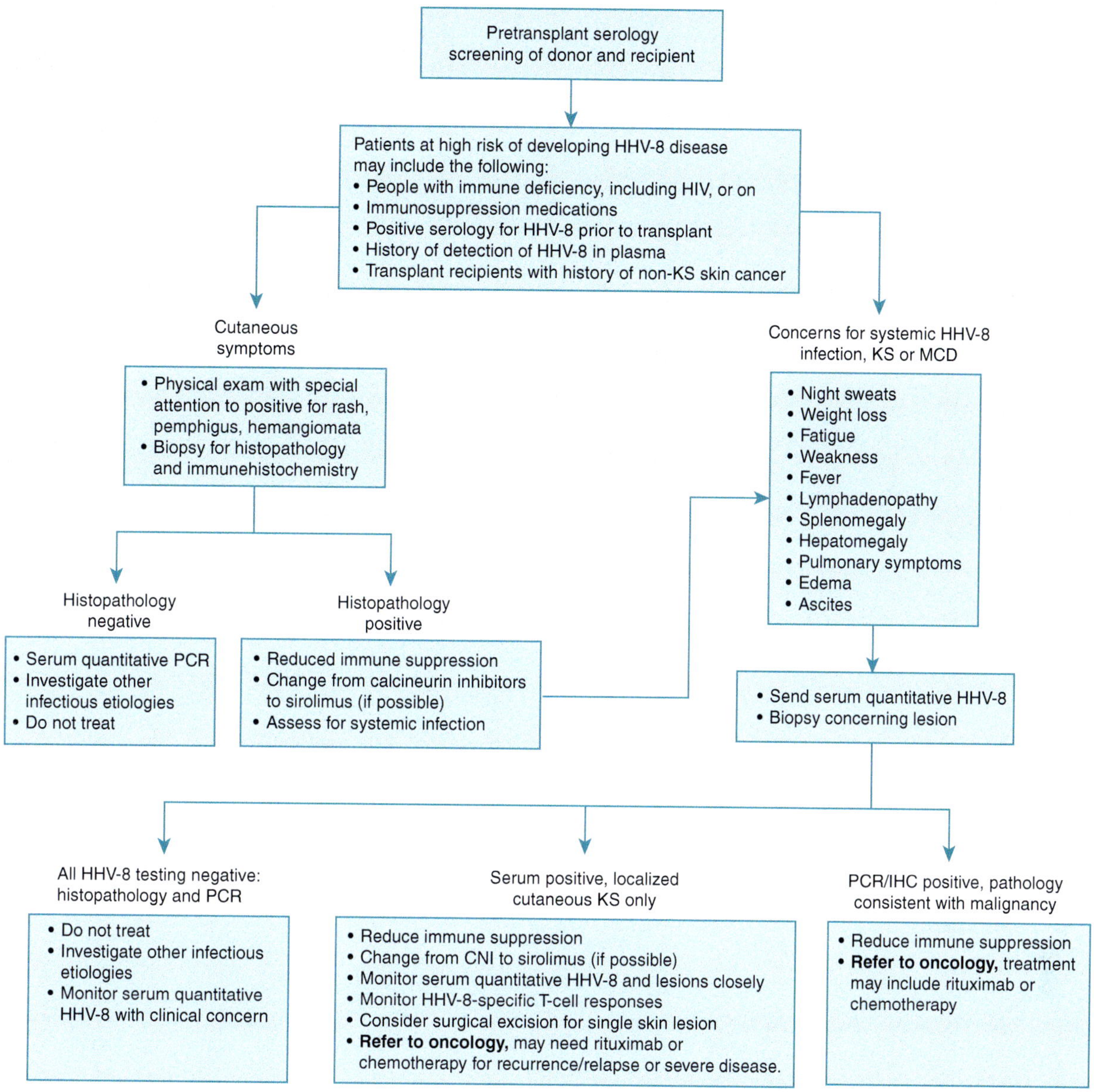

Fig. 20.3 Diagnosis of human herpesvirus 8 in solid organ transplant. *CNI*, calcineurin inhibitor; *CSF*, cerebrospinal fluid; *HHV*, human herpesvirus; *HIV*, human immunodeficiency virus; *KS*, Kaposi sarcoma; *LP*, lumbar puncture; *MCD*, multicentric Castleman's disease; *MRI*, magnetic resonance imaging; *PCR*, polymerase chain reaction.

TABLE 20.1 Treatment of HHV-6 in HSCT Patients

Indication	Medication	Dose	Duration	Monitoring
Treatment of HHV-6 disease, excluding encephalitis	*Foscarnet:* Active against HHV-6A, and HHV-6B *Ganciclovir:* active against HHV-6B, variable activity against HHV-6A	*Foscarnet:* 180 mg/kg per day divided q8h-q12h, can consider 90 mg/kg per day once daily if there is concern for renal insufficiency *Ganciclovir:* Induction: 5mg/kg IV q12h ×14-21 days *Maintenance:* 5mg/kg IV q24h	2 weeks, *OR* until improvement of end-organ disease	Repeat quantitative serum HHV-6 PCR weekly.
Treatment of HHV-6B infection, with encephalitis	Foscarnet *OR* Ganciclovir	*Foscarnet:* 180 mg/kg per day divided q8h *Ganciclovir:* 5mg/kg IV q 12h	3 weeks minimum	Recommend LP before initiation with quantitative CSF HHV-6 PCR. Consider repeat LP and quantitative CSF HHV-6 PCR if lack of improvement. Some experts would repeat the LP near the end of therapy to confirm viral clearance. Repeat quantitative serum HHV-6 PCR weekly.

CSF, cerebrospinal fluid; *h*, hour; JSCY, *IV*, intravenous; *LP*, lumbar puncture; *PCR*, polymerase chain reaction; *q*, every.

21

Respiratory Viruses

Alpana Waghmare, MD and Janet A. Englund, MD

EPIDEMIOLOGY AND RISK FACTORS

The seasonality of respiratory virus infections among immunocompromised children is similar to that in the community (Fig. 21.1). Respiratory syncytial virus (RSV) typically circulates in the community from November through March, with peak detection in January. Human metapneumovirus follows a similar pattern although often somewhat later. Influenza epidemiology can vary somewhat from year to year, with typical seasons lasting from December to March. Influenza A tends to be more predominant early in the season and influenza B is often seen later in the season. Up-to-date influenza surveillance data for the United States are published on the Centers for Disease Control and Prevention website (https://www.cdc.gov/flu/index.htm), and global surveillance data are maintained by the World Health Organization (https://www.who.int/influenza/surveillance_monitoring/updates/en/).

Parainfluenza viruses (PIVs) vary in seasonality by type. PIV-1 causes group epidemics in the autumn, generally every other year. PIV-2 infections usually follow the same pattern as PIV-1 and PIV-3 outbreaks, usually occuring in the spring. PIV-3 remains the most common PIV subtype detected in both hospitalized and outpatient studies, but newer molecular epidemiology suggests that either PIV-1 or PIV-4 may be the second most common PIV detected in children, depending on the year. PIV-4 may be detected year-round. Human rhinoviruses (HRVs) and human coronaviruses (HCoVs) are present at moderate levels year-round, although there may be peaks of certain strains over the course of the year.

Exposure to sick contacts is the single most well-described risk factor for respiratory viral acquisition in immunocompromised children. Respiratory viruses are typically transmitted by respiratory secretions through direct contact, via fomites, or by large droplet spread. Entry generally occurs through contact with nasal mucosa or eyes, in contrast to the less permissive oral route. Transmission by small-particle aerosols of RSV has not been proven and, if it occurs, it is an infrequent route. Clinical observations suggest PIVs and human metapneumovirus (HMPV) are transmitted similarly to RSV. Although PIV-1 and PIV-3 have been recovered from air samples collected in the vicinity of infected patients, direct contact and transmission via fomites are likely to be more important. The high initial and subsequent infection rates, as well as outbreaks reported in hematopoietic cell transplant (HCT) recipients in both inpatient and outpatient settings, demonstrate that these viruses spread readily and that a relatively small inoculum is likely able to cause infection.

Epidemiologic patterns of respiratory viral detection in children are roughly similar among HCT recipients, solid organ transplant (SOT) recipients, and oncology patients, although risk factors for viral detection are unique.

HCT Recipients. In a surveillance study of pediatric and adult HCT recipients in the first year after transplant, the most common viruses detected were HRV and HCoV, followed by PIV, adenovirus, RSV, influenza, HMPV, and human bocavirus.[1] In a separate multicenter retrospective study of pediatric HCT recipients, 16.6% of patient had at least one respiratory virus detected by PCR in the first year after HCT[2]; younger age was associated with viral detection in univariate analysis. Steroid exposure, neutropenia, and lymphopenia were commonly present in the week before respiratory viral onset.

SOT Recipients. In a large multicenter retrospective study of pediatric SOT recipients, the highest rates of inpatient respiratory virus infection occurred in intestine/abdominal multivisceral transplant recipients, followed by thoracic (heart/lung), liver, and kidney transplants.[3] HRV was the most common detected virus (45% of respiratory virus events), followed by RSV (22%), PIV (16%), HMPV (11%), and influenza (10%). Lymphopenia was present in 22% of patients with respiratory virus detected, although this was not evaluated as a risk factor for acquisition.

Oncology Patients. In a large cohort of pediatric cancer patients with fever and neutropenia, at least one respiratory virus was detected in 46% of subjects.[4] The most common respiratory viruses detected were HRV, RSV, PIV, influenza, adenovirus, and HMPV.

CLINICAL MANIFESTATIONS

In healthy individuals, most respiratory viral infections are associated with self-limited upper respiratory tract symptoms. Notable exceptions include a stronger association between RSV and bronchiolitis in young infants, PIV and laryngotracheobronchitis, and HRVs and reactive airway disease exacerbations. In immunocompromised patients, respiratory viral infections can be associated with prolonged shedding, lower respiratory tract disease, the need for supplemental oxygen, late airflow obstruction, and even death. Prolonged viral shedding can be associated with persistent respiratory symptoms or can be asymptomatic with durations up to 4 weeks (mean).[5] Persistent shedding of PIV in asymptomatic immunocompromised patients for many months has been noted using sensitive molecular detection methods,[6] and prolonged shedding has been described for HMPV, HCoVs, and HRVs.[7-9] Impairment of T-cell function appears to be commonly associated in children with prolonged shedding; additional risk factors in HCT recipients include initial high viral load, use of steroids, and myeloablative conditioning.[9]

Initial clinical symptoms related to RSV infection in immunocompromised hosts are similar to those in immunocompetent persons.

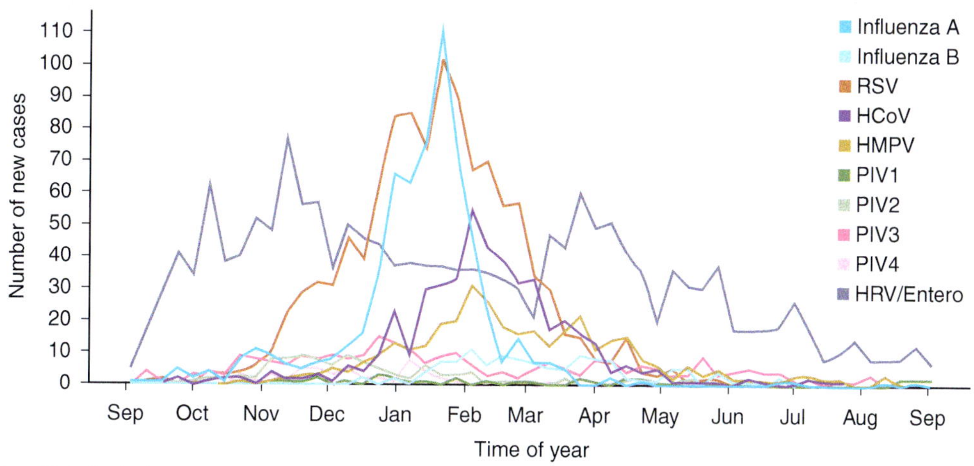

Fig. 21.1 Typical seasonal pattern of respiratory virus detection at a major pediatric medical center. *HRV/Entero,* human rhinovirus or enterovirus; *HCoV,* human coronavirus; *HMPV,* human metapneumovirus; *PIV,* parainfluenza virus; *RSV,* respiratory syncytial virus.

Upper respiratory tract infection may progress to lower respiratory tract disease, with likelihood of progression probably related to immune status. Over 1 to 2 weeks, lower respiratory tract involvement may become evident by increasing respiratory distress, worsening hypoxia, and potentially, the need for assisted ventilation. Children or adults who acquire RSV or HMPV during or shortly after chemotherapy for malignancy may also have severe, life-threatening disease.[10] Recovery after assisted ventilation for RSV and HMPV pneumonia occurs but remains uncommon despite advances in supportive care. The associated respiratory failure in severely immunocompromised patients may result in multiorgan system failure, with high mortality rates in patients requiring mechanical ventilation.[11,12] Severe and fatal infection attributed to HMPV has been reported in cancer patients, and HMPV is a relatively common cause of acute respiratory infection in children and adults with malignancy, HCT recipients or organ transplant recipients.[13] Risk factors for severe HMPV infection include lymphopenia.[7,10,13] Quantitative bronchoalveolar lavage (BAL) viral load has not been associated with mechanical ventilation or death for RSV, PIV, or HMPV in adult patients after HCT; however, the detection of respiratory virus RNA in serum has been associated with fatal outcomes.[11]

PIV infection with lower respiratory tract disease in immunosuppressed patients, particularly those in the immediate posttransplantation period, may result in a similar clinical picture, although the overall mortality rate may be less than that associated with RSV.[14,15] Many immunocompromised adults with PIV infection first present with symptoms of mild upper respiratory tract disease, but in contrast to RSV, influenza, and HMPV, detection of PIV-1 and PIV-3 in asymptomatic HCT recipients is relatively common, reported in 6 of 17 (35%) infection episodes in a prospective study.[6] Fewer than half of PIV-infected patients have a fever. In severely immunocompromised patients, such as allogeneic HCT recipients less than 100 days after transplant, PIV-3 is the most common PIV subtype detected, reported in 80% of 544 HCT recipients with PIV.[16] In all PIV-infected transplant recipients, infection may progress to lower respiratory tract disease with more serious disease linked to supplemental oxygen requirement, low monocyte counts, and high-dose steroid use. The detection of PIV in BAL or other lower respiratory tract specimens is associated with decreased survival overall in HCT recipients.[16] Higher pretransplant PIV-3 antibody levels were not protective against severe sequelae.[15] Concomitant infections with other viruses, fungi, or severe graft-versus-host disease are relatively common in adult patients with PIV pneumonitis.

Influenza remains a significant cause of morbidity and mortality in immunocompromised children and adults. In a recent multicenter review of immunocompromised children hospitalized with influenza, immunocompromised children were more likely to present with fever and less likely to present with respiratory distress. They were also less likely to require intensive care but were hospitalized longer.[17] In a study of adult and pediatric HCT and SOT recipients, 22.1% of subjects presented with pneumonia and 66.5% were hospitalized. Prior vaccination was associated with decreased disease severity.[18] Mortality after influenza was 2.9% in adults and 0% in pediatric patients in this study, although higher mortality rates have been previously reported.

With the increased use of molecular diagnostic assays, HRVs and HCoVs are now the most common respiratory viruses detected in immunocompromised patients. HRV can be detected in 20% to 30% of HCT recipients, with progression to lower respiratory tract infection occurring in 17% of patients.[1,19] Once HRV progresses, mortality rates can be similar to other respiratory viruses, including influenza, PIV, and RSV.[20] In addition to HRVs, other members of the *Enterovirus* genus, including Enterovirus-D68, can be associated with outbreaks and severe disease. Enterovirus D68 was associated with several hundred cases of severe respiratory illnesses in children in the United States in 2014 and 2018; severe disease was also seen in immunocompromised patients.[21] HCoVs can also be associated with severe disease in the lower respiratory tract and can result in death.[22] Specific considerations for HCT, SOT, and oncology patients are outlined in the following text.

HCT Recipients. HCT recipients of all ages may have a more fulminant course after respiratory viral infections, particularly if infection occurs around the time of transplantation. Risk factors for disease progression include lack of engraftment, decreased lymphocyte count, and older age. Evidence of pulmonary infiltrates on chest radiographs may be delayed or absent in patients with severe neutropenia but may become apparent after immune reconstitution or on chest computed tomography or magnetic resonance imaging. In a multicenter retrospective review of pediatric HCT recipients, the all-cause and attributable case-fatality rates within 3 months of hospitalized respiratory viral infection onset were 11% and 5.4%, respectively.[2] Lower respiratory tract infection was rare except in HMPV infections; fever was more common for influenza and HMPV. Multivariate models indicated that onset within 60 days of HCT, steroid use in the 7 days before onset, and the need for respiratory support at onset were associated with subsequent morbidity or death. Several risk scores have been proposed for adult HCT recipients with respiratory virus infections to predict the risk of progression to lower respiratory tract infection and mortality.[19]

SOT Recipients. In a large multicenter retrospective review, fever was the most common clinical sign detected, although a significant proportion had signs of lower respiratory tract infection at onset (35%).[3] Detection of any respiratory viral infection in SOT recipients was associated with an all-cause and attributable case-fatality rate of 4% and 0%, respectively. Receipt of an abdominal/intestinal multivisceral transplant was associated with increased risk of all-cause death in multivariable models. Overall, approximately 50% of patients with respiratory viral infections required some form of respiratory support.

Oncology Patients. Adults with leukemia and profound chemotherapy-induced myelosuppression are also at risk of fatal outcome from respiratory viruses. In pediatric patients with fever and neutropenia, episodes caused by different types of respiratory viruses had no differences in the clinical outcome (days of hospitalization, days of fever, oxygen requirement, admission to the intensive care unit, and death) and when comparing patients with a single virus versus coinfection.[4]

DISEASE PROPHYLAXIS/PREVENTION

Influenza Vaccination

The mainstay of influenza prevention in immunocompromised children is vaccination. Inactivated influenza vaccine (IIV) is recommended for all patients 6 months and older with hematologic malignancies by the Infectious Diseases Society of America (IDSA) guidelines. Vaccination is not recommended for in patients receiving intensive chemotherapy, such as induction or consolidation chemotherapy for acute leukemia, or those who have received anti–B-cell antibodies in the past 6 months.[23] Live attenuated influenza vaccine (LAIV) should not be used for immunosuppressed patients except in an outbreak setting when LAIV is determined to be a more effective option owing to strain type. Quadrivalent vaccine should be offered when available. Studies are ongoing to assess the immunogenicity and safety of high-dose influenza vaccination in immunocompromised adults and children.

Influenza vaccination is recommended for all family members, close contacts, and health care workers caring for immunocompromised patients. LAIV is not recommended for household contacts of HCT recipients (within 2 months after transplant), or those with severe immunosuppression as the result of graft-versus-host disease or severe combined immune deficiency.[23] If LAIV is given to persons caring for severely immunosuppressed patients, the Centers for Disease Control and Prevention guidelines recommend avoidance of contact for 7 days after vaccination.[24]

HCT Recipients. Immune responses to influenza vaccination are likely more effective further out from HCT. HCT recipients 6 months or older should receive IIV annually starting 6 months after transplant or starting 4 months after transplant during a community outbreak of influenza,[23] with second doses recommended for children depending on time from transplant. In reduced intensity HCT, pretransplant vaccination may be appropriate as host immunity is expected to extend into the early transplant period. High-dose vaccination is currently under study in pediatric and adult HCT recipients.

SOT Recipients. IDSA guidelines recommend against administering influenza vaccine during intensified immunosuppression, including the first 2-month posttransplant period, because of the likelihood of inadequate response. However, during a community outbreak, IIV can be administered 1 month or later after transplant.[23] Earlier vaccination has been supported by recent studies, and more data regarding high-dose vaccine and repeat vaccine dosing within a season are also becoming available.[25]

Oncology Patients. IIV is recommended for all patients older than 6 months with hematologic malignancies, although IDSA guidelines do not recommend vaccination in patients receiving intensive chemotherapy, such as induction or consolidation chemotherapy for acute leukemia, or those who have received anti–B-cell antibodies in the past 6 months.[23] Although immune responses are generally lower in children with malignancies, a recent Cochrane review demonstrated reductions in respiratory infections and hospitalization; however, the quality of evidence is low.[26]

Influenza Chemoprophylaxis

Postexposure chemoprophylaxis should be considered in immunosuppressed patients who are in close contact with confirmed influenza cases or during influenza outbreaks.[27] In outbreak settings, HCT recipients should receive vaccine immediately if they are 4 months or longer posttransplant. Chemoprophylaxis with oseltamivir or zanamivir should also be initiated for 2 weeks after vaccination while immunity develops.[27] Chemoprophylaxis is also recommended for HCT recipients who are less than 24 months posttransplant or those who remain substantially immunocompromised at 24 months or longer after HCT, regardless of vaccination history. For SOT, similar concerns regarding vaccine response in the early posttransplant period exist and chemoprophylaxis should be considered, although recommendations regarding the timing of this strategy are lacking.[28] Season-long prophylaxis has been evaluated in a randomized trial of SOT and HCT and showed reduction in culture- or polymerase chain reaction (PCR)-confirmed influenza, although this approach is not universally used and may be targeted to periods of high influenza virus circulation.[29] Antiviral resistance may emerge with widespread prophylaxis; drug resistance patterns of circulating strains should be considered when initiating prophylaxis and/or preemptive therapy.

Other Vaccines in Development

New advances in the understanding of RSV and HMPV, including the characterization of the RSV fusion (F) protein in its preinfusion and postfusion states, have contributed to the development of new RSV vaccines and monoclonal antibodies with the potential to be used for prophylaxis against RSV. Vaccines stimulating antibody directed to the F protein, and specifically to the pre-F protein, are now under development. RSV-specific serum-neutralizing antibodies are efficiently transferred from the mother to the newborn, and ongoing clinical trials may offer potential protection against RSV in family members and health care workers surrounding immunocompromised patients, with the potential to protect these patients. Candidate vaccines against PIV and HMPV, as well as chimeric vaccines containing genes from more than one virus, have also been tested in preclinical models.

Prophylaxis for Other Viruses

The identification of serum-neutralizing antibody as a correlate of protection against serious RSV lower respiratory tract disease has been an important advance. Although a humanized monoclonal antibody directed against the RSV F protein, palivizumab, has been licensed since 1998 to prevent RSV disease in young children with underlying cardiac or pulmonary disease, it is also currently used in children who are severely immunocompromised, such as infants with severe combined immune deficiency or congenital leukemia. Children younger than 24 months who are profoundly immunocompromised may be considered for palivizumab prophylaxis. The development of a potent and long-acting RSV monoclonal antibody directed against the pre-F protein of RSV is undergoing clinical trials in young infants. This, or similar products, may be available in the future to prevent RSV infection or disease in transplant candidates. Passive immunoprophylaxis against PIV and HMPV infection has not been studied in children.

DIAGNOSIS

Sample Type and Handling

The diagnosis of respiratory viral infections is critically dependent on the type and quality of the clinical specimen and proper handling of the specimen. The preferred specimens for the diagnosis of respiratory viruses in immunocompromised hosts are respiratory secretions obtained as a mid-turbinate or nasopharyngeal swab, nasal wash, nasal aspirate, or bronchoalveolar lavage. A nasal wash specimen is the classic sample used for viral diagnosis by culture and for obtaining samples to assess cytokines or antibodies.

Nasopharyngeal swabs and mid-turbinate swabs are not as sensitive as nasal washes for viral diagnosis using culture but have good diagnostic yields with molecular detection methods. In general, molecular methods of detection are preferred over fluorescent antigen-antibody detection or antigen detection tests in immunocompromised patients. Specimens from children are often more readily diagnosed than those from adults owing to higher viral loads. Other clinical specimens useful for the detection of respiratory viruses in patients of all ages include endotracheal aspirates collected from intubated patients, bronchoalveolar lavage, nasal mucosal epithelium collected by scraping, sputum, and lung tissue obtained by biopsy or at autopsy.

Nucleic Acid Detection

Molecular diagnostics, such as multiplex real-time PCR, have replaced cell culture, fluorescent antigen-antibody detection, and antigen detection methodologies because they have high sensitivity and specificity, excellent quality control procedures, and detect a large battery of viral and bacterial pathogens rapidly in a single sample. The use of molecular diagnostics has significantly improved the yield of detection. Numerous rapid multiplex PCR assays are now commercially available that can detect up to 18 or more viruses simultaneously. These assays are sensitive and specific and can detect RSV, HMPV, influenza, HRVs, and HCoVs and differentiate all four PIV subtypes.

TREATMENT

Supportive Treatment

The potential hypoxemia, apnea, and poor oral intake resulting from infection in young infants, both previously healthy as well as moderately or severely immunocompromised, requires close medical management. Hospitalization may be required for immunocompromised children younger than 1 year, particularly if intravenous (IV) fluid replacement and oxygen therapy are necessary. Systemic or inhaled steroids and bronchodilator therapies are not recommended for treatment of RSV, based on studies that failed to show decreased time in the hospital or improved outcomes.[30] Children with airway obstruction or signs of hypoxia require admission to an intensive care setting for close monitoring, and children with severe disease may require intubation. Supportive care for lower respiratory tract infections caused by PIV and HMPV in immunocompromised hosts similarly may require hospitalization and adjunct therapy, including IV fluids and oxygen support, as well as aggressive therapy of secondary fungal, bacterial, or viral infections.

Antiviral Treatment

Respiratory Syncytial Virus. Ribavirin, a synthetic guanosine nucleoside, has been licensed for the treatment of RSV respiratory disease in children since 1986 and for the treatment of RSV disease in patients undergoing mechanical ventilation since 1993. Ribavirin is the only approved drug for lower respiratory tract disease caused by RSV, but concerns regarding efficacy, difficulties in administration, and the extremely high cost of the drug have resulted in minimal current use of the drug.[31] Ribavirin is available in aerosolized, oral, and IV forms. Several retrospective studies, including a pooled analysis, have shown aerosolized or oral ribavirin is protective against disease progression to lower respiratory tract infection and mortality in HCT recipients; however, conclusive evidence of efficacy from randomized trials is not available.[32] In patients with leukemia, multivariate models demonstrated similar effects.[33] Oral ribavirin has been retrospectively evaluated in patients receiving chemotherapy or in HCT recipients, suggesting a possible effect of oral ribavirin; however, lack of randomized controls has been a limitation in all studies.[34]

In adult HCT and hematologic malignancy patients with RSV lower respiratory tract infection, use of aerosolized ribavirin was associated with decreased mortality. Oral or IV ribavirin although not statistically significant as the effect was smaller.[11,12] Of note, some data suggest pediatric HCT recipients with RSV have little morbidity and mortality even without ribavirin therapy.[35] Current international guidelines recommend aerosolized or systemic (oral or IV) ribavirin with intravenous immunoglogulin (IVIG) in patients with RSV upper respiratory tract infection undergoing allogeneic HCT, allogeneic HCT recipients with risk factors for progression to lower respiratory tract infection, and allogeneic HCT patients with lower respiratory tract infection.[36] Recommendations for ribavirin administration for HCT and SOT recipients, and oncology patients are outlined in Table 21.1. Most data and guidance for use of ribavirin are in HCT and oncology; few studies have clearly demonstrated efficacy in SOT recipients, and most data are in lung transplant when both oral and IV ribavirin have been used,[37] For HCT and oncology patients, high-risk situations include patients with lymphopenia; additional risk factors, such as smoking history and use of high-dose total body irradiation, could be used to further risk-stratify patients. In general, aerosolized ribavirin is reserved for subjects with virologically confirmed (BAL positive for RSV) lower respiratory tract infection. It is administered by small-particle aerosol from a solution containing the drug at a concentration of 20 mg/mL sterile water via aerosol for 2 to 20 hours/day, or at a concentration of 60 mg/mL water over 2 hours 3 times daily. Aerosol administration results in high levels of ribavirin in the secretions, with levels exceeding 1000 μM and little systemic absorption. The potential environmental release of ribavirin has caused concern in hospital personnel because of the potential teratogenicity of ribavirin and thus exposure is contraindicated in pregnant women because of its teratogenic potential. Administration of ribavirin via a ventilator, using a high-dose, short-duration method of drug delivery or with a vacuum-exhausted treatment hood, results in minimal or no detectable ribavirin in the rooms of treated children.

Oral ribavirin can be considered in patients weighing more than 15kg; hemolytic anemia is the most important side effect to consider, and patients should be monitored carefully.

Systemic antibody therapy, combined antibody therapy with ribavirin, and aerosolized antibodies have been used to treat RSV disease. The combination of high-titer RSV immunoglobulin and ribavirin has been associated with therapeutic success in uncontrolled studies in

TABLE 21.1 Prevention and Treatment of Respiratory Viral Infections for Pediatric Hematopoietic Cell Transplant Recipients, Solid Organ Transplant Recipients, and Oncology Patients

Virus	Prophylaxis	Asymptomatic Shedding	Upper Respiratory Tract Infection	Lower Respiratory Tract Infection
RSV	• Infection control procedures • Palivizumab for children ≤2 years (during season) undergoing HCT	• Isolation	• Isolation • HCT and Oncology: Ribavirin for high-risk situations[a,b,c] • SOT: limited data; consider oral ribavirin in lung transplant	• Isolation • Low-risk situations in HCT and oncology: consider oral ribavirin[b] • High-risk situations in HCT and oncology: consider aerosolized ribavirin initially followed by oral[b,c] • SOT: consider oral or aerosolized ribavirin in lung transplant • Supportive care
Influenza A/B	• Infection control procedures • Vaccination of contacts • Vaccination 2-3 weeks before HCT in non-immunodeficient recipients of nonmyeloablative conditioning • Vaccination of post-HCT recipients: starting 6 months after transplant or starting 4 months after transplant during a community outbreak • Vaccination of SOT recipients: 2 months after transplant, earlier if outbreak; guidelines may change • Vaccination of oncology patients: no vaccination in patients receiving intensive chemotherapy or those who have received anti–B-cell antibodies in the past 6 months	• Isolation • Oseltamivir or zanamivir	• Isolation • Oseltamivir or zanamivir	• Isolation • Oseltamivir or zanamivir • Consider combination therapy with baloxavir if ≥ 12 years, or rimantadine (only influenza A) and/or ribavirin • Consider IV peramivir if mechanically ventilated • Supportive care
PIV	• Infection control procedures	• Isolation	• Isolation • Consider reduction of steroid dose	• Isolation • Supportive care • Consider ribavirin if mechanically ventilated[b]
HMPV	• Infection control procedures	• Isolation	• Isolation	• Isolation • Supportive care • Consider ribavirin if mechanically ventilated[b]
HRV	• Infection control procedures	• Isolation	• Isolation	• Isolation • Supportive care
HCoV	• Infection control procedures	• Isolation	• Isolation	• Isolation • Supportive care

[a]Because of recent price increases, most centers have restrictions on the use of aerosolized ribavirin.
[b]Benefit and dosing of oral ribavirin not clearly understood.
[c]High risk: lymphopenia, smoking history, and use of high-dose total-body irradiation.
HCoV, human coronavirus; *HCT,* hematopoietic cell transplant; *HMPV,* human metapneumovirus; *HRV,* human rhinovirus; *IV,* intravenous; *PIV,* parainfluenza virus; *RSV,* respiratory syncytial virus; *SOT,* solid organ transplant.

severely immunocompromised adults with RSV disease but has not been confirmed in others. A small, nonrandomized unadjusted analysis in pediatric cancer patients with RSV lower respiratory tract infection suggested a beneficial effect of adjunctive palivizumab or IVIG.[38] Larger studies of HCT recipients with RSV lower respiratory tract infection were unable to demonstrate improved outcomes with adjunctive palivizumab[11,12]; palivizumab is not currently recommended for treatment of RSV infection in any immunocompromised patients.

The duration of ribavirin therapy in immunocompromised hosts is generally at least 3 days. Initiation of antiviral therapy at the stage of upper respiratory tract disease may decrease viral load and possibly reduce the risk of respiratory failure, although most data are based on retrospective uncontrolled data.

Influenza. Early influenza treatment is recommended for all immunocompromised individuals, although there may be benefit even with delayed treatment.[39] M2 inhibitors (amantadine and rimantadine) are currently ineffective, and neuraminidase inhibitors (NAIs) are now first-line therapy for prophylaxis and treatment of influenza. NAIs available in the United States include oral oseltamivir, inhaled zanamivir, IV peramivir, and baloxavir. Clinical efficacy with oseltamivir and inhaled zanamivir has been demonstrated in patients with leukemia or HCT recipients.[18] Many mutations causing oseltamivir and peramivir resistance, including the common *H275Y* mutation in A(H1N1)pdm09 influenza, do not confer resistance to zanamivir[40] and inhaled zanamivir may be used to treat these strains. IV peramivir used during the 2009 pandemic in severely ill patients was well tolerated, with evidence of recovery in most patients.[41] In a randomized trial comparing IV peramivir to oral oseltamivir in hospitalized adults, clinical outcomes were similar.[42] The optimal duration of peramivir therapy has not been determined for immunocompromised hosts. Longer treatment courses (10 days), although not higher doses, with oseltamivir or zanamivir have been suggested, given the potential for recurrence and the median time for progression to lower respiratory tract infection. Baloxavir was recently approved for treatment of uncomplicated influenza in adults and adolescents[43]; studies in younger children and immunocompromised hosts are underway.

Multidrug-resistant influenza strains have been identified in immunocompromised patients. Triple-combination antiviral therapy with amantadine, ribavirin, and oseltamivir has been proposed to treat immunocompromised patients with severe influenza A with resistance to oseltamivir. A randomized trial comparing triple-combination antiviral therapy with oseltamivir alone in high-risk adults demonstrated an effect on viral outcomes but no clinical benefit.[44]

Parainfluenza. In a retrospective study of patients with leukemia or HCT recipients with PIV infection, ribavirin had no impact on viral shedding, symptom and hospitalization length, progression to lower respiratory tract infection, or mortality.[45] A systematic review evaluated aerosolized or systemic ribavirin in 10 retrospective studies in this same population and found no difference in PIV-associated mortality or in progression to lower respiratory tract infection.[46] Given lack of evidence of clinical efficacy, ribavirin is not recommended for PIV infections. The impact of IVIG alone remains to be determined, although IVIG administration for PIV lower respiratory tract infection did not reduce mortality.[16]

Other Respiratory Viruses. The management of other respiratory viral infections in immunosuppressed patients is generally supportive (Table 21.2). Ribavirin has shown efficacy against HMPV in vitro and in mouse models, with anecdotal reports describing its use in severe infection in immunocompromised hosts (with and without IVIG). Lack of controlled studies of ribavirin and the known toxicities of therapy, including hemolytic anemia, limit its recommendation for HMPV. Currently, no approved antiviral agents exist for treatment of HCoV, HRV, HBoV, or enteroviruses, although some investigational agents are upcoming. The use of IVIG has not been evaluated prospectively and is not routinely recommended for treatment of respiratory viral infections. Some centers routinely check and replete immunoglobulins, but the impact on respiratory virus acquisition and severity is not known.

New Therapeutics Under Investigation

New RSV antiviral candidates have been investigated, including presatovir (Gilead Sciences , Foster City, CA), an oral RSV fusion inhibitor, and lumicitabine (Alios/Janssen, Titusville, NJ), an RSV nucleoside analog acting on the RSV viral polymerase. Both antivirals have been tested in human challenge models and have successfully demonstrated antiviral efficacy. Presatovir subsequently underwent two large placebo-controlled clinical efficacy trials for the treatment of RSV in placebo-controlled studies conducted in 185 and 60 adult HSCT patients with upper and lower respiratory tract infections, respectively. Clinical trial endpoints of efficacy were not met for presatovir; studies with lumicitabine have also been suspended. New studies of another nucleoside analog, JNJ-53718678 (Janssen), are underway in young children. Nanobodies, small antibody-like molecules derived from the heavy-chain variable Ig domains that occur naturally in camels, are being developed to be administered by inhalation for the treatment of RSV infection (Ablynx NV, Ghent, Belgium). Vaccines for RSV and PIV are under development, as discussed earlier.

A new potential antiviral therapy for PIV and other sialic acid–binding viruses targets the lung epithelial sialic acid receptor for PIV, thereby preventing viral entry. A novel recombinant sialidase fusion protein, DAS181 (Ansun Biopharma, San Diego, CA), first developed as an antiviral agent for influenza, functions by cleaving sialic acid from the host cell surface, thereby inactivating the host cell receptor recognized by PIV. Successful use of this agent in pediatric and adult transplant recipients under compassionate use has been reported, and clinical trials in immunocompromised subjects are ongoing.

Several studies of novel influenza therapeutics are under investigation, including the NAIs IV zanamivir and laninamivir, monoclonal antibodies, viral polymerase inhibitors, and nitazoxanide. The performance and safety of these newer agents remain to be seen in immunocompromised children.

TABLE 21.2 Diagnosis of Respiratory Viral Infections in Pediatric Immunocompromised Patients

Virus	Specimen Type	Real Time RT-PCR Assays	Enzyme-Based Immunoassay	Fluorescent Antigen Detection	Culture
Influenza A/B	Nasopharyngeal aspirate, nasal wash, nasal swab, bronchoalveolar lavage	Widely available	Widely available	Available	Limited availability
RSV			Widely available	Available	Limited availability
HMPV			Not available	Available	Limited availability
PIVs			Not available	Available	Limited availability
HRV			Not available	Not available	Limited availability
HCoVs			Not available	Not available	Not available
Test advantages		Sensitive, specific, and ability to be rapid (within 1 hour); typing, determination of viral load, and sequencing possible	Rapid but less sensitive (particularly for low viral loads); relatively inexpensive	Less expensive, rapid; assess quality of specimen; not as sensitive as RT-PCR	Becoming less available and increasingly expensive; not all viruses readily identified in culture (HRV, HCoV, PIV). Results take time but enable typing and analysis of viral strains

HCoV, human coronavirus; *HMPV,* human metapneumovirus; *HRV,* human rhinovirus; *PIV,* parainfluenza virus; *RSV,* respiratory syncytial virus; *RT-PCR,* reverse transcriptase polymerase chain reaction.

INFECTION PREVENTION AND ANTICIPATORY GUIDANCE

Nosocomial Outbreaks

RSV, PIVs, and HMPVs are common causes of nosocomial infections contributing to significant morbidity and mortality in pediatric wards. Nosocomial RSV and PIV infections in adults with leukemia and bone marrow transplants are associated with a high mortality rate.[5,14] The transmission of identical strains of RSV from the outpatient setting into the hospital has been documented, demonstrating the importance of infection control measures. Nosocomial transmission of HMPV also occurs, with outbreaks in both inpatient and outpatient units. In one study, 15 patients were diagnosed with HMPV within 7 weeks in a tertiary care cancer unit.[7] Molecular subtyping revealed infection with genotype A2a virus, implicating nosocomial transmission. Four patients (26.6%) died of HMPV-associated pneumonia and consequent multiorgan failure.

Nosocomial outbreaks characteristically occur from multiple introductions of community respiratory viral strains as well as patient-to-patient spread (perhaps with health care providers as intermediaries). For prevention of nosocomial transmission, contact isolation precautions are effective, provided that compliance with the policy is maintained among personnel. Hospital personnel may play a role in the transmission of RSV and other respiratory viruses to susceptible patients. Viral spreading can be limited by adherence to strict handwashing procedures and cohorting of infected and exposed individuals. Use of gloves, masks, and goggles in the hospital setting also limits spread. Such strict measures are appropriate in high-risk settings such as pediatric intensive care units or bone marrow transplant wards. Restriction of visitors, including young children, in hospital wards with patients at high risk for RSV infection may be necessary during epidemic periods in the community. Continued compliance through the respiratory virus season by all members of the health care team is critical.

The importance of isolation based on symptoms as opposed to positive viral test results has been shown, but prolonged shedding of respiratory viruses with even minimal symptoms may complicate efforts of infection control. Patients known or suspected to be infected with influenza, RSV, PIV, or HMPV should be kept in contact isolation or cohorted until symptoms have resolved and repeated sensitive diagnostic test results are negative.[27] PIV outbreaks may be difficult to bring under control owing to prolonged asymptomatic shedding, particularly in young children and immunocompromised hosts.[6]

Infections in HCT candidates

International guidelines recommend deferral of conditioning therapy in patients with respiratory infections prior to allogeneic HCT,[36,47] with low strength of evidence. The concern for progressive illness from respiratory viral infection needs to be balanced against concern for underlying disease progression and donor availability. In a large prospective study, respiratory viruses were detected in 116 of 458 HCT patients before transplantation, and viral detection was associated with prolonged hospitalization and lower survival at day 100.[48] This risk was also present in patients with HRV alone. A recent retrospective review of HRV detected in pediatric HCT recipients demonstrated that HRV detection without the presence of lower respiratory tract infection was not associated with decreased days alive and out of the hospital, suggesting the HCT delay is not always warranted.[49] These data should ideally be validated in larger, multicenter studies. The impact of other factors such as viral-specific risk scores, location of infection and viral load, need to be evaluated. In pediatric patients, diagnostic PCR should be considered on all transplant candidates, regardless of symptoms, and transplant delay should be considered, if feasible, with ongoing symptoms or evidence of lower respiratory tract infection.

Infections in SOT candidates

For SOT candidates, there are limited data examining clinical outcomes for pretransplant respiratory viral infections and often organ availability is a significant consideration on proceeding with transplantation. Specific clinical circumstances, such as duration of infection and severity of symptoms, should be considered. Donor transmission of influenza is of particular concern in lung or small bowel transplantation; however, non-lung and non–small bowel organs can be considered after donor antiviral treatment for 48 hours coupled with treatment of the recipient.[50] No clear guidance exists for other respiratory viruses, and decisions regarding organ use from infected donors should be evaluated on a case-by-case basis.

22

Adenoviruses

Diana F. Florescu, MD and Erica J. Stohs, MD, MPH

ADENOVIRUSES

In the past few decades, significant progress has been made in understanding the epidemiology of adenovirus infections and developing preventative and therapeutic strategies. However, adenovirus infections remain a clinical and diagnostic challenge. Isolation of adenovirus does not necessarily correlate with invasive disease because the virus may persist asymptomatically in lymphocytes.

Adenoviruses are classified within seven species (A through G) based on guanine and cytosine content in the DNA, ability to agglutinate red blood cells, and chemical and biophysical criteria; the species A through F circulate globally.[1] To date, 51 serotypes and 90 genotypes have been described; genomic variants can be identified within the same serotype.[1] About one-third of the known serotypes have been associated with disease in the immunocompetent pediatric population, with serotypes 1 through 5, 7, 21, and 41 most commonly identified. Adenoviruses display broad tissue tropism and can infect several cell types, but certain serotypes manifest as specific clinical infections (Table 22.1).[1] The predominant serotypes vary among different continents and countries and change over time as transmission of new strains replace existing dominant serotypes.[1]

Species C serotypes, commonly associated with respiratory tract infections in young children, can enter a latent phase that can last years with intermittent release of live virus in stool after resolution of the primary infection.[2] Small quantities of replicating and nonreplicating adenovirus DNA have been found in lung epithelial cells, the central nervous system, tonsils, and adenoids in the absence of acute infection; the majority of adenovirus DNA is isolated from the T-lymphocyte population.[2,3]

Latency is characterized by evasion from immune surveillance and expression of viral proteins by the host cell without complete replication of the adenovirus.[3] Several mechanisms contribute to latency: blockage by viral proteins of cellular apoptosis, cellular immune response, release of antiinflammatory and lytic cytokines, and down-regulation of major histocompatibility complex class I molecules.[3] Viral latency poses challenges in interpretation of detection of adenovirus DNA in stool and respiratory specimens. As humans are the only reservoir for adenovirus, the intermittent shedding of the virus in the airways and stool maintains the transmission of the viruses in the population.

Guidelines have established definitions of adenovirus infection and adenovirus disease.[4,5] Adenovirus infection is defined by detection of adenovirus in stool, blood, urine, or upper airway specimens by viral culture, antigen tests, or polymerase chain reaction (PCR) from asymptomatic patients.[4-6] Adenovirus disease is defined by detection of adenovirus in biopsy specimens (by immunohistochemical stain) or from bronchoalveolar lavage and cerebrospinal fluid (by culture, antigen detection, or PCR), in the absence of an alternative diagnosis, and in the presence of attributable signs and symptoms.[5,7] In leukemia and hematopoietic stem cell transplant (HSCT) patients, adenoviral disease may be classified as probable (adenovirus infection plus corresponding symptoms and signs without histologic confirmation) or proven (adenovirus infection plus corresponding symptoms related to the infection and histologic confirmation of the virus in the appropriate location).[4] Disseminated disease is defined by involvement of two or more organs, excluding DNAemia.[5,7] These definitions were developed mainly for consistency in outcome designation across research studies; however, the distinction between adenovirus infection and disease remains challenging in clinical practice.

EPIDEMIOLOGY AND RISK FACTORS

Adenoviruses are isolated more frequently in pediatric than adult solid organ and hematopoietic stem cell transplant recipients, with the highest incidence in children younger than 5 years and a decreased incidence toward adolescence.[1,8] As in the general population, adenovirus infections and disease in immunocompromised hosts do not have seasonal variability, although most are diagnosed in winter and spring.[9,10] Adenoviruses can be transmitted in several ways: (1) via the respiratory route by infected aerosols, by conjunctival inoculation, by person-to-person contact, by fomites, or by the fecal-oral route[11]; (2) through the transplanted organ[3]; or (3) through reactivation of a latent infection.[5,6] The majority of infections are community acquired in immunocompetent hosts, but nosocomial transmission has been described among hospitalized pediatric recipients.[6,12] The incubation period ranges from 2 days to 2 weeks, depending on the adenovirus serotype and mechanism of transmission.[3]

Solid Organ Transplantation

The incidence of adenovirus infections among solid organ transplant (SOT) recipients depends on the allograft type and degree of immunosuppression (Table 22.2). The majority of the infections are diagnosed within the first few months after transplantation,[3,6,12-14] but late infections have been described in pediatric SOT recipients.[13,15] Overall, infections are diagnosed early after transplantation at a median time of 1 month (0.5 to 10 months) in one study[12] and 1.64 months (0.03 to 153 months) in another study.[10] Early infections can suggest donor-derived infections, viral reactivation, or nosocomial infection.[1]

Risk factors for adenovirus disease are not well established in solid organ transplantation. Adenovirus serologic mismatch seems to be a potential risk factor, but standard screening of adenovirus serology and risk stratification based on donor and recipient serostatus are not

TABLE 22.1 Common Disease Association With Adenovirus Serotypes in Immunocompromised Patients

Adenovirus Serotype	Common Disease Association in Immunocompromised Patients
1-7; genotype 55	Respiratory tract infections
3; 7; 11; 21; 33-35	Urinary tract infection, hemorrhagic cystitis
12; 17; 31; 40; 41	Gastroenteritis
1; 3; 5; 7	Hepatitis
3-4; 7-8, 11; 14; 19; 37; genotypes 53, 54, 56	Keratoconjunctivitis

TABLE 22.2 Reported Adenovirus Incidence in Solid Organ Transplantation by Allograft Type

Allograft Type	Reported Adenovirus Incidence (%)
Kidney	11
Liver	3.5-38
Heart/lung/heart-lung	7-50
Intestinal, multivisceral	4.3-57.1

currently indicated.[5] Younger age seems to be an independent risk factor, especially children younger than 5 years, most likely because they are immunologically naïve and have higher exposure rate.[3,6,13] Pinchoff and colleagues reported adenovirus disease only in the pediatric intestinal transplant recipients in their cohort, whereas invasive disease did not develop in any of their adult intestinal transplant recipients during the same study period.[6] Adenoviruses persist in tonsillar lymphocytes in about 80% of children investigated, and the number of adenoviral genomes per lymphoid cell tends to decline with age.[16] Allograft type has an indirect correlation with the risk of adenovirus infections. Allografts with large amounts of lymphoid tissue (such as the intestine) pose a high risk of rejection, requiring more intense immunosuppressive regimens.[1,5] This lymphoid tissue could also be a reservoir of adenovirus. The degree of immunosuppression seems to be directly correlated with the rates of adenovirus infections; the highest prevalence of infections is reported early after transplantation.[1,5] Immunosuppression affecting more T-cell–mediated immunity, such as lytic therapy (OKT3 or ATG) for induction or steroid-resistant rejection[1,5,15] seems to be play an important role. The infections tend to resolve with reduction in immunosuppression.[5] A lower absolute lymphocyte count might be a risk factor for adenovirus disease but not adenovirus infection.[17]

Few risk factors for progression from asymptomatic infection to adenovirus disease have been described in solid organ transplant recipients:

1. Detection of the virus in the first months after transplantation
2. Repeated detection of adenovirus from the same site
3. Identification of adenovirus from two or more sites
4. Initial high adenovirus DNAemia, although a clear threshold has not been established
5. Intensification of immunosuppression, and
6. A more than 10-fold rise of viral load in the blood might be associated with fatal disease.[6,12,18]

Based on the available data, the latest American Society of Transplantation guidelines do not recommend routine screening for adenovirus DNAemia as it is unclear if asymptomatic DNAemia would require treatment, and the side effects associated with cidofovir use would outweigh the benefits.[5]

Hematopoietic Stem Cell Transplantation

Adenovirus infection rates between 8% and 28% have been reported in pediatric recipients of a HSCT,[19] considerably higher than in adults (3% to 15%).[3] Fifty percent of these infections progress to disease[4] with a case-fatality rate exceeding 50%.[19] Adenovirus in autologous HSCT patients is relatively rare,[4] whereas infection is more common in allogeneic HSCT patients, particularly in the first 100 days after transplant.[7] In 12 screening studies performed in children undergoing allogeneic HSCT, the incidence of adenovirus DNAemia ranged from 6% to 28%.[4] Younger age is associated with an increased risk of adenovirus infection and disease.[8,19,20] One retrospective study of 328 pediatric allogeneic HSCT patients found that children younger than 5 years 2.3 times as likely to develop adenovirus infection than those older than 5 years.[8]

Risk factors for adenovirus infection and disease are well established in pediatric allogeneic HSCT. They include the following: (1) use of T-cell depletion, (2) unrelated donor graft, (3) unrelated cord blood graft, (4) grades III and IV graft-versus-host disease (GVHD), and (5) severe lymphopenia (<300 CD3 cells/μL of peripheral blood).[3,4,11] Treatment with the anti-CD52 antibody alemtuzumab or antithymocyte globulin is also described as an independent risk factor of adenovirus infection.[3] Lack of adenovirus-specific T cells, and more generally, delayed recovery of lymphocyte count, is associated with delayed clearance of adenovirus infection.[3]

In pediatric allogeneic HSCT recipients, onset of invasive adenovirus infection and disseminated disease is often preceded by replication and detection of the virus in the gastrointestinal tract.[11,21] In one study of 138 pediatric recipients of a HSCT, rapidly increasing viral copies in serial stool specimens, particularly exceeding log 6.0, preceded onset of DNAemia by a median of 11 days.[21] Additional studies have confirmed the phenomenon of stool viral replication preceding DNAemia, although the threshold for stool copy number varies based on the molecular method used.[11] Another study correlated stool adenovirus copy number with histopathology for biopsy samples in pediatric HSCT patients and found that persistent adenovirus infection in gastrointestinal lymphoid tissue, particularly in the terminal ileum, correlated with adenovirus recurrence after transplant.[22] Critically high viral loads in stool appeared within the first 3 weeks after HSCT.[22] These data suggest that persistent adenovirus infection in the intestine represents an important risk factor for disease after transplant and serve as the basis for screening and preemptive treatment in high-risk pediatric HSCT recipients.

CLINICAL MANIFESTATIONS

In immunocompromised patients, adenovirus can be asymptomatic or cause varying disease manifestations, including conjunctivitis, acute respiratory illness, gastroenteritis, urinary tract infections, or disseminated disease.[11] These manifestations tend to be more severe in pediatric transplant populations, including respiratory failure as the result of pneumonitis, hemorrhagic cystitis, neurologic disease, and multiorgan failure.[3]

Solid Organ Transplantation

Similar to HSCT recipients, detection of adenovirus in SOT recipients can be without symptoms or be associated with local and disseminated disease. The risk for adenovirus disease is variable by type of allograft.[7] Published data suggest that detection of adenovirus in the blood in liver and intestine transplant recipients might be associated with increased risk of developing sepsis.[12] In a study by de Merzeville and colleagues, the most frequently involved site of disease was the gastrointestinal tract (75%), followed by respiratory tract (21%), blood (21%), and liver (7%); the most common clinical manifestations are diarrhea (68%) and fever (53%).[10]

In most SOT recipients, the allograft is the most likely site of disease.[1,5] It is possible that the allograft is more vulnerable, owing to the local immunologic environment (low-grade, subclinical GVHD and rejection) or reactivation of the virus from the donor or recipient lymphoid tissue.[13] In some studies, adenovirus detection has been linked with subsequent acute rejection, possibly caused by activation of the cytokine release by stimulating the cellular immune response and changes in immunosuppressive regimens.[5,23] However, not all studies support this association.[6,13,17]

In liver transplant recipients, infections tend to be diagnosed early, with severe disease seen predominantly in the first 2 months,[5,14] but late infections have been reported.[15] The median time to adenovirus infection after transplantation ranges from 25.5 days to 61 days.[5,14] Frequent symptoms on presentation noted in previous studies were fever, rhinorrhea, diarrhea, and blood in the stool.[5,12,24] Hepatitis was the most common presentation, with liver enzymes aspartate transaminase and alanine transaminase) peaking in thousands with aspartate transaminase higher than alanine transaminase.[5,12,24] However, patients can also present with stomatitis, rash, enteritis and/or colitis, hemorrhagic cystitis, nephritis, and pneumonitis and can progress to sepsis.[5,12,14,24] Pneumonitis is less common but can progress to adult respiratory distress syndrome and is associated with high mortality.[5,25] The case-fatality rate in patients with adenovirus hepatitis is high, approximately 63% reported in a small case series, including mainly pediatric patients; mild elevation of the liver enzymes and limited necrosis on the initial biopsy correlate with better survival.[24]

Intestinal transplant recipients present with fever, rhinorrhea, blood in the stool, and increase ostomy output; a significant proportion of these patients progress to disseminated adenovirus disease.[6,12,13,26] Not all patients in whom invasive disease develops have prior asymptomatic infection.[13] Median time from transplantation to adenovirus disease varies in different studies from 24 days to 113 days.[10,13] Adenovirus disease tends to be diagnosed more frequently in the first 6 months after transplantation at similar rates in isolated intestinal transplant and multivisceral transplant recipients.[13] Enteritis is a common presentation, and it can be challenging to distinguish it from acute cellular rejection, especially because adenovirus enteritis is often preceded by treatment for rejection.[5] In patients with increased stool output and blood in the stool, an endoscopy with biopsy to evaluate for rejection and stool testing to evaluate for gastrointestinal infections (including adenovirus) are indicated. The ileum is the most common site of infection, but jejunum and colon can also be involved.[6] Adenovirus ascending cholangitis seems to be a rare complication of the gastrointestinal infection.[27] Morbidity and mortality can be attributed to adenovirus disease and to bacteremia and sepsis owing to compromise of intestinal epithelium integrity.[6] Case-fatality rates have been reported as high as 45%.[12]

In lung transplant recipients, adenovirus can cause acute flu-like illness but patients often present with allograft infection, diffuse alveolar damage, or necrotizing pneumonia. In addition, adenoviruses have been associated with chronic allograft dysfunction owing to bronchiolitis obliterans, interstitial fibrosis or bronchiectasis, need for retransplantation, and death.[5] However, these associations have not been confirmed in large comparative studies.

In heart transplant recipients, detection of adenovirus genome in endomyocardial biopsy specimens was associated with adverse cardiac events in the short term, and it was an independent predictor of intermediate to long-term allograft dysfunction or loss.[23] Adenovirus has been associated with posttransplantation coronary vasculopathy, but the mechanism for this association has not been delineated. Based on the concern that persistence of adenovirus in the endomyocardium is responsible for subclinical inflammatory response, some have suggested that maintenance of steroid therapy and the use of intravenous immunoglobulin might reduce the infiltration and the complications; however, there are limited data to support this approach.

Adenovirus infections are infrequent in kidney transplant recipients and usually present with hematuria, dysuria, fever, or respiratory symptoms.[17] Adenovirus DNAemia was reported in 14.7% of pediatric kidney transplant recipients at a median of 173 days (interquartile range [IQR] 109 to 310 days); the median duration of DNAemia was relatively long 55 days (IQR 36 to 79 days).[17] Adenovirus disease in renal recipients seems to present later (at a median of 309 days after transplantation, IQR 258 to 360 days) and is associated with a longer duration of DNAemia (median of 79 days, IQR 55 to 97 days).[17] Hemorrhagic cystitis is the most common manifestation in pediatric populations and is generally a self-limited illness. Graft dysfunction is uncommon[18] and should be differentiated from BK virus nephropathy and rejection. Orchitis, gastroenteritis, and pneumonia have been described in renal transplant recipients.[18]

Hematopoietic Stem Cell Transplantation

In HSCT recipients, clinical manifestations vary based on the risk factors present, including age, type of graft, level of immunosuppression, and timing after transplant. Symptoms of adenovirus disease most often manifest within the first 100 days after transplant.[9,28] Fever and diarrhea are the most common symptoms reported,[20] followed by elevated liver enzyme levels and secondary pancytopenia.[4] Gastrointestinal symptoms range from mild diarrhea to hemorrhagic colitis[9,29]; diarrhea can mimic gastrointestinal GVHD, causing diagnostic uncertainty in allogeneic transplant patients.[20] Respiratory symptoms can vary from mild, nonspecific cold-like symptoms of the upper tract to severe pneumonia.[9,29] Urothelial involvement usually manifests as hemorrhagic cystitis, which rarely progresses to disseminated infection.[9] Additional reported symptoms include nephritis, hepatitis, encephalitis, myocarditis, pancreatitis, and multiorgan involvement, the latter of which is frequently associated with hepatic failure.[4] Fatal adenovirus disease is reported in 13 to 50% of infected patients.[4]

DISEASE PROPHYLAXIS/PREVENTION

Because of the high mortality from localized and disseminated disease in high-risk allogeneic HSCT patients, guidelines exist to direct screening and preemptive therapy for adenovirus in high-risk groups.[4,11,30] Monitoring in autologous and standard-risk allogeneic HSCT patients, such as those receiving human leukocyte antigen–identical sibling transplants, is not routinely recommended. Defining which allogeneic HSCT patients are at high risk varies slightly among guidelines, but generally includes pediatric recipients of T-cell–depleted grafts, unrelated donor grafts, cord blood grafts, severe GVHD, severe lymphopenia, and treatment with alemtuzumab and antithymocyte globulin (Fig. 22.1).[4,11,30] An algorithm for adenovirus surveillance and treatment is provided (Fig. 22.2). As adenovirus screening of stool specimens is not widely available, weekly monitoring of serum adenovirus PCR

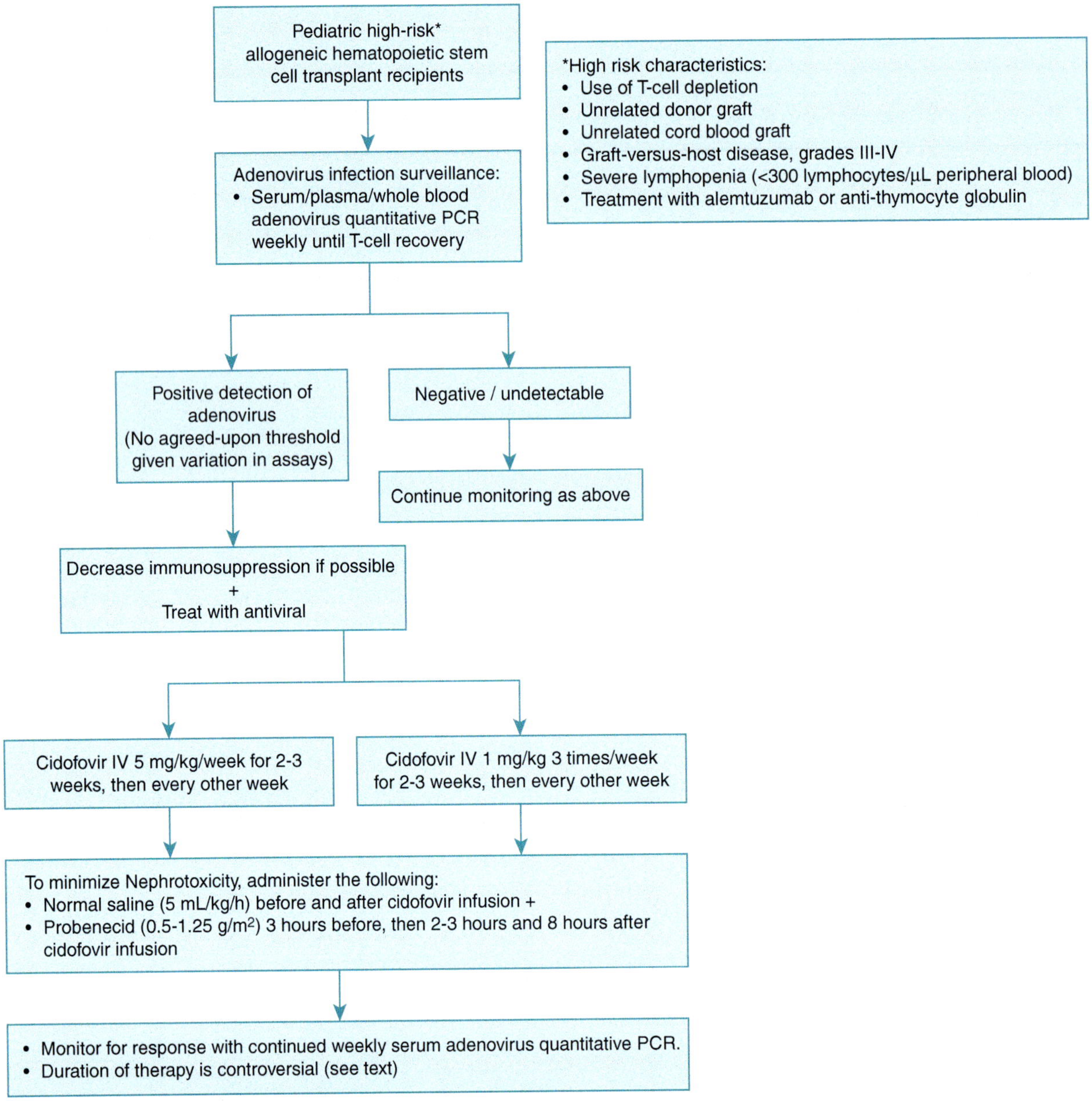

Fig. 22.1 Algorithm for Adenovirus Surveillance and Treatment in Pediatric Hematopoietic Stem Cell Transplant Recipients. *PCR,* polymerase chain reaction; *IV,* intravenous; *mg,* milligram; *kg,* kilogram; *mL,* milliliter; *h,* hour; *g,* gram; *m*^{2}, meter squared.

immediately after transplant is recommended until immune reconstitution (Fig. 22.1).[4,11] Preemptive treatment when DNAemia is detected is discussed in the treatment section.

Surveillance strategies and interventions in SOT patients require a better understanding of the timing of adenovirus infections after transplantation and the natural course of the infection. At present, donors and recipients are not screened for adenovirus serologies. In addition, there are many adenovirus serotypes and cross-reactive cellular immune responses among the different serotypes and long-term protection is not completely elucidated.[31] Currently, there are no data regarding the value of monitoring for adenovirus in the stool or other specimens in SOT recipients as a predictor of subsequent disease, and there is no set threshold values or specific algorithm when antiviral therapy should be started. Prolonged detection of adenovirus by PCR in blood in the absence of any symptoms has been described, but the clinical significance remains unclear.

In the SOT patient population, the focus of disease surveillance should be in liver, intestinal, and lung transplant recipients, mainly in the first 6 to 12 months after transplant. DNAemia is detected before detection in other fluids, secretions (sputum, pericardial fluid, pleural fluid, stool), and tissues, suggesting that DNAemia precedes adenovirus disease by 1 to 3 weeks.[3,12] Early identification of adenovirus by DNA detection rather than other diagnostic techniques may be associated with lower mortality.[12] Serial quantitative PCR may be useful to decide when to initiate therapy and to monitor response to therapy. However, the initial viral load in SOT recipients most likely would not predict progression to adverse outcomes.[15]

DIAGNOSIS

Several diagnostic methods are available for identification of the adenovirus: viral culture, direct antigen detection, molecular methods, and histopathology. Electron microscopy is also available but is mainly used in research settings.[7] Molecular detection via quantitative PCR is the most common diagnostic method used in clinical practice because of its high sensitivity.[7] Serotyping of adenoviruses is available through the Centers for Disease Control and Prevention and is best done by sequencing amplified virus. Such testing is often reserved for enhanced outbreak response or to help guide prevention and control measures. Sequencing can be used to identify coinfections with different serotypes; however, at this time there is no clear individual clinical benefit of serotyping.

To differentiate between infection and disease, results of the culture, antigen testing, or molecular testing should be correlated with clinical presentation and histopathology when available. Interpretation of any positive adenovirus test result (culture, direct antigen detection, or a molecular test) requires assessment of clinical signs and symptoms to determine the likelihood of adenovirus being the causative agent and the correlation with histopathologic findings. A positive test result at one site may prompt the search for detection of the virus from other sites to more comprehensively assess virus presence in various compartments.

Although viral culture is the gold standard for detection of adenovirus, the results can be affected by inappropriate sampling and poor transport conditions.[25] Viral cultures are usually performed from fresh stool and urine samples, pharyngeal and conjunctiva swabs, and bronchial and nasal wash. All adenovirus serotypes except serotypes 40 and 41 grow well in human epithelial cells and produce a characteristic cytopathic effect after 2 to 28 days.[7] Because viral culture takes at minimum several days to yield a positive result, it is less useful in clinical practice. Faster detection techniques have been developed such as centrifugation in shell vial assays with immunofluorescent monoclonal antibody staining, rapid antigen detection kits, and molecular assays. Direct fluorescent antibody tests are used in nasopharyngeal swabs and respiratory specimens, whereas enzyme immunoassays are used mainly for stool samples.[7] The commercially available rapid antigen detection kits yield rapid and specific results. Most of these assays detect the common adenovirus serotypes, but their sensitivity and specificity in the immunocompromised population has not been studied.

PCR is widely used in clinical practice and is accepted as the standard method for identification and quantification of adenovirus in immunocompromised hosts. This is because this testing platform has high sensitivity (the lower limit of detection is 100 to 1000 copies/mL, depending on the assay used) and it can be performed on different specimens (blood, respiratory secretions, and stool). Although PCR is considered to be the standard of care for adenovirus detection, clinicians should be aware of several factors that can influence the results of the assay: the type of the specimen, how the specimen is processed, DNA extraction, the primers used, and the amplification platform. Even though adenovirus-specific assays target conserved regions within the genome and should be able to detect all adenovirus serotypes,[3] there are reports of sequence polymorphisms leading to underestimation of adenovirus viral loads.[32] Multiplex PCR assays for stool or respiratory samples have been developed, but they are less sensitive and specific than the assays specifically targeting adenovirus and test only for a selected number of adenovirus serotypes.[33] In addition to detection of infection, PCR is often performed for serial quantification of adenovirus load at a specific source to guide either timing of initiation of therapy or for monitoring response to therapy. As the PCR platforms used by each laboratory often vary, testing results cannot be easily compared from one laboratory to the next. Therefore when trending viral loads, the same laboratory should be used. Decreasing viral loads with or without antiviral treatment could correlate with clinical improvement.[18,34]

Histopathology is the gold standard for the diagnosis of tissue invasive adenoviral disease. The classic histopathologic finding for adenovirus disease are "smudge cells," confirmed through immune-peroxidase and in situ hybridization staining. The smudge cells are easy to identify because of large nuclei with basophilic inclusions and a thin rim of cytoplasm.[7] However, other histopathologic findings can denote adenovirus disease even in the absence of smudge cells. The most common histologic finding of adenovirus hepatitis is necrosis, which can be focal, spotty, or extensive. In most cases, there is no inflammation, but if present, it is periportal, focal, and lymphohistiocytic; granulomas are rarely noted. Smudge intranuclear inclusions tend to be more numerous at the periphery of the necrotic areas.[24] In intestinal biopsies, villous blunting with hyperplasia, disorganization of the superficial epithelium, focal mixed inflammatory infiltrate (especially in the lamina propria), crypt apoptosis, and focal necrosis can be seen; rarely smudge cells can be identified. Viral inclusions are frequently seen in the surface enterocytes but can also be seen in the crypts in patients with high viral loads.[26] The myocardial biopsies do not show significant inflammatory infiltrate or necrosis.[26] Kidney biopsies in patients with adenovirus interstitial nephritis would demonstrate tubule-centric, sometimes granulomatous inflammation; focal necrosis is not common. Tubular epithelial cells with smudge cell morphology can rarely be seen. The distal nephrons are mainly affected in the medulla and the corticomedullary junction.[26]

TREATMENT

The most important part of therapy is supportive care, with antimotility agents for severe diarrhea, antiemetics for nausea and vomiting, and oral or intravenous fluid and electrolytes, depending on the severity of volume depletion.[5,35] In addition, three therapeutic approaches can be used, alone or in combination: reduction of immunosuppressive therapy, antiviral therapy, and immunotherapy. In many cases, it is difficult to determine if clinical improvement or resolution of the disease could be attributed to antiviral therapy, reduction of immunosuppression, immunotherapy, or some combination of these.[36]

Some immunocompromised patients clear adenovirus DNAemia without any intervention.[17] In most cases, however, reduction of immunosuppressive therapy should be the first step.[5,11,35] At present, guidelines regarding how to adjust immunosuppressive therapy are unavailable, including which immunosuppressive agent to adjust or which to stop to allow immune reconstitution. The ability to monitor immunocompromised patients for the presence or development of adenovirus-specific immune response would be useful for identifying patients in need of antiviral therapy.[36] Close collaboration with infectious diseases, oncology, and/or transplant services is recommended to identify options to reduce immunosuppression.

Antiviral Agents

No antiviral agent has been approved by the U.S. Food and Drug Administration for the treatment of adenovirus infection or disease. With the exception of brincidofovir, there are no prospective randomized clinical trials of antiviral drugs for the management of adenovirus. Clinicians need to recognize that recommendations for any of the currently available agents are predominantly founded on case reports, case series, and expert opinion. Furthermore, the decision to initiate antiviral therapy needs to be made with an understanding of the potential toxicities of the antiviral agent to be started.

Cidofovir. Cidofovir is often initiated at the time of asymptomatic detection of adenovirus (i.e., preemptive therapy) in high-risk

HSCT recipients or at the time of diagnosis of severe, progressive, or disseminated adenovirus disease (i.e., definitive therapy) in solid organ and HSCT recipients.[4,11,35,37-39] Cidofovir is a nucleotide analog of cytosine with in vitro activity against all adenovirus serotypes.[7,9,18] Cidofovir is converted intracellularly to the active metabolite cidofovir diphosphate, which is subsequently incorporated by the DNA polymerase into newly synthesized viral DNA, leading to termination in chain elongation. The misincorporated cidofovir diphosphate is resistant to excision from the new DNA chain.[40] Cidofovir, as per the package insert, is associated with significant drug toxicities, including up to 50% nephrotoxicity and up to 20% neutropenia.[5,7] Cidofovir causes nephrotoxicity by uptake into renal proximal tubules via the human organic anion transporters (hOAT), more specifically hOAT1.[11,41] Several small studies in pediatric allogeneic HSCT and SOT recipients suggest that cidofovir is associated with minimal to no renal toxicity; however, other reports have documented a 17% rate of acute renal failure and 71% with some degree of renal tubular dysfunction.[11,13,37] In a series of 25 pediatric SOT patients treated with cidofovir, 24% required renal replacement therapy because of fluid overload while cidofovir was used.[37]

Two dosing regimens of cidofovir tend to be used for the treatment of adenovirus disease: 1 mg/kg 3 times per week or 5 mg/kg per week for 2 weeks followed by 5 mg/kg every other week.[35,42] Of note, the safety and efficacy of either regimen has not been confirmed via comparative studies nor have there been any studies to directly compare the two regimens. Probenecid (0.5 to 1.25 g/m^2) should be administered 3 hours before and then 2 to 3 hours and 8 hours after the administration of cidofovir to decrease the risk of nephrotoxicity.[5,13,34,43] Hydration with normal saline solution (5 mL/kg per hour) before and after cidofovir dosing should be also administered to minimize the risk of nephrotoxicity.[4,5,11,13,43] The first regimen (1 mg/kg thrice weekly) has been perceived as less nephrotoxic.[11,38,43] The dosage of cidofovir needs be adjusted based on creatinine clearance; if creatinine clearance is less than 0.3 mL/min per kilogram, the dose should be decreased to 0.5 mg/kg 3 times per week; for patients undergoing hemodialysis, the hemodialysis should be stopped 1 hour before and 4 hours after cidofovir administration to allow intracellular distribution of the drug.[5,13] Data from a small study did not demonstrate any statistical difference in the increase of blood urea nitrogen and creatinine when comparing the two regimens, probably owing to good monitoring and aggressive renal-protective strategies.[15]

The duration of therapy is not well established. For adenovirus disease some have suggested continuing therapy until complete resolution of the signs and symptoms of disease and documentation of one to three negative adenovirus samples taken 1 week apart from the sites that were originally positive.[5,13,15,34] There does not seems to be a faster virologic clearance based on the cidofovir dosing regimen in a study of both pediatric HSCT and SOT patients.[15] However, the thrice-weekly regimen may be associated with breakthrough cytomegalovirus and herpes simplex infections and the emergence of antiviral resistance.[38] A temporal decrease in viral load after cidofovir administration has been associated with clinical improvement and survival,[34] although the lack of a decline in viral load (≥1.0 log) after 2 weeks of therapy has been associated with disease progression and death.[34] It has been hypothesized that a poor response to cidofovir might result from a longer interval between the onset of symptoms and initiation of treatment and with a high initial adenovirus viral load before starting therapy.[34]

Brincidofovir. Brincidofovir (CMX001, Chimerix) is an oral lipid conjugate derivative of cidofovir with in vitro activity against adenoviruses and other double-stranded DNA viruses.[41,44] Brincidofovir has several advantages over cidofovir:

1. It is orally bioavailable.
2. It achieves higher intracellular levels of active drug compared with cidofovir.
3. It is associated with less nephrotoxicity as it is not a substrate for hOAT and hence it does not accumulate in renal tubules.
4. It is more potent than cidofovir against adenoviruses based on the inhibitory concentration of 50%.

Preliminary studies have evaluated the use of brincidofovir as preemptive therapy for adenoviremia in pediatric HSCT patients. The largest study randomly assigned 48 pediatric and adult allogeneic HSCT recipients with asymptomatic adenoviremia 1:1:1 to receive oral brincidofovir 100 mg (or 2 mg/kg if weight <50 kg) twice weekly; brincidofovir 200 mg (or 4 mg/kg if weight <50 kg) once weekly; or placebo for 6 to 12 weeks. Treatment failure (progression to probable or definitive adenovirus disease or increasing adenoviremia) was the primary endpoint. Although the proportion of subjects receiving twice-weekly brincidofovir encountered less treatment failures (21%) compared with the once-weekly brincidofovir group (38%) and placebo (33%), results were not statistically significant. In seven patients with DNAemia greater than log 3.0 at baseline, 86% receiving twice-weekly brincidofovir achieved undetectable DNAemia compared with 25% of those receiving placebo.[41] Meanwhile, retrospective multicenter data from the UK Paediatric BMT Group, compared viremic kinetics and toxicities between cidofovir and brincidofovir in children with HSCT with similar viral burden, lymphopenia, and immune reconstitution. They observed improved virologic response (≥1 log reduction in 2 weeks) in adenoviremia episodes treated with brincidofovir (83%) compared with cidofovir (83% vs. 9%, $P < .001$) and concluded that brincidofovir was highly effective and well tolerated.[44]

Brincidofovir was used as salvage therapy for 13 immunocompromised patients (one with severe combined immunodeficiency, one small bowel transplant recipient, and 11 allogeneic HSCT recipients) with adenovirus disease and a 10-fold or greater drop in viral load was noted in approximately two-thirds of the patients after 1 week of therapy. After 8 weeks, 70% of patients responded to treatment with brincidofovir. Virologic response correlated with survival advantage, which could not be explained by immune recovery alone.[45]

Gastrointestinal symptoms, particularly diarrhea, are the most commonly reported adverse events associated with brincidofovir.[41] Abdominal pain, nausea, and vomiting were also reported, but it is important to distinguish these symptoms from concomitant mucositis, GVHD, drug toxicity, and other infections (i.e., cytomegalovirus, norovirus, *Clostridium difficile*).[11] In certain cases, histologic examination of intestinal biopsy specimens demonstrated epithelial apoptosis, gland and crypt architectural distortion or dropout, lymphoplasmacytic and neutrophilic inflammation, and lamina propria edema, all overlapping features for several diagnoses.[46] Despite the effectiveness of brincidofovir in controlling adenoviremia and its limited toxicity profile, it remains available only through clinical studies or for compassionate use. Additionally, it is currently available only as an enteral formulation, which can be a major barrier to administration for a patient population with frequent gastrointestinal complications.

Ribavirin. Ribavirin, a nucleoside analog of guanosine that inhibits the viral polymerase, has antiviral activity limited to species C adenoviruses (serotypes 1, 2, 5, and 6).[3,5] The main side effect is hemolytic anemia, but safety and efficacy in pediatric patients younger than 5 years have not been established. Treatment with ribavirin was not associated with a significant decrease in the adenovirus viral loads,[3,5] and it is not recommended for treatment of adenovirus infections in immunocompromised patients.[5,11,35]

Ganciclovir. Ganciclovir has limited activity against adenovirus because it requires phosphorylation by an enzyme called thymidine kinase to convert the agent from a prodrug to its active form that would subsequently inhibit viral replication. Adenoviruses lack thymidine kinase and human kinases are not efficient at phosphorylating ganciclovir to its active state.[28]

Nitazoxanide. Nitazoxanide, a thiazolide and its active metabolite tizoxanide, has a low toxicity profile and may have antiviral activity by targeting cellular pathways involved in the syntheses of viral proteins.[47] Clinical data are limited to adult studies that suggest nitazoxanide may shorten the duration of adenovirus enteritis of mild to moderate severity.[47]

Immunotherapy

Immunotherapy for invasive adenovirus infection is a promising therapeutic strategy but is not widely available. The role of T-cell–mediated immunity in controlling adenovirus is demonstrated by (1) poor outcomes in HSCT recipients with absolute lymphocyte counts less than 300/ dL, (2) resolution of adenovirus detection with reduction in immunosuppression, and (3) clearance of DNAemia in correlation with increased lymphocyte counts and detection of adenovirus-specific $CD4^+$ and $CD8^+$ T cells.[36] Adoptive transfer of adenovirus immunity using donor lymphocyte infusion or using adenovirus-specific T cells has been attempted in HSCT recipients with adenovirus, but these strategies have been limited by toxicity of donor-derived alloreactive cells.[11] More recent manufacturing processes have led to development of cytotoxic T-lymphocyte cell lines generated by third-party seropositive donors with a response rate of more than 70% for HSCT patients with severe, refractory adenovirus infections.[11]

Intravenous immunoglobulin administration has been postulated as adjunctive therapy for adenovirus in SOT patients. Acquired hypogammaglobulinemia (immunoglobulin G levels <350 mg/dL) has been associated with increased risk of infectious complications, morbidity, and mortality in SOT patients, but maintaining immunoglobulin G levels above this threshold has not generally resulted in changes in patient or graft survival. Intravenous immunoglobulins have been administered in the setting of adenovirus disease, especially for severe cases, with mixed results.[5,15] Data from a small study did not demonstrate that adjunctive therapy with intravenous immunoglobulin affected the virologic response in SOT recipients.[15]

INFECTION PREVENTION AND ANTICIPATORY GUIDANCE

Isolation and hand hygiene measures for patients shedding adenovirus should be enforced. Adenovirus outbreaks in hospital or institutional settings have been reported.[48] Centers for Disease Control and Prevention/Healthcare Infection Control Practices Advisory Committee guidelines recommend contact and droplet precautions during hospitalization for the duration of illness to prevent nosocomial transmission; however, in immunocompromised hosts, the duration might need to be extended because of the potential for prolonged and intermittent shedding of the virus.[48]

Adenoviruses are resistant to many common disinfecting agents, allowing for persistent viability in the environment.[49] Ethyl alcohol, at concentrations of 60% to 80%, is a virucidal agent that can inactivate hydrophilic viruses such as adenoviruses.[49] Adenoviruses are resistant to inactivation by ultraviolet light and may survive for prolonged periods in water; maintaining adequate levels of chlorine in swimming pools is important to prevent outbreaks of conjunctivitis owing to adenovirus.[49]

Vaccination for the general public is not available. A newly Food and Drug Administration–approved live oral vaccine is available for U.S. military trainees; the vaccine covers adenovirus serotypes 4 and 7. It is formulated in two tablets to be taken at the same time. The vaccine has 99.3% efficacy (95% confidence interval 96.0% to 99.9%; $P < .001$)[50] Because this vaccine offers immunity limited to two serotypes that are not the most common in transplantation, the vaccine has not been studied in the peritransplant period and would be contraindicated after transplantation because it is a live vaccine.

23

BK and Other Polyomavirus Associated Diseases in Children

Benjamin L. Laskin, MD, MSc and Hans H. Hirsch, MD, MSc

Polyomavirus (PyV) infections were first described in mice in 1952 as a cause of tumors in newborn animals. Since then, PyVs have been found in virtually all vertebrates, including primates, monkeys, cows, rabbits, birds, and fish.[1] BK polyomavirus (BKPyV) was isolated in 1971 from a kidney transplant patient shedding decoy cells in the urine. The isolation of JC polyomavirus (JCPyV) was also reported in 1971 from postmortem tissues of patients with progressive multifocal leukoencephalopathy (PML), but PyV particles had been noted by electron microscopy in PML tissue sections as early as 1965. Since then, more than 10 human polyomaviruses (HPyVs) have been characterized molecularly, and there is serologic evidence that healthy adults are concurrently infected with at least six to seven different HPyVs.[2] Clinical and histopathologic evidence of disease is currently available for six HPyVs (Table 23.1), which almost exclusively affect immunocompromised patients.[3,4] This chapter reviews the recent literature on HPyVs in immunocompromised children undergoing cancer/chemotherapy, solid organ transplantation (SOT), or hematopoietic cell transplantation (HCT).

VIRAL STRUCTURE AND LIFE CYCLE

PyVs share a common morphology of non-enveloped icosahedral virion particles of 40 nm to 45 nm that contain a double-stranded DNA genome of approximately 5000 base pairs wrapped around histones.[3] PyV genomes can be divided into three regions called the non-coding control region (*NCCR*), early viral gene region (*EVGR*), and late viral gene region (*LVGR*).[3] After virion uptake and delivery of the viral genome to the nucleus, the *NCCR* coordinates, together with host cell factors,[5] the start of the PyV replication cycle by initiating expression of the *EVGR*-encoded regulatory large T-antigen (LTag) and small-antigen (sTag). LTag and sTag inactivate tumor suppressor proteins pRB and p53 and shift cells into G_1/S phase to provide necessary building blocks and recruit the host cell DNA polymerase complex for efficient bidirectional replication of the viral DNA genome from the *NCCR ori*. This is followed by *NCCR*-driven expression of the *LVGR*-encoded capsid proteins Vp1, Vp2, Vp3, and the regulatory agnoprotein. The *LVGR* also encodes viral micro-ribonucleic acids (miRNAs).[6-8] Vp1 forms the outer shell of the virions consisting of 72 pentamers and assembles spontaneously in virus-like particles used for serologic studies. Vp2 and Vp3 are minor capsid proteins inside the particles adjacent to the viral DNA genome. Enlarged nuclei with prominent intranuclear inclusions consisting of densely packed PyV particles are the hallmark of PyV replication in the late phase of the viral life cycle. Immunohistochemistry for LTag using cross-reactive monoclonal antibody raised originally against the monkey SV40 LTag protein is commonly used for proven BKPyV or JCPyV pathology erroneously called "SV40 positive," but detection of Vp1 or in situ hybridization has also been used by some centers. Although the principal virology of PyVs is conserved, there are significant differences which permit concurrent infections and mediate differences in host cell tropism, virus biology, and pathology. Thus the outer part of the Vp1 virions is more diverse, and is responsible for primary host cell tropism as judged from selective binding to gangliosides carrying differently branched sugar residues.[9] These Vp1 domains are also the target of neutralizing antibodies. Conversely, the inner parts seem more conserved and mediate interactions between Vp1 pentamers or to Vp2. Binding of immunoglobulin G (IgG) are more frequently cross-reactive between different HPyVs and have less frequently neutralizing activity. The *NCCRs* of HPyVs differ in length, type, and number of transcription factor binding sites, and are critical for the secondary host cell tropism, which is realized inside the host cell nucleus by the exact timing of *EVGR* and *LVGR* expression.[5] PyV micro-RNAs 5p and 3p target the *EVGR* transcripts and downregulate natural killer cell targets on the cell surface, thereby facilitating immune escape and latency.[6] Taken together, HPyV biology subverts and hijacks the host cell metabolism without offering classic antiviral targets of high selectivity.

EPIDEMIOLOGY AND RISK FACTORS

General Population

The exact mode of natural BKPyV and JCPyV transmission is undefined but most likely involves contact with mucosal surfaces in the oral/pharyngeal, gastrointestinal, or respiratory tract.[3] Seroprevalence studies indicate that primary infection with BKPyV occurs in toddlers, reaching IgG positivity rates of greater than 90% between the ages of 2 and 4 years. There are no known symptoms associated with primary BKPyV infection and a nonspecific, constitutional illness cannot be excluded. Primary JCPyV infection appears to occur significantly later as only 35% of adolescents have JCPyV-specific IgG antibodies compared with 60% of blood donors.[10] In a study of 18 patients undergoing thymectomy in children owing to congenital heart surgery, the IgG seroprevalence of BKPyV and JCPyV was 70% and 25%, respectively.[11] However, some differences in seroprevalence rates across different studies reflect patient age and waning antibody responses over time, but particular attention should be paid to the different antigens used (e.g., Vp1 monomers or fusion proteins, Vp1-pentamers or Vp1-virus-like particles).[12-14]

HPyVs have been detected in the urine of 30% of healthy children and adults as well as 40% of stool samples from hospitalized children.[15] Detection of BKPyV and JCPyV in human sewage systems supports the possibility of secondary indirect environmental exposures other than the direct transmission route (e.g., from child to child). Indeed, PyV particles are fairly resistant to environmental inactivation and can withstand heating to 60°C for 30 minutes and many disinfectants.[16] Other routes of transmission are less well defined and even controversial (e.g., via transfusion, transplacental, seminal fluids, or organ transplantation), with the notable exception of kidney transplantation, where transmission has been shown to occur from donor to recipient.

TABLE 23.1 Human Polyomaviruses Associated With Disease in Immunocompromised Patients[3]

Common Name	Genus	Taxonomic Name	Organ of Latency	Human Disease
BK polyomavirus	*Betapolyomavirus*	Human polyomavirus 1	Kidney and urinary tract	Nephropathy, hemorrhagic cystitis
JC polyomavirus	*Betapolyomavirus*	Human polyomavirus 2	Kidney, brain, blood cells	Progressive multifocal leukoencephalopathy
Merkel cell polyomavirus	*Alphapolyomavirus*	Human polyomavirus 5	Skin	Merkel cell carcinoma
Trichodysplasia spinulosa	*Alphapolyomavirus*	Human polyomavirus 8	Skin	Trichodysplasia spinulosa
New Jersey polyomavirus	*Alphapolyomavirus*	Human polyomavirus 13	Unknown	1 pancreatic transplant patient with muscle, skin, and eye disease
Human polyomavirus 7	Deltapolyomavirus	Human polyomavirus 7	Skin	Pruritic hyperproliferative keratinopathy in lung transplant patients

From Greenlee JE, Hirsch HH. Polyomaviruses. In: Richman DD, Whitley RJ, Hayden FG, eds. *Clinical Virology*. 4th ed. Washington, DC: ASM Press; 2017:599-623.

TABLE 23.2 Clinical Manifestations of Polyomavirus Infection in Children With Solid Organ Transplant, or Hematopoietic Cell Transplant or other Immunocompromised Conditions[a]

Pediatric Population	Clinical Manifestation (Reported Pediatric Rates)
BKPyV	
Kidney transplant	Nephropathy (5%-15%)
	Hemorrhagic cystitis (rare)
Hematopoietic cell transplant	Hemorrhagic cystitis (8%-25%)
	Nephropathy (rare)
Liver Transplant	Nephropathy (rare)
Heart transplant	Nephropathy (rare)
Lung transplant	Hemorrhagic cystitis (rare)
Malignancy	Hemorrhagic cystitis (rare)
JCPyV	
HIV/AIDS, refractory multiple sclerosis	Progressive multifocal leukoencephalopathy
Kidney transplant	Nephropathy (rare)
	Progressive multifocal leukoencephalopathy (very rare)
Malignancy	Progressive multifocal leukoencephalopathy
Less common clinical manifestations: gastrointestinal, pulmonary, ophthalmologic, hepatic, neurologic, cancer	

[a]Nephropathy and hemorrhagic cystitis associated with BKPyV are the predominant clinical manifestations affecting kidney transplant and hematopoietic cell transplant recipients, respectively. Progressive multifocal leukoencephalopathy associated with JCPyV is the predominant clinical manifestation affecting patients with human immunodeficiency virus/AIDS and refractory multiple sclerosis.

BKPyV, BK polyomavirus; *HIV*, human immunodeficiency virus; *JCPyV*, JC polyomavirus.

After primary infection, BKPyV and JCPyV reach the renourinary tract presumably by DNAemia, where they preferentially infect the renal tubular and bladder epithelial cells in the case of BKPyV and the urothelial cells of the renal pelvis and the bladder in the case of JCPyV.[3,17] Moreover, detection of JCPyV DNA has been reported in tonsils, bone marrow, and the central nervous system. Taken together, large parts of the general human population have been infected with HPyVs, including BKPyV and JCPyV, but neither primary infection, persistence, nor shedding has been linked to significant pathology or disease in immunocompetent persons. Conversely, as outlined in Table 23.2, immunocompromise appears to be a *conditio sine qua non* for HPyV disease, but the differences in incidence rates in the respective clinical settings strongly suggest that specific risk signatures beyond mere immunodeficiency appear to play a role. Thus BKPyV-associated nephropathy is most frequently diagnosed in adult and pediatric kidney transplant recipients at rates of 1% to 15%, but only rarely in non-kidney SOT or allogeneic HCT, despite similar or higher intensity of immunosuppression as evidenced by other opportunistic infectious diseases caused by *Pneumocystis jirovecii* or cytomegalovirus (CMV) replication. Conversely, hemorrhagic cystitis is most frequently seen after allogeneic HCT, but only rarely after kidney transplantation, wherein local toxic damage of the bladder urothelia from conditioning and impaired immune control are followed by increased inflammatory responses postengraftment.[18] JCPyV-mediated PML has reached the highest rates in human immunodeficiency virus/AIDS before the availability of combination antiretroviral therapy or in refractory relapsing multiple sclerosis treated with natalizumab, but less data are available for treatment with dimethyl fumarate or fingolimod, or in SOT or HCT. Accordingly, risk-adapted consultation, screening, and intervention are currently recommended for these respective patients.

Kidney Transplantation

The key steps of BKPyV reactivation to nephropathy have been described in detail, but they were mostly derived from adult patients after kidney transplantation. These include the following:

1. Low-level viruria in approximately 5% to 10% of patients with residual urine production before kidney transplantation
2. High-level replication with urine BKPyV loads greater than 10 million copies/mL and decoy cell shedding in 20% to 50% of patients after transplantation
3. Detection of BKPyV DNA in plasma in 10% to 40% of patients after transplantation
4. Histologically proven BKPyV-associated nephropathy with little inflammation and baseline allograft function (PyVAN-A)
5. Increasing allograft damage due to BKPyV replication and inflammation decreasing kidney allograft function (PyVAN-B1, -B2, -B3); and
6. Irreversible fibrosis and tubular atrophy causing decline in allograft function (PyVAN-C).

Accordingly, screening for high-level viruria and/or DNAemia using nucleic acid testing (NAT) is recommended to identify patients with persistent DNAemia who would benefit from preemptive reduction in immunosuppression.[19]

Most of the literature describing BKPyV infection replication and disease in children has been published in the past decade. In a prospective clinical and laboratory study from 2002 to 2005 in Italy, Ginevri and colleagues followed up with 62 children who received basiliximab and standard maintenance triple therapy with a calcineurin inhibitor, mycophenolate mofetil, and corticosteroids.[20] Only 3 of the 62 patients received induction that included antithymocyte globulin. Blood and urine samples were collected at months 1, 3, 6, 9, 12, 18, 24, 36, and 48 after transplant for NAT testing (458 samples, average of 7 samples per patient after transplant). The cumulative risk of viruria was 64% (95% confidence interval 53% to 78%) and that of DNAemia was 22% (95% confidence interval 13% to 35%), and was first detected at a median of 3 months (range 1 to 24 months for viruria and 1 to 18 months for DNAemia) after transplant. Using a protocol to reduce immunosuppression, no cases of BKPyV-associated nephropathy occurred in this series.

Risk factors for BKPyV replication after kidney transplant have included the depth and type of immunosuppression, including the use of antithymocyte globulin for induction or rejection treatment and the level of exposure to tacrolimus and mycophenolate mofetil. Other reported risk factors include human leukocyte antigen (HLA) mismatches, deceased donation, older age, male gender, donor antibody high/recipient antibody low, and ureteral stents.[19] In their analysis of 313 children receiving a kidney transplant in Europe, Höcker and colleagues reported the cumulative incidence of DNAemia and biopsy-proven nephropathy after kidney transplant (Fig. 23.1). In a multivariate model, they found that a higher degree of immunosuppression (odds ratio [OR] 1.3, $P < .01$), tacrolimus use (vs. cyclosporine) (OR 3.6 $P < .01$), younger recipient age (OR 1.1 per year, $P < .001$), and obstructive uropathy (OR 12.4, $P < .01$) were associated with higher risk of BKPyV infection.[21]

The serostatus of the donor and recipient may also contribute to posttransplant BKPyV risk.[19] Ali and colleagues conducted a retrospective analysis of pediatric kidney transplant patients at their center in Canada from 1986 to 2007.[22] All patients had follow-up for at least 1 year after transplant. Using an enzyme-linked immunosorbent assay to detect IgG against the BKPyV Vp1 virus-like particle, the authors tested stored blood samples from donors and recipients. An antibody titer of 1:2560 or less was categorized as a low titer and a titer of 1:10,240 or more was defined as a high titer. Of the 94 included transplant recipients, 34% had low anti-BKPyV IgG serostatus and 66% had high serostatus before transplant. Consistent with published reports for healthy children, pretransplant antibody titers were higher with increasing age, especially after the age of 6 years. Blood was also available to test 40 donors, 73% of whom had antibody titers in the high anti-BKPyV IgG serostatus group. Recipients with a low serostatus had a significantly higher risk of BKPyV DNAemia in the first year after transplant. The highest risk of BKPyV DNAemia was found in children with high donor serostatus and low recipient serostatus. Although BKPyV-specific IgG mediate part of the antiviral immune response, a higher antibody status may be a surrogate of recent exposure or reactivation, and hence reflect a higher tissue BKPyV load in the allograft that cannot be countered by sufficient immune effector functions in the recipient with low BKPyV-specific immunity evidenced by low antibody titers.[19] Although the numbers were small, BKPyV DNAemia occurred in 4 of 7 (57%) transplants from a high donor serostatus to a low serostatus recipient, in none of the 3 transplants in which both the donor and the recipient had low serostatus, and in only 1 of 26 (4%) transplants in which the recipient had high serostatus before transplant. Unlike CMV and Epstein-Barr virus (EBV), it is not standard to test for donor and recipient antibodies against BKPyV before kidney transplant in children or adults. This may change, however, as more research becomes available on the functional and surrogate role of antibody titers and specificities in donor-recipient pairs, and may help to better determine the posttransplant risk of uncontrolled BKPyV replication and disease.[19]

This notion may be extended to differences in BKPyV subtype antibody titers. BKPyV can be divided into four major subtypes (I, II, III, and IV) and each subtype can be further divided in subgroups yielding a total of 12 different categories of BKPyV strains.[23] BKPyV subtype I is found in patients worldwide, whereas subtype IV is found in patients mostly from East Asia and Europe. Subtypes II and III are rarely reported. Subtypes II, III, and IV and subgroups Ib1 and Ib2 are also known to be distinct serotypes.[24] Thus a subtype mismatch arising from transplanting of a donor graft harboring BKPyV subtype IV into a recipient with antibody titers to Ib may be followed by preferential replication of the donor BKPyV subtype. Momynaliev and colleagues examined BKPyV subtypes among 6 pediatric kidney transplant recipients and 10 adult controls at their center in Russia from 2008 to 2009.[25] They found that 66% of the identified BKPyV isolates were Ib2 and 24% were IVc2. More research is needed to determine the role of BKPyV genotypes and serotypes in

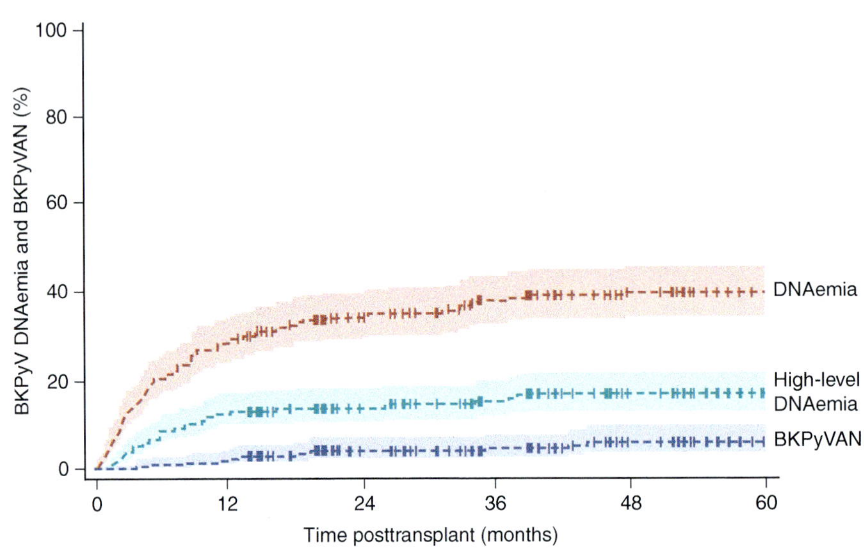

DNAemia	311	223	146	101	69	48
High-level DNAemia	311	273	199	114	99	64
BKPyVAN	311	305	202	121	101	68

Fig. 23.1 BKPyV DNAemia (>0 copies/mL), high-level DNAemia (>10,000 copies/mL), and biopsy-proven nephropathy in 311 children who received a kidney transplant in Europe. (Modified from Hocker B, Schneble L, Murer L, et al. Epidemiology of and risk factors for BK polyomavirus replication and nephropathy in pediatric renal transplant recipients: an International CERTAIN Registry Study. *Transplantation.* 2019;103(6):1224-1233.)

children with respect to posttransplant high-level viruria, DNAemia, and disease, and the risk-benefit of BKPyV mitigation and graft survival through informed screening and organ allocation.

Nonrenal Solid Organ Transplantation

Few studies have examined the risk of BKPyV replication in children after nonrenal SOT with most of the literature limited to cross-sectional analyses of patients who were several years after transplant, when the risk of BKPyV replication events is presumably lower. In a study of 59 pediatric liver transplant recipients in Israel by Amir and colleagues, blood and urine samples were tested at a single time point at least 1 month after transplant and retested if they were positive.[26] At a median of 5 years after liver transplant, 9 of 59 (15.3%) had viruria, and 1 of 59 patients (1.7%) had low-level DNAemia. In all 9 of the patients with viruria, BKPyV replication was transient and there was no longer evidence of DNAemia or viruria by their next clinic visit 5 months later. In Germany, Brinkert and colleagues tested 100 pediatric liver transplant recipients for BKPyV and JCPyV in urine, and plasma was tested only if the initial urine result was positive above 100,000 copies/mL.[27] Of the 100 included patients in this cross-sectional analysis, 15 (15%) had isolated BKPyV viruria at a median of 6 years after transplant, but no DNAemia was identified.

In contrast to liver transplantation, recipients of thoracic transplants (heart and lung) typically receive higher doses of immunosuppression to prevent rejection, placing them at greater risk for infectious disease events. Ducharme-Smith and colleagues conducted a cross-sectional analysis of pediatric heart transplant recipients in the United States by collecting urine samples at regular clinic appointments.[28] Since 2006, urine testing was performed only in patients with a history of chronic kidney disease and all patients were screened starting in 2012. Blood testing for BKPyV DNA was performed only if urine testing was positive. Of the 83 patients screened for viruria at a median of 3.3 years after transplant, 28 (34%) had viruria. Of these 28 patients, 7 had test results for DNAemia (representing 8% DNAemia among the total study population). In multivariate analysis, patients in whom BKPyV viruria developed were significantly more likely to have evidence of EBV detection in the blood. In a follow-up study, the authors prospectively collected urine and blood samples from 10 consecutive pediatric heart transplant recipients from 2013 to 2015.[29] Samples were collected before transplant and at 1 week and months 3, 6, 9, 12, and 15 after transplant. Quantitative blood and urine NAT was only performed if the result of the initial qualitative urine NAT was positive. The 10 subjects had follow up for 15 months after transplant, during which time viruria developed in 2 of 10 and 1 of 10 (10%) had DNAemia.

Several reviews have summarized the literature describing cases in adults and children with BKPyV replication after heart or lung transplant.[30,31] In adults after heart transplant, studies have reported a viruria risk of 19% and a DNAemia risk of 5%. After lung transplant, 33% of recipients have been found to have viruria, with less data available on the risk of DNAemia.[30] No studies have systematically examined the risk of BKPyV replication after pediatric lung transplant or in children with cancer. As summarized in later text, there are mainly case reports of BKPyV nephropathy in children after nonrenal SOT, especially in those receiving heart or lung transplants. However, the exact risk of nephropathy in the native kidneys of children with SOT remains unknown.

Hematopoietic Cell Transplantation

After HCT, BKPyV is typically associated with hemorrhagic cystitis, leading to significant morbidity and possibly an increased risk of death. Less commonly, BKPyV nephropathy was diagnosed in the native kidneys of HCT recipients, and presented similar to what is seen in patients after kidney transplantation. Risk factors for BKPyV replication after HCT include the type of graft, HLA mismatch, recipient CMV serostatus, and conditioning with antithymocyte globulin.[18] In a time-varying analysis including 88 children undergoing allogeneic HCT, graft-versus-host disease (GVHD) was not associated with the subsequent development of hemorrhagic cystitis.[32]

In the most comprehensive study to date assessing BKPyV replication in children after HCT, Cesaro and colleagues prospectively examined patients younger than 18 years after allogeneic HCT at their center in Italy from 2005 to 2012.[33] Plasma and urine samples were collected for BKPyV NAT at baseline, weekly until day 30, then at days 45, 60, 90, and 100 after transplant. Of the 107 patients enrolled, 20 patients (18.7%) had hemorrhagic cystitis, 90% of whom had BKPyV viruria and 80% of whom had BKPyV DNAemia. Among the 87 patients in whom hemorrhagic cystitis did not occur, 64% had viruria and 47% had DNAemia after transplant. Gaziev and colleagues assessed children younger than 17 years undergoing allogeneic HCT for sickle cell anemia or thalassemia at their center in Italy from 2004 to 2009.[34] They enrolled a total of 117 patients over the study period, including 64 of whom were monitored prospectively for BKPyV DNA in the blood and urine weekly until day 100 after transplant. Of the 64 patients monitored prospectively, 60 (94%) had at least one sample positive for viruria and 52 (81%) had at least two samples positive for viruria. Regarding DNAemia, 34 (53%) had at least one positive sample and 18 (28%) had at least two samples positive for DNAemia. These studies support findings that BKPyV viruria, DNAemia, and hemorrhagic cystitis are common in children undergoing HCT. No studies have systematically evaluated the epidemiology of hemorrhagic cystitis in children with cancer who have not undergone HCT.

CLINICAL MANIFESTATIONS

Clinical disease associated with HPyV in children is almost exclusively limited to immunocompromised patients (see Table 23.2). In fact, one of the first cases of BKPyV-associated nephropathy presenting as interstitial nephritis occurred in a child with hyper-IgM syndrome (CD40 ligand/CD40 deficiency).[35] BKPyV is most commonly associated with direct kidney injury (nephropathy) after kidney transplant or hemorrhagic cystitis after allogeneic HCT. However, in HCT recipients, nephropathy of their native kidneys can also develop, even in the absence of hemorrhagic cystitis, but there are no reliable data about the incidence. Conversely, it is undefined why hemorrhagic cystitis rarely develops in kidney transplant patients, non-kidney SOT recipients, and children undergoing treatment for cancer. It is possible that a urotoxic insult damaging the urothelial cells may cause rarefication of the mucosal cell layer, on top of which high-level BKPyV replication promotes progression to hemorrhagic cystitis. Less commonly, PyV infections have been linked with gastrointestinal, pulmonary, ophthalmologic, hepatic, and neurologic disease. JCPyV has been much less associated with clinical manifestations in SOT, HCT, or children with cancer, among which the diagnosis of PML is the most devastating one. Of interest, only rare cases of JCPyV nephropathy have been seen in adult and pediatric kidney transplantation at rates of less than 1% to 5%, respectively.[4,21,36] This is notable because the rate of serologic mismatch between donor and recipient, and hence specific immune effector mismatch, would be predicted to occur in approximately 20% among adults and 50% in children assuming average seroprevalence rates of 60% and 35%, respectively. Thus as yet undefined factors must be involved in mitigating JCPyV-mediated pathology in the kidney as opposed to the brain, despite the high homology and similarity between JCPyV and BKPyV. Both viruses have been associated with malignant transformation and cancer, including the demonstration of chromosomal integration and *NCCR* alteration in BKPyV variants detected in urothelial carcinoma in kidney transplant patients.[37,38]

Nephropathy

Proven BKPyV nephropathy is diagnosed in about 5% of pediatric renal transplants and is associated with chronic graft damage, premature decline in function, and an at least 10% attributable risk of graft loss. Most cases of BKPyV nephropathy occur in the first year after kidney transplant. Graft outcomes appear to be worse in patients with a later diagnosis of nephropathy and in those who did not respond to preemptive reductions in immunosuppression.

BKPyV is also recognized as a cause of nephropathy in the native kidneys of children who have received an HCT, mostly published as case reports. Verghese and colleagues described two children in whom biopsy-proven BKPyV nephropathy developed after HCT.[39] A 10-year-old was found to have a serum creatinine level of 1.5 mg/dL 3 years after cord blood transplant for chronic myelogenous leukemia. Severe GVHD was treated with intense combination immunosuppression, including corticosteroids, mycophenolate mofetil, tacrolimus, infliximab, and photopheresis. Without signs of hemorrhagic cystitis, the serum creatinine eventually rose to 3 mg/dL, at which point BKPyV viruria and DNAemia were detected. Five years after transplant, the patient had chronic kidney disease with a serum creatinine level of 1.7 mg/dL. The second patient was a 13-year-old presenting with acute kidney injury, hypertension, and edema 16 months after allogeneic HCT for Fanconi anemia. At that time the serum creatinine level was 1 mg/dL and the patient was being treated with amphotericin for fungal disease and immunosuppression for GVHD. The serum creatinine peaked level at 2.3 mg/dL 2 years after HCT in conjunction with BKPyV viruria and DNAemia. The patient's kidney function worsened and died after declining dialysis.

BKPyV has also been reported in the native kidneys of children after nonrenal SOT, primarily in heart transplant recipients. Lorica and colleagues reviewed six children in whom BKPyV nephropathy developed after heart transplant including a 14-year-old presenting with posttransplant lymphoproliferative disorder 12 years after heart transplant. The serum creatinine concentration rose to 3 mg/dL and the patient had a positive test result for BKPyV DNAemia and viruria with a kidney biopsy demonstrating nephropathy and positive immunohistochemistry for the SV40 LTag.[40] The patient started dialysis but died. In their cross-sectional study of 83 pediatric heart transplants, Ducharme-Smith and colleagues identified 1 patient in whom biopsy-proven BKPyV nephropathy *developed and who required* a kidney transplant for subsequent end-stage kidney disease.[28] They also noted that patients with BKPyV viruria had lower estimated glomerular filtration rates compared with those heart transplant recipients without viruria. So far, there are no reported cases of BKPyV nephropathy after pediatric liver transplant. In their cross-sectional study of 59 pediatric liver transplant recipients, Amir and colleagues[26] found no difference in renal function between recipients with or without viruria, similar to the findings reported by Brinkert and colleagues in their cohort of 100 pediatric liver transplant recipients.[27]

Hemorrhagic Cystitis

Hemorrhagic cystitis associated with BKPyV infection is most commonly reported in children undergoing allogeneic HCT. Hemorrhagic cystitis can develop early after transplant (<1 week), typically related to conditioning chemotherapy, and cyclophosphamide in particular. Late-onset hemorrhagic cystitis (>1 week) is more often secondary to infections. Although it is believed that BKPyV contributes to most cases of late-onset hemorrhagic cystitis after HCT, it is important to note that the exact mechanism for BKPyV-associated hemorrhagic cystitis remains unknown. It is also unclear why hemorrhagic cystitis is largely limited to the allogeneic HCT population, whereas kidney transplant recipients, who have similarly high urine BKPyV loads, rarely have hemorrhagic cystitis. Many have hypothesized that cystitis occurs from some combination of residual urothelial damage to the bladder from conditioning chemotherapy, BKPyV replication from primary or reactivation infection in the face of immunosuppression, and inflammation from engraftment after transplant.[18] BKPyV-associated hemorrhagic cystitis is much less common in children with cancer who have not received an HCT, primarily reported as cases. In one of the larger series, Cheerva and colleagues described 14 nontransplant pediatric oncology patients treated with high-dose cyclophosphamide or ifosfamide, in whom cystitis developed in 4 (29%) despite hyperhydration and mesna prophylaxis.[41] Three of the four patients with cystitis had positive test results for BKPyV viruria and hematuria persisted for 10 to 16 weeks.

The all-cause incidence of hemorrhagic cystitis after HCT is reported to be about 25% and is associated with morbidity from prolonged inpatient lengths of stay and severe urinary discomfort. Early hemorrhagic cystitis is typically associated with conditioning chemotherapy, whereas later-onset cystitis (>1 week after transplant) can be associated with other causes, including viral and bacterial infection.[18] In its most severe form, hemorrhagic cystitis can lead to life-threatening bleeding complications requiring aggressive surgical interventions. Reported risk factors for late-onset hemorrhagic cystitis after HCT include high-level BKPyV viruria (>7 $\log_{10}$), myeloablative conditioning, unrelated mismatched donors, cord blood transplant, peripheral blood stem cells, cyclophosphamide, busulfan, antithymocyte globulin, total body radiation, CMV, human herpesvirus 6 (HHV-6) infection, and older age (>7 years).[18,32,34]

The prospective analysis by Cesaro and colleagues has provided the strongest evidence for the association between BKPyV replication and hemorrhagic cystitis in children after HCT.[33] In addition to collecting plasma and urine samples during the first 100 days after transplant, routine urinalyses to screen for hematuria were performed daily while patients were hospitalized and weekly after discharge until day 100. Hemorrhagic cystitis was defined as gross hematuria plus clinical signs of cystitis. Of the 107 patients enrolled, cystitis developed in 20 (18.7%) at a median of 25 days after HCT (range 7 to 98 days). The duration of gross hematuria was a median of 13 days (range 2 to 71 days). About half of the cases of cystitis occurred before platelet or neutrophil engraftment. The authors examined how viruria and DNAemia predicted cystitis in the first 30 days after transplant. Viruria greater than 7 $\log_{10}$ had a positive predictive value of 14% and a negative predictive value of 98% for later cystitis. DNAemia greater than 1000 copies/mL performed slightly better, with a positive predictive value of 39% and a negative predictive value of 100% for later cystitis. In a multivariate model, BKPyV DNAemia greater than 1000 copies/mL predicted hemorrhagic cystitis with an adjusted hazard ratio (HR) of 6.1 (2.2 to 17.1, $P < .001$). After a median 2.5 years of follow-up, hemorrhagic cystitis was associated with higher risk of overall mortality (HR 2.6, 1.2 to 5.8, $P < .02$).

Other studies in children have supported that BKPyV DNAemia can predict subsequent hemorrhagic cystitis after HCT. Laskin and colleagues analyzed samples from a previously enrolled prospective cohort of 88 allogeneic HCT transplant recipients in Cincinnati from 2010 to 2011.[32] Cystitis was identified by chart review and subjects also had routine urine analyses weekly while hospitalized. Hemorrhagic cystitis was defined as gross hematuria. BKPyV DNAemia results obtained on clinical request were combined with an analysis of stored samples obtained days 0 to 14, days 15 to 85, and day 100 after transplant. Of the 88 subjects, hemorraghic cystitis developed in 17 (19%) at a median of day 25 (interquartile range 18 to 42 days) after transplant. There was no difference in the maximum grade of acute GVHD, platelet engraftment, neutrophil engraftment, or absolute lymphocyte counts between those with and without hemorrhagic cystitis. A time-varying analysis showed that peak DNAemia (1 to 9999 copies/mL) had an HR of 5.3 (2 to 14.6, $P < .01$) and more than 100,000 copies/mL had an HR of 34.3 (4.6 to 256.1, $P < .01$) for later cystitis. HHV-6 DNAemia and older age were also independently associated with hemorrhagic cystitis.

DISEASE PROPHYLAXIS/PREVENTION

There are currently no agents that have demonstrated efficacy in preventing BKPyV replication. Knoll and colleagues conducted a double-blind, placebo-controlled, randomized trial of 3 months of levofloxacin starting 5 days after kidney transplant in 154 adults.[42] Levofloxacin did not decrease the risk of BKPyV viruria or DNAemia, but it did increase the risk of quinolone-resistant bacterial infections and possibly tendinitis. Intravenous immunoglobulin preparations contain high concentrations of anti-BKPyV antibodies. Although some have hypothesized that immunoglobulin formulations could prevent BKPyV infection, no trial data are available to support its use. Despite the fact that many patients receive immunoglobulin infusions for hypogammaglobulinemia after HCT, the risk of BKPyV infection and cystitis remains high. In the future, development of a BKPyV vaccine may allow recipients to be immunized before transplant to prevent infection.[19,43]

Pretransplant Approaches to Prevent Infection

More research is needed to determine optimal strategies for assessing prior to transplantation the posttransplant risk of BKPyV replication and disease. Before transplant, it is standard to test donors and recipients for EBV and CMV antibody status, but there is not enough evidence to support similar testing for BKPyV antibodies. Children who are seronegative for BKPyV may have a higher risk of developing DNAemia and nephropathy after transplant, but replication and disease has been shown to develop in seropositive patients.[22] As mentioned earlier, in a retrospective analysis of pediatric kidney transplant recipients, Ali and colleagues found that recipients with a low serostatus had a significantly higher risk of BKPyV DNAemia in the first year after transplant, and the highest risk of BKPyV DNAemia was found in children with low antibody titers who received transplants from donors with high antibody titers.[22] Finally, Koskenvuo and colleagues reported that among six children in whom hemorrhagic cystitis developed after allogeneic HCT, five were seronegative for BKPyV IgG and IgM before transplant.[44] Of note, the response to intravenous and intravesical cidofovir coincided with mounting a serologic response, raising the possibility that previous cidofovir-attributable effects were actually confounded by emerging BKPyV-specific antibody and cellular immune responses.

Posttransplant Screening to Prevent Infection

Awaiting the development of an effective prophylactic medication or vaccine against BKPyV, prevention of viral disease currently relies on screening for BKPyV viruria and/or DNAemia after transplant to permit timely reduction of immunosuppression, whenever possible.[19] Ginevri and colleagues demonstrated that a stepwise protocol to lower immunosuppression in response to asymptomatic DNAemia prevented the development of any cases of BKPyV nephropathy, without corresponding increase in rejection, in 62 children after kidney transplant.[20] Specifically, in response to increasing BKPyV DNAemia, a patient's calcineurin inhibitor was first reduced by 15% to 20%. If DNAemia persisted, the mycophenolate mofetil was then decreased by half and then discontinued. The optimal screening protocol for BKPyV replication after kidney transplant remains unknown.[19] Pape and colleagues conducted a survey among 90 pediatric nephrologists in Europe and found 26% of providers performed screening for viruria alone, 37% screened both urine and blood, and another 37% screened only for DNAemia.[45] Most physicians (47%) screened patients at months 1, 2, 3, 6, 9, and 12 after transplant.

In support of screening for viruria first, urine samples may be easier to obtain and a negative test result has a very high negative predictive value for BKPyV DNAemia and nephropathy. On average, viruria usually precedes DNAemia by 4 weeks and DNAemia precedes nephropathy by 8 weeks. In favor of screening for DNAemia first, the specificity of BKPyV viruria for nephropathy is low and pediatric transplant patients are frequently already having blood sampling. Most centers have determined their own screening protocols depending on the laboratory resources and expertise available.[19] A screening algorithm for children after kidney transplant is shown in Fig. 23.2. Because most cases of BKPyV nephropathy occur in the first 2 years after kidney transplant, it is reasonable to screen more frequently early after kidney transplant or after treatment for rejection. There is no current evidence or guidelines to suggest screening for BKPyV after nonrenal transplant.[30] However, this may change if more research demonstrates that BKPyV DNAemia can predict hemorrhagic cystitis after allogeneic HCT or if the risk of BKPyV replication and disease after nonrenal SOT is comparable to that seen after kidney transplant.

DIAGNOSIS

Nephropathy

The diagnosis of proven BKPyV nephropathy after kidney transplant or in the native kidneys of nonrenal transplant patients requires a kidney biopsy. On kidney biopsy, BKPyV nephropathy is diagnosed when the tissue shows positive staining for polyomavirus proteins (typically by antibodies to the SV40 LTag), cytopathic changes in renal tubules, and associated interstitial nephritis. Patients with persistent BKPyV DNAemia greater 10,000 copies/mL are often classified as having presumptive nephropathy in the absence of biopsy. However, data supporting the implications of persistent BKPyV DNAemia are from adult studies, and differences in NAT assays across centers can make comparisons difficult.[19]

Although a biopsy is considered the gold standard, false-negative results can occur secondary to sampling errors resulting from the focal replication and associated tissue damage. It is therefore recommended to obtain at least two biopsy cores containing medullary tissue.[19] It is unknown if all patients with persistent DNAemia (or any level of DNAemia) require a kidney biopsy in the absence of graft dysfunction, especially in children. Kidney biopsy findings can sometimes be difficult to interpret because the inflammatory infiltrate seen with BKPyV nephropathy can be similar to that seen with acute rejection.[19] Highlighting some of these uncertainties, Pape and colleagues reported that only 50% of nephrologists perform kidney biopsies in children with high-level BKPyV DNAemia whose kidney function is at baseline before prescribing changes in immunosuppression or other interventions.[45] Outside the pediatric kidney transplant population, there are no recommendations to guide diagnosing BKPyV nephropathy in other high-risk patients. Nonrenal solid organ transplant and allogeneic HCT recipients are at risk for chronic kidney failure, which is frequently attributed to calcineurin inhibitor toxicity. Although there are no recommendations for screening these patients for BKPyV replication, clinicians should consider checking a blood BKPyV DNAemia by quantitative NAT in any immunosuppressed patient with unexplained chronic kidney disease.[30]

There are several novel diagnostic approaches in patients with concern for BKPyV nephropathy. First, monitoring for BKPyV-specific T-cell numbers or function may help predict the course of BKPyV replication. Ginevri and colleagues performed ELISPOT assays in their prospective cohort of children after kidney transplant.[20] Specifically, patients' peripheral blood mononuclear cells were stimulated with BKPyV peptides and the amount of interferon-gamma release was measured after *in vitro* expansion as an indicator of the presence of BKPyV-virus specific T cells. In their study, patients with BKPyV DNAemia had lower ELISpot (Mabtech, Stockholm, Sweden) counts compared with healthy controls, and after reduction of immunosuppression patients with BKPyV DNAemia had increases in ELISpot counts. Recent advances suggest that LTag-specific T cells in pediatric and adult kidney transplant patients may recognize HLA class 1–dependent immunodominant 9mer epitopes, which correlated with clearance of BKPyV DNAemia.[46,47] Second, Laskin and colleagues reported

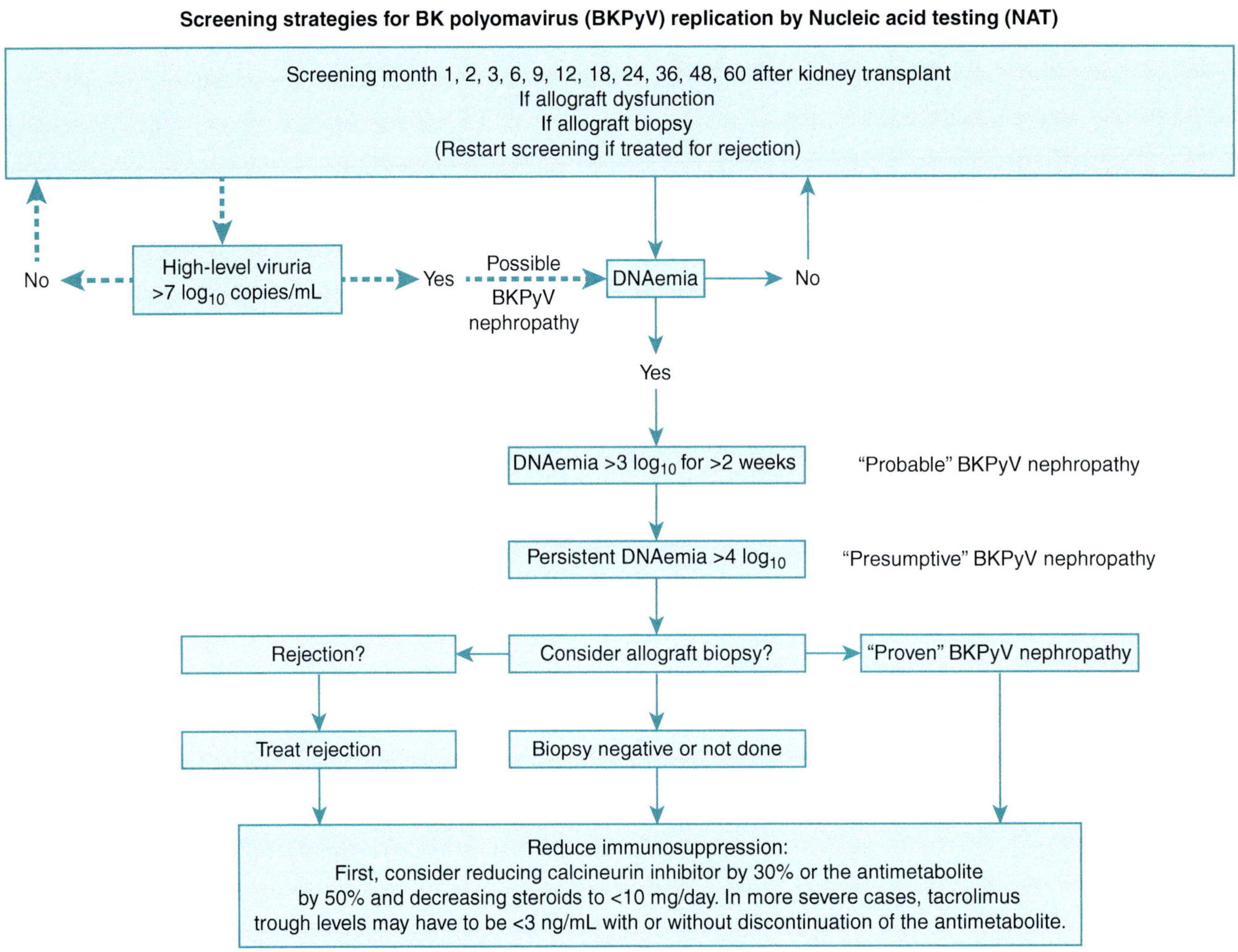

Fig. 23.2 Screening and treatment protocol for BKPyV replication in children after kidney transplant. No similar screening or treatment guidelines exist for hematopoietic stem cell, nonrenal solid organ transplant recipients, or children with cancer. However, it is reasonable that immunosuppressed patients be checked for BKPyV DNAemia if they develop increases in creatinine, chronic kidney disease, or proteinuria. Reduction of immunosuppression, should be considered as first-line treatment if feasible. (Data from Hirsch HH, Randhawa P, AST Infectious Diseases Community of Practice. BK polyomavirus in solid organ transplantation. *Am J Transplant.* 2013;13(suppl 4):179-188.)

that a novel, noninvasive urinary test detecting BKPyV aggregates by routine electron microscopy (so-called PyV-Haufen) may be able to diagnose BKPyV nephropathy in children after HCT.[48] If validated in larger studies, these tests may help guide therapy without the need for biopsy.

Hemorrhagic Cystitis

Table 23.3 summarizes the diagnostic criteria and severity grading for BKPyV-associated hemorrhagic cystitis after HCT. In patients presenting with signs and symptoms of cystitis, it is important to rule out other causes, including adenovirus, JCPyV, CMV, bacteria, parasite, malignancies and mechanical including catheter-associated bleeding.[18] In patients with concern for hemorrhagic cystitis, BKPyV urine NAT should first be obtained. It is unclear if testing the blood or repeat urine samples for BKPyV DNA in patients with established hemorrhagic cystitis is useful, or if patients should simply have follow-up for resolution of clinical signs and symptoms. Few studies have examined if markers of immune function may predict the course of hemorrhagic cystitis, similar to

TABLE 23.3 Grading of Hematuria and Diagnostic Criteria of BKPyV-Associated Hemorrhagic Cystitis

Grading of hematuria	Grade I	Microscopic hematuria
	Grade II	Macroscopic hematuria
	Grade III	Urinary clots
	Grade IV	Urinary obstruction
Diagnostic criteria for BKPyV-associated hemorrhagic cystitis	Clinical symptoms of dysuria, urgency, lower abdominal pain, frequency	
	At least macroscopic (grade II) hematuria	
	BKPyV viruria >10 million copies/mL (7 $\log_{10}$)	

Modified from Haley SA, O'Hara BA, Nelson CD, et al. Human polyomavirus receptor distribution in brain parenchyma contrasts with receptor distribution in kidney and choroid plexus. *Am J Pathol.* 2015;185(8):2246-2258.

findings in patients with nephropathy after kidney transplant. Koskenvuo and colleagues reported that among six children in whom hemorrhagic cystitis developed after allogeneic HCT, BKPyV antibody titers increased in the four subjects with resolution of cystitis and DNAemia, whereas antibodies against BKPyV did not developed in the remaining two subjects, who had had persistent BKPyV DNAemia and symptoms.[44]

TREATMENT

The only established treatment for BKPyV replication or disease is to reduce immunosuppression.[19] However, it is not always possible to lower immunosuppression in some patients owing to the risk of rejection or GVHD. Moreover, despite lowering immunosuppression, BKPyV infection persists in many patients. Finally, BKPyV replication and disease may develop in some patients as the result of underlying immune deficiency or poor immune reconstitution including those who are not receiving any immunosuppression that can be reduced.

Other therapies for BKPyV replication are of unproven benefit and have not been systematically tested in clinical trials. Therapies with in vitro activity against BKPyV include fluoroquinolones, cidofovir, leflunomide, and intravenous immunoglobulin. There are many studies in the literature reporting the presumably use of these therapies, all of which are flawed by their retrospective and uncontrolled nature.[19]

As described earlier, fluoroquinolones have not been shown to be effective as BKPyV prophylaxis in a randomized controlled trial in adults after kidney transplant, and it is therefore unlikely to assume efficacy when treating ongoing BKPyV replication and disease.[42] Cidofovir is an antiviral agent that has been administered intravenously and/or through bladder instillation in patients with clinically significant BKPyV replication. Doses studied are 0.5 to 1.5 mg/kg per week intravenously without probenecid and 3 to 5 mg/kg per week with probenecid to prevent renal tubular damage. Without probenicid, cidofovir Cidofovir is taken up by the renal tubular cells in which BKPyV replicates, but then causes nephrotoxicity, limiting its use in patients with kidney disease. Similarly, cidofovir may also associated with uveitis. Leflunomide is a pyrimidine synthesis antagonist with antiinflammatory properties used in rheumatoid arthritis, which inhibits BKPyV replication in vitro in the absence of exogenous uridine. The drug requires periodic screening of drug levels and is associated with hepatitis, myelosuppression, and anemia.[19]

In patients with severe hemorrhagic cystitis, other reported therapies include hyperbaric oxygen, fibrin glue, and estrogens. Treatment is typically supportive with hydration, bladder irrigation, transfusions, and pain control.[18]

The optimal approach to lowering immunosuppression, when feasible, is also unknown. Most studies recommend either reducing the calcineurin inhibitor dosing or the antimetabolite (mycophenolate mofetil) first. Specific protocols have included some combination of a 30% reduction in calcineurin inhibitor, 50% reduction in antimetabolite, and decreasing steroids to less than 10 mg per day. In patients with low-level DNAemia, tacrolimus trough levels less than 6 ng/mL, cyclosporine trough levels less than 150 ng/mL, sirolimus levels less than 6 ng/mL, and/or mycophenolate mofetil less than 1000 mg/day should be first considered. In patients with persisting high-level or refractory replication, tacrolimus trough levels may have to be decreased to less than 3 ng/mL with or without discontinuation of mycophenolate mofetil.[19,20] After intervention, it can take 1 to 2 months before BKPyV DNAemia starts to decrease. In their survey of pediatric nephrologists, Pape and colleagues noted that the first intervention performed by pediatric nephrologists was decreasing mycophenolate mofetil (40% of providers), decreasing calcineurin inhibitor dosing (29% of providers), or both (31% of providers).[45] Most providers reserved changing immunosuppressive agents for patients with biopsy-proven nephropathy, and specific interventions included discontinuation of mycophenolate mofetil (75% of providers) and switching to mechanistic target of rapamycin inhibitors (52% of providers) for these situations. Cidofovir, intravenous immunoglobulin, leflunomide, and fluoroquinolones were used by less than one-third of providers. Importantly, 66% of providers saw a need for new antiviral drugs, new immunosuppressive strategies, and vaccine development.

Although it has generally been assumed that the overall degree of immunosuppression is the primary risk factor for BKPyV replication and disease, emerging evidence suggests that tacrolimus may itself be associated with a higher risk compared with other agents. Hirsch and colleagues compared the effects of mechanistic target of rapamycin inhibitors and calcineurin inhibitors on BKPyV replication in primary human renal tubular epithelial cells.[49] Sirolimus and cyclosporine were found to decrease BKPyV replication. However, tacrolimus increased BKPyV replication and even reversed sirolimus inhibition by competing for the intracellular FK-binding protein 12. Egli and colleagues used interferon gamma ELISpot assays to study the associations between immunosuppressive drug levels and BKPyV-specific T-cell responses in kidney transplant patients and healthy controls.[12] In kidney transplant patients, BKPyV-specific T-cell responses were inversely correlated with tacrolimus trough levels ($R = 0.28$, $P < .002$), but not with mycophenolate levels, prednisone, or overall immunosuppressive dosing. The BKPyV-specific interferon-gamma release was inhibited by calcineurin inhibitors affecting T-cell signal-1, but not affected by antiproliferative and signal-3 inhibitors. Tacrolimus concentrations above 6 ng/mL inhibited BKPyV-specific T cells more than 50%, whereas less than 30% inhibition was observed at tacrolimus concentrations below 3 ng/mL. These studies suggest that tacrolimus is associated with a higher risk of BKPyV infection and support targeting trough levels below 6 ng/mL as the initial intervention in patients.[19] Long-term follow-up data in adult kidney transplant patients indicate that clearance in more than 95% of patients can be obtained, and that graft survival is not significantly different from patients with high-level viruria or no BKPyV replication if reducing immunosuppression is guided by a standard operating procedure.[50]

A new promising novel therapy for BKPyV infection is the infusion of BKPyV-specific T cells, either generated in vitro directly from the patient (autologous), from the transplant donor, or from a third party. Tzannou and colleagues generated a bank of virus-specific T cells capable of recognizing EBV, adenovirus, CMV, BKPyV, and HHV6.[51] They conducted a phase II trial in 38 patients after HCT. Thirteen of 14 patients treated for BKPyV replication orassociated hemorrhagic cystitis experienced complete resolution of gross hematuria 6 weeks after infusion. The treatments were deemed safe as only two cases of mild GVHD occurred. The third-party T cells persisted in the recipient for up to 12 weeks. More research is needed, especially in children, to determine the safety and efficacy of infusing BKPyV-specific T cells for prevention or treatment of disease after SOT and HCT.

INFECTION PREVENTION AND ANTICIPATORY GUIDANCE

Current guidelines recommend standard precautions for patients admitted to the hospital who also have BKPyV replication. It is unknown how BKPyV is spread.[19] Interestingly, in their study after HCT, Koskenvuo and colleagues conducted a genetic analysis of the viral isolates and showed there was possible nosocomial transmission of BKPyV between two patients who roomed close together during hospitalization.[44] More research is needed to determine the pathogenicity of different BKPyV strains and if more restrictive preventative measures could prevent BKPyV exposure of highly susceptible patients admitted to the hospital or in the community.

24

Aspergillosis

William J. Steinbach, MD

Aspergillus is a ubiquitous organism with an ecological niche in the soil. Most disease is primarily caused by *A. fumigatus*, *A. flavus*, *A. niger*, *A. terreus*, and *A. nidulans*, and classification of the genus has been revised multiple times to incorporate newer molecular definitions. *A. fumigatus* causes approximately 70% to 80% of cases of invasive aspergillosis (IA), but it is difficult to differentiate from the other closely related species based solely on morphology. *A. fumigatus* is also responsible for most pulmonary disease, whereas isolated sinus disease is often caused by *A. niger* and *A. flavus*. Specific determination of the infecting species of *Aspergillus* is clinically important as there is a variation in therapeutic susceptibility profiles between and within species. Although there is an estimated global incidence of more than 300,000 cases of IA per year, there are significantly more cases of chronic pulmonary aspergillosis (estimated 3,000,000 per year) and allergic *Aspergillus* disease (many millions per year).

EPIDEMIOLOGY AND RISK FACTORS

Although not rigorously defined, most experts define a patient group as high risk for IA if the incidence of IA in that group is reported to be 5% to 10% or higher. Following this approach, pediatric populations falling into this high-risk category are those with new-onset or relapsed acute myelogenous leukemia (AML), relapsed acute lymphoblastic leukemia (ALL), and new-onset ALL using aggressive treatment protocols (i.e., high-risk ALL). Other high-risk patients include those with bone marrow failure syndromes (e.g., myelodysplastic syndrome); hematopoietic stem cell transplant (HSCT) recipients and especially those with allogeneic donors; solid organ transplant (SOT) recipients and especially those undergoing lung, heart-lung, or high-risk liver transplant; patients with underlying chronic granulomatous disease (CGD); and patients receiving prolonged courses of corticosteroids or other immune modifiers.

A prospective French study of all three major populations at risk for IA found that time to development of IA after transplantation was similar in different transplantation settings, with 68% of IA after HSCT diagnosed more than 100 days after transplant, and the majority (18 of 27) of SOT recipients with IA diagnosed at least 100 days after transplant.[1] Multivariate analysis showed that factors independently associated with increased risk of death from IA included older age, diagnosis based on positive culture results with two positive galactomannan (GM) assays, and the presence of pleural effusion or central nervous system (CNS) involvement. The case-fatality rate of IA in patients with acute leukemia was 38%, whereas allogeneic HSCT recipients had a staggering 56% overall case-fatality rate.

The Transplant-Associated Infection Surveillance Network (TRANSNET) study sponsored by the Centers for Disease Control and Prevention evaluated largely adult HSCT and SOT recipients from 23 U.S. medical centers (2001 to 2005) and included a total of 642 cases of IA.[2] The 12-month cumulative incidence of IA in all HSCT recipients was 1.6% compared with 0.63% in SOT recipients. Twelve-week all-cause mortality was 57.5% among HSCT recipients and 34.4% among SOT recipients. Multivariable analysis demonstrated that neutropenia, renal insufficiency, hepatic insufficiency, early-onset (<30 days) IA, proven IA, and methylprednisolone use (often for graft-versus-host disease [GVHD]) were independently associated with mortality. Analysis for SOT recipients revealed that hepatic insufficiency, malnutrition, and CNS disease were independently associated with increased risk of death. Among both HSCT and SOT recipients, receipt of voriconazole as part of the initial antifungal therapy was more common among survivors.

The epidemiology and further risk factors specific to HSCT recipients, SOT recipients, and children with malignancy or bone marrow failure syndromes are discussed in more detail in the following sections.

Hematopoietic Stem Cell Transplant

IA was the most common invasive mold disease in a review of approximately 5500 patients who underwent HSCT. Whereas more than 7% of HSCT recipients had mold infections, *Aspergillus* infections were the most common, followed by *Fusarium*, mucormycosis, and *Scedosporium* infections.[3] The incidence of IA in HSCT recipients has ranged from 3% to 7%, but the true incidence is likely dependent on multiple factors, the most important of which is the type of transplantation (allogeneic vs. autologous). In one study of HSCT recipients with IA, the risk of developing the disease was 12.8 times higher among recipients of allogeneic than autologous HSCT.[4] A prospective French study analyzed 424 cases of IA and found an incidence of 0.9% in autologous and 8.1% in allogeneic HSCT patients, respectively,[1] highlighting a consistent finding that IA occurs much more readily in the allogeneic HSCT recipient.

In allogeneic HSCT recipients, three periods of risk for IA occur: (1) neutropenia after the conditioning regimen; (2) exogenous immunosuppression for prevention or treatment of acute GVHD; and (3) exogenous immunosuppression for treatment of chronic GVHD (after day 100 after transplant). The level of allogeneic donor and recipient HLA disparity is the major determinant for GVHD severity and intensity of immunosuppression to control GVHD, which, in turn, is the major predisposing factor for IA during this risk window. There is a well-characterized bimodal distribution of IA in HSCT recipients that correlates with pre-engraftment neutropenia (median of 16 days after transplantation) and the peak of GVHD (median of 96 days after transplantation).[5] Most patients (86%) with autologous transplants were diagnosed with IA while neutropenic, whereas patients with allogeneic transplants were at greatest risk after engraftment or during impairment of cell-mediated immunity owing to cytomegalovirus (CMV) or GVHD.

A subanalysis of the TRANSNET study data focused on only the 875 largely adult HSCT recipients and found IA was the most common (43%) of all invasive fungal diseases, followed by invasive candidiasis (28%).[6] The median time of developing IA after HSCT was 99 days. Of the 80 cases of IA in autologous HSCT, 50% occurred within 1 month after receipt of transplant, whereas in allogeneic HSCT recipients only 22% occurred within 1 month after transplantation. Autologous HSCT recipients had all-cause mortality of 13% at 12 months, whereas allogeneic recipient mortality was higher at 36% at 12 months. The 12-month cumulative incidence for IA in all HSCT recipients was 1.6% compared with 1.1% for invasive candidiasis, and the overall 1-year survival among HSCT recipients with IA was only 25.4%.

Another large database, the Prospective Antifungal Therapy Alliance also found IA most frequent among the largely adult HSCT recipients studied, and approximately 70% of those HSCT recipients with IA were allogeneic transplants. The median time to develop IA after HSCT was similar (82 days), with a diagnosis of a median of 51 days after autologous transplant and 83 days after allogeneic transplantation.[7]

In several HSCT patient risk factor studies, only moderate-to-severe GVHD, steroid prophylaxis for GVHD, or total body irradiation were significant variables in the multivariate analyses. In one study several parameters in the period from HSCT to diagnosis of fungal disease were found to influence survival, each of which was related to the cumulative dose of prednisolone. In the multivariate analysis, there was a relative risk (RR) of 8.78 of death from IA in patients with acute active GVHD (grade II or more) or extensive chronic GVHD combined with a cumulative total prednisolone dose of more than 7 mg/kg in the week before diagnosis.[8]

Solid Organ Transplant

In SOT recipients, the intensity of immunosuppression to prevent or treat allograft rejection and coinfection with CMV all influence the risk of IA. Data from the TRANSNET database specific to SOT recipients found IA to be the second most common source of invasive fungal disease (19%) behind invasive candidiasis (53%).[9] The median time to onset of IA was 184 days after SOT, with a 1-year cumulative IA incidence of 0.65% and a 12-month survival of 59%. Data on SOT recipients from the Prospective Antifungal Therapy Alliance analysis also found IA (25%) second to invasive candidiasis. IA was most frequently found in lung transplant recipients (60%).[10] IA developed a median of 400 days after any type of SOT; however, this varied by transplant type. The median time from SOT to IA in liver transplantation was 100 days compared with 504 days and 384 days in lung and heart transplant recipients, respectively. Most cases of IA in liver transplant recipients occurred less than 6 months after transplant, whereas 62% of lung transplant recipients with IA developed disease less than 1 year after transplant. This contrasted to a retrospective review of 158 cases of IA in Spanish SOT recipients that found that 57% had early-onset IA (first 3 months after transplantation).[11] The overall incidence of IA in those SOT recipients was 1.4%, including a similar distribution among specific organ transplants with an incidence of 3% (lung), 2.4% (heart), 2% (liver), and 0.2% (kidney). The overall case fatality rate was 77%, with no significant differences between SOT groups. Risk factors for developing early-onset IA included complicated postoperative period, repeated bacterial infections or CMV disease, and renal failure.

In a large prospective mostly adult French study[1] among those SOT recipients with IA, the highest incidence of IA was for heart transplant recipients (4.8%), followed by lung (4.1%), and significantly dropping for liver (0.8%) and kidney (0.3%). Pediatric-specific data on SOT recipients confirmed the highest incidence for all invasive fungal diseases is in pediatric heart-lung and lung recipients, followed by liver and kidney recipients.[12]

Oncology

In patients with malignancy, myelodysplastic syndrome, and other diseases associated with marrow failure (e.g., aplastic anemia), neutropenia is the most important risk factor for IA. Furthermore, assessing the intensity and duration of neutropenia can help the clinician further refine the risk of IA in a patient. In a large case series of IA events, the majority (59%) of patients had a hematologic or solid tumor malignancy with neutropenia as their primary risk factor. Among the remaining 41%, most of the patients had steroid-reliant chronic obstructive pulmonary disease, asthma, or rheumatologic disorders but did not have neutropenia. The clinical presentation of the two groups differed; the latter group was less likely to have typical symptoms of IA and more likely to have frequent intercurrent pneumonia with another microorganism. The case-fatality rates of both patient types were high; nonneutropenic patients had a case-fatality rate of 89% compared with 60% in neutropenic patients.[13]

The risk of IA is estimated to increase from 1% per day after the first 3 weeks of neutropenia to 4% to 5% per day after 5 weeks.[14] Prolonged or marked macrophage dysfunctions that occur as a result of underlying disease and its treatment can also predispose patients to IA. Therefore the risk of infection is higher with advanced underlying disease, transplantation during relapse of malignancy or chemotherapeutic rescue therapy, GVHD, or concurrent infection such as CMV.

In the French prospective study,[1] the majority of patients with IA had a hematologic malignancy and the largest group had acute leukemia (35%), but the second largest group had chronic lymphoproliferative disorders (22%). For those with acute leukemia, IA occurred for 68% during the induction phase of chemotherapy, when cytotoxic agents are generally the most intense, and for 27% during the consolidation phase.

Corticosteroids are also a well-known major risk factor for the development of IA and can suppress the ability of monocytes/macrophages to kill conidia through inhibition of nonoxidative processes and impairment of lysosomal activity. Corticosteroids also inhibit polymorphonuclear neutrophils in their chemotaxis, oxidative bursts, and activity against hyphae. Generally, corticosteroids suppress macrophages, whereas cytotoxic chemotherapy decreases neutrophil number and function.

Pediatric-Specific Invasive Aspergillosis Epidemiology

There is little information on the fundamental epidemiology of pediatric IA, and most overall epidemiologic investigations do not offer pediatric-specific analyses. Analysis of a large U.S. pediatric inpatient database found an annual incidence of 0.4% of IA among all immunocompromised children, and the highest incidence of IA was seen in children who had undergone allogeneic HSCT (4.5%) and those with AML (4%), whereas autologous HSCT had a lower incidence of 0.3%. Specifically, the incidence of IA in patients with AML was significantly greater than the incidence in patients with ALL (RR 5.6, 95% confidence interval [CI] 4.6 to 7.0). Lung SOT recipients had the greatest incidence among those pediatric SOT recipients (5%). Comparing mortality in pediatric patients with specific underlying diseases with and without IA revealed the relative risk (RR) of death was increased in CNS tumors (RR 21.6), ALL (RR 14.9), and lymphoma (RR 13.5), showcasing the overall good survival rates of those common pediatric malignancies and the devastating effect of adding IA to reasonably curable underlying pediatric malignancies.[15] The largest pediatric case series was a retrospective multicenter review of 139 children with IA. *A. fumigatus* was the species most frequently recovered (52.8%), and the majority of the children had a malignancy with or without HSCT. Significant risk factors that affected survival were immunosuppressive therapies and allogeneic HSCT.[16]

The largest international, prospective case series of any invasive mold disease in children (2007 to 2011)[17] included 98 children with IA. Children with IA and those with other types of invasive mold diseases had similar underlying risk factors, except that children with infections caused by non-*Aspergillus* species were more likely to have received mold-active antifungal agents preceding diagnosis. Among 43 patients who underwent HSCT, 27 (63%) underwent myeloablative conditioning. Of the 36 HSCT recipients who had complete information regarding the timing of diagnosis of invasive mold disease relative to transplantation, 5 (14%) were diagnosed before or on the day of HSCT and 31 (86%) were diagnosed at a median of 168 days following HSCT (interquartile range 25 to 247 days).

CLINICAL MANIFESTATIONS

Aspergillus species are relatively unique among pathogens as they are responsible for a gamut of infections extending across the clinical spectrum to include primary allergic reactions, saprophytic involvement, chronic disease, and acute invasive disease. The type of *Aspergillus* infection generally depends on the immunologic background of the infected host, and the focus here is exclusively on immunodeficient patients in whom acute invasive disease develops. The clinical manifestations of these infections in immunocompromised patients can be subtle, nonspecific, and commonly occur late in the course of disease. As a result, a high index of suspicion should be maintained to implement treatment in the early stages of disease.

Invasive Pulmonary Aspergillosis

Aspergillus species are ubiquitous in the environment and one major portal of entry is the respiratory tract. In some immunocompetent patients, this inhalation could result in nonpathogenic saprophytic colonization; however, in immunocompromised patients, this conidial acquisition will likely result in establishment of invasive disease. Invasive pulmonary aspergillosis (IPA) is the most frequently documented form of IA.

The clinical manifestation of IPA is heterogeneous; typically it may include fever unresponsive to broad-spectrum antibiotics, dry cough, shortness of breath, pleuritic chest pain, hemoptysis, and pulmonary nodules or infiltrates on radiography. Although neutropenic patients more commonly present with fever, in some patients the fever and cough are not present for the first several days of infection, specifically in patients receiving high-dose corticosteroid therapy. Progression of infection is characterized by invasion of small vessels leading to hemoptysis as a leading symptom of IPA in some neutropenic patients. Two patterns of hemorrhage may be identified—hemorrhagic infarction as the result of vascular invasion or formation of mycotic aneurysms during recovery from neutropenia that can rupture and result in fatal hemoptysis.

Invasive *Aspergillus* Sinusitis

Fungal sinusitis can manifest as allergic, saprophytic, or invasive disease. Invasive *Aspergillus* sinusitis is likely underdiagnosed because of its variable clinical presentation and difficulty in establishing the diagnosis, possibly owing to a decreased inflammatory response in affected patients. Patients can present with nasal congestion, discharge, headache, facial pain or swelling, and abnormal findings of the nasal cavity, such as pallor of the nasal septum or turbinate mucosa. Epistaxis, orbital swelling, and high fever can also be present. However, definitive diagnosis can be established only by endoscopic evaluation and biopsy. Common findings on endoscopy include pallor of the mucosa, discoloration or granulation of the mucosa owing to ischemia as a result of angioinvasion, and as the disease progresses, a blackened necrotic focus can be found. Extension into bony structures can occur at the site of necrosis. leading to spread of disease into adjacent structures, such as the orbit and the brain, which carries high morbidity and mortality. Although imaging is not diagnostic, it can aid in establishing the diagnosis because it can be used as a road map for endoscopy by showing which sinuses are involved. Lack of bony destruction on imaging should not deter pursuit of a diagnosis of IA, as bony destruction is a late manifestation of this process.

Cerebral Aspergillosis

IA most commonly involves the lungs, but disease can disseminate via the bloodstream and involve distant organs. One of the most frequent sites of dissemination is the CNS. Cerebral aspergillosis may also be a result of direct extension through the sinuses. As with other *Aspergillus* infections, *A. fumigatus* is the most frequently encountered species in cerebral aspergillosis, but other implicated species are *A. flavus*, *A. niger*, and *A. nidulans*. More classical symptoms for an intracranial process, such as headache, nausea, or vomiting, are often absent in cerebral aspergillosis. Instead patients present with mental status alteration, convulsions, hemiplegia or hemiparesis, ophthalmoplegia and loss of consciousness. Severely immunocompromised patients may not display these symptoms and disease progresses more rapidly.

Aspergillus hyphae are angioinvasive and thrombose arteries to create hemorrhagic infarcts, and as a result, CNS aspergillosis can present as solitary or multiple abscesses, and less commonly, as mycotic aneurysms and carotid artery invasion. Cerebral aspergillosis can also appear as meningitis or granuloma. Cerebral aspergillosis presents as multiple areas of low density and no enhancement even with contrast on computed tomography (CT), and lesions are usually located within the basal ganglia and gray-white matter junction. On magnetic resonance imaging (MRI), these same abnormalities appear as foci of intermediate T2 signal surrounded by a rim of higher signal. Aspergillosis of the CNS carries an extremely high case-fatality rate, so prompt diagnosis and treatment are key to survival. Unfortunately, definitive diagnosis requires biopsy and typically these patients are often too coagulopathic to undergo such a procedure.

Cutaneous Aspergillosis

Cutaneous aspergillosis can be primary, as is more often seen in children via a result of direct skin injury or traumatic inoculation, or secondary, as a result of hematogenous spread or extension from infected underlying structures. Primary cutaneous aspergillosis has been associated with intravenous access devices, adhesive dressings, and sites of skin compromise such as from GVHD or surgery. Cutaneous disease can also develop from secondary hematogenous seeding from a primary source, usually the lungs. This has been described particularly among HSCT recipients. Lesions often begin as erythematous, indurated papules that progress to ulcerative, painful, and necrotic lesions.

DISEASE PROPHYLAXIS/PREVENTION

Two main strategies exist for managing patients at high risk for IA, primary prophylaxis or no antifungal prophylaxis with close monitoring (generally twice weekly) using biomarkers. The latter is often referred to as a preemptive therapy approach in which a positive fungal biomarker, such as GM antigen or a chest CT scan with pulmonary infiltrates, triggers the use of antifungal treatment while a more confirmatory diagnosis is undertaken. The preferred approach is the source of much debate and likely depends on local epidemiology and the ability to access rapid fungal diagnostics. Notably, there are limited pediatric-specific data on primary prophylaxis or preemptive therapy approaches in children.

In adult guidelines, primary prophylaxis for IA is recommended for patients with hematologic malignancy or those undergoing allogeneic HSCT during periods of neutropenia and at times of GVHD treatment.[18] Posaconazole is recommended as first-line prophylaxis, with other agents such as lipid amphotericin B products, echinocandins, or voriconazole considered as less desirable alternatives. The 2019 ESCMID-ECMM pediatric-specific guidelines for IA[19] state that primary antifungal prophylaxis should be considered during the granulocytopenic phase of allogeneic HSCT. Suggested agents for prophylaxis include itraconazole, posaconazole (for patients ≥13 years), and voriconazole (for patients ≥2 years). Alternative agents include liposomal amphotericin B and micafungin, and less recommended options include aerosolized amphotericin B and caspofungin. In the absence of GVHD, antifungal prophylaxis can continue after engraftment until discontinuation of immunosuppression and signs of immune recovery, but in the presence of GVHD requiring augmented immunosuppression, continuation of antifungal prophylaxis is recommended. These guidelines also recommend IA prophylaxis in children with neutropenia during periods of new-onset or relapsed AML, relapsed ALL, and for bone marrow failure syndromes. In children undergoing SOT, antifungal prophylaxis is recommended in those undergoing lung, heart-lung, heart alone with a high-risk profile, and high-risk liver transplant. It is important to note that there are limited pediatric data from either randomized trials or comparative observational studies on the effectiveness of prophylaxis. As such, most of the aforementioned recommendations for pediatric IA prophylaxis are based on expert opinion.

A preemptive approach with surveillance testing results dictating initiation of antifungal therapy represents an alternative approach to primary prophylaxis. There are no data to compare preemptive and primary prophylaxis approaches in children. However, a randomized trial compared the preemptive versus the empirical antifungal approach (initiation of antifungal therapy after prolonged period of fever and neutropenia) in 149 children with high-risk febrile neutropenia demonstrated that the preemptive approach using molecular biomarkers was associated with similar rates of invasive fungal disease and mortality, and resulted in a significant reduction of antifungal use compared with the empirical therapy approach.[20] Unfortunately, this study does not inform about the effectiveness of this approach compared with primary prophylaxis.

DIAGNOSIS

The diagnosis of IA is not straightforward, and involves integration of clinical, radiologic, and microbiologic data (Fig. 24.1). Because of myriad clinical presentations, IA diagnosis is categorized as "proven," "probable," or "possible" disease based on meeting certain clinical, microbiologic, and radiologic criteria designed and later revised by the European Organization for the Research and Treatment of Cancer and the Mycoses Study Group.[21] These criteria have served as a standard in clinical trials and observational studies to segregate patients with similar disease characteristics, but it should be noted that these criteria are not perfect and the designers have specifically cautioned against their implementation in routine clinical practice. Nonetheless, these distinctions have served the community well to establish a common framework for discussion about disease in the complicated high-risk patient. Generally, "proven" and "probable" IA can be considered as one entity, as numerous clinical trials have shown their general equivalency in patient outcomes.

Cultures

A proven diagnosis of IA requires isolation of an *Aspergillus* spp. from a culture specimen taken from an otherwise sterile site in association with histologic evidence of invasive disease. Although the histopathologic appearance of hyphae can provide a proven invasive fungal disease [IFD] designation, confirmation of IFD as IA requires detection of *Aspergillus* by culture or nonculture technique. This is necessary because *Aspergillus* cannot be distinguished histopathologically from other filamentous fungi, such as *Fusarium* spp. and *Scedosporium* spp.

Unfortunately, the requirements for proven IA diagnosis are challenging to meet, especially because biopsy specimen procurement is often considered too invasive and is complicated by bleeding or secondary infection in high-risk patients. Detection of *Aspergillus* in noninvasive specimens, such as sputum, allows for designation of probable IA in association with radiographic findings, but sputum culture is complicated by the fact that the presence of *Aspergillus* may represent colonization and not disease. The sensitivity of sputum culture for *Apsergillus* is poor likely because IPA is predominantly infiltrative and does not have aerial growth in the bronchial tree. In one study of heart transplant recipients, during a 10-year study period, *Aspergillus* species were recovered from 30 episodes from 27 heart transplant recipients (incidence 10.5%). The overall positive predictive value was 60% to 70%, but this increased to 88% to 100% when it was recovered from a respiratory specimen other than sputum, and decreased to 50% to 67% when it was recovered from sputum.[22] Taking all of this into consideration, it is likely that the incidence of IA is underestimated in many published cohorts.

Isolation of *Aspergillus* spp. from the blood is difficult, and thus any positive blood culture result for *Aspergillus* spp. is often presumed to be a laboratory contaminant and not a true infection. The difficulty in detecting *A. fumigatus* in blood culture stands in contrast to other angioinvasive filamentous fungi (e.g., *Fusarium* spp., *Paecilomyces lilacinus, Scedosporium prolificans, Acremonium* spp.) that have the ability to discharge a steady series of unicellular spores into the bloodstream, which are more likely to be captured in a blood sample. This ability to sporulate in tissue and blood has been termed adventitious sporulation. As *A. terreus* also displays adventitious sporulation, a positive blood culture with *A. terreus* or another mold that demonstrates adventitious sporulation should not be ignored.

Radiology

In high-risk patients when there is concern for IFD (e.g., in a child with persistent fever and neutropenia despite broad-spectrum antibacterial treatment), further investigation with radiographic imaging is warranted. The focus of this section is on the radiographic findings of the lungs, brain, and sinuses, as these are the most likely sites of IA. However, *Aspergillus* can disseminate hematogenously to any location of the body from one of these primary sites. Therefore imaging of the abdomen or musculoskeletal system may be warranted in some settings. High-resolution CT scan is considered the imaging modality of choice for the lungs and sinuses,[18] whereas MRI is preferred for evaluation of the brain.

Pulmonary Imaging. IPA characteristically manifests as multiple, ill-defined, 1- to 3-cm peripheral nodules that gradually coalesce into larger masses or areas of subsegmental and segmental consolidation. Lobar, pleural-based wedge-shaped, alveolar, or diffuse pulmonary consolidation are also common findings.[18,23] Plain chest radiographs can detect some of these pathologies, but they are insensitive and can

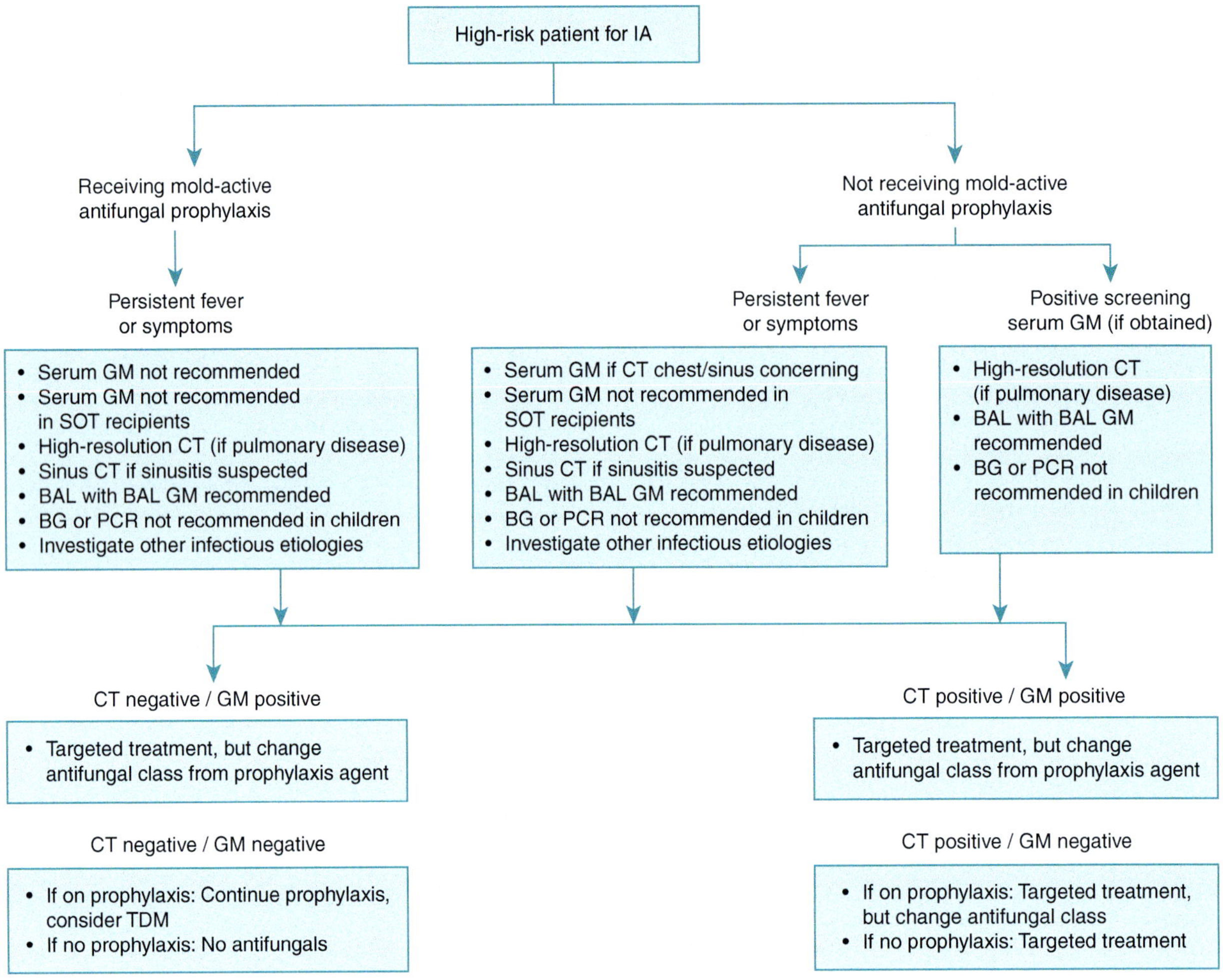

Fig. 24.1 Diagnosis of invasive aspergillosis. *BAL*, bronchoalveolar lavage; *CT*, computed tomography; *GM*, galactomannan; *IA*, invasive aspergillosis; *PCR*, polymerase chain reaction; *SOT*, solid organ transplant; *TDM*, therapeutic drug monitoring.

result "normal" in patients even in the week preceding death. The aforementioned findings are relatively nonspecific findings; however, there are two radiologic signs—the halo sign and the air crescent sign—that were previously thought to be considered highly suggestive of IPA. The halo sign occurs in neutropenic patients with a hemorrhagic nodule owing to angioinvasion. An early CT finding of the halo sign is a rim of ground-glass attenuation opacity surrounding the nodule. These early lesions subsequently change into a cavitary lesion or lesion with an air crescent sign 2 to 3 weeks later when neutropenia recovers. Cavitation of the nodules or masses occurs in about 40% of patients and is characterized by an intracavitary mass composed of sloughed lung and a surrounding rim of air. Although the halo sign can be seen in patients with biopsy-proven IPA, it is nonspecific and can be seen in patients with mucormycosis, organizing pneumonia, or pulmonary hemorrhage.

A long-term CT follow-up in 40 immunocompromised patients with IPA showed that formation of cavitation most strongly predicted time until radiologic remission and beneficial outcome. In that study, the natural history of early IPA lesions was evaluated and it was found that 90% of patients experienced an increase in lesion size and number followed by a plateau in size and a decrease in number. Cavitation of the lesions developed in 55% of patients and complete radiologic remission, within a median 80 days, was observed in 42.5% of patients. The number of days until remission without cavitation (50 days) was less than for those with cavitation (95 days), so formation of no cavitation was strongly predictive of radiologic remission.[24] Repetition of a CT scan before 2 weeks after the start of treatment is not usually recommended unless the patient experiences clinical deterioration. An exception is the presence of a nodule close to a large vessel because of the risk for massive hemoptysis if lesions continue to increase in size. Routine use of contrast with CT is not recommended.

There may be radiologic differences for IA in adult and pediatric patients. In adult series of IPA, approximately 50% of cases show cavitation and 40% air crescent formation. In one 10-year review of pediatric patients (mean age 5 years), there was central cavitation of small nodules in only 25% of children and no evidence of air crescent formation within any area of consolidation.[25] The largest series of contemporary pediatric IA cases found the most common radiologic finding for IPA was nodules (34.6%). Importantly, only 2.2% of the children showed the air crescent sign, 11% demonstrated the halo sign, and cavitation was seen in 24.5% of patients.[16] Other pediatric series with higher mean ages have slightly higher rates of cavitation and air crescent formation, suggesting that there may be a spectrum of radiologic disease presentation that is directly related to age, with cavitation and air crescent formation more likely in the older child and adult than in the younger child.

A review of serial radiographs of 27 HSCT pediatric recipients with IFD highlights how radiographic findings can change over time.

Although this study was not exclusive to IPA, it highlighted the wide range of possible radiographic findings on lung imaging and the change in appearance over time. At initial detection, unilateral infiltrates (52%) were slightly more common than bilateral infiltrates, and the infiltrates were interstitial (41%), alveolar (41%), and mixed (18%). Hilar or mediastinal lymphadenopathy and pleural effusion/thickening were rare. On follow-up, the infiltrates were more commonly bilateral (66%) and alveolar or nodular (74%), including 22% of patients who had cavitary lesions.[26]

In selected patients in whom CT is not feasible, thoracic MRI is an alternative but findings are not as characteristic as chest CT findings, and the typical MRI sign is the target sign, a nodular lesion with a lower signal in the center compared with a higher, contrast-enhancing signal intensity in the rim on T1-weighted images.

Brain Imaging. MRI is the modality of choice for diagnosing cerebral aspergillosis and is preferred over CT for sensitivity. Findings often show multiple lesions located in the basal ganglia that include an intermediate signal intensity, lack of contrast enhancement, and absence of mass effect. Although MRI is preferred for its ability to more completely assess the brain, CT of the head can still be useful, especially if an MRI is not attainable. The head CT scan often reveals one or multiple hypodense, well-demarcated lesions. Hemorrhage and mass effect are unusual, but for patients with adequate peripheral white blood cell counts a ring enhancement and surrounding edema are more frequent.

Sinus Imaging. Although imaging is not diagnostic, it can aid in establishing the diagnosis because it can be used as a road map for endoscopy by showing which sinuses are involved. In a review of 25 patients with rhinosinusitis, 44% showed evidence of invasion beyond the sinus cavities on CT scan. In the same study, however, 12% of patients had negative CT scan results, again highlighting that a high index of clinical suspicion must guide establishment of the diagnosis to ensure the best outcome.

Galactomannan Antigen

GM is a major cell wall component of *Aspergillus*. An enzyme-linked immunosorbent assay (ELISA) technique was developed using a rat anti-GM monoclonal antibody, EB-A2, which recognizes the 1→5-β-D-galactofuranoside side chains of the GM molecule. A sandwich ELISA technique was introduced in 1995 and by using the same antibody as both a capture and detector antibody in the sandwich ELISA (Platelia *Aspergillus*, Bio-Rad, Hercules, CA) the threshold for detection was lowered to 1 ng/mL. This technique is used in the currently commercially available GM assay for diagnosis of IA.

Serum Galactomannan Testing. The latest U.S. guidelines[27] support serum GM as an accurate marker for the diagnosis of IA in adult and pediatric patients when used in certain patient subpopulations (hematologic malignancy, HSCT). This recommendation includes serial screening in patients with prolonged neutropenia not receiving mold-active prophylaxis and is founded on predominantly adult data showing a high sensitivity and negative predictive value for IA in this clinical setting. More recent pediatric data, however, suggest that surveillance testing in pediatric patients is not as useful as it is in adults even in the absence of mold prophylaxis. In adult populations, serum GM is advocated to be sampled twice weekly (every 3 to 4 days), with the highest test accuracy requiring two consecutive positive samples (optical density index [ODI] $\geq$ 0.5) or retesting the same sample. Currently, pediatric-specific data do not support this broad of an approach.

It is well accepted that routine serum GM screening should not be performed in patients receiving mold-active antifungal therapy or prophylaxis owing to the low prevalence of IA in this setting with a consequently low positive predictive value of the serum GM assay.[18]

Neutropenia also affects GM utility, and the sensitivity of serum GM is significantly lower in nonneutropenic versus neutropenic patients.[18] GM values in adult patients with an absolute neutrophil count (ANC) less than 100 cells/μL and not receiving antifungal therapy were statistically higher than those patients with an ANC greater than 100 cells/μL. However, GM values were not statistically different in patients with an ANC less than 100 cells/μL and receiving antifungal therapy versus those with an ANC greater than 100 cells/μL.[28] It is possible that this neutropenia effect is due to fungal burden higher at the time of initial IA in neutropenia or that IA lesions are more extensive and possibly result in angioinvasion in the setting of neutropenia.

The specific patient population tested is critical to optimizing GM utility. Although GM has been extensively validated in patients with hematologic malignancy and those who have undergone HSCT, for unclear reasons GM appears less useful in SOT recipients. The U.S. guidelines do not recommend GM for screening in SOT recipients because of the low predictive value and high false-negative rates, respectively.[27] In liver transplant recipients, there was a high false positivity, especially in patients with autoimmune liver disease or dialysis, and in lung transplant recipients, there was a greatly decreased sensitivity, perhaps owing to the pathophysiologic differences in *Aspergillus* tracheobronchitis or anastomotic disease seen in these patients.

False-positive results with GM can hamper its clinical utility and are seen in patients concurrently receiving some β-lactam antibacterials. Importantly, piperacillin-tazobactam, once the major cause of this false-positive reaction, is now no longer cross-reactive. Several years ago, there were concerns of a supposed increased false positivity in children, and one theory suggested it was due to (1) *Bifidobacterium bifidum* spp. in the gut microflora, which mimics the epitope recognized by the EB-A2 in the ELISA kit, and (2) GM-positive infant formula used in pediatric patients. False positivity is likely due to the ELISA testing itself cross-reacting with specific antigens, likely not all of which have been defined, and this phenomenon appears irrespective of the patient's age.

Diagnosis of pediatric IA with GM, although originally reported to be less useful owing to a higher false-positive rate, has been validated to also be effective in children when used in the correct patient population. Multiple pediatric GM studies for focused testing, not surveillance, were reviewed to highlight the current knowledge of this assay in children, and it was determined that the GM assay has similar operating characteristics in pediatric as well as in adult patients.[29]

Bronchoalveolar Lavage. Guidelines state that bronchoscopy with bronchoalveolar lavage (BAL) is recommended in patients with a suspicion of IPA.[27] The yield of BAL is low for peripheral nodular lesions, so that percutaneous or endobronchial lung biopsy should be considered. BAL should include routine culture and cytology, and most importantly non–culture-based methods (e.g., GM), as routine culture alone can have a low sensitivity. BAL is often useful in diagnosing IA, but a negative BAL culture result does not conclusively rule out disease.

The ability to detect *Aspergillus* in BAL samples may be increased by use of GM, thus increasing the yield of bronchoscopy and possibly avoiding the need for further invasive procedures. Although the GM cutoff value in sera is 0.5, the cutoff is best used at 1.0 for BAL GM to increase the accuracy of the test. A retrospective analysis of 99 high-risk hematology patients, including 58 with IA, who underwent BAL for the diagnosis of new pulmonary infiltrates found that a BAL GM value of 1.0 or higher yielded an increased sensitivity (91.3%) compared with BAL culture (50%) or BAL microscopy (53.3%). The combined sensitivity of all three BAL methodologies was 98.2%.[30] Further analyses in that study found that the mean BAL GM value was not different in neutropenic versus nonneutropenic patients.

A meta-analysis of BAL GM studies found the sensitivities between 59% and 100% and specificities between 76% and 100%, and most importantly, that antifungal therapy did not significantly affect sensitivity as it does with serum GM.[31] A retrospective study in hematologic malignancy patients and HSCT recipients also found that BAL GM was more sensitive than serum GM for diagnosing IA, and found that BAL GM was not affected by mold-active antifungals, suggesting that this may be due to the levels of antifungals found in sera versus alveolar fluid.[32] A retrospective pediatric BAL GM found an optimal BAL GM cutoff value of 0.98 to yield the best sensitivity (78%) and specificity (92%). Using a BAL GM value of 1.0 or higher and a concurrent serum GM value of 0.5 or higher yielded the best sensitivity (89%) and specificity (90%).[33]

(1,3)-β-D-Glucan

(1,3)-β-D-Glucan is an integral cell wall component and, in contrast to GM, is not normally released from the fungal cell. Factor G, a coagulation factor of the horseshoe crab, is a highly sensitive natural detector of (1,3)-β-D-glucan. The G test detects (1,3)-β-D-glucan via a modified limulus endotoxin assay but does not identify the genus of the fungi detected. Unlike the GM assay, this assay is nonspecific as (1,3)-β-D-glucan is present in several different fungi, including *Aspergillus* spp., *Candida* spp., *Fusarium* spp., *Trichosporon* spp., *Saccharomyces cerevisiae, Acremonium, Coccidioides immitis, Histoplasma capsulatum, Sporothrix schenckii*, and *Pneumocystis jirovecii*. The (1,3)-β-D-glucan assay does not detect *Cryptococcus* and the yeast form of *Blastomyces dermatididis* (which produce low levels of (1,3)-β-D-glucan) or organisms from the Mucorales Order (which produce no (1,3)-β-D-glucan). Importantly, this assay does not identify the genus of the fungi detected, only the presence of the fungal call wall component.

False-positive results can occur in a variety of contexts, such as through glucan-contaminated blood collection tubes, gauze, depth-type membrane filters for blood processing, intravenous immunoglobulin, and various drugs (e.g., antibiotics, including some cephalosporins, carbapenems, and ampicillin-sulbactam and possibly chemotherapeutics such as pegylated asparaginase). The Fungitell assay (Associates of Cape Cod, East Falmouth, MA) for detection of (1,3)-β-D-glucan is cleared by the U.S. Food and Drug Administration for the diagnosis of invasive mycoses, IA, and has been evaluated in high-risk patients with hematologic malignancy and allogeneic HSCT.

In one study comparing (1,3)-β-D-glucan and GM, the sensitivity, specificity, and positive and negative predictive values for GM and (1,3)-β-D-glucan were identical. False-positive reactions occurred at a rate of 10.3% in both tests, but the patients with false-positive results were different in each test. Both tests anticipated the clinical diagnosis and CT abnormalities, but the (1,3)-β-D-glucan result tended to become positive earlier than GM. A combination of the two tests improved the specificity (to 100%) and positive predictive value (to 100%) of each individual test without affecting the sensitivity and negative predictive values.[34] A meta-analysis of cohort studies of (1,3)-β-D-glucan for IA revealed that using a single test resulted in a pooled sensitivity of 57% with a specificity of 97%.[35]

Recent guidelines state serum assays for (1,3)-β-D-glucan are recommended for diagnosing IA in high-risk patients (hematologic malignancy, allogeneic HSCT) but are not specific for *Aspergillus*.[27] Current guidelines for children recommend against (1,3)-β-D-glucan testing for screening or evaluation of suspected IA because of the limited data in children and the unknown optimal cutoff value in pediatric patients.[19,29,36]

Polymerase Chain Reaction

The exact clinical utility of blood-based polymerase chain reaction (PCR) in diagnosing IA is currently unclear, and experts debate the present utility for standard clinical practice of this diagnostic modality until conclusive validation of standardized commercially available assays. Recent guidelines state that direct comparison studies have shown *Aspergillus* PCR to be substantially more sensitive than culture.[27] In a meta-analysis of clinical trials evaluating the accuracy of serum or whole-blood PCR assays for IA for various indications, sensitivity and specificity were 84% and 76%, respectively.[37] These values are promising, but PCR of blood or serum is unable on its own to confirm or exclude suspected IA in high-risk patients. The sensitivity of *Aspergillus* PCR on BAL fluid was higher than within blood, but in many instances its specificity was lower. In a systematic review of nine studies using reference IA definitions strictly adherent to the European Organization for the Research and Treatment of Cancer and the Mycoses Study Group criteria, the sensitivity and specificity of PCR of BAL were 77% and 94%, respectively.[38] The lower specificity in BAL has been attributed to the fact that lungs are often colonized by *Aspergillus* (particularly in many high-risk populations, such as lung transplant recipients), and that PCR is not able to differentiate colonization from disease or to distinguish different *Aspergillus* spp. The high negative predictive value of BAL PCR (usually ≥95%) suggests a role in ruling out IPA. To date, data suggest that the diagnostic performance of blood or BAL PCR is comparable to that of serum and BAL GM index and that sensitivity for both tests is affected by antifungal use. Using both PCR and GM in serum resulted in improved sensitivity with no sacrifice of specificity.

Despite these promising results, *Aspergillus* PCR cannot yet be recommended for routine use in clinical practice because few assays have been standardized and validated, and the role of PCR testing in patient management is not established. Initiatives such as the European *Aspergillus* PCR Initiative have made significant progress in developing a consensus standard protocol for blood-based *Aspergillus* PCR. At present, this diagnostic method is not commercially available, and reports can be difficult to interpret because of the lack of experimental standardization between centers. Owing to the ubiquitous nature of the mold, it is likely that the value of this test will be its high negative predictive value. Because of the lack of sufficient pediatric data, there is no guideline recommendation for PCR in the diagnosis of IA for children.[19,29,36]

TREATMENT

Overall success in treating IA is dependent on numerous factors, not simply the choice of a specific antifungal therapy (Fig. 24.2). As with all immunocompromised patients, detailed knowledge of host factors, underlying disease, concomitant infections, and the degree and duration of immunosuppression are key to overall management. It is well known that immune reconstitution is paramount to successful IA therapy, and continued exposure to certain immunosuppressive medications, such as corticosteroids, is known to worsen IA. Any antifungal prophylaxis used before the diagnosis of IA could also have an effect on the ultimate choice of empiric or targeted therapy. The diagnostic workup needs to be aggressive to confirm disease, but it should never delay antifungal therapy in the setting of true concern for IA. The cornerstone of antifungal therapy for IA is prompt and aggressive institution of antifungal therapy, based not only on diagnostic results but also on clinical suspicion of infection if diagnosis is not immediate. Antifungal resistance is now slowly increasing among *Aspergillus* isolates and continues to have specific geographic trends that could

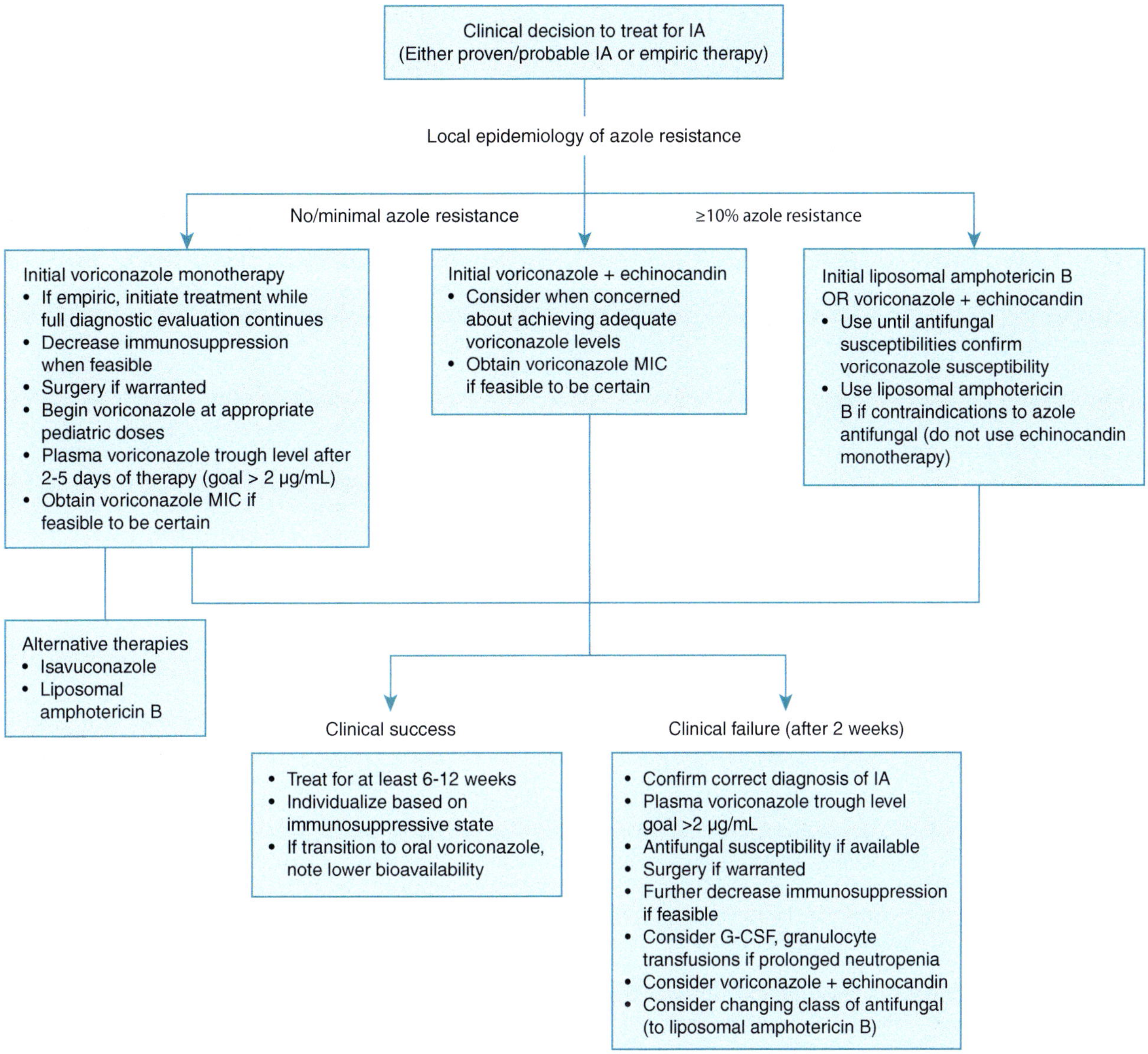

Fig. 24.2 Treatment of invasive aspergillosis. *IA*, invasive aspergillosis; *G-CSF*, granulocyte colony-stimulating factor; *MIC*, minimum inhibitory concentration.

influence antifungal choice. For the moment, resistance among *Aspergillus* isolates isolated from patients in the United States is rare. There is also the question of using antifungal monotherapy or combination antifungal therapy, and if so, which classes of agents. Finally, although immune reconstitution is paramount, the role and real benefit of adjunctive immunotherapy remains somewhat unclear. Treatment for most forms of IA follows the recommendations made for the more common invasive pulmonary aspergillosis.[27]

Primary Antifungal Therapy for Invasive Aspergillosis

There are multiple published guidelines for IA from different regions of the world, but the 2016 Infectious Diseases Society of America treatment guidelines,[27] the 2017 European Society for Clinical Microbiology and Infectious Diseases (ESCMID)/European Confederation of Medical Mycology (ECMM)/European Respiratory Society joint clinical guidelines,[18] and the 2017 ECIL-6 (European Conference on Infections in Leukemia) guidelines[39] are the most referenced. The newer ESCMID-ECMM pediatric guidelines for IA[19] are similar and highlight some of the pediatric dosing nuances.

The latest U.S. guidelines recommend primary (initial) treatment with voriconazole. These recommendations mirror guidelines from multiple other international groups that recommend voriconazole for the primary treatment of IA regardless of the location of the infection. Alternative therapies include liposomal amphotericin B, isavuconazole, or other lipid formulations of amphotericin B. Both the European ESCMID and ECIL guidelines recommend isavuconazole and voriconazole for treatment of pulmonary disease with a similar strength of recommendation, mentioning fewer adverse effects with isavuconazole than voriconazole, and liposomal amphotericin B as an alternative.[18,39] Treatment of extrapulmonary disease is similar to the U.S. recommendations, with voriconazole based on the preponderance of experience.[18] The European guidelines specifically recommend voriconazole as the agent of choice in children in any population other than neonates, followed by alternatives of liposomal amphotericin B and then caspofungin. In neonates, liposomal amphotericin B is recommended.[18]

The U.S. guidelines state that combination primary antifungal therapy with voriconazole plus an echinocandin may be considered in select patients with documented IA; however, this is not a universal recommendation.[27] The ECIL-6 guidelines graded combination therapy with voriconazole plus anidulafungin as lower, with all other combinations even less recommended.[39] Importantly, primary therapy with an echinocandin is not recommended, but an echinocandin can be used in the settings in which azole or polyene antifungal are contraindicated. Treatment of IA in children uses the same recommended agents as in adult patients; however, the dosing is often very different and for some antifungals, the exact dosing in children is unknown.

Treatment of IA should be continued for a minimum of 6 to 12 weeks; however, the ultimate duration of any patient depends on the degree and duration of immunosuppression, site of disease, and evidence of disease improvement. Patients treated successfully who require subsequent immunosuppression should receive secondary prophylaxis to prevent recurrence. Many experts believe that treatment should continue until complete clinical and radiographic resolution of disease. If a patient remains substantially chronically immunosuppressed because of ongoing cytotoxic chemotherapy or lack of engraftment after HSCT, it is advisable to continue the antifungal therapy for IA until there is no evidence of disease, often 3 months or longer. Surgical therapy may be an important adjunctive therapy in the management of IA. In particular, surgery should be considered in patients with single lesions, especially if they have cavitated, or lesions contiguous with the great vessels or pericardium to avoid fatal hemoptysis. Surgery to debulk disseminated pulmonary lesions is generally not advised, but debridement of sinus disease (often technically easier to access) is suggested to decrease disease burden. Treatment of cutaneous disease involves debridement and excision of necrotic tissue, which provides diagnostic material, and systemic intravenous antifungal agents as well as topical preparations. The role of topical antifungals alone is unclear, as often the cutaneous aspergillosis is a harbinger for underlying undiagnosed systemic disease, so relying on topical antifungal coverage alone is likely inadequate.

More recent epidemiologic studies have also shown the benefit of voriconazole versus the decades of data with amphotericin B. A French epidemiology study analyzed 393 adult patients with IA and found that any treatment regimen containing voriconazole, alone or in an antifungal combination, was superior in terms of survival to any antifungal regimen without voriconazole.[1] There are limited comparative data of voriconazole versus other antifungal agents for treatment of IA in children. A case series of 42 children treated for IA with voriconazole for refractory IA demonstrated a 43% complete or partial response.[40] Voriconazole was also shown in these studies to be better tolerated and to have less toxicity than amphotericin B in both adults and children.

The fundamental pharmacokinetics of voriconazole are different in children (linear) than in adults (nonlinear). For instance, although the recommended starting dose of voriconazole in adult patients is 6 mg/kg per dose twice daily for the first day and then a maintenance dosing of 4 mg/kg per dose twice daily, the preferred pediatric dosing is substantially higher. Population pharmacokinetic analyses of voriconazole in children, adolescents, and adults reveal that, based on the area under the concentration-time curve, children should be given an intravenous 9 mg/kg per dose twice-daily loading dose to be comparable to the 6 mg/kg per dose twice daily given to adults.[41] Maintenance intravenous dosing in children at 8 mg/kg per dose twice daily was comparable to 4 mg/kg per dose twice daily in adults, and the oral dosing of 9 mg/kg per dose twice daily was found to be similar to adults receiving 200 mg oral voriconazole twice daily. The majority of adolescents can be dosed as adults, but in younger adolescents (12 to 14 years), the analysis found that body weight was more important than age in predicting voriconazole pharmacokinetics in this age. Therefore during this age transition period, adolescents 12 to 14 years old should be dosed as children if their weight is less than 50 kg, and dosed as adults if their weight is 50 kg or more.[41] Additionally, the oral bioavalability of voriconazole, although believed to be greater than 95% in adults, is lower in children at approximately 50% to 65%. This oral bioavailability in dosing is important, especially for those patients receiving oral voriconazole after hospital discharge during the second bimodal peak of disease at approximately day 100 after transplantation.

The triazole antifungals require therapeutic drug monitoring. Effective management of IA requires obtaining a voriconazole trough level. Trough-level measurements are well known to have high interpatient variability, limiting their extrapolation to a larger population on similar dosing, but much lower intrapatient variability, allowing successive trough levels to be used to monitor dose adjustments in the individual patient. The exact voriconazole trough level for clinical effectiveness against IA is somewhat unknown, as there have been several clinical studies in which occasional individual patients have had undetectable voriconazole levels and still shown a clinical response. However, it is commonly believed that a serum trough level at least greater than the usual minimal inhibitory concentration (MIC) of the infecting *Aspergillus* species would be preferable. Although individual studies have debated the exact cutoff, it is clear that the serum level should be a true trough level and not a random drug level. Most experts today would advocate for a serum trough voriconazole level of at least more than 2.0 μg/mL (2 to 6 μg/mL), and stress the importance of individualized therapy for each patient. Levels should be monitored between 2 and 5 days after initiation of therapy and repeated the following week to confirm the patient's levels remain in the therapeutic range and 4 days after change of dose.[18] Inherent in the individualized treatment approach is the understanding that different populations also metabolize voriconazole uniquely, with three major genotypes owing to allelic polymorphisms in the human cytochrome P450 isoenzymes (largely CYP2C19) responsible for voriconazole metabolism. When posaconazole is used for treatment, a trough level of more than 1.0 μg/mL is recommended, and when feasible the extended-release tablet is preferred over the oral suspension because of greater consistency in achieving a therapeutic target and less affect by gastrointestinal-dependent interactions.[18] Although there are no firm data to suggest a therapeutic drug monitoring range for isavuconazole, some experts recommend targeting a serum trough level of 2 to 3 μg/mL.[18]

A more recent concern is the choice of antifungal therapy in the setting of a possible azole-resistant isolate, often pan–azole-resistant. This concern is growing in specific geographic regions of the world. An international (largely European) surveillance study of approximately 4000 isolates from 19 countries found the azole resistance rate in *A. fumigatus* was 3.2%, and azole resistance was documented in 5.1% of cases of IA.[42] Of particular concern is that approximately 70% of patients with azole-resistant IA have never received an azole antifungal. Of the many genotypes uncovered in azole-resistant species, TR_{34}/L98H and TR_{46}/Y121F/T289A are responsible for 80% of azole-resistant IA. These genotypes denote mutations in the *CYP51A* gene, which encodes the target enzyme of the azoles, as well as a tandem repeat of 34 of 46 base pairs in the *CYP51A* promoter region. Epidemiologic cutoff values have been established for determining likely clinical resistance for itraconazole (1 μg/mL), voriconazole (1 μg/mL), posaconazole (0.25 μg/mL), and preliminarily for isavuconazole (1 μg/mL). An international expert opinion panel recommended azole susceptibilities be performed for all isolates of *Aspergillus* spp. If an isolate is determined to be azole resistant, the panel recommends therapy with liposomal amphotericin B, combination voriconazole plus echinocandin, or monotherapy with an echinocandin.[43] In the case of empiric therapy, if the rate of environmental resistance is 10% or higher, then voriconazole plus echinocandin or liposomal amphotericin B should be used initially. European guidelines suggest that the probability of voriconazole treatment failure may be higher against isolates with a voriconazole MIC > 2 μg/mL; thus for those isolates, initiation of liposomal amphotericin B is preferable over a voriconazole plus echinocandin approach.[18]

Alternative Antifungal Therapy for Invasive Aspergillosis

An alternative for primary therapy of IA is a lipid formulation of amphotericin B. Although voriconazole was found to be more effective than conventional amphotericin B, there have been no randomized trial comparisons of lipid formulation amphotericin B to voriconazole for primary treatment of IA. However, a number of studies support the utility of lipid formulation amphotericin B as a second-line agent. One clinical trial evaluated liposomal amphotericin B at either 3 mg/kg per day (n = 107 patients) versus 10 mg/kg per day (n = 94 patients).[44] The favorable overall response for the lower dose (50%) and the higher dose (46%) were similar, with no demonstrable additional benefit to higher amphotericin B dosing and only higher rates of nephrotoxicity. However, although these response rates are generally similar to the favorable response seen earlier with voriconazole, most of the amphotericin B responses were partial responses and not complete treatment responses, suggesting that the triazole was overall more effective in disease eradication. These results suggest that lipid formulation amphotericin B be considered as alternative primary therapy in some patients, especially in situations in which hepatic toxicities or drug interactions warrant nonazole alternatives, and when voriconazole-resistant molds (e.g., mucormycosis) remain a concern. Because conventional amphotericin B was shown to be inferior to voriconazole, few experts recommend conventional amphotericin B for IA management.

A pivotal randomized trial compared voriconazole and isavuconazole and demonstrated noninferiority in treatment of IPA.[45] This multicenter, randomized, double-blind study in patients 18 years and older showed noninferiority in terms of the primary endpoint of all-cause mortality at 6 weeks (isavuconazole 19%, voriconazole 20%) in the intent-to-treat population of patients with possible, probable, and proven aspergillosis. There were also fewer drug-related adverse events in people who received isavuconazole (42% vs. 60%). Based on these data, isavuconazole was approved by the Food and Drug Administration for first-line therapy of IA and is recommended as an alternative primary therapy for IA. There are no currently approved pediatric dosing recommendations for isavuconazole, and as such, the utility of this agent in children is limited.

Salvage Antifungal Therapy for Invasive Aspergillosis

Salvage therapy is defined as therapy after primary therapy, often owing to the perception that therapy is ineffective or the patient is intolerant. Assessing patient response 2 weeks after treatment initiation generally allows prediction and recognition of impending clinical failure.[18] In general, guidelines recommend an individualized approach that takes into consideration the rapidity, severity, extent of infection, patient comorbidities, and need to exclude the emergence of a new pathogen.[27] Importantly, there should be an aggressive and prompt attempt to establish a specific correct diagnosis, including bronchoscopy and/or CT-guided biopsy, if needed. For example, mucormycosis and aspergillosis appear radiographically similar, yet treatment of mucormycosis with voriconazole will not result in success. Assuming that the diagnosis of IA is correct, the first step in refractory disease should be to establish that the correct dose of voriconazole is being used. Documentation of serum azole levels should also be verified if therapeutic drug monitoring is available, as this has historically been a common etiology of antifungal failure. Antifungal susceptibility testing of available isolates is paramount, especially in examining for azole resistance. Other salvage approaches include examination for poor vascular supply in the area of the infection that would inhibit antifungal agent delivery. In this setting, surgical resection of the vascularly compromised area may be necessary for clinical improvement.

The general strategies for salvage therapy typically include (1) changing the class of antifungal; (2) tapering or reversal of underlying immunosuppression when feasible; (3) susceptibility testing of any *Aspergillus* isolates recovered from the patient; and (4) surgical resection of necrotic lesions in selected cases. In the context of salvage therapy, an additional antifungal agent may be added to current therapy, or combination antifungal drugs from different classes other than those in the initial regimen may be used. In patients currently receiving an antifungal and exhibiting an adverse event attributable to this agent, it makes sense to change to an alternative class of antifungal or to use a second agent with a nonoverlapping side effect profile. For salvage therapy, agents include lipid formulations of amphotericin B, micafungin, caspofungin, posaconazole, or itraconazole.

When deciding on therapy choices, a patient's prior azole (antifungal prophylaxis before diagnosis) exposure is important to consider as it may increase concerns of resistance among identified fungal pathogens. Itraconazole resistance was first described in 1997, and antifungal resistance to echinocandins is currently largely due to modulation of the *FKS1* gene (target of echinocandins) in *A. fumigatus*. In general, azole resistance is now increasing, and often resistant isolates are multi-azole resistant or pan-azole (voriconazole, posaconazole, itraconaozle)-resistant strains.

Speciation of an identified isolate can also provide insights into antifungal choice. An increasing number of *Aspergillus* species, such as *A. lentulus*, *A. udagawae*, and *A. pseudofischeri*, with reduced antifungal susceptibility, are being isolated. In the case of *A. pseudofischeri* and *A. udagawae*, susceptibility to amphotericin B and itraconazole is somewhat controversial. For voriconazole, on the other hand, there is a general consensus that these species are less susceptible than *A. fumigatus*. Importantly, *A. calidoustus* is known to be resistant to all azoles. *A. lentulus* is overall less susceptible than *A. fumigatus* to amphotericin B, itraconazole, and voriconazole based on its high MICs.

Certain *Aspergillus* species have intrinsic resistance to antifungals. *A. terreus* and *A. alliaceus* (*A. flavus* complex) should be considered resistant to amphotericin B, and *A. nidulans* often has elevated MICs to amphotericin B. In addition to *A. calidoustus*, other *Aspergillus* spp. such as *A. tubingensis* (*A. niger* complex) and *A. niger* have higher azole MICs.[18]

There are no randomized studies examining posaconazole for primary therapy of IA, but numerous in vitro and in vivo data suggest that this triazole will be as effective as voriconazole as a potential first-line agent against IA. A multicenter salvage therapy study evaluated 107 patients with IA treated with posaconazole versus 86 historic controls (treated largely with amphotericin B) and found a response rate of 42% versus 26%, respectively, as well as improved survival at 30 days (74% vs. 49%).[46] This study was significant as the posaconazole recipients were all receiving it as salvage therapy (generally after failure of amphotericin B products or itraconazole), demonstrating that triazoles are indeed the best treatment option for IA.

Three echinocandins are currently approved in the United States: caspofungin, micafungin, and anidulafungin. Several in vitro antifungal susceptibility studies have shown the general equivalency of all three echinocandins against *Aspergillus* species. The echinocandin are fungistatic against *Aspergillus*, compared with the triazoles which are fungicidal. Echinocandin activity causes blunting of the hyphal tip of *Aspergillus*, which impedes but does not kill the organism. Caspofungin was first studied in an open-label, noncomparative salvage therapy in immunocompromised patients with proven or probable aspergillosis.[47] Caspofungin produced a complete or partial response in 45% (37 of 83) of patients, which is again significant because these patients who were either refractory or intolerant to previous antifungal therapy.

The largest study with micafungin was a noncomparative, open-label, multicenter study in adult and pediatric patients to examine the safety and effect of micafungin in the treatment of patients with IA whose disease had failed to respond to prior therapy or who could not tolerate other therapy. Of the 225 patients who met diagnostic criteria, a favorable response rate was seen in 35.6% (80 225), and of those treated with only micafungin, a favorable response was seen in 6 of 12 (50%) of the primary and 9 of 22 (40.9%) of the salvage therapy group.[48] Anidulafungin has been approved in the United State for treatment of candidemia and esophageal candidiasis, and although in vitro studies show activity against Aspergillus species isolates, there are no clinical studies against IA as primary or salvage monotherapy.

Combination Antifungal Therapy for Invasive Aspergillosis

Clinicians are desperately seeking new strategies for improved outcome and sometimes turn to combination antifungal therapy. With the surge in the development of newer antifungals for IA, there are now more permutations of new potential combination antifungal therapies. Drawing from other infectious diseases such as human immunodeficiency virus, tuberculosis, and cryptococcal meningitis, a combination therapeutic approach for IA seems like a reasonable consideration to optimize outcomes. Unfortunately, there have been numerous in vitro and animal model studies as well as small clinical series and a large randomized clinical trial that provide conclusions ranging from synergy to antagonism or ineffectiveness to effectiveness. This conundrum actually parallels the wide range of unproven treatment practices used by clinicians today searching for the best care for patients who have illnesses with high morbidity and mortality.

Before data availability from clinical trials, clinicians often derive clinical strategy information from experimental in vitro or in vivo data. Unfortunately, given the extensive heterogeneity of both experimentation and interpretation, one cannot accurately draw a firm conclusion as to the clinical relevance of the combination antifungal experiments. Perhaps the greatest usefulness for in vitro combination is to screen antagonistic interactions before investigating animal model or clinical studies.

The prevailing expert opinion is that if a combination antifungal therapy approach is beneficial to treating IA, it is likely best taken with the combination of a cell membrane–active triazole with a cell wall–active echinoncandin. It is unclear if any combination therapy will have the great advance observed when monotherapy with voriconazole was shown to be better than monotherapy with conventional amphotericin B. There was a recent large adult randomized antifungal trial that compared voriconazole monotherapy to voriconazole plus anidulafungin combination for primary therapy of IA.[49] A total of 454 hematologic malignancy patients age 16 years and older were randomly assigned 1:1 in this double-blind, placebo-controlled study and given voriconazole alone versus combination therapy for a minimum of 2 weeks, followed by voriconazole monotherapy to complete 6 weeks of treatment. The primary efficacy endpoint was 6-week all-cause mortality in the patients with confirmed proven/probable IA. Mortality at 6 weeks was 19.3% for combination recipients and 27.5% for monotherapy recipients (P = .087, 95% CI 19 to 1.5). Although these results with combination therapy identified a potentially meaningful clinical benefit, this difference did not achieve the prespecified threshold for statistical significance. In a post hoc analysis of the subgroup of patients who were diagnosed as having probable aspergillosis based on radiographic abnormalities and positive GM assays, the mortality rate difference was statistically significant (15.7% combination vs. 27.3% monotherapy, P =.037, 95% CI 22.7 to −0.4). However, global clinical responses at 6 weeks were lower in the combination group (33% vs 43%), which was attributed to more patients in the combination group being unevaluable for this secondary endpoint owing to missing data. Based on these data, the latest guidelines[27] suggest consideration, but not a definitive indication, for an echinocandin with voriconazole for primary therapy in the setting of severe disease, especially in patients with hematologic malignancy and those with profound and persistent neutropenia.

Adjunctive Therapies for Invasive Aspergillosis

Reducing doses of, or eliminating, immunosuppressive agents, when feasible, is always strongly recommended. However, IA is not an absolute contraindication to additional chemotherapy or transplantation, and the risks and benefits of the antineoplastic treatment of any underlying disease must be weighed against the risk of progressive IA if treatment is delayed. According to the latest guidelines,[27] colony-stimulating factors may be considered in neutropenic patients, but there is insufficient evidence regarding the value of granulocyte colony-stimulating factor versus granulocyte-macrophage colony-stimulating in this setting. Granulocyte transfusions can be considered for neutropenic patients with IA that is refractory or unlikely to respond to standard therapy, and/or if the anticipated duration of neutropenia is going to be more than 1 week. However, the effectiveness of granulocyte transfusions has not been proven and also likely depends on the methods of harvesting from the donors to deliver a larger cell dose.[50] Recombinant interferon gamma, although recommended as prophylaxis in patients chronic granulomatous disease, is of unclear benefit as adjunctive therapy for IA. Surgery for aspergillosis should be considered for localized disease that is easily accessible to debridement (e.g., invasive fungal sinusitis, localized cutaneous disease, or solitary cavitary lung lesions). The benefit for IA in other settings, such as in the treatment of endocarditis, osteomyelitis, or focal CNS disease, appears rational. Other indications are less clear and require consideration of the patient's immune status, comorbidities, confirmation of a single focus, and the risks of surgery.

INFECTION PREVENTION AND ANTICIPATORY GUIDANCE

Inhalation of fungal spores is the most common route of entry, but one can also develop IA via ingestion of contaminated items. As such, provision of a protected environment for severely immunocompromised patients to reduce exposure to such fungal spores is recommended. The challenge is that there are limited to no data on how to reduce such exposures. Guidelines for inpatient care suggest that patients need to be segregated from construction or renovation, should not have potted plants or cut flowers in their rooms, and should have filters in place for the water supply (especially in showers). Frequent cleaning of all surfaces in the patient room is also advised to reduce the presence of mold spores. This can be challenging in patients who have prolonged hospital stays during which they have accumulated many personal items in the room. In the outpatient setting, patients and families should be advised to avoid activities such as gardening and composting (mulching), as this can result in significant exposures.[18,27] The effectiveness of surgical masks to protect against IA exposure is unknown.

25

Mucormycosis, Fusariosis, Scedosporiasis, and Other Invasive Mold Diseases

Rachel L. Wattier, MD, MHS and William J. Steinbach, MD

Although invasive aspergillosis is the most common invasive mold disease (IMD), mucormycosis and other non-*Aspergillus* opportunistic mold infections are increasingly associated with significant morbidity and mortality among highly immunocompromised patients. Early clinical suspicion is critically important to accurately distinguish, diagnose, and appropriately treat these life-threatening infections. Their relative rarity compared with other infections in these patient populations makes diagnosis and treatment challenging because of the lack of large-scale available data; therefore current clinical outcomes remain far from ideal.

MUCORMYCOSIS

Mucormycosis refers to IMD caused by members of the order Mucorales. "Mucormycosis" is now preferred to the historical term "zygomycosis" owing to an updated understanding of fungal phylogenetic relationships. It is the second most common IMD in immunocompromised hosts, after invasive aspergillosis.

Epidemiology and Risk Factors

Causative genera of mucormycosis are listed in Box 25.1. Organisms within the genera *Rhizopus, Mucor,* and *Lichtheimia* (formerly *Absidia*) account for the majority of reported cases. Organisms causing mucormycosis are ubiquitous in the natural environment. Spores can be inhaled into the upper and/or lower airways, inoculated at sites of skin trauma, or rarely, ingested via the gastrointestinal tract. Disease develops primarily in hosts with significant impairment of innate and/or cellular immunity.

Major predisposing factors across multiple types of immunocompromised populations include profound and prolonged neutropenia and high-dose corticosteroid exposure. Additionally, iron overload, hyperglycemia, and ketoacidosis increase risk for mucormycosis even in the absence of other immunosuppressive conditions and can further compound risk when they occur in transplant recipients and oncology patients.

Increasing Incidence and Breakthrough Infections. The overall incidence of mucormycosis-related hospitalizations in the United States doubled from 1.7 per million in 2000 to 3.4 per million persons in 2013.[1] Breakthrough infection in patients receiving voriconazole, which has anti-*Aspergillus* activity yet no activity against mucormycosis, has been noted more often among patients with mucormycosis than controls and patients with other IMDs.[2,3] Although there may be some selective effect favoring emergence of non-*Aspergillus* IMD in patients receiving mold-active antifungal therapy, there has also been substantial growth in the at-risk population and improved survival from other opportunistic infections. For example, some studies have found a stable incidence of mucormycosis over time among hematopoietic stem cell transplant (HSCT) recipients, but an increase in the absolute number of cases corresponding to patients who receive transplants.[1,4,5] Signs or symptoms concerning for an IMD in a patient already receiving a mold-active antifungal agent without mucormycosis coverage (e.g., voriconazole) should increase suspicion for mucormycosis or another rare, potentially antifungal-resistant IMD.[3] Additionally, it is important to maintain consideration of invasive aspergillosis, especially an azole-resistant isolate or an azole-resistant species (e.g., *Aspergillus calidoustus*) in the differential diagnosis for breakthrough IMD. Breakthrough IMD could occur because of intrinsic or acquired antifungal resistance, suboptimal antifungal exposure owing to inadequate dosing, nonadherence, high inoculum burden, or host immune factors. Table 25.1 summarizes reported breakthrough IMDs on various antimold prophylaxis agents.

Hematopoietic Stem Cell Transplant. Table 25.2 summarizes the key epidemiologic features of mucormycosis in HSCT recipients, solid organ transplant (SOT) recipients, and oncology patients. The majority of data are derived from adult studies. Among HSCT recipients in the Transplant-Associated Infection Surveillance Network (TRANSNET) study from 2001 to 2006, mucormycosis represented 77 (8%) of 983 invasive fungal disease (IFD) cases, whereas invasive aspergillosis represented 43% of IFDs.[6] Mucormycosis is more likely to occur in allogeneic HSCT recipients than autologous HSCT recipients. The median time of onset of mucormycosis in the TRANSNET study was 135 days after transplant versus 99 days after transplant for invasive aspergillosis.[6]

Solid Organ Transplant. Among primarily adult SOT recipients in the TRANSNET study, mucormycosis represented only 2% of all IFDs versus 19% caused by invasive aspergillosis.[7] Compared with other types of SOT recipients, liver transplant recipients present earlier after transplant and have a higher frequency of disseminated disease; their risk is hypothesized to be related to iron overload.[7,8] Mucormycosis is rare among pediatric SOT recipients.

Oncology. Hematologic malignancy (with or without HSCT) is the most common underlying condition reported among adult and pediatric patients with mucormycosis, accounting for 45 to 60% of cases in large series.[9-11] Patients undergoing therapy for hematologic malignancy often share multiple concurrent risk factors for mucormycosis.

Prognosis and Modifying Factors. Mucormycosis is a highly fatal disease; however, specific mortality estimates vary widely depending on the clinical population and duration of follow-up. A recent pediatric case series reported a case fatality rate of 33.3% at last follow-up.[11] Risk factors for death include disseminated disease, hematologic malignancy,

BOX 25.1 Genera of Organisms Causing Mucormycosis

Rhizopus
Mucor
Rhizomucor
Actinomucor
Lichtheimia
Cunninghamella
Apophysomyces
Saksenaea
Syncephalastrum
Cokeromyces

TABLE 25.1 Breakthrough Invasive Mold Infections Reported[a] on Antifungal Prophylaxis[b]

Antifungal Agent/Class	Predominant Reported Breakthrough Invasive Mold Disease	Other Breakthrough Infections Reported
Voriconazole	Mucormycosis	Aspergillosis Fusariosis Penicilliosis Scedosporiasis *Acremonium* infection
Posaconazole	Aspergillosis	Mucormycosis Fusariosis Scedosporiasis Penicilliosis *Rasamsonia (Geosmithia) argillacea* infection
Isavuconazole	Mucormycosis Aspergillosis[c]	Aspergillosis Fusariosis Scedosporiasis
Itraconazole	Aspergillosis	Fusariosis Mucormycosis Scedosporiasis
Echinocandins	Aspergillosis	Mucormycosis Fusariosis *Exserohilum* infection *Hormographiella aspergillata* infection
Amphotericin B deoxycholate or lipid formulation of amphotericin B	Aspergillosis	Undetermined etiology (probable pulmonary invasive mold disease)

[a]Reports based primarily on data from adults with hematologic malignancy and/or hematopoietic stem cell transplantation.
[b]Includes primary or secondary prophylaxis.
[c]Based on 2 studies only; one reported mucormycosis most commonly and the other reported aspergillosis most commonly.
Adapted from Lionakis MS, Lewis RE, Kontoyiannis DP. Breakthrough invasive mold infections in the hematology patient: current concepts and future directions. *Clin Infect Dis.* 2018;67(10):1621-1630.

HSCT, monocytopenia at diagnosis, and lymphopenia at diagnosis.[10,12,13] In some studies, higher mortality has been noted with infection caused by *Cunninghamella* species.[14] Favorable prognostic factors include localized cutaneous disease, surgical resection of disease, early amphotericin B–based therapy, and neutrophil recovery.[8,11,12,15]

Clinical Manifestations

Table 25.3 lists the major clinical syndromes of mucormycosis with their relative frequency in transplant recipients and oncology patients. The clinical manifestations of mucormycosis are nonspecific and similar to those of other IMDs. Individual patients may present with subtle or few symptoms initially, requiring a high index of suspicion from the clinician. Pulmonary infection is the predominant clinical syndrome in transplant recipients and oncology patients, as opposed to rhinocerebral infection in patients with diabetic ketoacidosis and cutaneous infection in patients in whom mucormycosis develops after trauma. Disseminated mucormycosis refers to involvement of 2 or more noncontiguous sites. Regardless of the site of disease, vascular invasion is a characteristic feature of disease and can lead to thrombosis, septic emboli, and rapid progression.

Pulmonary Mucormycosis. The presenting symptoms and signs of pulmonary mucormycosis are similar to those of other pulmonary IMDs. Radiographic findings can include nodules, consolidation, cavitary lesions, and/or wedge-shaped lung infarcts. Despite the clinical similarities, case series evaluating radiographic findings of mucormycosis in patients with hematologic malignancies have identified certain findings more frequently in patients with pulmonary mucormycosis as opposed to pulmonary aspergillosis. These include multiple pulmonary nodules (>10), pleural effusion(s), and the reverse halo sign. The reverse halo sign (Fig. 25.1) is a focal area of ground-glass opacity surrounded by a ring of consolidation; among patients with hematologic malignancies it is strongly associated with mucormycosis.[16] However, there are other potential etiologies of the reverse halo sign, so it should be interpreted based on pretest probability. The reverse halo sign is uncommon in nonneutropenic patients with mucormycosis.[17]

Rhinocerebral Mucormycosis. Different literature sources refer variably to rhino-orbital, sino-orbital, sinus, rhinocerebral, or rhino-orbito-cerebral mucormycosis. In this chapter we use the term "rhinocerebral mucormycosis" to describe infection involving any of the following structures: the palate, the sinuses, the orbit and any adjacent structures, with or without extension via contiguous or hematogenous routes to the brain. Manifestations depend on the specific sites and the extent of disease involvement. Features that distinguish rhinocerebral mucormycosis from rhinocerebral aspergillosis include a propensity to involve the orbit, involvement of the ethmoid sinuses, and pansinusitis.[18] Concurrent pulmonary and rhinocerebral/sinus involvement should also prompt suspicion for mucormycosis as opposed to aspergillosis.

Cutaneous Mucormycosis. Cutaneous lesions seen in mucormycosis can be primary, developing after localized inoculation at sites of trauma, intravascular catheters or adhesive tape, or secondary owing to hematogenous dissemination from another site of disease.

Other Forms of Mucormycosis. The gastrointestinal tract is the least commonly involved primary site of mucormycosis; its manifestations are described in Table 25.3. One exception is in neonatal disease, but the pathogenesis is likely different than mucormycosis in transplant recipients or oncology patients. Mucormycosis can involve any organ or tissue, either via hematogenous dissemination, deep contiguous extension from the primary focus, or inoculation at sites of trauma or surgery.[14] The brain is one of the most common sites involved via hematogenous dissemination.

Disease Prophylaxis

Guidelines for diagnosis and management of mucormycosis have been developed jointly by the European Society for Clinical Microbiology

TABLE 25.2 Epidemiologic Features of Mucormycosis by Immunocompromised Population

Feature	Hematopoietic Stem Cell Transplant	Solid Organ Transplant	Oncology
Incidence estimates	Cumulative incidence during first year after transplant: 0.29% in autologous and allogeneic cohort (TRANSNET) 0.60% in allogeneic only cohort (CIBMTR)	Cumulative incidence during first year after transplant: 0.07% (TRANSNET)	72.0 mucormycosis-related hospitalizations per 100,000 hematologic malignancy hospitalizations[1]
Timing of onset	Median, 4.4 months after transplant (TRANSNET) Median, 75 days after transplant (CIBMTR)	Median, 5 months after transplant, earlier in liver transplant recipients[8]	Median, 8.8 months after diagnosis[10]
Risk factors for disease	Allogeneic transplantation Unrelated donor Acute graft-versus-host disease grade II-IV Prior aspergillosis	Lung transplantation Liver transplantation Recent organ rejection episode Diabetes mellitus Renal failure before transplant	Hematologic malignancy, particularly acute myelogenous leukemia Active malignancy Prolonged (>7 days) neutropenia
Mortality/case-fatality rate estimates	72% at 1 year after diagnosis of mucormycosis (TRANSNET) 85% at 1 year after diagnosis of mucormycosis (CIBMTR)	38% at 90 days[8]	52% during course of mucormycosis (follow-up period undefined)[9]

CIBMTR, Center for International Blood and Marrow Transplant Research[5]; *GVHD*, graft-versus-host disease; *TRANSNET*, Transplant-Associated Infection Surveillance Network.[7]

TABLE 25.3 Frequency and Clinical Manifestations of Mucormycosis Clinical Syndromes

Syndrome	Percentage of Cases[a]	Clinical Manifestations
Pulmonary	50-60	Fever, cough, chest pain, dyspnea, hemoptysis
Rhinocerebral	15-30	Facial swelling, pain, proptosis, headache, nasal congestion, nasal discharge, necrotic lesions of palate or nasal septum, cranial neuropathies With brain involvement: seizure, stroke, focal neurologic deficit(s), encephalopathy
Cutaneous	10-20	Erythematous, indurated lesion, progression to ulcer, then necrotic eschar
Gastrointestinal	<5	Abdominal pain, nausea, vomiting, gastrointestinal bleeding, obstruction, perforation
Disseminated	15-25	Variable based on site of dissemination

[a]Based on series in hematopoietic stem cell transplant, solid organ transplant, and oncology patients.[7,8,10,14]

Data combined from Park BJ, Pappas PG, Wannemuehler KA, et al. Invasive non-*Aspergillus* mold infections in transplant recipients, United States, 2001-2006. *Emerg Infect Dis*. 2011;17(10):1855-1864; Singh N, Aguado JM, Bonatti H, et al. Zygomycosis in solid organ transplant recipients: a prospective, matched case-control study to assess risks for disease and outcome. *J Infect Dis*. 2009;200(6):1002-1011; Lanternier F, Dannaoui E, Morizot G, et al. A global analysis of mucormycosis in France: the RetroZygo study (2005-2007). *Clin Infect Dis*. 2012;54(suppl 1):s35-s43; Roden MM, Zaoutis TE, Buchanan WL, et al. Epidemiology and outcome of zygomycosis: a review of 929 reported cases. *Clin Infect Dis*. 2005;41(5):634-653.

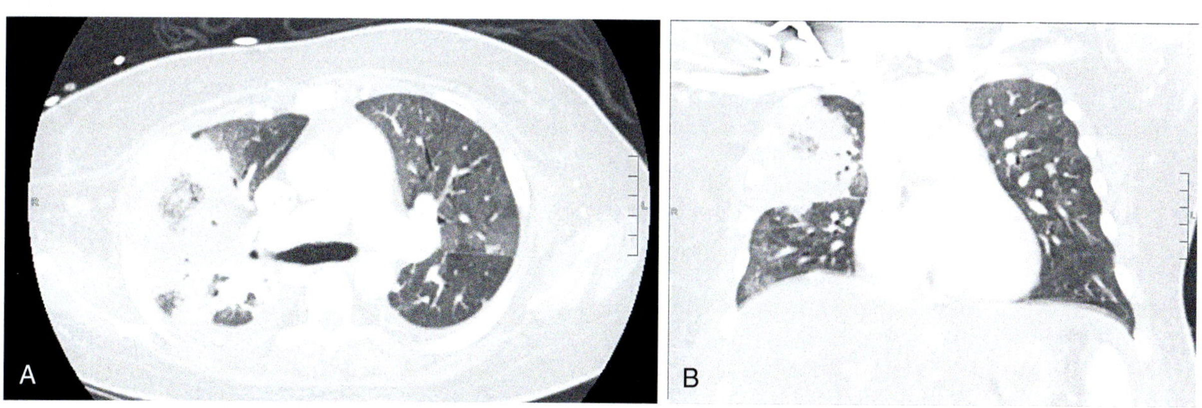

Fig. 25.1 Reverse halo sign in a patient with pulmonary mucormycosis. **(A)** Axial and **(B)** coronal views of a large consolidation with central hypodensity in the right upper lobe.

and Infectious Diseases (ESCMID) and the European Confederation of Medical Mycology (ECMM).[19] These guidelines, based primarily on adult data, offer a marginal recommendation for primary prophylaxis with posaconazole during periods of graft-versus-host disease (GVHD) with augmented immunosuppression and during outbreak situations. Use of posaconazole as secondary prophylaxis is recommended during ongoing immunosuppression in patients who have previously been diagnosed with mucormycosis. Guidelines developed for diagnosis and treatment of mucormycosis in patients with hematologic malignancy from the third European Conference on Infections in Leukemia (ECIL-3), and subsequently updated (ECIL-6), do not provide recommendations on primary prophylaxis but support the use of posaconazole for secondary prophylaxis.[20,21] Available pediatric dosing data for are limited to children 13 years and older, limiting use of this medication in younger patients. It is important to recognize that patients receiving posaconazole prophylaxis can still develop mucormycosis as a breakthrough infection (see Table 25.1).

Diagnosis

The diagnosis of mucormycosis can be challenging and relies on early clinical suspicion and aggressive pursuit of diagnostic samples. A suggested diagnostic approach is outlined in Fig. 25.2. Multidisciplinary coordination is recommended between transplant and oncology specialists, infectious diseases and surgical specialists, along with clinical pathologists, clinical pharmacists, and microbiologists. Empiric antifungal therapy should be started promptly and concurrently with attempts to establish the diagnosis, because delay in treatment has been associated with increased mortality.[12]

Diagnostic Sampling. Obtaining clinical samples from the affected site(s) is essential as there are currently no standardized diagnostic biomarkers or other well-validated noninvasive tests to diagnose mucormycosis. Results of serum galactomannan and (1,3)-β-D-glucan tests are usually negative in mucormycosis as these antigens are not

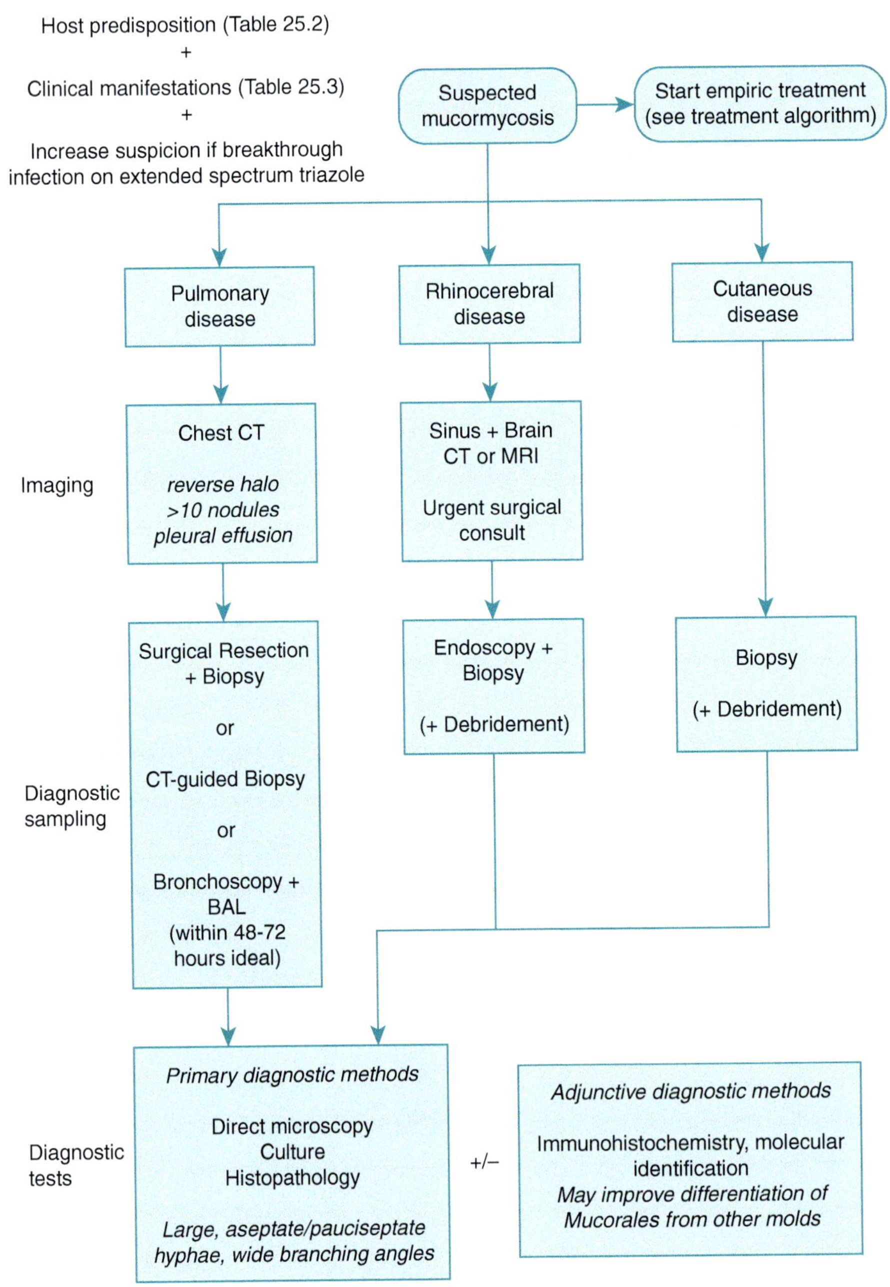

Fig. 25.2 Diagnostic algorithm for mucormycosis. The approach refers to the most common disease presentations but could be applied similarly to other localized disease presentations. Similar diagnostic strategies could be applied as well to other uncommon invasive molds. *BAL*, bronchoalveolar lavage; *CT*, computed tomography; *MRI*, magnetic resonance imaging.

released or not released in detectable quantities by the Mucorales. The ideal sample for diagnostic evaluation is tissue from the affected site(s) for histologic verification. Tissue samples are more readily obtainable in the setting of rhinocerebral and cutaneous disease but are challenging to obtain from the lungs. Unfortunately, the lungs are the predominant site of mucormycosis in transplant recipients and oncology patients. Recovery of Mucorales from sputum and bronchoalveolar lavage (BAL) samples is low (25% from BAL in one study); however, BAL may be useful in evaluating for other etiologies of pneumonia in an immunocompromised patient, and experts have suggested higher potential yield in the first 48 to 72 hours from symptom onset.[18] Computed tomography (CT)-guided lung biopsy has shown utility in establishing the diagnosis of pulmonary mucormycosis. Correction of coagulopathy and/or transfusion of platelets may be required to reduce bleeding risk before a patient can undergo biopsy. Correcting any identified coagulopathy is of particular importance in this setting given the angioinvasive nature of these pathogens, which may further predispose the patient to bleeding during or after a biopsy procedure. Although clinicians may be reluctant to pursue invasive procedures, the value of an invasive intervention should be emphasized given its influence on antifungal therapy choice (e.g., different antifungal classes for invasive aspergillosis versus mucormycosis), the likelihood for earlier initiation of appropriate directed therapy, and the opportunity for improved source control with removal of necrotic tissue that might diminish antifungal effectiveness.

Primary Diagnostic Tests. Direct microscopy of clinical samples with an optical brightener such as calcofluor white can provide early confirmation of the diagnosis.[19,20] Causative organisms of mucormycosis can be visualized on histopathology via commonly used tissue stains. Hyphae of Mucorales are large with variable width (6 to 25 μm), irregular, and ribbon-like in appearance, contain few or no septations, and demonstrate wide-angle (90-degree) branching. As histology often offers the first clues to pathogen identification, it is critical to recognize these morphologic characteristics of Mucorales and to identify how they differ from other fungi. For example, hyphae in invasive mucormycosis differ from invasive aspergillosis (regularly septate, smaller hyphae). In some cases, damage to tissue or a paucity of organisms precludes differentiation of Mucorales from other molds via conventional histopathology. Therefore additional methods for identification of the organism are necessary. This can include a constellation of diagnostic testing, including immunohistochemistry, conventional culture, and more contemporary molecular methods. Practitioners should also be aware of the possibility of co-infection with other molds.

Owing to the lack of septations, the organisms are prone to shearing during tissue processing, and culture results may be negative even with organisms visualized on histopathology. Mincing of tissues rather than grinding is recommended to improve recovery in culture. Speciation of the Mucorales is difficult using conventional microbiology methods, but can be improved using adjunctive molecular methods. The ESCMID/ECMM and ECIL guidelines for mucormycosis recommend identification to the genus and species level, if possible, primarily for epidemiologic understanding.[19-21] It is not clear at this time that identification of the genus and species is important to guide clinical management. Standardized methods of microdilution susceptibility testing for the Mucorales are guided by the European Committee on Antimicrobial Susceptibility Testing and Clinical & Laboratory Standards Institute, but no validated susceptibility breakpoints have been established. Methodologies for determining an epidemiologic cutoff value have been developed and used for common species. These cutoffs can provide a guide to the clinician regarding the relative susceptibility of an organism. However, despite the terminology, epidemiologic cutoffs are not correlates of clinical effectiveness.

Adjunctive and Emerging Diagnostic Tests. Novel methods show potential to supplement conventional diagnostic methods for mucormycosis. Immunohistochemistry on histopathology samples and molecular detection methods, including polymerase chain reaction–based strategies and matrix-assisted laser desorption ionization time-of-flight mass spectrometry have been demonstrated in small clinical cohorts. Few molecular diagnostic tests are currently available commercially, and there is a lack of standardized approaches. To the extent that these tests are available, they may be useful in providing genus- and species-level identification when Mucorales are detected via conventional methods, in differentiating Mucorales from other molds when histopathologic findings are ambiguous, or improving detection of Mucorales from lower-yield clinical samples such as BAL fluid.[19-21] When molecular detection methods are used, fresh clinical samples are preferred over formalin-fixed paraffin-embedded samples.

Some of the most promising strategies are those that may establish the diagnosis of mucormycosis without invasive diagnostic sampling. Such strategies include detection of circulating Mucorales DNA in the blood via polymerase chain reaction, detection of Mucorales-specific host immune responses, and detection of a characteristic metabolite signature in exhaled breath.[22] Unbiased pathogen detection via circulating cell-free nucleic acids has also shown potential to detect IMD including mucormycosis. Such methods are promising and may change the future diagnostic strategy for mucormycosis and other IMDs. However, before they are comprehensively validated against conventional diagnostic methods, they should not be considered a replacement for diagnostic biopsy in patients with suspected mucormycosis.

Treatment

Mucormycosis is a rare disease and thus it is difficult to study therapeutic options via robust clinical trials. The only randomized controlled trial of mucormycosis therapy enrolled just 20 patients and focused on adjunctive therapy, largely in patients with diabetes mellitus.[23] Most treatment recommendations are therefore based on observational data, small single-arm clinical trials, animal models, and expert opinion. The treatment algorithm outlined in Fig. 25.3 is based on a synthesis of European and Australian clinical guidelines, expert opinion reviews, and pediatric considerations for drug therapy.[18-21,24] Mucormycosis is life-threatening and can be a rapidly progressive condition, yet favorable outcomes are achievable and most likely to occur when antifungal therapy is combined with surgery and reversal of predisposing conditions. An expeditious and multidisciplinary approach to therapy is recommended.

Primary Antifungal Therapy

Amphotericin B–based monotherapy. Amphotericin B–based therapy is recommended as first-line treatment of mucormycosis in all age groups based on a preponderance of observational data demonstrating its impact on survival.[19-21,24] Although conventional amphotericin B deoxycholate has been used historically, its use is discouraged outside the neonatal period because of poor tolerability. Among the lipid formulations of amphotericin B, liposomal amphotericin B (L-AmB) is favored, especially for central nervous system (CNS) disease and for patients with renal insufficiency. Amphotericin B lipid complex (ABLC) is also an option. It is important to initiate therapy upon suspicion of mucormycosis, as delay of more than five days from onset of symptoms has been associated with near doubling of mortality.[12] The optimal dose of L-AmB is not

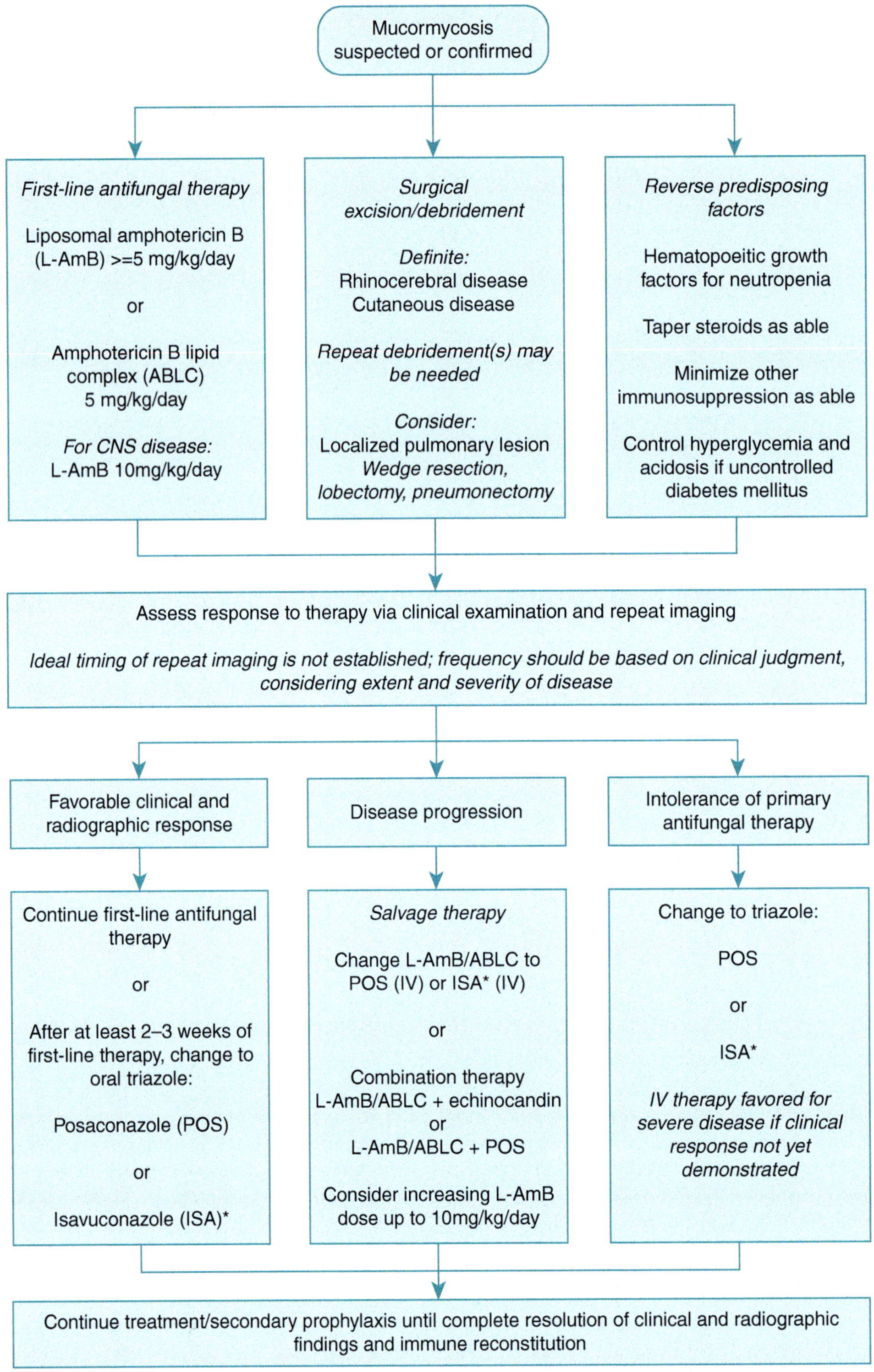

Fig. 25.3 Treatment algorithm for mucormycosis. The approach is based on the authors' synthesis of clinical guidelines, expert opinion reviews, and the available pediatric literature. *Isavuconazole is currently licensed for adults 18 years and older; off-label use in pediatric patients should be based on clinical judgement and pharmacotherapy expertise. *IV*, intravenous.

well-defined; at least 5 mg/kg per day is recommended. Escalation of the dose up to 10 mg/kg per day increases drug exposure and improves disease response in animal models, but it is not clear that it alters clinical response in humans. A single-arm trial of L-AmB at 10 mg/kg per day in 40 patients showed clinical response rates similar to those reported in observational literature, but creatinine doubling occurred in 40% of participants.[25] Nonetheless, clinical guidelines recommend L-AmB at 10mg/kg per day for treatment of CNS mucormycosis, primarily based on animal model and case report data.[19-21,24]

Triazole monotherapy. Isavuconazole is an extended-spectrum triazole antifungal now licensed for primary therapy of mucormycosis in adults based on a single-arm trial (VITAL) of 37 patients 18 years and older with mucormycosis, including 21 receiving the drug as primary therapy.[26] The 6-week all-cause mortality of 33% in primary treatment cases was comparable to 39% in amphotericin B–treated matched controls from a registry. A pediatric pharmacokinetic and safety study of isavuconazole is in progress. Given the current lack of pediatric data and limitations in the methodology of the VITAL study, clinicians should use caution in considering isavuconazole for primary therapy for mucormycosis in children. Potential pitfalls reported are breakthrough mucormycosis in patients receiving isavuconazole (see Table 25.1), and high minimum inhibitory concentrations to isavuconazole among some causative pathogens, particularly *Mucor circinelloides*.[3] No other monotherapy regimens, including posaconazole, have been systematically studied for primary therapy of mucormycosis.

Combination antifungal therapy. Some experts recommend routine use of combination antifungal therapy with L-AmB and an echinocandin as primary therapy for mucormycosis.[18] The rationale is based on in vitro and animal model studies. Although echinocandins lack activity against the Mucorales when given as monotherapy, their target enzyme, (1,3)-β-D-glucan synthase, is expressed at least by some species, and animal studies indicate they may be beneficial when combined with lipid formulations of amphotericin B. Small retrospective case series have shown better outcomes in patients treated with combination therapy versus monotherapy.[27] The studies are limited by small size, retrospective design, and lack of clear comparability between the combination therapy and monotherapy-treated patients with respect to surgical management or other important factors influencing outcome. Generalizability to transplant and oncology patients is also unclear based on combination therapy data derived from patients with rhinocerebral mucormycosis in the setting of diabetic ketoacidosis.

Larger observational studies incorporating methods to control for confounding, including "natural experiment" analysis based on era of treatment, or propensity score adjustment, have conversely not shown a benefit to combination therapy.[4,28] Clinical guidelines for mucormycosis conclude that there is insufficient evidence at this time to recommend primary combination therapy.[19-21,24] Some experts advocate for primary combination therapy based on theoretical benefit with modest impact on cost or toxicity of treatment, but more data are needed to support these conclusions.

Animal studies have shown conflicting results regarding additional benefit of posaconazole when added to lipid-formulated amphotericin B for primary treatment of mucormycosis. Clinical studies supporting this combination for primary therapy are lacking. Some experts recommend this combination as empiric treatment when the etiology of a breakthrough IMD is undetermined.[3] The primary rationale is to broaden the spectrum of empiric treatment in case of a relatively drug-resistant species of *Aspergillus*, Mucorales, or another breakthrough IMD.

Salvage Antifungal Therapy. Responses to primary antifungal therapy in mucormycosis are characteristically poor, slow, and often very dependent on host immunologic status. Even in cases with an ultimate favorable outcome, there may be initial disease progression before improvement (especially if there has been evidence of immune recovery such as resolution of neutropenia), and disease control can take several weeks. Therefore clinicians must resist desires for early transition to salvage therapy. Unfortunately, knowing when to adjust a therapeutic plan can be challenging, and often initial disease progression prompts modification to a salvage therapy approach. Clinical trials of salvage antifungal therapy typically enroll patients considered to have refractory disease after at least 7 days of primary antifungal therapy. Additionally, intolerance of amphotericin B–based therapy, primarily because of nephrotoxicity, may prompt modification of therapy to an alternative agent. Posaconazole has demonstrated favorable effectiveness as salvage therapy for mucormycosis, with response rates of 60% to 80%.[29] It is important to avoid overinterpreting salvage therapy response rates as indicating potential responses to primary therapy. Patients who receive salvage therapy have survived long enough since diagnosis to be eligible for salvage therapy, and they may have benefited already from initial surgery and first-line antifungal therapy. Given favorable data for posaconazole, clinical guidelines recommend it as an option for salvage therapy in patients with refractory disease or life-threatening intolerance of first-line therapy.[19-21,24] Isavuconazole has also been studied in adults for salvage therapy of mucormycosis.[26]

Salvage therapy because of intolerance of primary therapy. In our treatment algorithm (Fig. 25.3), we suggest differentiation of patients who switch to salvage therapy because of intolerance of primary therapy from those who switch because of disease progression. Changing to posaconazole (or off-label isavuconazole in selected adolescents) is reasonable for clinically stable patients with life-threatening intolerance to amphotericin B–based therapy if they do not show disease progression and do not have CNS disease. Although initial studies of posaconazole used the suspension formulation, the delayed-release tablet formulation is preferred now for patients age 13 years or older owing to improved bioavailability. Intravenous (IV) formulations of posaconazole and isavuconazole are also available and initial use of IV therapy is favored in patients with severe disease. Optimal dosing of posaconazole for younger children (<13 years) is not well-established, and the oral suspension has poor and highly variable bioavailability. Posaconazole therapeutic drug monitoring is recommended, with a suggested target trough of > 1 mg/L based primarily on expert opinion and extrapolation from other invasive fungal diseases.

Salvage therapy because of refractory or progressive disease. Switching to posaconazole (or off-label isavuconazole in selected adolescents) is an option for salvage therapy in patients with refractory or progressive disease; however, caution should be exercised against early abandonment of guideline-recommended amphotericin B–based therapy. Compared with triazole agents, amphotericin B is active against a wider spectrum of causative agents of mucormycosis. Animal models raise concern for failure of posaconazole against *Rhizopus arrhizus* (formerly known as *Rhizopus oryzae*) and *Mucor circinelloides*, 2 of the most common causative organisms. The potential gaps in the spectrum with isavuconazole are not well characterized, but breakthrough mucormycosis has been reported in patients receiving isavuconazole. Posaconazole is a P-glycoprotein substrate and thus achieves poor concentration in the CNS. Owing to unknowns and potential limitations with these agents as monotherapy, clinicians may wish to continue L-AmB and add posaconazole or isavuconazole for refractory or progressive mucormycosis. Although there has been concern about antagonism between these agents in other fungal diseases, in vitro data have not supported antagonism when used in combination for Mucorales organisms. Some clinical guidelines have suggested salvage therapy with combination L-AmB and an echinocandin, whereas some experts have offered the suggestion of escalating the dose of L-AmB up to 10 mg/kg per day for refractory disease.[18-21] Unfortunately, there are limited data to support or refute these recommendations. Likewise, there has been no systematic evaluation of triple-combination therapy, including L-AmB, posaconazole and an echinocandin, but this regimen is sometimes used in clinical practice.[2]

Given the limited evidence for an ideal approach, treatment of the patient with refractory or progressive mucormycosis should be individualized, considering the potential risks and benefits of the therapy based on the patient's age, comorbidities, and concurrent medications. Clinicians should familiarize themselves with the antifungal agents, their pharmacokinetic characteristics in children, drug interactions and adverse effects, and ideally work closely with a multidisciplinary team to plan and monitor therapy. It is also critical to pursue surgical debridement and reversal of predisposing factors to the extent possible.

Step-Down Therapy and Duration. Response to therapy should be assessed by clinical evaluation and repeated imaging of the affected site(s). The optimal timing of reassessment and optimal duration of initial therapy are not established. More frequent repeat imaging (weekly) is suggested for patients with severe and/or extensive disease, or those with potential invasion of vital structures such as the thoracic vasculature or CNS. Patients who show a favorable clinical response and have well-controlled localized disease may not require such frequent repeat imaging. Amphotericin B–based primary therapy should be continued until at least a partial response is demonstrated clinically and radiographically; this usually takes several weeks.[18] Patients who demonstrate a response may either continue with amphotericin B–based therapy or switch to oral posaconazole (or off-label isavuconazole, in selected adolescents) for long-term maintenance therapy. Transition to an azole regimen in children younger than 13 years is challenging as there are limited dosing recommendations for these agents in this age group. Therefore continued use of amphotericin B–based therapy even after initial clinical response is favored by some experts. Amphotericin B–based therapy toxicity or intolerance may necessitate use of posaconazole or isavuconazole in these patients. In such situations, guidance from an experienced pediatric pharmacist, along with input from the members of the multidisciplinary team, is important. Guidelines for mucormycosis recommend continuation of antifungal therapy until complete resolution of clinical and radiographic findings, and reconstitution of immune function.[19-21,24] Clinicians should be aware of the potential for recrudescence of mucormycosis in patients receiving oral triazoles.[3] Therapeutic drug monitoring is recommended to ensure adequate posaconazole exposure, with a suggested target trough of more than 1 mg/L. Currently there are no recommendations for therapeutic drug monitoring of isavuconazole, but this may change with additional experience as it did with other agents in the azole class.

Surgical Management. Surgical debridement in combination with antifungal therapy improves survival and is strongly recommended for patients with the rhinocerebral and cutaneous forms of mucormycosis.[19-21,24] The goals of surgery are to remove devitalized tissue that is poorly penetrated by antifungals, to limit local extension of disease, and to potentially prevent hematogenous dissemination. Rhinocerebral mucormycosis is considered a surgical emergency. Repeated debridement is often needed and should be guided based on repeated endoscopic examination and imaging. Input from a surgical specialist with experience in debriding rhinocerebral mucormycosis can further optimize care. Similar to invasive aspergillosis, the role for surgical resection of localized pulmonary lesions via wedge resection, lobectomy, or pneumonectomy is not as well established but should be considered as it may be associated with a survival benefit.[18,20]

Reversal of Predisposing Conditions and Adjunctive Therapy. Measures to reverse predisposing conditions are recommended for all patients with mucormycosis because ongoing immune dysfunction is consistently associated with poor outcomes.[19-21] Hematopoietic growth factors (granulocyte colony-stimulating factor or granulocyte-macrophage colony-stimulating factor) are recommended to reverse neutropenia. Steroids should be tapered as possible and other immunosuppressive therapies should be reduced. Control of hyperglycemia and acidosis is important for patients with uncontrolled diabetes mellitus.

If the patient is receiving the iron chelator deferoxamine, it should be discontinued because it increases the risk for disseminated mucormycosis. Deferoxamine serves as a siderophore and makes iron available for fungi to use metabolically; other iron chelators do not serve as siderophores and their use has been considered for adjunctive therapy to reduce available iron. A clinical trial (Deferasirox-AmBisome Therapy for Mucormycosis) of the iron chelator deferasirox as adjunctive therapy for mucormycosis showed unexpectedly increased mortality among patients with hematologic malignancy in the deferasirox arm.[23] Although this result could have occurred because of imbalance of baseline risk factors in the 2 treatment arms, the study results have led to recommendation against use of adjunctive deferasirox.[19-21]

Other adjunctive strategies, predominantly described in case reports, include the use of hematopoietic growth factors to augment immune response in patients without neutropenia, use of granulocyte transfusions in patients with refractory neutropenia and fungal disease, and use of interferon gamma to enhance the immune response. None of these strategies are routinely recommended because of limited supporting evidence.[19-21] Hyperbaric oxygen therapy has shown benefit in case reports and series of patients with diabetes mellitus and rhinocerebral mucormycosis, but limited data in patients with hematologic malignancy have not supported a benefit and it is not routinely recommended in immunocompromised patients with mucormycosis.

Infection Prevention and Anticipatory Guidance

Mucormycosis can be transmitted as a nosocomial infection in the context of hospital construction activities or contaminated supplies. Procedures for air filtration and recirculation should be used in oncology, hematology, and HSCT wards to limit environmental mold exposure. Given the rarity of mucormycosis, clustering of cases should trigger investigation for a potential nosocomial source. Patients should be counseled to avoid activities with risk for high inoculum exposure to inhaled aerosolized fungal spores, such as construction activities or soil excavation. If such exposure is unavoidable, then a mask may be worn in high-risk areas.

FUSARIOSIS AND *SCEDOSPORIASIS*

Fusarium and *Scedosporium* are genera of hyaline molds that are usually the third and fourth most common IMDs in immunocompromised hosts, after invasive aspergillosis and mucormycosis. The causative species are morphologically similar to *Aspergillus* and cause a similar spectrum of disease; fusariosis and scedosporiasis can be rapidly progressive and challenging to treat owing to multidrug resistance.

Epidemiology and Risk Factors

Causative organisms of fusariosis and scedosporiasis are grouped into species complexes encompassing member species that can be differentiated via molecular methods. The majority of human cases of fusariosis are caused by members of the *F. solani*, *F. oxysporum*, and *F. fujikuroi* species complexes, with the *F. solani* species complex demonstrating greater pathogenicity.

Nomenclature of the organisms causing scedosporiasis can be confusing and has undergone recent changes. The genus name *Pseudallescheria* applies to the sexual state (teleomorph), whereas *Scedosporium* applies to the asexual state (anamorph) of these organisms. *S. apiospermum* was once thought to be the anamorph of *Pseudallescheria boydii*, but they are now known to be distinct species. The *S. apiospermum* species complex encompasses *S. apiospermum*, *S. boydii*, *S. aurantiacum*, *S. dehoogli*, and *S. minutispora*. The organism formerly known as *S. prolificans* is now renamed *Lomentospora prolificans* and is phylogenetically distinct from the *Scedosporium* species. *L. prolificans* is categorized by some sources as a dematiaceous (pigmented, melanized) mold rather than a hyaline mold (akin to *Aspergillus*, *Fusarium*, and *Scedosporium*). However, it is usually grouped clinically with the *Scedosporium* species and the former nomenclature may be seen in clinical references.

In addition to the usual airborne and cutaneous inoculation routes of acquisition common to other invasive molds, *Fusarium* can be transmitted via contaminated water sources (e.g., shower heads) and can cause infection associated with IV catheters. Both *Fusarium* and *Scedosporium/Lomentospora* species can cause infection in immunocompetent hosts, primarily localized infections such as keratitis or onychomycosis. In immunocompromised patients, *Fusarium* can disseminate from initially localized infections such as onychomycosis or intertrigo.[30] The major predisposing factors for invasive disease are profound and prolonged neutropenia and severe cell-mediated immunodeficiency.

Although fusariosis and scedosporiasis are generally less common than invasive aspergillosis and mucormycosis, their relative incidence varies geographically. For example, a multicenter study in Brazil identified invasive fusariosis more commonly than invasive aspergillosis in HSCT recipients and patients with hematologic malignancy, and the incidence of invasive fusariosis there increased over 10-fold up to 10 cases per 1000 hospitalizations from 2000 to 2010.[30,31]

Hematopoietic Stem Cell Transplant. Among HSCT recipients in the TRANSNET study, fusariosis accounted for 3% of IFDs.[6] The estimated incidence among allogeneic HSCT recipients from the Center for International Blood and Marrow Transplant Research registry from 1995 to 2008 was 4.34 cases per 1000 patients who had transplants.[5] The incidence of fusariosis was lower between 2002 and 2008 compared with the 1995 to 2002 period; the difference is hypothesized to be related to voriconazole prophylaxis and empiric therapy in the later period. Identified risk factors for fusariosis in HSCT recipients include history of CMV infection, receipt of an umbilical cord blood transplant (compared with other stem cell sources), receipt of antithymocyte globulin, and hyperglycemia.[5,32] Risk factors specific to the development of fusariosis beyond day 40 after transplant include GVHD and prior IMD.[32] Scedosporiasis is less common among HSCT recipients compared with fusariosis, with only 16 cases identified in the TRANSNET study compared with 31 cases of fusariosis and 77 cases of mucormycosis.[7] Specific risk factors for scedosporiasis among HSCT recipients are not well described.

Solid Organ Transplant. Among 1208 invasive fungal infections in the TRANSNET study of SOT recipients, there were 6 cases of fusariosis and 11 cases of scedosporiasis, compared with 28 cases of mucormycosis.[7] In a literature review of *L. prolificans* cases, SOT recipients constituted 8.6% of cases.[33] Scedosporiasis is most common among lung transplant recipients, in whom colonization of the airways can occur before transplantation (particularly in patients with cystic fibrosis) or after transplantation, and may progress to invasive infection. Some centers consider colonization with *Scedosporium* species to be a contraindication to lung transplantation, given the risk for dissemination and high mortality after transplantation, but this practice varies. Disseminated scedosporiasis can develop in immunocompetent persons after drowning, and transmission of scedosporiasis from SOT donor to multiple recipients has been described in the context of the donor's death caused by drowning.[34]

Oncology. Among patients undergoing therapy for cancer, fusariosis primarily occurs in those with hematologic malignancy, especially acute myelogenous leukemia (AML). In Brazil, where fusariosis is a relatively common cause of IFD, the 1-year cumulative incidence of fusariosis in patients with AML or myelodysplastic syndrome was 5.2%.[31] In a single-center study of 44 cases, the most commonly identified risk factors for fusariosis in patients with hematologic malignancy were active leukemia, prolonged and profound neutropenia, and high-dose corticosteroid exposure.[35] Smoking has been identified as a risk factor for fusariosis in adults.[32] Pediatric case series have described fusariosis occurring in children with AML, acute lymphoblastic leukemia, and juvenile myelomonocytic leukemia.[36,37] Scedosporiasis is less common overall, but malignancy, primarily hematologic, was the most common underlying risk factor in a review of reported cases of scedosporiasis.[33]

Prognosis and Modifying Factors. Fusariosis and scedosporiasis confer high mortality, with the ultimate outcome dependent on the extent of disease, the causative species complex, and the degree to which immune function is reconstituted. A multinational study of fusariosis cases (predominantly in adults, but inclusive of children) showed a 43% survival rate at 90 days between 2001 and 2011, an improvement from 22% at 90 days between 1985 and 2000.[38] Treatment with voriconazole was associated with higher probability of survival; receipt of corticosteroids and lack of neutrophil recovery were associated with lower probability of survival. Disseminated fusariosis with fungemia carries a particularly high case-fatality rate with one series reporting only 6% survival at 6 weeks.[35] Overall mortality resulting from infection with *L. prolificans* was 46.9% in one series; however, the study included immunocompetent patients with localized disease; the case-fatality rate was 87.5% in those with disseminated disease.[33]

Clinical Manifestations

The clinical manifestations of invasive fusariosis and scedosporiasis are similar in many respects to those of invasive aspergillosis, as described in detail in Chapter 24, with distinctive features outlined in the following text.

Fusariosis. The most common sites of invasive fusariosis in immunocompromised persons are the skin (60% to 80% of cases), lungs (50% to 80% of cases), and sinuses (20% to 30% of cases).[35,38] *Fusarium* can develop yeastlike adventitious sporulation within infected tissue, which facilitates dissemination, seen in 70% of cases.[35-38] Unlike other molds that infrequently cause detectable fungemia and are difficult to recover in standard blood culture media, blood culture results are positive for *Fusarium* in 40% to 50% of cases.[35-38]

Radiographic series comparing findings of pulmonary fusariosis with those of invasive aspergillosis and mucormycosis note that the halo sign (a nodule surrounded by ground-glass opacity) is frequently absent in cases of fusariosis.[39] However, children with IMDs of all types often lack characteristic radiographic features such as the halo sign, so this distinction may not be applicable to younger patients.

Cutaneous lesions of invasive fusariosis (Fig. 25.4) are distinctive, consisting of painful, circular macules or papules, usually with central necrosis and surrounding erythema, similar in appearance to ecthyma gangrenosum.[36] The appearance of cutaneous lesions in invasive fusariosis is usually secondary to hematogenous dissemination to the skin, rather than direct inoculation into the skin. A solitary lesion may develop initially, usually with progression to multiple lesions, mostly distributed on the extremities.

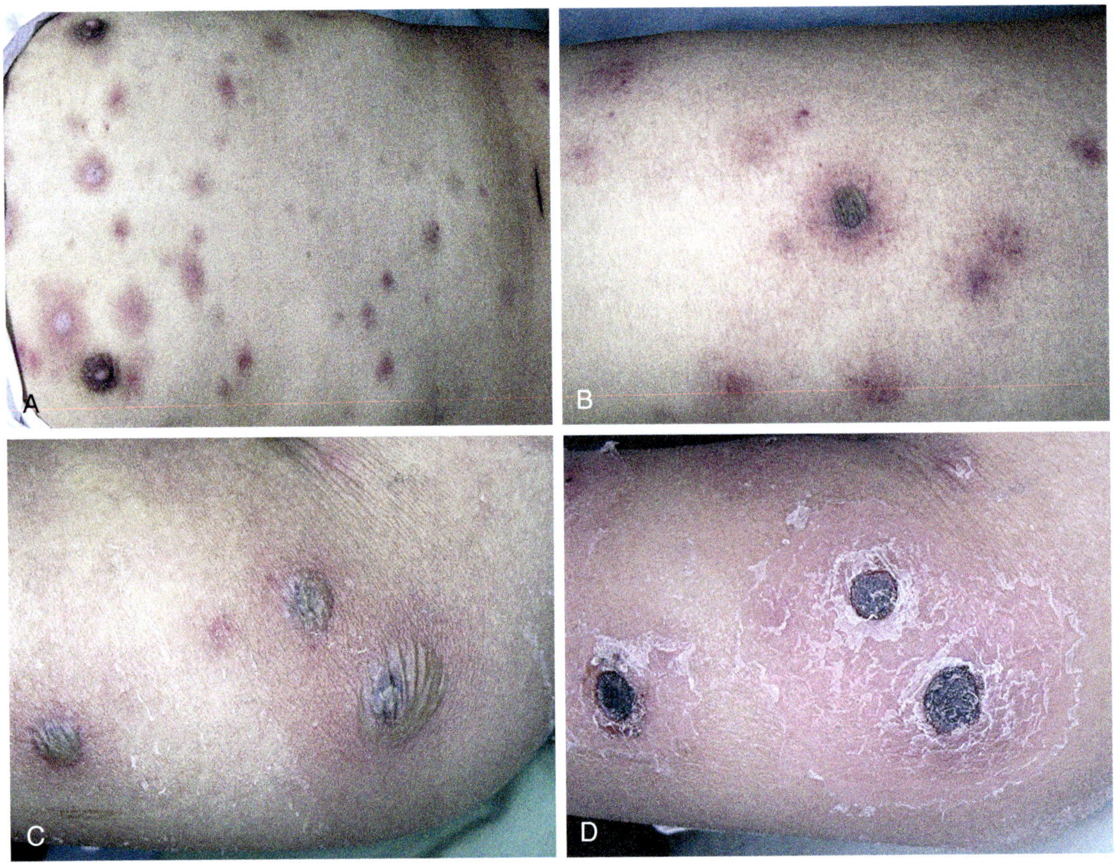

Fig. 25.4 Cutaneous lesions of invasive fusariosis. **A,** Multiple cutaneous lesions on the trunk. **B,** Early-stage lesions. C and D, Later-stage lesions with progression to bullae and eschars. (From Yeh Y-W, Wang W-M. Multiple erythematous nodules with a necrotic center in a patient with acute lymphoblastic leukemia. *Dermatologica Sinica*. 2012; 30[3]:117-118.)

Scedosporiasis. Invasive scedosporiasis can involve any organ and is frequently disseminated owing to sporulation within tissues akin to *Fusarium*. Invasive disease caused by *S. apiospermum* species complex most frequently involves the skin, lungs, and CNS. CNS disease develops in the context of hematogenous dissemination and can manifest as brain abscess(es) or meningoencephalitis. Other manifestations include sinusitis and endogenous endophthalmitis. Skin lesions of *S. apiospermum* species complex can manifest as nodules, erythematous or violaceous papules, or bullae, which may develop necrosis. They are usually secondary to hematogenous dissemination rather than primary cutaneous lesions from direct inoculation of the skin. Lymphangitic or sporotrichoid spreading patterns have been described. Blood culture results are positive in approximately 30% of cases of invasive infection with *S. apiospermum* species complex. Similar manifestations are seen in invasive *L. prolificans* infections, but the propensity to disseminate is higher and positive blood culture results are reported in over 50% of cases.[33] Hematogenous dissemination of *L. prolificans* to the CNS is common.

Disease Prophylaxis

Prophylaxis against fusariosis and scedosporiasis is not routinely indicated because of the relative rarity of these infections. However, voriconazole or posaconazole used for prophylaxis against other IFDs may be beneficial. Initiation of voriconazole or posaconazole in patients with hematologic malignancy who have *Fusarium* identified from superficial skin lesions has been associated with a lower risk of subsequent invasive disease.[40]

Diagnosis

Diagnosis of fusariosis or scedosporiasis requires isolation and identification of the causative organism from the affected site(s). Imaging and diagnostic sampling can be performed as outlined in the diagnostic algorithm for mucormycosis (see Fig. 25.2). The causative organisms have thin septate hyphae with acute angle branching; they are not morphologically distinguishable from *Aspergillus* when examined in tissue. Culture is necessary for definitive identification of these organisms, although distinguishing between *Fusarium* species complexes may be difficult using conventional methods. As with the Mucorales, molecular identification methods can facilitate species-level identification but are not yet widely available or validated. Organisms causing fusariosis and scedosporiasis can be detected in conventional blood cultures; however, they may be initially reported as "yeast" because of the appearance of conidia produced via adventitious sporulation.

The *Aspergillus* serum galactomannan assay result is positive in approximately half of patients with invasive fusariosis, and detection of serum galactomannan above threshold has been shown to precede diagnosis of invasive fusariosis in a high-prevalence setting.[41] It is possible that a subset of patients diagnosed with probable invasive aspergillosis via the galactomannan assay actually have fusariosis. The serum galactomannan assay is usually negative in patients with scedosporiasis. The result of serum (1,3)-β-D-glucan assay is frequently positive in the setting of invasive fusariosis or scedosporiasis, but the test does not distinguish these infections from other IMDs, and the appropriate cutoff for positivity is not well established in children.

Treatment

Treatment recommendations for fusariosis and scedosporiasis are provided in ESCMID and ECMM joint guidelines and in Australian consensus guidelines.[24,42] The optimal therapy is unknown; recommendations are primarily based on case reports, clinical experience, and in vitro data given a lack of clinical trials for these rare diseases.

Antifungal Therapy for Fusariosis. The ESCMID/ECMM guidelines recommend voriconazole or a lipid-based amphotericin B formulation for treatment of fusariosis, with preference for voriconazole.[42] Australian guidelines do not state a preference for either agent on the basis of inadequate data.[24] Voriconazole treatment has been associated with higher treatment responses and improved survival in era-based studies, although these should be interpreted with caution because of potential confounding by earlier diagnosis or other interventions.[38,43] Therapeutic drug monitoring of voriconazole is recommended given its high intrapatient and interpatient pharmacokinetic variability. Because in vitro susceptibility of *Fusarium* isolates to both voriconazole and to amphotericin B varies widely, some experts routinely use combination therapy with voriconazole and lipid-based amphotericin B to ensure that at least one agent is active.[35] Some reports describe successful combination therapy with terbinafine and either L-AmB or voriconazole, and in vitro data show synergy between terbinafine and voriconazole. There are no systematic comparative studies of combination antifungal therapy for *Fusarium*.

Posaconazole has been used as salvage therapy with an approximately 50% favorable response rate.[44] Isavuconazole has been studied in few adult cases; based on in vitro susceptibilities it appears to be less active than voriconazole. *Fusarium* species are resistant to the echinocandins and to itraconazole.

As with other IMDs, the duration of therapy is individualized, with continuation until a complete clinical and radiographic response is achieved and immune function is restored. Ongoing secondary prophylaxis is advisable for patients who remain immunocompromised.

Antifungal Therapy for *S. apiospermum* Species Complex. The activity of antifungal agents against members of the *S. apiospermum* species complex is variable and there are species-based differences in susceptibility pattern. Amphotericin B–based therapy is not recommended because of in vitro resistance and poor clinical responses. Voriconazole is the most active agent and the recommended first-line therapy.[24,42] In a large observational study, the response rate to voriconazole therapy for *S. apiospermum* infections was 66%.[45] Voriconazole has good CNS penetration, which is important in treating *Scedosporium* infections given their propensity to disseminate to the CNS. The echinocandins, itraconazole, and posaconazole have variable activity. Isavuconazole is active in vitro but so far has been studied in only a handful of adults with scedosporiasis, limiting conclusions about its utility. Combination therapy has been reported, including voriconazole and either terbinafine or caspofungin, but systematic comparative data are lacking. Therapy should be adjusted based on antifungal susceptibility testing when available.

Antifungal Therapy for *L. prolificans*. *L. prolificans* is highly resistant to all antifungal agents currently available. Successful treatment of infections caused by this organism depends on reversal of predisposing conditions and aggressive surgical debridement. Voriconazole is the antifungal with the best demonstrated activity, but minimum inhibitory concentrations tend to be high and clinical responses to voriconazole therapy are suboptimal. In one case series, 16 of 36 patients with *L. prolificans* infection had a favorable outcome when treated with voriconazole in addition to surgery and reversal of predisposing conditions.[45] Combination therapy is typically used including voriconazole and other agents; successful outcomes have been reported with voriconazole or posaconazole and terbinafine, or voriconazole with an echinocandin. Australian guidelines recommend the combination of voriconazole with terbinafine.[24] However, terbinafine is highly protein bound with distribution primarily to skin and adipose tissue, leading some experts to doubt its utility in treating systemic fungal infections. There have been reports of combination therapy including miltefosine, which is typically used in the treatment of leishmaniasis but demonstrates some in vitro antifungal activity against *L. prolificans*. It is important to recognize that publication bias likely affects the reporting of outcomes, and no particular antifungal regimen has convincing evidence to support efficacy against *L. prolificans*. The majority of patients surviving in case series demonstrated recovery of neutropenia or other predisposing condition(s), or had localized disease that was fully resectable.[33]

Surgical Management of Fusariosis and Scedosporiasis. Surgical debridement of infected and necrotic tissue is recommended to facilitate cure, particularly in *L. prolificans* infection where surgery and immune reconstitution are the primary effective therapies. Surgery is recommended for skin and soft tissue infections, osteoarticular infections, and cerebral abscesses when possible.[42] As with other IMDs, surgery for pulmonary disease is more challenging and likely to be less effective when there is multifocal pulmonary involvement. Resection of a single cavitary lung lesion is recommended in the setting of hemoptysis or radiographic progression on antifungal therapy.[42] Surgery is also recommended for lesions that infiltrate the pericardium, great vessels, bone, or thoracic soft tissue. Removal of intravenous IV catheters is recommended for catheter-associated fusariosis.

Adjunctive Therapy. The outcome of fusariosis or scedosporiasis in immunocompromised hosts is highly dependent on the extent of recovery of immune function, particularly recovery from neutropenia.[33,35] Treatment with hematopoietic growth factors to reverse neutropenia and reducing other immunosuppression, to the extent possible, are recommended.[42] The role of other adjunctive therapies such as granulocyte transfusions is undetermined, but their use in patients with refractory fusariosis and scedosporiasis has been reported.

Infection Prevention and Anticipatory Guidance

Strategies to reduce exposure of immunocompromised patients to airborne molds are recommended as for prevention of invasive aspergillosis and mucormycosis. Hospital outbreaks of *Fusarium* have also been linked to contaminated water, including tap water and standing water (for example, in showers). Highly immunocompromised patients with significant disruption of skin integrity (e.g., extensive cutaneous GVHD) should consider avoiding contact of skin to tap water. Any sites of skin breakdown, onychomycosis, paronychia, or other localized infection should be treated appropriately to reduce the risk of subsequent invasive infection.

OTHER INVASIVE MOLD DISEASES

The remaining IMDs can be categorized broadly as either hyalohyphomycoses—infections caused by hyaline (colorless, translucent) molds with septate hyphae—or phaeohyphomycoses— infections caused by pigmented or melanized molds, sometimes called dematiaceous molds. The hyalohyphomycoses include *Aspergillus, Fusarium,* and *Scedosporium* as well as the much rarer genera *Acremonium, Paecilomyces, Purpureocillium, Scopulariopsis,* and *Trichoderma*. There are more than

70 genera and 150 species of fungi known to cause phaeohyphomycosis. These fungi are characterized by melanin pigment, which lends them a dark appearance in tissue and culture. This pigment is hypothesized to also serve as a virulence factor. It is not uncommon for organisms within this group to be newly reported as a source of human disease after previously being thought to be nonpathogenic. However, it is likely that any of these organisms can be opportunistic pathogens and isolation of any in an immunocompromised patient should raise concern for true infection. There are also frequent nomenclature changes and species reclassifications, which can make it challenging to understand their clinical epidemiology.

Epidemiology and Risk Factors

Most of the rare invasive molds, including organisms causing hyalohyphomycosis and phaeohyphomycosis, are found commonly in environmental settings, associated with soil and/or decaying organic material. Some organisms causing phaeohyphomycosis are geographically restricted, but members of the group can be found worldwide. Infection with these organisms is thought to be acquired through similar means as other IMDs, primarily via inhalation or cutaneous inoculation at sites of minor trauma. Some infections can be associated with intravascular catheters or peritoneal dialysis catheters. Table 25.4 provides distinguishing epidemiologic features for some of the most frequently described rare molds.

Historically, organisms causing phaeohyphomycosis have been largely associated with cutaneous and subcutaneous infections occurring mostly in immunocompetent persons in tropical and subtropical regions. However, they have emerged with increasing frequency as causes of invasive disease in immunocompromised persons worldwide.

Hematopoietic Stem Cell Transplant. In the multicenter TRANSNET study, 26 cases of phaeohyphomycosis were identified in HSCT recipients, representing 2.6% of reported IFDs in the HSCT cohort.[46] The median time from transplant to diagnosis was 100 days, and 92% of cases were seen in allogeneic HSCT recipients. The mortality rate was 42% at 90 days after diagnosis. There was a higher incidence of phaeohyphomycosis noted from transplant centers in the southern United States versus other regions of the country.

Solid Organ Transplant. Phaeohyphomycosis represented 2.5% of overall IFD in SOT recipients in the TRANSNET study, a proportion similar to HSCT recipients.[46] The median time from transplant to diagnosis was 18 months, and 53% of cases were diagnosed in lung transplant recipients. There was a 10% mortality rate at 90 days after diagnosis.

Oncology. A case series from a large cancer center reported an increasing incidence of invasive phaeohyphomycosis from 1989 to 2008, up to 3.1 cases per 100,000 patient-days in the later time period.[47] The majority (82%) of affected patients were in intensive phases of therapy for hematologic malignancy. The mortality rate among all patients was 33% at 12 weeks, with a higher risk of death in patients with disseminated infection and/or without recovery of neutropenia.

Clinical Manifestations

The spectrum of clinical disease caused by uncommon hyaline and pigmented molds ranges from localized to invasive manifestations. Although the focus of this section is on invasive disease, it is important for the clinician to be aware of the common localized manifestations of phaeohyphomycosis, because immunocompromised persons are at increased risk for both forms.

Localized Manifestations. The melanized fungi most frequently cause indolent cutaneous and subcutaneous infections, which can occur in either immunocompetent or immunocompromised persons. Distinct clinical syndromes include chromoblastomycosis, a chronic subcutaneous infection characterized by sclerotic bodies in tissue, and mycetoma, characterized by involvement of cutaneous and subcutaneous tissue, fascia, and bone with fungal granules and draining sinus tracts. Other cutaneous manifestations are varied, with single or multiple subcutaneous nodules, ulcerative, macular, or papular lesions, usually on the extremities, sometimes with sporotrichoid or lymphangitic patterns of spread. Immunocompromised patients may have more extensive and refractory disease and are at greater risk for dissemination of initially localized infections.

Invasive Manifestations. Invasive clinical syndromes associated with some of the more frequently identified rare molds are listed in Table 25.4. Most of the invasive syndromes are not easily distinguishable from those of other IMDs. Notably, several uncommon invasive molds can cause fungemia, sometimes catheter-associated, and several demonstrate tropism to the CNS. In particular, *Cladophialophora bantiana* is almost exclusively associated with CNS infections, which can occur in either immunocompetent or immunocompromised hosts, and is the most common cause of CNS phaeohyphomycosis. Other neurotropic organisms include *Rhinocladiella mackenziei* (geographically restricted to the Middle East), *Verruconis* (formerly *Ochroconis*) *gallopava*, and *Exophiala dermatitidis*. The most common CNS manifestation is a solitary brain abscess. Although the pathophysiology is not well understood, these are thought to originate via hematogenous dissemination from occult pulmonary or cutaneous foci.

Disease Prophylaxis

Although many commonly used prophylactic agents may be active against rare molds, none of these infections are sufficiently common to require primary prophylaxis.

Diagnosis

Diagnosing any of the rare mold infections requires isolation of the pathogen from the site of infection. Clinical isolates from nonsterile sites should be interpreted cautiously; in one series only 39 of 348 (11%) dematiaceous mold isolates from a single center were associated with proven or probable IMD using strict diagnostic criteria.[47] By direct microscopy or histopathology, pathogens causing hyalohyphomycosis appear similar to *Aspergillus*, *Fusarium*. and *Scedosporium*; culture or molecular-based methods are required to identify them to the genus and species level. The dematiaceous/melanized molds are darkly pigmented and can be stained with the Fontana-Masson stain, which is specific for melanin. Their hyphae have irregular septations, may be branched or unbranched, and appear more fragmented in tissue than those of *Aspergillus*. Associated yeastlike forms may also be visualized. Genus and species identification is important to guide optimal therapy of hyalohyphomycosis and phaeohyphomycosis, as antifungal susceptibility can vary substantially by species.[48] Sometimes the organisms fail to sporulate in culture, precluding species identification by conventional methods. As with other fungi, molecular methods are emerging and can be useful in such cases, but further clinical validation is needed. Susceptibility testing is often requested to guide therapy, but as with other molds breakpoints of susceptibility correlating with clinical success are not available.[48]

Treatment

Treatment recommendations for the rare molds causing hyalohyphomycosis and phaeohyphomycosis are primarily based on in vitro

TABLE 25.4 Clinical and Epidemiologic Features of Rare Invasive Molds

Genus/Key Species	Invasive Syndromes[a]	Epidemiologic Features
Organisms Causing Hyalohyphomycosis		
Acremonium	Pulmonary, osteoarticular, endocarditis, CNS, peritonitis, fungemia, disseminated	Fungemia may be intravenous catheter associated; peritonitis is dialysis catheter associated
A. kiliense[b]		
Paecilomyces	Pulmonary, soft tissue, sinus, pyelonephritis, osteoarticular, fungemia, disseminated	May be transmitted via contaminated fluids
P. variotii		
Purpureocillium	Pulmonary, sinus, soft tissue, pyelonephritis, fungemia, disseminated	May be transmitted via contaminated fluids.
P. lilacinum[c]		
Scopulariopsis	Pulmonary, soft tissue, cardiac, CNS, disseminated	Extremely high mortality
S. brevicaulis		
Trichoderma	Pulmonary, soft tissue, CNS, disseminated	Associated with contaminated water, aerosols
T. longibrachiatum		
Organisms Causing Phaeohyphomycosis		
Alternaria	Subcutaneous, sinus, CNS, disseminated	Most common agent of phaeohyphomycosis
A. alternata		
Aureobasidium	Fungemia, ocular, CNS	Fungemia usually catheter associated
A. pullulans		
Bipolaris	Sinusitis, ocular, pulmonary, peritonitis, CNS, disseminated	Peritonitis is dialysis catheter associated
B. australiensis[d]		Frequent cause of allergic sinusitis, may precede invasive sinusitis
B. hawaiiensis[d]		
B. spicifera[d]		
Cladophialophora	CNS infections almost exclusively	Global distribution, more case reports from India, may occur in immunocompetent hosts
C. bantiana		
Curvularia	Sinusitis, CNS, peritonitis, endocarditis, disseminated	Peritonitis is dialysis catheter associated.
C. aeria		Frequent cause of allergic sinusitis, may precede invasive sinusitis
C. geniculata		
C. lunata		
Exophiala	Pulmonary, CNS, fungemia, disseminated	Fungemia may be catheter associated
E. dermatitidis[e]		
E. xenobiotica		
E. oligosperma		
Exserohilum	CNS, osteoarticular, disseminated	Outbreak of *E. rostratum* meningitis from contaminated steroid injections in 2012
E. rostratum		

[a]Most organisms causing phaeohyphomycosis are also associated with indolent cutaneous and subcutaneous infections; invasive infectious syndromes that may occur in immunocompromised hosts are emphasized here.
[b]*Alternaria kiliense* is now renamed *Sarocladium kiliense*.
[c]*Purpureacillium lilacinum* was previously named *Paecilomyces lilacinus*.
[d]These 3 common species of *Bipolaris* have been reclassified in the *Curvularia* genus.
[e]Formerly *Wangiella dermatitidis*.
CNS, Central nervous system.

susceptibility data, case reports, and expert opinion. Recommendations can be found in European and Australian guidelines and the American Transplant Society Infectious Diseases Community of Practice Guidelines.[24,42,48,49] In many cases the guidelines do not strongly recommend one therapy of choice, given a lack of evidence.

Antifungal Therapy. A summary of antifungal susceptibilities and guideline-recommended therapy of selected rare molds is provided in Table 25.5. For phaeohyphomycosis, there is substantial variability in susceptibility both between and within species of a given genus, making correct species identification and susceptibility testing especially critical in guiding therapy for these infections. The optimal therapy of invasive syndromes is unknown and, in some cases, no specific recommendation is made in guidelines, but empiric approaches can be devised from predicted susceptibility. Combination therapy is suggested in some circumstances for disseminated or CNS infection and for organisms for which no single agent has predictably favorable activity.

For most of the localized manifestations of phaeohyphomycosis, antifungal therapy with an oral triazole (voriconazole, posaconazole, or itraconazole) is recommended, guided by susceptibility testing.[24,48,49] Localized phaeohyphomycosis with a single cutaneous or subcutaneous lesion can sometimes be cured by surgery alone, but antifungal therapy is recommended for immunocompromised patients to prevent dissemination.

Therapy for CNS infections with *C. bantiana* is often unsuccessful despite susceptibility of this organism to several antifungal agents, and it is unclear whether antifungal therapy alters outcome as survival

TABLE 25.5 Antifungal Susceptibility[a] and Primary Guideline-Recommended Therapy of Rare Invasive Molds

Genus/Species	AMB	VCZ	POSA	ITRA	5-FC	ECHIN	TER	Recommended[b]
Organisms Causing Hyalohyphomycosis								
Acremonium spp.	−/+	−/+	−/+	−/+	−	−		VCZ,[c,d] AMB[d,e] For AMB, guidelines recommend using lipid formulations for treatment.
Paecilomyces variotii	++	−/+	++	++	−/+	−		AMB,[c,f] POSA[d,f]
Purpureocillium lilacinum	−	++	++	+/++	−	−		VCZ or POSA[c,d]
Scopulariopsis brevicaulis	−/+	−/+	−/+	−/+	−	−/+	−/+	Combination VCZ or POS and TER or CAS[e]
Trichoderma longibrachiatum	v	++	+	−/+		+		Combination AMB + VCZ or POSA[f]
Organisms Causing Phaeohyphomycosis								
Alternaria spp.	+/++	−/+	+/++	+/++	−	−/+	−	Combination therapy if disseminated[g]
Aureobasidium pullulans	−/+	−/+	−/+	−/+	−/+	−/+		AMB[g]
Bipolaris spp.	+/++	−/+	+/++	+/++	−	−		AMB or triazole[g]
Cladophialophora spp.	+/++	+/++	+/++	+/++		−/+	++	VCZ or combination therapy[g]
Curvularia spp.	−/+	−/+	++	−/+	−	−/+		
Exophiala spp.	+/++	+/++	++	++	−/+	−	++	VCZ, POSA, or ITRA[f]
Exserohilum spp.	++	+/++	++	++	−	−/+	++	AMB[g] or VCZ[g]

[a]Typical in vitro susceptibility patterns as described in guidelines.[42,48]
[b]Recommendations left blank where guidelines do not make a specific recommendation or organism not addressed in guidelines.
[c]Guideline source: European Society for Clinical Microbiology and Infectious Diseases and the European Confederation of Medical Mycology.[42]
[d]Guideline source: Australian Consensus Guidelines.[24]
[e]Guidelines recommend using lipid formulations of amphotericin B for treatment.
[f]Guideline source: American Society of Transplantation, Infectious Diseases Community of Practice.[49]
[g]Guideline source: European Society for Clinical Microbiology and Infectious Diseases and the European Confederation of Medical Mycology.[48]
5-FC, flucytosine; *AMB,* amphotericin B; *CAS,* caspofungin; *ECHIN,* echinocandins; *ITRA,* itraconazole; *POSA,* posaconazole; *TER,* terbinafine; *VCZ,* voriconazole.
−, Not active or poorly active; +, some activity; ++, good activity. Blank cells indicate that susceptibility is poorly characterized.

without complete abscess resection is exceedingly rare. Some experts recommend voriconazole because of its favorable CNS penetration, and the combination of L-AmB with flucytosine has been used in reported cases.[48,50] Some have suggested combination therapy including multiple active agents, particularly for cases in which the abscess cannot be completely resected.

Surgical Management and Other Source Control Measures. Surgery is recommended for debridement or removal of localized cutaneous and subcutaneous infections.[48] Indications for resection of pulmonary lesions are generally similar to those for other IMDs. Surgery is particularly important for brain abscesses caused by *C. bantiana*; regardless of host immune status and antifungal therapy, survival is extremely poor if the abscess is not completely resected.[48,50] If an invasive mold infection is associated with an IV catheter or a peritoneal dialysis catheter, removal of the catheter is recommended.

Adjunctive Therapy. As with other IMDs, treatment of invasive infections caused by rare molds should generally include reversal of neutropenia and other predisposing conditions to the extent possible.

Infection Prevention and Anticipatory Guidance

Very little is known about preventive strategies for rare invasive molds, although in the hospital setting strategies that are effective in preventing exposure to other airborne molds are recommended. Table 25.4 includes notable nosocomial and device exposure risks for some of the more frequently identified rare molds.

Candidiasis

Jennifer E. Schuster, MD, MSCI and Brian T. Fisher, DO, MPH, MSCE

The *Candida* genus represents a group of more than 200 species present in both human flora and the environment. Of these, approximately 20 have been implicated in human disease. Typically, the pathogens from this genus are divided into *C. albicans* and non-*albicans Candida* species. The epidemiologic distribution of *Candida* spp. in children differs somewhat from that of adults. *C. albicans* is the most common species, and contemporary studies suggest that this species accounts for 30% to 35% of all invasive candidiasis (IC) cases. *C. parapsilosis* represents the second most common species, causing approximately 15% of IC events, followed by *C. glabrata*, *C. tropicalis*, and *C. krusei*. This is in contrast to the epidemiology of adult patients, in which *C. glabrata* is the second most common species. Collectively, these five species account for more than 90% of all identified isolates of candidemia.[1] The remaining 10% of IC cases are caused by a variety of less commonly identified species, such as *C. lusitaniae*, *C. dubliniensis*, *C. guilliermondii*, *C. stellatoidea*, *C. keyfr*, *C. pseudotropicalis*, and *C. intermedia*. More recently, significant attention has been focused on *C. auris*. This species is still relatively uncommon but is important as it has the potential to harbor multidrug resistance.

Candida spp. are often a component of the normal commensal flora in children, but they can cause both superficial and invasive disease in specific clinical settings. Children with malignancy and hematopoietic stem cell transplant (HSCT) and solid organ transplant (SOT) recipients in whom IC develops often have at least one predisposing risk factor for candidiasis beyond their underlying condition.

Understanding the epidemiology of *Candida* spp. in these high-risk children is important because treatment strategies are dependent on the *Candida* spp., location of disease, and immune status. Although the epidemiology and prophylactic strategies for *Candida* spp. infections differ among clinical manifestations, diagnostic and treatment strategies remain similar.

EPIDEMIOLOGY AND RISK FACTORS

The rate of IC in hospitalized children has been decreasing.[2] This decline is likely multifactorial and been attributed to improvements in infection control measures, such as managing central venous catheters (CVCs) and prophylaxis in high-risk patient groups. Although these efforts have helped to reduce the frequency of IC, IC persists as the most common form of invasive fungal disease (IFD) for children receiving chemotherapy for malignancy and those undergoing transplantation, resulting in significant morbidity and mortality. A number of factors can predispose children to candidiasis, including compromise of anatomic barriers (e.g., the presence of CVCs or peritoneal catheters and recent surgery or trauma); disturbance of the normal flora with gastrointestinal insufficiency or after antimicrobial exposures; compromise of the immune system in the setting of primary or acquired immunodeficiencies; and iatrogenic compromise of the immune system secondary to receipt of chemotherapy or immune-modulating agents. The epidemiology and risk factors specific to oncology, pediatric HSCT, and SOT populations are discussed in the following sections.

Hematopoietic Stem Cell Transplant

Candida infections account for nearly 10% of all infections and 60% of all IFDs in the first year after HSCT in children.[3] IC has been reported as either the most common or second most common source of IFDs in pediatric allogeneic HSCT patients.[4] The epidemiology of the different species has varied over time. From 1991 to 1996, *C. albicans* and *C. parapsilosis* dominated as the cause of IC in pediatric HSCT patients. However, rates of *C. glabrata* and *C. tropicalis* have increased in more recent years, exceeding rates of *C. albicans* and *C. parapsilosis* in some cohorts.[3] The timing of IC can differ by HSCT-related factors, but typically these infections occur early with a median onset of 20 days after allogeneic HSCT.[5] Rates of IC are higher in allogeneic versus autologous (8% vs. 5%) transplant recipients, likely related to immunosuppression and graft-versus-host disease (GVHD). The presence of GVHD can prolong the risk period, with some cases of IC presenting 8 months after transplantation in the setting of chronic GVHD.[4] Other studies describe the majority of *Candida* infections occurring within the first 30 days after transplant. In pediatric recipients of an autologous or matched sibling allogeneic HSCT, IC tends to develop early after HSCT, compared with children undergoing haploidentical, umbilical cord blood, or matched unrelated transplants presumably owing to the reduced risk of GVHD in the former patient groups.[3]

Solid Organ Transplant

Recent publications have begun to better define the epidemiology of IC in each respective SOT groups.[6-13] IC appears to have the most significant burden in children undergoing small bowel transplant. In a cohort of 98 small bowel recipients, 25 (25.5%) patients had 59 episodes of IC. Candidemia was the most common presentation, but patients also had urinary tract and abdominal involvement, with presentations including abscess or peritonitis. In small bowel recipients, non-*albicans Candida* species predominate, with *C. albicans* accounting for only 25% to 38% of the events. Risk factors for IC after small bowel transplantation include administration of total parenteral nutrition and receipt of antibiotics during the 7 days preceding infection.

Although less common than in small bowel transplant recipients, IC is still relatively common after pediatric liver transplantation, occurring in 2.5% to 7% of all liver recipients. The majority of IC in this organ group occurs in the first 3 weeks after transplant. Interestingly, *C. albicans* is the most common species, accounting for more than 50%

of IC events. Candidemia is the most common presentation of IC, although hepatic abscesses and surgical site infections have also been described. Intensive care unit admission before liver transplant and prolonged operative time have been associated with IC in univariate analyses, with intensive care unit admission remaining associated in multivariate modeling.

Pulmonary fungal disease has been reported in approximately 10% of pediatric lung transplant recipients. *Aspergillus* species are the most common pathogen identified, followed by *Candida* species, with *C. albicans* as the predominant *Candida* species isolated. However, identification of *Candida* from a sputum or bronchoalveolar specimen may represent colonization and not true infection, and thus clinicians must take caution in ascribing *Candida* as the true pathogen of pulmonary disease. *Candida* species do not typically cause a primary pulmonary process but can result in lung parenchymal involvement upon dissemination from the bloodstream.

In a pediatric cardiac transplant cohort of 1854 patients, the rate of all IFDs was estimated at 5.9%. *Candida* species were the most common etiology of IFD in this cohort, accounting for more than 75% of IFD events. Of note, the majority of *Candida* species isolated in patients designated as IC were from nonsterile sites, which calls into question whether these were true IC events versus colonization. Thus the frequency of IC in pediatric cardiac transplant recipients may be overestimated from this cohort. Similar to the epidemiology of liver and pulmonary transplant recipients, *C. albicans* (55%) was the most common detected species. The majority of IC infections occurred early after transplant, within the first 2 months.

Candida infections in pediatric renal transplant patients are uncommon. A 13-year retrospective review of 234 pediatric kidney transplants revealed no cases of IC. In a mixed, but predominantly adult cohort of renal transplant patients, 11% of subjects had candiduria. However, the majority (54%) were asymptomatic, and only 5% had concomitant candidemia.

Oncology

IC is a leading cause of IFD and infection-related mortality in pediatric oncology patients. The frequency of IC can vary by malignancy type, which is likely a function of the variation in the intensity of chemotherapy regimens across cancer types. When considering a cohort inclusive of all pediatric cancers, the incidence of IFD was 4.9% and *Candida* spp. accounted for 69% of these events. The overall case-fatality rate in the children with IC was 63%, which rivaled the rate of 85% in children with invasive aspergillosis.[14] In children with acute myelogenous leukemia (AML), the incidence of IC has ranged from 6% to 13%, with incidence varying based on intensity of treatment.[15] The overall case-fatality rate of these children with AML and IC was 17.6%. In cohorts of pediatric acute lymphoblastic leukemia, lower rates (3.5%) of IC have been described during the induction chemotherapy period.[16] The distribution of *Candida* species varies by study and malignancy and may be a function of the local hospital epidemiology. Although some studies suggest that *C. albicans* accounts for the majority of cases, other studies have found a predominance of *C. parapsilosis.*[17]

Data on risk factors for IC within cohorts restricted to oncology patients are limited. Generally, IC is more common in children with a hematologic malignancy compared with those with a solid tumor. In a study of children in an intensive care unit, the presence of a malignancy increased the odds of candidemia by 4-fold. The presence of a CVC, recent receipt of vancomycin, or recent receipt of anaerobic antimicrobials, all common in children with malignancy, further increased the risk of candidemia.[18] However, predictive models have been difficult to validate.[19]

As chemotherapy protocols and SOT immunosuppressive induction and maintenance regimens are adapted to include novel immunosuppressive agents, and as supportive care measures are optimized (e.g., administration of antifungal prophylaxis and more judicious use of antibiotics), the rates of IC in children with a specific SOT or malignancy will continue to vary. Recommendations on certain supportive care measures are provided in later text, but clinicians need to remain vigilant to changes in care protocols that will affect the risk of IC in these patient groups.

CLINICAL MANIFESTATIONS

Candida species can cause superficial and invasive infections. The former are often identified at mucosal surfaces. The latter can involve the bloodstream (i.e., candidemia), be limited to one organ (i.e., focal candidiasis), or have multiple foci (i.e., disseminated candidiasis). These clinical entities have signs and symptoms that are often similar across children with malignancy or transplant recipients.

Superficial and Mucosal Infections

Dermatitis. *Candida* dermatitis occurs in both oncology and transplant patients, similar to non-immunocompromised children. It commonly occurs in the distribution of a diaper and presents as an erythematous rash with or without satellite lesions. Use of broad-spectrum antibiotics, either as prophylaxis or treatment, is often a predisposing factor. Other locations of infection include areas of skin overlap (e.g., inguinal and axillary regions or areas of skin breakdown or breech, particularly at surgical incision or CVC sites). Compared with immunocompetent children, these children are at higher risk to develop secondary IC from a superficial *Candida* dermatitis infection.

Mucosal Infections. Infection of the oropharynx, esophagus, or vulvovaginal mucosa typically occurs secondary to changes in normal flora after exposure to broad-spectrum antibiotics and/or after receipt of chemotherapeutic or conditioning agents that can also result in dysbiosis or breakdown of the mucosa. Oropharyngeal and esophageal candidiasis can occur in isolation or concurrently. Oropharyngeal candidiasis (thrush) is characterized by a white pseudomembrane on the oral mucosa, including buccal regions, gums, tongue, palate, tonsils, and uvula. Children typically present with pain and dysphagia, leading to decreased oral intake. Rarely, lesions are reported to be painless. The lesions are apparent on physical examination and can be removed by scraping. Underlying mucosa may be erythematous or normal in appearance.

Candidal esophagitis typically presents with dysphagia or odynophagia. In patients without oropharyngeal candidiasis, the diagnosis often requires invasive testing to confirm candidiasis or to evaluate for other infectious causes of esophagitis (e.g., cytomegalovirus or herpes simplex virus), which can present similarly or in tandem with candidal esophagitis. Gross inspection on endoscopy may reveal erythematous, edematous, and ulcerated mucosa as well as white plaques. Rarely, strictures have been reported. In cases of severe disease, mucosal changes may be seen on barium esophogram.

Similar to other mucosal areas of involvement, candidal vulvovaginitis may be asymptomatic, pruritic, or painful. Dysuria and vaginal discharge may also occur. White plaquelike lesions are often present on examination.

Suspicion for mucosal candidiasis is often based on direct visualization of the affected area along with reported symptoms. However, isolation of a *Candida* spp. may be desired to confirm the diagnosis or to differentiate from other possible processes on the differential (e.g., herpes simplex virus esophagitis). Culture of mucosal surface scrapings can be performed, but it must be recognized that isolation of *Candida* from these cultures may represent only colonization rather than definitive evidence of infection. Nonetheless, isolation of a *Candida* spp. may be helpful in directing therapy, especially if a patient is not responding to initial empiric antifungal therapy. *C. albicans* is the most commonly identified species in the setting of mucosal disease, although children receiving antifungal prophylaxis may present with a non-*albicans Candida* species.

Invasive Candidiasis

IC most commonly presents as a bloodstream infection (i.e., candidemia) with potential for dissemination to multiple organs, often referred to as disseminated candidiasis. It is also possible to have IC of a single organ system or body compartment that may result from local inoculation of *Candida*, such as with intraabdominal candidiasis in the setting of a peritoneal catheter.

Candidemia. Candidemia can present with nonspecific findings that mimic the clinical presentation of bacteremia. Signs and symptoms range from fever without localizing symptoms to septic shock. Focal symptoms (e.g., dyspnea, abdominal pain) may be present in cases with dissemination to end organs. This would include extension to the skin and soft tissues that may be clinically evident as erythematous macular, papular, or pustular lesions. Laboratory findings such as hyperglycemia and thrombocytopenia may be present but are not sensitive or specific. The presence of a CVC is common and is often considered as the portal of entry. However, translocation from the commensal flora across a compromised alimentary track without mucosal infection is also possible.

Genitourinary and Renal Candidiasis. *Candida* spp. can result in both lower and upper genitourinary tract involvement. The presence of *Candida* in the bladder, candiduria, can be either asymptomatic or symptomatic. Asymptomatic candiduria often occurs in association with an indwelling bladder catheter in contrast to symptomatic candiduria, or cystitis, in which children may report dysuria. *Candida* can infrequently ascend the genitourinary tract to involve the renal parenchyma, similar to bacterial pyelonephritis. In this clinical scenario, signs and symptoms are similar to that of a bacterial pyelonephritis, including fever, vomiting, dysuria, and flank discomfort. Alternatively, *Candida* spp. can hematogenously disseminate to the kidneys, resulting in renal parenchymal involvement. For this process, patients may be asymptomatic but may also have signs and symptoms consistent with pyelonephritis, including fever and flank pain, in addition to hypertension and an elevated creatinine level. Radiographically, disseminated candidiasis that involves the kidney appears as numerous small nodular lesions, similar to that of hepatosplenic candidiasis (see next section). Less commonly, a mycelial mass (fungal ball) may be present and cause symptoms of urinary obstruction.

Hepatosplenic (Chronic Disseminated) Candidiasis. Hepatosplenic candidiasis primarily occurs in neutropenic patients. It can present with gastrointestinal symptoms, such as abdominal pain, nausea, and/or vomiting. However, neutropenic patients may be asymptomatic or present with only fever. Fever often persists until and even well beyond neutrophil recovery, at which time abdominal symptoms may develop. Disease may be identified in patients with candidemia undergoing abdominal imaging for evaluation of disseminated disease; however, the majority (>80%) of children with hepatosplenic disease do not have *Candida* detected in the bloodstream by culture. It has been postulated that in the setting of neutropenia, *Candida* spreads to the liver and spleen from the gastrointestinal tract via the hepatoportal circulation. Thus hepatosplenic disease is not dependent on antecedent candidemia. This would explain the rarity of positive blood culture results for *Candida* spp. in these patients. Laboratory findings and imaging may be unrevealing during the neutropenic period. After neutrophil recovery, elevations in the alkaline phosphatase level and abnormalities on imaging (e.g., computed tomography [CT] or ultrasound) can be identified. The majority of patients have lesions identified in both the liver and spleen, although isolation to one organ is possible. Classic CT findings include multiple small lesions that may appear as a "wheel within a wheel" or bull's-eye pattern. This radiographic appearance correlates with a histologic inner circle of necrotic fungal elements, a middle circle of inflammatory cells, and an outer circle of fibrosis. Other imaging findings include hypoechoic lesions, or later in the course of disease, echogenic foci, which may be due to calcifications or fibrosis.[20]

Intraabdominal Candidiasis. Intraabdominal candidiasis is a distinct entity from hepatosplenic candidiasis. Intraabdominal disease is typically related to surgery (e.g., anastomotic leaks after liver transplantation or bowel perforation) or the presence of a foreign body (e.g., peritoneal dialysis catheter or drain). Peritonitis and/or intraabdominal abscess may develop. Both *Candida* peritonitis and intraabdominal abscess are clinically similar to their bacterial counterparts; fever and abdominal pain are common. Intraabdominal abscesses may be polymicrobial. In patients with postsurgical infections, the surgical site may become erythematous or tender, and purulent drainage may be present. Alternatively, a nonhealing wound or wound dehiscence should raise suspicion for *Candida* infection in high-risk patients. Identification of *Candida* from a peritoneal catheter or drain culture may represent colonization rather than true infection. Thus the diagnosis is made from aspiration of peritoneal fluid or intraabdominal abscess in conjunction with clinical signs and symptoms consistent with intraabdominal candidiasis. Similarly, surgical sites may also be colonized with *Candida*, so the presence on a surgical site swab does not confirm *Candida* as a pathogen and clinical correlation is important.

Osteoarticular Candidiasis. *Candida* osteoarticular disease presents with signs and symptoms similar to those in bacterial osteoarticular disease. Disease is typically secondary to hematogenous dissemination, and the long bones are the most commonly involved foci. Focal findings of bone pain and/or limited joint range of motion or pain are often present. *Candida* osteoarticular disease more frequently involves multiple bones compared with bacterial disease.[21] Additionally, because *Candida* osteoarticular disease often presents in an immunocompromised host, symptoms may be less apparent than bacterial osteoarticular disease. This is of particular concern in the neutropenic patient, who may have absence of significant bone discomfort or micromotion tenderness typically associated with osteomyelitis or septic arthritis. However, with neutrophil count recovery, these signs or symptoms may become more apparent.

Endovascular Candidiasis. Endovascular disease, including endocarditis and suppurative thrombophlebitis, most commonly occurs in the presence of persistent candidemia. Children presenting with endocarditis may have a history of predisposing cardiac lesions, cardiac surgery, or prosthetic cardiac material. Persistent fever is common but is not absolute. Fever may be the only sign of endovascular infection. Other signs or symptoms of endovascular disease include chest pain, dyspnea, evidence of embolic phenomena (e.g., wedge-shaped lesions on imaging of other organs, nodular lesions in distal extremities or skin), new heart murmur, or signs of heart failure. Notably, these signs and symptoms are not specific for *Candida* endovascular disease versus other infectious causes of endocarditis. Suppurative thrombophlebitis may present with focal tenderness, overlying erythema, or a palpable cord at a previous or current CVC site.

Ocular Candidiasis. *Candida* endophthalmitis is typically endogenous, secondary to candidemia, although traumatic exogenous disease can occur. Endogenous endophthalmitis is often asymptomatic and is recognized only upon a dedicated ophthalmologic examination. Symptoms may present as the disease progresses and include unilateral or bilateral vision loss. Pain is uncommon. In patients with neutropenia, examination findings, such as chorioretinal lesions, may be present only after neutrophil recovery. Chorioretinitis presents with focal, white lesions on the retina. In cases of vitreal involvement, fluffy white balls in the vitreous can be seen. Anterior chamber involvement, sometimes as a hypopyon, occurs with significant inflammation.

Central Nervous System Candidiasis. Central nervous system (CNS) disease typically results from hematogenous dissemination in the presence of candidemia. CNS disease after hematogenous spread may be asymptomatic, but it also can be associated with altered mental status, meningismus, seizures, or headache. The size and location of the lesions influence clinical manifestations. The radiographic appearance of CNS candidiasis can be quite varied and include meningeal enhancement, vasculitis, and/or parenchymal foci that are nodular in appearance. The latter can range from multiple small lesions to a single large mass. Histopathologically, these nodular lesions can appear as granulomas or abscesses. Pediatric patients requiring surgical interventions, such as resection of a tumor or placement of a shunt, are at risk of *Candida* surgical site or device-related infections.

Pulmonary Candidiasis. *Candida* species do not typically cause primary pneumonia. In fact, identification of *Candida* spp. from a respiratory tract specimen (e.g., sputum culture or bronchoalveolar lavage) almost always represents airway colonization and not true disease. However, pulmonary candidiasis can result from hematogenous spread to the lungs. This is of particular concern when candidemia exists in the presence of prolonged neutropenia. Pulmonary involvement after dissemination may be asymptomatic but can also cause cough, dyspnea, and hypoxemia. Imaging findings most commonly include a diffuse, nodular pattern, representative of microabscesses. Less commonly, lobar infiltrates, ground-glass opacities, or empyemas are reported.

DISEASE PROPHYLAXIS AND PREVENTION

The comparative effectiveness of antifungal prophylaxis has been variably studied and thus inconsistently used as a preventative measure against IC in children with malignancy and recipients of either an SOT or HSCT. Because the risk of IC and evidence for prophylaxis varies among the three groups of immunosuppressed children, recommendations are discussed separately for each high-risk group. Studies evaluating the use of antifungal prophylaxis are most commonly performed in adults and many use any IFD, rather than IC, as the outcome of interest, limiting the ability to development informed decisions on prophylaxis for individual risk groups.

Hematopoietic Stem Cell Transplant

In HSCT recipients, there are two primary risk periods for IC: the period of neutropenia sustained from conditioning, and in relevant patients, the period of GVHD. The sentinel adult antifungal prophylaxis study was completed in 1992 by Goodman and colleagues, who randomly assigned patients to fluconazole versus placebo through the posttransplant neutropenia period. Fluconazole recipients had significantly decreased rates of superficial (33.3% vs. 8.4%, $P < .001$) and invasive (15.8% vs. 2.8%, $P < .001$) fungal disease in HSCT patients.[22] Meta-analyses consistently demonstrate a decrease in mortality and IFD in HSCT patients receiving antifungal therapy.[23] These predominantly adult data have reasonably been extrapolated to include pediatric HSCT populations. Current pediatric HSCT-specific antifungal prophylaxis guidelines support the use of fluconazole prophylaxis in children undergoing allogeneic HSCT and children undergoing autologous HSCT with an anticipated duration of neutropenia more than 7 days. Prophylaxis should be initiated at the start of conditioning and continue until engraftment. Echinocandins are an alternative when fluconazole is contraindicated (e.g., busulfan administration).[24] A recent randomized trial in children comparing either voriconazole or posaconazole to fluconazole during the neutropenic period after allogeneic HSCT was stopped early for futility, suggesting that fluconazole should still be the prophylactic agent of choice in children during neutropenia after HSCT.

A substantial subset of children have engraftment after allogeneic HSCT but subsequently have either acute or chronic GVHD, necessitating systemic immunosuppressive therapy. This is a second period of risk for IFD in general, and IC specifically, for HSCT patients. Unfortunately, there are limited pediatric specific data on the utility and choice of antifungal prophylaxis during GVHD. One trial, consisting predominantly of adults with only a small number of children, did not find a benefit of voriconazole compared to fluconazole for prevention of IFD during periods of GVHD.[25] A second trial of predominantly adults with a small number of adolescents found that posaconazole reduced rates of proven and probable IFD as well as IFD-related mortality when given during periods of GVHD.[26] Although this study was not specific to an outcome of IC, posaconazole was associated with an overall reduction in the rates of proven and probable IFD as well as IFD-related mortality. Based on these data, posaconazole should be favored in children 13 years and older during acute grade II to IV or chronic, extensive GVHD, not because of enhanced IC protection but rather to prevent invasive mold disease (IMD). In the absence of posaconazole pharmacokinetic data for children younger than 13 years, fluconazole is recommended as the prophylactic agent in this younger age group.

Even with routine antifungal prophylaxis, breakthrough mucosal candidiasis and IC occurs. Thus clinicians should continue to be suspicious for IC in children receiving antifungal prophylaxis. If breakthrough infection is identified, then an antifungal agent with a different mechanism of action should be strongly considered.

Solid Organ Transplant

Determining the benefit of antifungal prophylaxis in SOT recipients is more challenging as the period of risk is less discrete than that in HSCT recipients, and thus the necessary duration of antifungal prophylaxis is often less clear. This factor has likely contributed to the limited comparative data in these patient groups to establish the effectiveness or efficacy of antifungal prophylaxis. However, the epidemiology can inform the risk by organ and timing of IC onset that can help guide prophylaxis decisions. The rate of IC has been shown to be highest in liver, small bowel, and pancreas transplant recipients and lowest in lung, heart, and renal transplant recipients. Most infections occur within the first 3 months after transplant.[6] The impact of IC has been most comprehensively studied in pediatric liver transplant recipients, in whom IC develops in approximately 3% and 5% of recipients during the first 30 and 180 days after transplant, respectively. Mortality rates in this population are overall low, unlike those in their adult counterparts.[6,8] In meta-analyses of primarily studies of adult patients, fluconazole has been associated with a reduction in IFD and IFD-attributable mortality.[27] Based on these studies, guidelines for adult patients recommend antifungal prophylaxis in patients with specific risk factors for IC, including prolonged operation time, renal failure, and large transfusion requirements, among others.[9] Because the rates of IC in children after liver transplant appear to be lower than in adults, it is difficult to generalize fluconazole prophylaxis recommendations to all pediatric liver transplant recipients. It is reasonable to consider fluconazole prophylaxis in liver transplant recipients with risk factors associated with IC, including prolonged operation time or need for hospitalization in the intensive care unit immediately before transplantation.[8]

Data supporting the utility for antifungal prophylaxis against IC in other pediatric SOT groups are less convincing. A recent retrospective assessment of IC in lung, heart, and renal transplant recipients at a single children's hospital found rare events of IC despite lack of routine antifungal prophylaxis use at that center. This finding suggests that antifungal prophylaxis directed at IC is not universally necessary in these transplant groups. Some SOT recipient groups, particularly lung transplant recipients, may warrant antifungal prophylaxis against other fungal pathogens, such as molds, based on patient specific risk factors such as prior mold infection or colonization. These cases should be assessed individually, as the need for antimold prophylaxis would supersede the need for IC prophylaxis.

The epidemiology for IC in pediatric pancreas and small bowel transplant recipients is not known. The number of pediatric patients receiving these organs each year is small, and thus the ability to establish IC incidence in these populations is limited. Because cumulative incidence of IC in adult pancreatic and small bowel transplant recipients is higher than in liver recipients, it may be prudent to extrapolate adult recommendations, which recommend fluconazole prophylaxis for all small bowel transplant recipients and for a subset of pancreatic transplant recipients with specific risk factors for IC.[9]

In patients who are not tolerant of fluconazole or have concerns for drug-drug interactions, alternative antifungal agents can be considered. A randomized trial of anidulafungin versus fluconazole prophylaxis in high-risk adult liver transplant recipients found no significant difference in IFD rates.[28] Therefore echinocandins may be considered second-line agents in this setting, although this would necessitate intravenous administration, which may present unnecessary risks in maintaining a CVC. Selective bowel decontamination, with the use of enteral nystatin, has not been shown to decrease IFD.[29]

The optimal duration of prophylaxis is not known, but guidelines for adult patients have suggested from 14 days to 4 weeks or until resolution of risk factors. Whether this duration is appropriate for children is not known and should be assessed in future studies. It is likely the duration of therapy would need to be adjusted according to ongoing risk factors, including need for follow-up surgical procedures, retransplantation, persistent transfusion requirement, and until healing of the surgical site (e.g., anastomotic healing in a small bowel recipient).

Oncology

The etiology of IC in oncology patients is typically multifactorial, but the highest risk period is during prolonged neutropenia, often defined as more than 7 days after receipt of intensive chemotherapy. Most studies assessing the effectiveness of antifungal prophylaxis during prolonged neutropenia periods in patients with an oncologic diagnosis have been focused on adults. These studies are not specific to IC but rather are considerate of all IFD outcomes. Multiple meta-analyses revealed that fluconazole was effective at significantly reducing the risk of IFD versus placebo or no prophylaxis, presumably via the reduction in IC events. The largest effect has been noted during periods of intensive chemotherapy.[23] Based on these data, the adult fever and neutropenia guidelines endorsed fluconazole prophylaxis during periods of prolonged neutropenia (i.e., ≥7 days) secondary to chemotherapy for acute leukemia with the intention of reducing the rate of IC.[30] These same guidelines for adult patients support the use of posaconazole prophylaxis in patients with AML, in whom the risk of IMD is higher.[30]

Although the studies that informed the meta-analyses had limited pediatric patients, pediatric-specific guidelines have used these data to reasonably support the administration of antifungal prophylaxis in children with neutropenia secondary to AML or myelodysplastic syndrome chemotherapy.[24] Retrospective observational data in pediatric AML cohorts have corroborated this recommendation to use antifungal prophylaxis, noting a decreased hazard in induction mortality in patients receiving antifungal prophylaxis. The current recommended agent for antifungal prophylaxis in children with AML is fluconazole, as dosing recommendations for posaconazole are not available. In centers with concern for increased rates of IMD, posaconazole can be substituted for fluconazole in children 13 years and older, but this prophylaxis regimen would be to target mold prevention rather than just for prevention of candidiasis.

Studies are currently in progress to compare the efficacy of other agents with both anti-*Candida* and anti-mold activity (e.g., echinocandins) to fluconazole in pediatric AML cohorts. Should a broader spectrum agent be found more efficacious, it would likely be due to prevention of IMD rather than improved IC prevention. At this time, the risk of IFD, and specifically IC, in other oncology cohorts is not considered high enough to warrant routine recommendation of antifungal prophylaxis in those populations.[24] As chemotherapy regimens change, the risk profile for IFD, including IC, may also change. Close monitoring of these rates is important, and comparative effectiveness studies to establish the utility of prophylaxis will be necessarily based on specific malignancies and chemotherapy regimens.

DIAGNOSIS

Signs and symptoms of IC are often nonspecific and frequently consistent with a bacterial infection or a noninfectious etiology (e.g., mucositis, surgery, medication toxicity). Furthermore, clinical findings may be subtle or absent in patients with neutropenia, which makes the diagnosis of IC difficult. Findings that should prompt consideration for additional diagnostic testing for IC include presence of prolonged fever despite broad-spectrum antibiotics in a high-risk patient. Specific clinical findings suggestive of IC include multiple erythematous, pustular, or nodular skin lesions or chorioretinitis on fundoscopic examination. These entities should lead to immediate diagnostic evaluation for IC.

Regardless of the clinical presentation, if IC is suspected, diagnostic testing is necessary to establish a diagnosis. Testing options include traditional culture and histopathologic procedures as well as radiographic studies; however, these options are limited by the prolonged time to results and/or the requirement for invasive procedures. More recently, there has been optimism regarding an evolution of non–culture-based technologies, but pediatric evidence on the utility of these studies is less than convincing or not yet available. It is important for the clinician to understand that the operating characteristics of a diagnostic tool may vary in pediatric patients and in certain clinical scenarios. It is key to have this understanding before using the diagnostic test in practice as the results can be misleading if tests are ordered in the wrong setting.

Laboratory Findings

Nonspecific laboratory values, such as leukocytosis, thrombocytopenia, acidosis, and hyperglycemia, may be present but are not sensitive or specific for the diagnosis of IC. Neutropenia, although not a sign of IC, is a predisposing factor and may be present before or at the time of clinical symptoms.

Culture

Blood culture is the gold standard for the diagnosis of candidemia. *Candida* spp. will grow readily in commercially available blood culture systems. In one study, the median time to growth was 36 hours, and 97% of positive cultures grew within the first 72 hours.[31] *C. glabrata* may require additional time for growth. Although *Candida* spp. take longer to trigger a positive blood culture than many bacterial pathogens, a blood culture in the setting of candidemia often becomes positive within the standard 5 days that blood culture bottles are incubated. Therefore dedicated fungal blood cultures are not routinely recommended for identification of candidemia as they will not improve the yield of blood culture for *Candida* spp. However, IC often occurs in the absence of a positive blood culture for *Candida*. Studies demonstrate that blood culture positivity varies from 25% to 71% in cases of autopsy-proven IC.[32] Thus clinicians should not assume that IC is excluded if blood cultures are negative for *Candida*.

Direct assessment of material from the site of local infection by Gram stain, potassium hydroxide, histopathology, or culture can be useful for superficial, mucosal, and invasive infections. Skin and mucosal scrapings can be obtained in the outpatient setting in subjects with superficial or mucosal disease. *Candida* spp. are identified as a budding yeast (with or without hyphae) on Gram stain or potassium hydroxide preparation. Interpretation of these results for superficial specimens should be done with caution as the presence of *Candida* spp. from a superficial specimen can represent colonization rather than true disease.

For tissue-invasive disease, a biopsy of focally involved tissue may be necessary for the diagnosis because *Candida* is not always successfully isolated from the blood in invasive disease even when hematogenous dissemination is assumed. The likelihood of candidemia does increase with the number of organs involved. The decision to pursue a diagnostic biopsy should be considerate of the potential yield of the biopsy, the potential effect of the biopsy results on clinical decision making, and the possible risks of a biopsy. For instance, hepatosplenic candidiasis is a diagnosis often supported by multiple small nodules on radiographic studies in the absence of positive blood cultures. A biopsy can be performed in this setting, but frequently the biopsy results reveal the presence of yeast on histopathology but with negative cultures because the patient is already receiving antifungal therapy. Risks of biopsy may include bleeding, particularly in patients with thrombocytopenia. Therefore a biopsy in this setting does not often change clinical management. When a biopsy is performed, specimens should be obtained for both histopathology and fungal culture. Histopathology may demonstrate microabscesses or budding yeast, hyphae, or pseudohyphae. The latter can often be seen on special stains, including Gomori methenamine silver or periodic acid–Schiff staining. Identification of fungal elements from histopathologic specimens may be useful in cases where *Candida* does not grow from culture specimens (e.g., pretreatment with antifungals). Culture allows for possibility of determining specific *Candida* spp. and performance of antifungal susceptibilities testing.

Determination of *Candida* species after culture has yielded an isolate is important for guiding therapeutic decisions. Traditionally the first step for dichotomizing an isolate as *C. albicans* or non-*albicans Candida* was incubation in proteinaceous liquid at 35°C. *C. albicans* forms germ tubes when incubated in this way. The remainder of *Candida* spp. were then identified by kits that included a panel of biochemical tests. Performing the assays from these kits, which included a variety of temperature, culture medium, and carbohydrate tests, could take days. More recently, a number of techniques have improved the time to species identification, including polymerase chain reaction (PCR) platforms, fluorescence in situ hybridization, and matrix-assisted laser desorption ionization time-of-flight mass spectrometry, which can more rapidly identify *Candida* spp. compared with biochemical testing.

Non-Culture Detection Methods

Even with the advancement in species detection from cultured material, there remains a prolonged period of time from culture attainment until identification. Additionally, the less than optimal yield of blood cultures for *Candida* and challenges for obtaining invasive specimens from focal disease sites have resulted in pursuit of alternative detection methods for the diagnosis of IC in high-risk populations. Unfortunately, for many of these diagnostic texts, there are few pediatric-specific data, limiting conclusions on their clinical utility. As time evolves and pediatric data become available, these technologies will likely become pertinent to pediatric care.

Non-Culture DNA-Based Diagnostic Tests

PCR for *Candida* detection can be highly sensitive, identifying as few as four genome copies/mL.[33] In a cohort of both oncologic and non-oncologic patients with IC, multiplex *Candida* PCR testing identified eight patients with candidemia who were also identified by standard blood culture. The test identified five additional patients with negative blood cultures, and control samples were negative.[33] In a meta-analysis of adult and pediatric patients with IC, PCR testing demonstrated high sensitivity (0.95) and specificity (0.92). PCR had higher sensitivity than routine blood culture for proven or probable IC (85% vs. 38%).[34] Unfortunately, numerous PCR assays have been studied with little standardization across assays. Furthermore, limited pediatric data exist and none are approved by the U.S. Food and Drug Administration. At this time, routine clinical use of PCR for *Candida* detection cannot be endorsed.

A novel magnetic resonance platform, T2Candida (T2 Biosystems, Lexington, MA), has been developed for detection of certain species of *Candida*. This system works by amplifying *Candida* DNA directly from a whole blood sample followed by agglomeration of species-specific magnetic resonance particles that can then be measured. In an adult population, the platform was 91% sensitive and 99% specific compared with blood culture. The median time to identification of *Candida* spp. was approximately 4 hours. Detection limits are sensitive down to one colony forming unit/mL for some species.[35] Based on these data the test has been approved by the Food and Drug Administration, but the utility in children is still not clear. One study in pediatrics did demonstrate high correlation with blood culture results for *C. albicans*, *C. tropicalis*, *C. parapsilosis*, and *C. glabrata*, but this study included only 24 blood cultures, and therefore more data are needed to support routine use in children.[36] Particular challenges for T2Candida include clarification of the required blood volume for children. The adult protocol requires 4 mL of blood starting material, which can be a challenge to obtain routinely in children. Additionally, T2Candida identifies only five species of *Candida* (the previously reported species and *C. krusei*) and does not distinguish between *C. albicans* and

C. tropicalis or *C. glabrata* and *C. krusei*. Susceptibility results are also not provided. Both of these issues are important, especially recognizing the increasing presence of other resistant *Candida* species, such as *C. auris*.

Non-DNA and Non-Culture Diagnostic Tests

These non-DNA and non-culture diagnostic studies, often referred to as fungal biomarkers, are founded on a principle of identifying a component of *Candida* spp. (e.g., a metabolite or part of the fungal cell wall) or identifying a patient's response to *Candida* spp. (e.g., antibody). These studies include arabinitol, mannan antigen and antibody, and (1,3)-β-D-glucan (BDG). Arabinitol is a metabolite produced by some *Candida* spp. Evaluation of this assay revealed low specificity; it is not currently commercially available and thus is not discussed further.

Both antigen and antibody tests for mannan, a component of the fungal cell wall, have been assessed. The highest sensitivity (83%) and specificity (86%) occurred when both assays were used together, but significant variability can occur among *Candida* spp. Data suggest these assays may have a role in early detection of IC. Positive test results have been reported before blood culture positivity in candidemic patients and before radiologic detection of lesions in patients with hepatosplenic candidiasis.[37] Assessment in pediatric populations has primarily been in neonates. In one small study of neonates and children with malignancies, the mannan antigen assay detected two of five oncologic patients with candidemia, and none (zero of five) of the patients with *C. parapsilosis*.[38]

BDG is another fungal cell wall component that is present in *Candida*, as well as other fungal genera such as *Aspergillus*. Four different assays available, but each assay has a different cutoff value; therefore tests cannot be compared and are not interchangeable. Currently, the Fungitell BGD assay (Viracor Eurofins, Lee's Summit, MO) is the only commercially available BDG test in the United States. In a meta-analysis, the performance of the BDG assay on blood specimens had a sensitivity of 77% and specificity of 85% for the detection of IFD.[39] Based on these studies, the package insert for the Fungitell assay recommends a threshold for positivity of more than 80 pg/mL for blood testing, but the optimal threshold has been questioned with some studies proposing sequential monitoring and alternative cutoff values. Additionally, the BDG assay has been used successfully to detect *Candida* spp. presence in other specimens such as cerebrospinal fluid, but the optimal threshold for positivity from these specimens is not known.

In pediatrics, the utility of the BDG assay is challenged by higher baseline levels of BDG in the blood among healthy children, which has the possibility of more false-positive results.[40] Assessment of varying cutoffs has been attempted to improve sensitivity and specificity with little success. In a cohort of Italian children, the test had a specificity of more than 0.90 for a high cutoff value (≥200 pg/mL) but had low sensitivity at all cutoff values assessed (40 to 400 pg/mL) with overall low positive predictive values.[41]

Several additional limitations for BDG testing exist. It is not known whether or how the use of prophylactic antifungals interferes with the test. Limited data exist in the pediatric and SOT populations, and the majority of studies assessing BDG in oncology and HSCT patients have been in the context of IFD as the outcome measure rather than specifically IC. This is because the test is not specific for *Candida* spp., and BDG is found in the cell wall of other fungi, including *Aspergillus* spp., *Fusarium* spp., *Histoplasma capsulatum*, *Sporothrix schenckii*, *Pneumocystis jirovecii*, *Coccidioides immitis*, *Trichosporon* spp., *Acremonium* spp., and *Saccharomyces cerevisiae*. Lastly, false-positive results have been attributed to blood products, hemodialysis, surgical gauze, immunoglobulin, albumin, and β-lactam antibiotics, specifically piperacillin-tazobactam. Based on the poor positive predictive value and limited data in pediatrics, BDG is not recommended as a routine diagnostic test for detection of IC in children with cancer or those undergoing HSCT.[42]

TREATMENT

Several available antifungal agents for empirical and definitive therapy of IC in children are available. These include echinocandins (anidulafungin, caspofungin, and micafungin), triazoles (e.g., itraconazole, fluconazole, voriconazole, and posaconazole), and amphotericin B formulations (e.g., amphotericin B deoxycholate, lipid amphotericin B complex, and liposomal amphotericin B). The echinocandins and amphotericin B formulations are both fungicidal against *Candida* spp., whereas the triazoles are considered fungistatic. In choosing an antifungal agent for treatment of IC, pathogen-specific factors (e.g., species identified, resistance testing), host-specific factors (e.g., age of the child, the location of the infection, other therapeutic agents being received), and medication-specific factors (e.g., pharmacokinetics/pharmacodynamics of the agent) all need to be considered. With this context, recommendations for definitive antifungal therapy are provided. The choice and duration of antifungal therapy is often dependent on the clinical presentation, location of infection, and *Candida* spp., and as such the recommendations should be consistent across oncology patients as well as SOT and HSCT recipients.

Definitive Therapy Based on *Candida* Species

Species identification and susceptibility testing should be performed on all invasive *Candida* isolates. Resistance testing should be considered on isolates from superficial specimens in certain scenarios (e.g., the initial therapeutic choice is not effective). When a patient is known to have IC but susceptibility testing is not yet available, the choice of initial antifungal therapy should take into account the patient's history (e.g., prior *Candida* infections, prior antifungal exposure), the hospital's antibiogram for *Candida* spp., and published data on resistance profiles for a given species (Table 26.1). Importantly, if a child is receiving antifungal prophylaxis and IC develops, a different antifungal class should be used until results of antifungal susceptibility testing are available.

In a large study of more than 5000 IC isolates, only 1.2% of *C. albicans* isolates were resistant to fluconazole, and less than 0.5% of *C. parapsilosis*, *C. tropicalis*, and *C. lusitaniae* isolates were fluconazole resistant.[43] Therefore fluconazole remains a primary therapeutic option after definitive identification of *C. albicans* and these additional species.[21] Fluconazole resistance in *C. glabrata* isolates approached 6%, with higher rates of reduced susceptibility in other studies.[42] Most fluconazole-resistant *C. glabrata* isolates are cross-resistant to voriconazole, and an alternative class of antifungals should be used. Some experts advocate the use of higher-dose azoles in patients with *C. glabrata*–susceptible isolates owing to reduced susceptibility. These isolates are often referred to as susceptible dose-dependent. *C. krusei* is inherently resistant to fluconazole, but almost all isolates retain susceptibility to the echinocandins, amphotericin B, and voriconazole.[21,43] For *C. parapsilosis* isolates, the minimum inhibitory concentration (MIC) of 90% of isolates to echinocandins was 1 μg/mL, indicative of dose-dependent susceptibility.[43] However, despite the elevated MIC, the use of an echinocandin in cases of *C. parapsilosis* was not associated with worse outcomes as compared to other therapeutic options.[21,44]

C. auris has recently emerged as a multidrug-resistant species.[45] Although cases are primarily in adults, reports of *C. auris* infection in children have occurred, including one child with leukemia. *C. auris*

TABLE 26.1 **Common Susceptibility Patterns of *Candida* Species**

Species	Fluconazole	Voriconazole	Amphotericin B	Echinocandins
C. albicans	+	+	+	+
C. tropicalis	+	+	+	+
C. parapsilosis	+	+	+	+[a]
C. glabrata	+/−[b]	+/−[b]	+	+
C. krusei	−	+	+	+
C. lusitaniae	+	+	−	+
C. auris	−	+/−	+/−	+/−

[a]*C. parapsilosis* demonstrates a higher minimum inhibitory concentration to the echinocandins; however, outcomes are similar between patients treated with fluconazole and echinocandins.
[b]Some experts advocate using a higher dose of azoles for *C. glabrata*.
+, susceptible, +/−, susceptible to resistant; −, resistant.

species demonstrate elevated MIC to azoles, polyenes, and echinocandins, significantly limiting treatment options. Limited data from collected specimens demonstrate that 41% of isolates were resistant to two or more classes of antifungals. Overall, more than 90% of isolates are resistant to fluconazole and 64% were resistant to voriconazole. Approximately one-third of isolates were resistant to amphotericin B. Thus echinocandins are recommended to be the empirical drug of choice; however, 7% of isolates are resistant to echinocandins. Additionally, echinocandins may not appropriately penetrate the site of infection.[46]

Definitive Therapy Based on Location of Infection

Superficial Candidiasis. Superficial candidiasis can be treated with nonsystemic agents. Oral nystatin is effective against oropharyngeal candidiasis. Superficial dermatitis (i.e., skin disease not associated with IC) can be treated topically, including with topical nystatin or topical azoles such as clotrimazole, miconazole, or ketoconazole. These topical azoles can also be used to treat vulvovaginitis. Topical therapy for these conditions is an appropriate first therapeutic approach in children with malignancy or transplant recipients if they otherwise appear well. However, occasionally these superficial infections are recalcitrant to topical therapy and thus transition to a systemic agent may be necessary. Fluconazole is a reasonable systemic agent for superficial candidiasis, assuming *C. krusei* or *C. glabrata* is not the etiology. If these species are identified, a different therapeutic class, such as an echinocandin or amphotericin B formulation, should be considered. Children with evidence of both superficial and IC should be treated as recommended based on location of IC.

Invasive Candidiasis: Candidemia. Comparative data for treatment of candidemia in children are limited. The few studies available suggest that echinocandins, amphotericin B formulations, and azoles have similar effectiveness.[47] However, randomized controlled trial data in adult patients support the superiority of echinocandins to azoles and amphotericin B formulations.[48] Based on these data, guidelines for adult candidiasis recommend echinocandins as first-line therapy.[21] These guidelines do not clearly apply to children, and the aforementioned pediatric data suggest that the different classes of therapy may be similarly effective. The concern for children with cancer or pediatric transplant recipients is that the risk of poor outcomes from candidemia may be greater than the overall pediatric population and closer to that observed in adults. There is an ongoing observational study by the International Pediatric Fungal Network underway that will help inform pediatric-specific decision making. Until these data are available, it is reasonable to extrapolate the adult data to these high-risk pediatric populations and start therapy for candidemia with an echinocandin (Fig. 26.1). Fluconazole can be considered as initial therapy in patients who are not critically ill and unlikely to have a fluconazole-resistant organism (e.g., those without previous azole exposure and in health settings with low rates of fluconazole-resistant organisms). Voriconazole and posaconazole are not considered more effective than fluconazole, with the exception of *C. glabrata* and *C. krusei* isolates that may be resistant to fluconazole but susceptible to these newer azoles. An amphotericin B formulation may be an alternative option, but toxicities from these agents are a concern.

The duration of therapy for uncomplicated candidemia (i.e., no disseminated disease) is typically 14 days from clearance of fungemia and resolution of symptomatology.[21] Some experts would advocate for extension of therapy beyond 14 days until resolution of neutropenia in neutropenic patients.[21,49] When disseminated disease is present, a longer duration of therapy is needed, based on the location of dissemination.

Because of the high risk of *Candida* dissemination, particularly in neutropenic patients, patients should undergo evaluation for foci of IC (see Fig, 26.1). An ophthalmologic examination should be performed in patients with and without neutropenia. The ideal timing for the eye evaluation is not known. Some advocate for early assessment after candidemia detection as it might affect the choice of antifungal therapy, whereas others suggest waiting until resolution of candidemia so that a second examination is not necessary if the result of the first is negative but candidemia persists. In neutropenic patients, it is often desirable to have neutrophil recovery before ophthalmologic assessment as lesions may be missed in the setting of neutropenia.

Additional imaging, specifically of the gastrointestinal tract and the heart, may be warranted, particularly in neutropenic patients and/or in patients with persistent candidemia. The exact duration of candidemia to dictate abdominal imaging or echocardiogram is not known but should be considered if more than one culture result is positive and should always be performed when certain symptoms or signs are present, such as abdominal pain or new heart murmur. The ideal modality for abdominal imaging is not clear. Abdominal ultrasound of the viscera can be helpful in identifying disseminated *Candida* to these organs. However, IC lesions are not always found by ultrasound, so CT scan with contrast or magnetic resonance imaging with gadolinium may be necessary. Finally, if dissemination to multiple abdominal viscera is identified or if eye lesions are found, further imaging with a brain magnetic resonance imaging scan and a chest CT scan are warranted. Identifying lesions in all affected organs can be important in guiding total duration of therapy.

In addition to antifungal therapy and workup for disseminated disease, additional adjunctive measures should be considered. CVCs should be removed, when feasible, in patients with candidemia

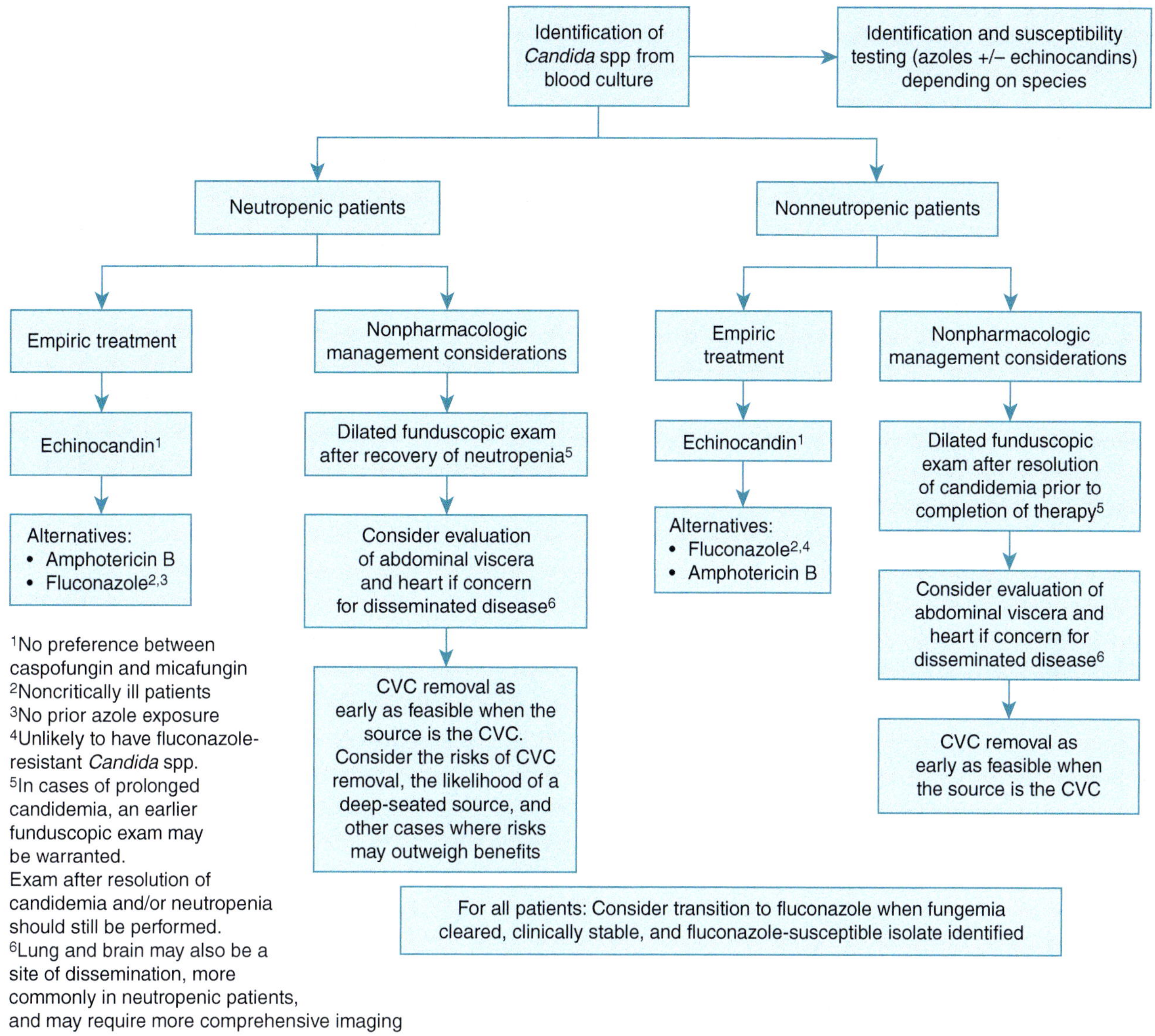

Fig. 26.1 Evaluation and management of candidemia.

because the organism has a propensity to form biofilms that are difficult to eradicate. In fact, for many patients, particularly nonneutropenic patients, the CVC is the focus of infection and CVC removal is necessary for clearance. Amphotericin B formulation lock therapy has been reported, although it is not routinely recommended for catheter salvage, when needed. CVC removal should be considered in all patients with persistent candidemia despite appropriate therapy regardless of the presumed source.[21] Data to support adjunctive therapy with granulocyte transfusions in children with neutropenia and IC are limited and thus are not routinely recommended. Combination therapy for candidemia is not recommended for routine care. It can be considered in severe infections or in areas of limited drug penetration (e.g., central nervous system [CNS] infection), but little evidence is available to support combination therapy.[49]

Invasive Candidiasis: Focal Disease. The antifungal agent of choice should be chosen based not only on *Candida* spp. but also on the location of infection (Table 26.2). For example, although echinocandins may be recommended for first-line therapy in immunocompromised children with candidemia, they have decreased penetration into the CNS and excretion into the urine, limiting their use in meningitis and/or when the lower genitourinary tract is involved. Any of the lipid amphotericin B formulations are generally the preferred amphotericin B product with a few exceptions: liposomal amphotericin B is preferred for CNS disease and endophthalmitis. However, lipid formations have limited penetration of the kidney and thus should not be used when the kidney or genitourinary tract is involved. For that clinical situation, an azole or amphotericin B deoxycholate should be used.

In many cases of either isolated candidemia or disseminated disease, step-down therapy is appropriate after an initial period of treatment and clinical improvement. The choice for the step-down agent should be based on the isolated species, resistance profile, location of infection, and probability for patient adherence. The latter is important as both the echinocandins and amphotericin B formulations require parenteral administration. Additionally, therapeutic changes may be necessary based on toxicities and drug-drug interactions with other agents. Adjunctive and local therapy may also be recommended in some disease states (Table 26.3). Amphotericin B deoxycholate or voriconazole intravitreal injections may be used in cases of *Candida*

TABLE 26.2 Preferred Initial Empiric Therapy for *Candida* Infection Based on Location of Disease[a]

Site of Infection	Initial Therapy	Second-Line Therapy	Step-Down Therapy
Candidemia	Echinocandin	Azoles or amphotericin B[b]	
Central nervous system	Amphotericin B[c]		Azoles
Endocarditis	Echinocandin or amphotericin B		Azoles
Endophthalmitis	Azoles	Amphotericin B[c]	
Esophagitis	Echinocandin or azoles	Amphotericin B	
Hepatosplenic (chronic disseminated)	Echinocandin or amphotericin B	Azoles	
Intraabdominal	Echinocandin	Azoles or amphotericin B	
Osteoarticular	Echinocandin or azoles	Amphotericin B	
Suppurative thrombophlebitis	Echinocandin or azoles or amphotericin B		
Urinary tract	Azoles	Amphotericin B[d]	

[a]Recommendations are for initial empirical therapy. Results of species identification and sensitivity testing should inform additional management decisions.
[b]Unless otherwise specified, any lipid amphotericin B formulation is preferred.
[c]Liposomal amphotericin B is preferred for central nervous system infections and endophthalmitis.
[d]Amphotericin deoxycholate is preferred for urinary tract infections.

TABLE 26.3 Adjunctive Therapy and Duration of Therapy Based on Site of Infection

Site of Infection	Duration of Therapy	Additional Treatment Considerations
Candidemia	• 14 days from clearance of positive cultures and resolution of symptoms • A longer duration may be needed in patients with persistent neutropenia	• Consider transition to fluconazole after clinical improvement in patients with susceptible isolate. • Recommend CVC removal early, especially if this is the suspected source.
Central nervous system	• Resolution of signs and symptoms and normalization of CSF parameters and imaging	• Consider flucytosine with amphotericin B • Hardware (i.e., shunt material) should be removed if present. • Consider ventricular amphotericin B deoxycholate in patients who cannot have an intraventricular device removed and have persistent positive culture results. • Consider step-down to fluconazole, if susceptible, after significant clinical improvement and with guidance from an infectious diseases expert.
Cystitis	• 14 days	• Indwelling catheter should be removed
Endocarditis	• ≥6 weeks after valve replacement; longer in complicated cases	• Consider flucytosine if amphotericin B is used. • Surgical intervention is recommended. • Consider step-down to fluconazole, if susceptible, after significant clinical improvement. • Indefinite suppressive therapy may be needed in cases with retained hardware or without valve replacement.
Endophthalmitis		
Chorioretinitis (without vitritis)	• ≥4-6 weeks dependent on resolution of lesions	• Both fluconazole and voriconazole have good penetration into the posterior eye. • Consider flucytosine if amphotericin B is used.
Chorioretinitis (with macular involvement or vitritis)	• ≥4-6 weeks dependent on resolution of lesions	• Intravitreal amphotericin B deoxycholate or voriconazole should be used in conjunction with systemic therapy. • Consider vitrectomy.
Esophagitis	• 14-21 days	• If therapy initiated is based on clinical presentation and symptoms persist on empirical therapy, an endoscopy for direct visualization and culture may be necessary.
Hepatosplenic (chronic disseminated)	• Resolution of lesions and through period of high risk	• Occasionally, fevers persist despite neutrophil count recovery and appropriate antifungal therapy. In this setting immune modulation may be necessary for symptom relief.
Intraabdominal candidiasis	• Based on source control and response to therapy	• Appropriate drainage and source control is recommended.
Osteomyelitis	• 6-12 months	• Consider step-down to fluconazole, if susceptible, after significant clinical improvement. • Surgical debridement may be needed.

TABLE 26.3 Adjunctive therapy and Duration of Therapy Based on Site of Infection—cont'd

Site of Infection	Duration of Therapy	Additional Treatment Considerations
Septic arthritis	• ≥6 weeks	• Surgical drainage is recommended. • Consider step-down to fluconazole, if susceptible, after significant clinical improvement. • Removal of prosthetic device, if present. • Longer duration and chronic suppressive therapy may be needed if prosthetic material remains in place.
Suppurative thrombophlebitis	• ≥2 weeks after resolution of candidemia • Therapy may be extended until thrombus resolution	• Consider step-down to fluconazole, if susceptible. • Catheter removal is recommended. • Incision and drainage is recommended.

CSF, cerebrospinal fluid; *CVC,* central venous catheter.

chorioretinitis with macular involvement or vitritis. Amphotericin B deoxycholate may also be administered intraventricularly in cases when a ventricular device remains in place or through nephrostomy tubes in cases of mycelial masses in the renal parenchyma. In some cases, surgery is warranted for drainage or removal of focal infection to achieve source control. Examples include vitrectomy in cases of *Candida* chorioretinitis and vitreal involvement or removal of mycelial masses in renal or urinary disease. Cardiac valve replacement, including native valves, is recommended for cases of *Candida* endocarditis.[21] Each of these adjunctive interventions is in addition to systemic antifungal therapy.

The duration of therapy for focal disease varies based on disease location (see Table 26.3). For patients with multiple sites of dissemination, the longest recommended duration of therapy should be considered. Initiation or continuation of chemotherapy or progression to HSCT or SOT should not necessarily be delayed because of IC. Ideally, IC-directed therapy should be promptly started and clinical symptoms improved or stabilized before progressing with chemotherapy or conditioning. If immunosuppressive agents are given while a child is receiving antifungal therapy for IC, the antifungal therapy should be continued through the subsequent period of immunosuppression. In some patients with frequent or persistent neutropenia, such as those undergoing allogeneic HSCT or receiving chemotherapy for acute leukemia, therapy is continued until immune function is improved and there is evidence of radiographic resolution of previously identified disseminated foci. It is possible that radiographic lesions may persist even after appropriate durations of therapy, and imaging findings may wax and wane based on the presence of neutropenia. This is especially true in hepatosplenic candidiasis. Additionally, children with hepatosplenic candidiasis may present with findings similar to immune reconstitution inflammatory syndrome with high, persistent fevers that can be incapacitating. In such cases, a short course of nonsteroidal antiinflammatory drugs or glucocorticoids may be considered to modulate the immune system.[21] Relapse may occur if antifungal therapy is discontinued too early.

Therapeutic Drug Monitoring

Therapeutic drug monitoring (TDM) is not recommended for fluconazole. However, TDM is necessary and integral to IC treatment when using itraconazole, voriconazole, posaconazole, and flucytosine. Target concentrations for the azoles do not differ for *Candida* spp. versus other IFDs. Flucytosine TDM is recommended within 72 hours of drug initiation and any dose adjustments. Monitoring is also recommended when signs of toxicity are present or when the potential exists for drug interactions.

INFECTION PREVENTION AND ANTICIPATORY GUIDANCE

Standard precautions are recommended for patients with IC. However, infection prevention measures differ for *C. auris,* owing to high rates of antifungal resistance. Both standard and contact precautions with both daily and terminal cleans are recommended for patients who are colonized or infected with *C. auris*, and patients should be placed in single rooms. Contact precautions are recommended for the length of colonization, and no data exist on the effectiveness of decolonization strategies. *C. auris* detection, even in the setting of colonization only, should be reported to public health authorities. Local requirements may also require reporting of other multidrug-resistant *Candida*. Hand hygiene is crucial to decrease the spread of *C. auris* and other multidrug-resistant *Candida*.[50]

Limiting unnecessary antibiotic use, particularly broad-spectrum antibiotics, is important for prevention of IC. Although not always feasible, minimizing the presence and duration of CVCs as well as periods of neutropenia decreases the risk of IC. Prophylaxis, when appropriately indicated, is important. Lastly, high suspicion for IC in high-risk patients is important given the limitations in diagnostics.

Prevention of Recurrent Infections

Prevention of recurrent *Candida* spp. infections is generally related to correction of the underlying predisposing factor. In immunocompromised patients, this may not be an achievable goal. Prophylaxis against recurrent episodes of IC has been used in select situations. In patients with prosthetic valve endocarditis, chronic suppressive antifungal therapy, typically with fluconazole, is recommended to prevent recurrent infection, particularly in patients who cannot have surgical removal of the valve. Thrice-weekly chronic suppressive therapy can be considered in patients with recurrent oropharyngeal or esophageal candidiasis after treatment has been completed. Once-weekly fluconazole dosing is recommended for recurrent vulvovaginitis. However, the majority of these studies were conducted in patients with human immunodeficiency virus, and thus the generalizability to pediatric oncology and transplant patients is not clear.[21] Although secondary prophylaxis with fluconazole has been used in high-risk patients after an episode of IC, no clear data support this practice outside the specific prophylaxis indications documented earlier.

27

Cryptococcosis and Other Rare Invasive Yeasts Infections

Philip Lee, PharmD and David L. Goldman, MD

The vast majority of invasive yeast infections in organ transplant recipients and patients with malignancy are caused by *Candida* species. However, a variety of other yeasts are important opportunistic pathogens for these patients and are reviewed in this chapter. This includes the *Cryptococcus neoformans–Cryptococcus gattii* complex, which is the second most common cause of invasive yeast infections in this cohort and an important cause of fungal meningoencephalitis and pneumonia. It also includes a collection of other yeasts that as a group cause a small minority of invasive fungal disease. Disease caused by these pathogens can be difficult to treat because of anti-fungal resistance and is often associated with a high mortality.

CRYPTOCOCCOSIS

Background

Cryptococcus neoformans and *Cryptococcus gattii* are encapsulated basidiomycetous yeasts that are responsible for the syndrome of cryptococcosis. As these two species share many biologic characteristics and clinical presentations, they are often discussed together as the *C. neoformans– C. gattii complex.* However, there are notable differences in the epidemiology, risk factors, and clinical presentations of the 2 species. As such, throughout the chapter there is discussion that is generalizable to both species of the *C. neoformans* and *C. gattii* complex with distinction between the species highlighted. Although these pathogens can be opportunistic to a wide range of immunocompromised hosts, the focus is on pediatric oncology patients and recipients of solid organ or hematopoietic stem cell transplantation. Diseases secondary to other cryptococcal species (i.e., C. *albidus* and *C. laurentii*) are much less commonly reported and are not discussed further.

C. neoformans and *C. gattii* exhibit several virulent traits, which have been hypothesized to have evolved as an adaptive response to environmental stressors.[1] The polysaccharide capsule of *Cryptococcus* plays an essential role in promoting disease by helping the organism evade and limit the host inflammatory response. The capsular material is actively shed during infection and detection of this polysaccharide in bodily fluids serves as an important diagnostic tool. Antibodies to the capsular polysaccharide can be used to serotype the organism. A variety of other cryptococcal virulence factors have been elucidated, including melanization, urease production, ability to grow at 37°C, and phenotypic variation.

Epidemiology and Risk Factors

In the environment, *C. neoformans* is often localized to areas contaminated by pigeon droppings and decaying trees. The ubiquitous nature of this pathogen makes it a possible pathogen regardless of geographic location. *C. gattii* has been classically associated with the red gum eucalyptus tree, which results in a more focused geographic distribution of this pathogen. Until recently, *C. gattii* disease was primarily restricted to the tropical and subtropical areas, especially Australasia, where the disease is endemic. Beginning in the late 1990s, an outbreak of *C. gattii* disease was recognized in British Columbia. This outbreak quickly spread to other areas of the Pacific Northwest, including parts of the Northwest United States. Sporadic disease has also been reported in Europe. The regional distribution of the pathogen can help quantify a patient's risk for *C. gattii*; however, clinicians should be aware that prior travel to these regions can place a patient a risk.[2]

Exposure to both species is thought to be via the inhalation of aerosolized organisms from the environment. Subsequent to exposure, a person can develop either a primary progressive symptomatic infection or have an asymptomatic immunologic response. In the latter scenario, the organism can establish latency with risk for reactivation later in life. Person-to-person spread is not thought to occur. Symptomatic disease is uncommon in young children even though serologic studies suggest that exposure occurs in most children by 3 years of age.[3] This increasing risk for symptomatic disease with increasing age is highlighted in specific immunocompromised populations. For example, in children with AIDS, cryptococcosis is more common in adolescents and preadolescents than younger children.[4]

Cryptococcosis can occur in both immunocompetent and immunocompromised children. Interestingly, *C. neoformans* is much more common in children with defects in immunity, especially cellular immunity; whereas *C. gattii* tends to primarily cause disease in healthy individuals, although subtle defects in the host immune response may be present such as auto-antibodies to granulocyte-macrophage colony-stimulating factor, corticosteroid use, and chronic lung disease.[5] As *C. neoformans* is a more ubiquitous pathogen, the epidemiologic data for cryptococcosis are primarily dependent on reports focused on this species. There was a sharp rise in the incidence of cryptococcosis in association with the human immunodeficiency disease epidemic, but this incidence has dramatically waned with the advent and availability of highly active antiretroviral therapy (HAART). *C. neoformans* remains an important cause of disease in children with primary and secondary immunodeficiencies, especially children who have undergone organ transplantation.

Transplant Recipients

Cryptococcosis is significantly more common among solid organ transplant (SOT) recipients compared with stem cell transplant recipients for whom this infection is relatively rare. Among SOT recipients it is the third most common invasive fungal disease (after candidiasis and aspergillosis). Cryptococcosis accounts for approximately 7% of fungal infections in adult SOT recipients, with mortality rates on the order of 30%.[6] In SOT recipients, cryptococcosis typically occur several months to years after transplantation and may result from primary infection or from reactivation of a latent infection. Infections within 30 days of transplantation are well described and appear to be caused by reactivation of a latent infection in the transplanted organ.[7] The majority of SOT recipients have disseminated cryptococcosis, although as many as one-third have isolated pulmonary disease.[8]

Malignancies

A range of hematologic malignancies, including chronic lymphocytic leukemia, acute lymphoblastic leukemia (ALL), acute myeloid leukemia (AML), and lymphoma, have been reported in association with cryptococcosis. Among adults, cryptococcosis is most common in patients with chronic lymphocytic leukemia and lymphoma.[9] In contrast to invasive candidiasis and aspergillosis, neutropenia is generally not considered a risk factor for cryptococcosis. Instead, risk factors include advanced disease, lymphopenia, and prior chemotherapy.[10] Infection most commonly presents as disseminated disease. In children with soft tissue malignancies, *C. neoformans* pulmonary disease may be detected as a result of imaging done to exclude pulmonary metastasis.[11]

Other Risk Factors for Cryptococcosis

A variety of immunosuppressive regimens, (i.e., corticosteroids, chemotherapeutics) have been associated with an increased susceptibility to cryptococcosis. Biologic agents can also be a risk factor for cryptococcosis. This is especially true of tumor necrosis factor antagonists and T-cell–depleting therapies. More recently several cases of cryptococcosis have been reported in patients receiving ibrutinib, a Bruton's tyrosine kinase inhibitor.[12] As the number of novel chemotherapeutic and biologic agents available for use increases and their indications for use broadens, clinicians need to be aware that the populations at risk for cryptococcosis will also increase.

Clinical Manifestations

The *C. neoformans-gattii* complex can cause disease in most organ systems, although the most common presentations are meningoencephalitis, disseminated disease, and pneumonia. These organisms are highly neurotropic and can enter the central nervous system (CNS) via several different mechanisms.[13] Compared with *C. neoformans*, *C. gattii* more commonly causes pulmonary disease without CNS involvement. Furthermore, *C. gattii* disease is more likely to be characterized by the presence of cryptococcomas, which are mass-like lesions containing large number of organisms.

Meningoencephalitis. Cryptococcal meningoencephalitis (CME) is a subacute to chronic disease (Fig. 27.1). The precise manner of presentation depends both on the underlying immune status of the host and the infecting cryptococcal species/strain. Symptoms are nonspecific but most commonly include headache, neck stiffness, and fever, which can last for weeks to months before diagnosis. Personality changes, lethargy, along with cranial nerve palsies, nausea, vomiting, and visual changes, may also occur. Meningismus is not a reliable sign and is absent in the majority of patients. Parenchymal brain lesions occur in the minority of patients, but when present are associated with higher mortality.[14] Increased intracranial pressure (ICP) is a hallmark feature of CME.[15] The basis of increased ICP is not completely understood, but it may be related to impaired cerebrospinal fluid absorption caused by the viscous capsular polysaccharide that is shed by the organism. Increased ICP is an important contributor to the acute morbidity and mortality of CME and should be managed aggressively.

Pneumonia. Pulmonary cryptococcosis can occur alone or in the context of CME (Fig. 27.2). Concomitant CNS disease occurs more commonly in patients with AIDS compared with SOT recipients, which is believed to be due to the anti-cryptococcal activity of calcineurin inhibitors.[8] Nonetheless, any patient with cryptococcal lung disease and an underlying immunocompromising condition should be evaluated for evidence of dissemination, which would include a lumbar puncture, fungal blood culture, serum antigen testing, and physical examination. Pulmonary disease is often asymptomatic and may be

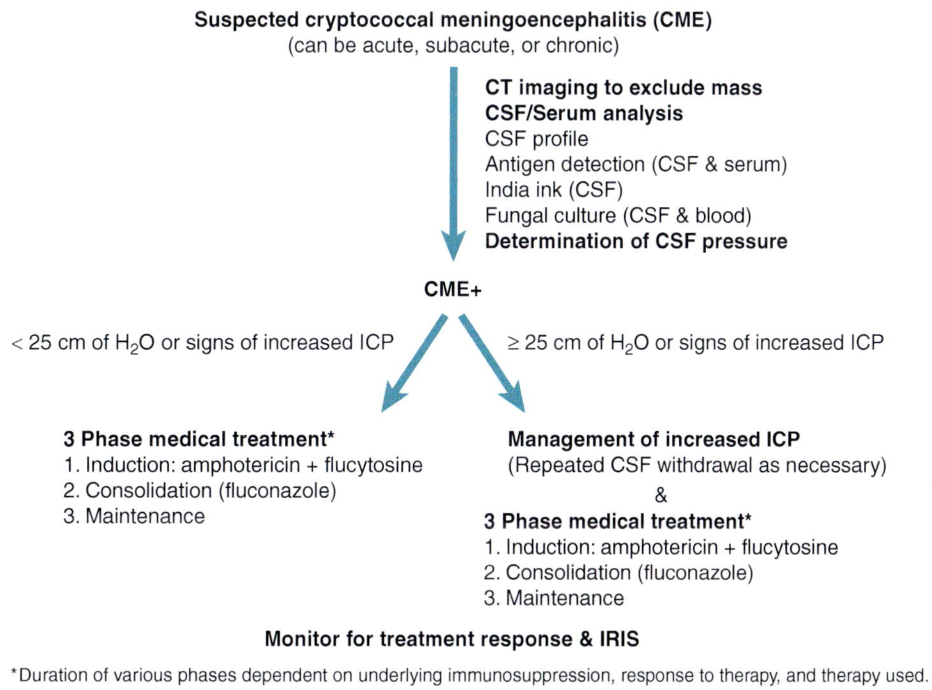

Fig. 27.1 Algorithm for the diagnosis and management of cryptococcal meningoencephalitis. *CSF*, cerebrospinal fluid; *CT*, computed tomography; *ICP*, intracranial pressure; *IRIS*, immune reconstitution inflammatory syndrome.

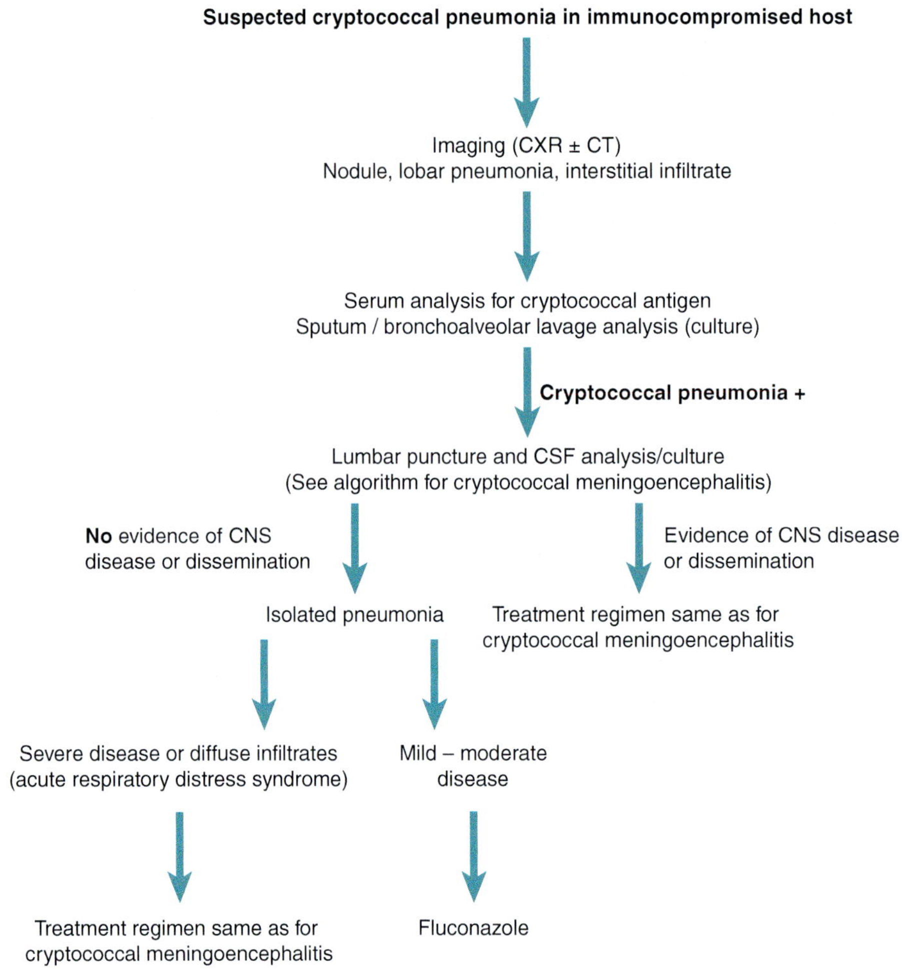

Fig. 27.2 Algorithm for the diagnosis and management of cryptococcal pneumonia. *CSF,* cerebrospinal fluid; *CNS,* central nervous system; *CT,* computed tomography; *CXR,* chest x-ray.

only recognized as a result of imaging studies done for other purposes. Symptoms, when present, are nonspecific and include cough, dyspnea, increased sputum production (in older children), hemoptysis, and pleuritic chest pain. Rarely, pulmonary cryptococcosis can present with rapid respiratory decompensation. The imaging findings of pulmonary cryptococcosis are variable and include singular and multiple nodules, consolidation, and masses. Interstitial infiltrates have also been described and are often the result of secondary dissemination from other sites of lung involvement. Finally, cavitation and pleural effusions have been described, although they are not common.[16]

Other Forms of Disease. Skin involvement in cryptococcosis is typically the result of hematogenous spread and may be the initial clinical sign of disseminated disease. Because skin disease rarely results from direct inoculation, all patients with skin manifestations of cryptococcal disease should be evaluated for disseminated disease and CME. Skin manifestations include papules, nodules, molluscum, acneiform rash, and cellulitis.[17] Because of the high variability and nonspecificity of skin disease, a high degree of suspicion is needed to make the diagnosis (see later text). Cryptococcosis can cause disease in most organ systems, including bones, joints, eyes, prostate, liver, kidneys, and spleen.

Diagnosis

The diagnosis of cryptococcosis can be made by growing the organism in culture. The same diagnostic assays can be used for both *C. neoformans* and *C. gattii infections.* Most colonies are white to cream colored and may have a mucoid appearance owing to the capsule. Diagnosis is also made by visualization using microscopy or detection of the cryptococcal polysaccharide in body fluids. The utility of these techniques varies depending on the host and organ system involved. Growth in specialized media and matrix-assisted laser desorption/ionization time-of-flight mass spectrometry (MALDI-TOF) can be used as necessary to distinguish *C. neoformans* from *C. gattii.*[18] For CME, cerebrospinal fluid (CSF) examination generally reveals a lymphocytic pleocytosis, although the actual cell number may be low or normal in patients with severe immune dysfunction. CSF protein levels tend to be elevated, whereas glucose levels are depressed. Cryptococcus can be readily isolated from the CSF by standard fungal culture, although growth may take several days. India ink staining of the CSF allows for rapid detection of the organism because the capsular polysaccharide excludes ink, which allows the unstained organisms to be visualized. The sensitivity of this stain depends on the cryptococcal burden, which is related to the underlying immune status of the host. In SOT recipients, the sensitivity may be as low as 50%.[19]

Several different antibody-based methods are available for polysaccharide antigen detection, including latex agglutination, enzyme-linked immunosorbent assay (ELISA), and a lateral flow assay. The sensitivity of these assays in CSF testing has been reported to range between 93% and 100% (reviewed in Perfect and Bicanic[20]). The sensitivity of serum antigen testing in patients with CME is lower than CSF testing and in SOT recipients has been reported to be 90%.[19] False-negative reactions for these tests are very uncommon, but can be seen early in disease and with extremely high antigen levels when the latex antigen assay is used. False-positive reactions are also very uncommon, but cross-reactivity with the polysaccharides of other organisms, such as *Trichosporon* and *Capnocytophaga*, can occur. Antigen detection assays provide semi-quantitative measurements of polysaccharide antigen within the CSF and serum. High initial CSF antigen levels are generally associated with higher fungal burdens and a worse prognosis.[21] Unfortunately, antigen detection assays have limited utility in measuring response to therapy. Cryptococcal polymerase chain reaction (PCR) assays as part of multiplex meningitis assays are also commercially available, but experience with these diagnostic assays is limited.

Cryptococcal pneumonia can be diagnosed by culture of the sputum and bronchoalveolar lavage fluid. Blood cultures and serum cryptococcal antigen test results are typically negative, especially with isolated pulmonary disease.[22] Latex agglutination testing of bronchoalveolar lavage fluid has been described, although the assay has not been formally studied, nor is it licensed for this purpose.[23] Evaluation for CME including a lumbar puncture should be done in all immunocompromised patients with cryptococcal pneumonia. A complete physical examination along with serum cryptococcal antigen and fungal blood cultures should be performed to evaluate for dissemination. For pulmonary nodules and masses a biopsy may be necessary to establish a diagnosis. Mucicarmine staining highlights the capsule of the organism and helps distinguish this organism from other yeasts.

In skin disease, biopsy and culture of the affected area are generally needed to make a diagnosis. Skin lesions are generally a manifestation of disseminated disease and affected patients often have elevated serum antigen levels. All immunocompromised patients with skin disease should have a complete evaluation to exclude dissemination, including a lumbar puncture to rule out CNS involvement.

Treatment

Because of the rarity of disease in children, many of the recommendations regarding pediatric cryptococcosis are based on extrapolations from adult data, in particular from adults with human immunodeficiency virus/AIDS. Treatment approaches must consider the underlying immune status of the host as well as the organ system involved. In addition to antifungal therapy, attempts should be made to lessen immunosuppression as possible.

The treatment of CME as established by the Infectious Diseases Society of America consists of 3 consecutive phases: induction, consolidation, and maintenance. For the initial induction phase, patients are treated with a combination of amphotericin and flucytosine.[24] Most of the original treatment studies were performed with conventional amphotericin. However, recent studies suggest that lipid preparations of amphotericin are therapeutically equivalent and may be better tolerated in individuals with or at risk for renal disease.[25] Thus strong consideration should be given to use of lipid or liposomal preparations in patients who are at risk for renal dysfunction, including transplant recipients who are receiving calcineurin inhibitors, and for those who cannot tolerate conventional amphotericin.

The duration of induction is typically 2 weeks. Longer durations (i.e., 4 to 6 weeks) should be considered in the following circumstances: (1) in patients who did not receive flucytosine as part of their initial therapy; (2) in those with complicated neurologic disease (including those with cryptococcomas), and (3) failure to sterilize CSF at 2 weeks. Induction therapy is followed by an 8-week consolidation with fluconazole and concluded with a maintenance course of fluconazole. In patients with AIDS the minimal duration of total antifungal therapy is 12 months. After this time, discontinuation of maintenance fluconazole can be considered in the context of immune reconstitution (in adults >100 $CD4^+$ T cells/μL) and undetectable DNAemia. For SOT recipients the maintenance phase of fluconazole should be 6 to 12 months.

The treatment of pulmonary cryptococcosis depends on the extent of disease and underlying immune status of the host. Patients with severe pulmonary disease (i.e., acute respiratory distress syndrome) or with evidence of dissemination should be treated as those with CME. For patients with localized pulmonary disease (i.e., extrapulmonary disease has been excluded), fluconazole therapy for 6 to 12 months is recommended.[24]

Management of Increased Intracanial Pressure

Increased ICP often accompanies CME and plays a significant role in the early morbidity and mortality of this disease. According to Infectious Diseases Society of America guidelines, CSF pressure should be lowered by CSF drainage to less than 20 cm of H_2O or decreased by 50 % if very elevated. CSF pressure should be monitored daily until CSF pressure has normalized for 2 consecutive days.[24] Mannitol is not helpful in the management of increased ICP in CME and corticosteroids (in the absence of IRIS and cryptococcomas) are generally contraindicated. Some authors have reported the utility of corticosteroid in the treatment of CME caused by *C. gattii*, although this literature is limited to case reports and series.[26]

Immune Reconstitution Inflammatory Syndrome

Immune reconstitution inflammatory syndrome (IRIS) was first recognized in AIDS patients with a variety of opportunistic infections, for whom disease symptoms recurred with improvement in immune function secondary to HAART. For patients with CME, IRIS results in an enhanced, but detrimental inflammation, often within the brain. This inflammation is characterized by an exaggerated proinflammatory response (i.e., Th1 and Th17 immunity) that begins days to weeks after the initiation of HAART.[27] *Cryptococcus*-associated IRIS has also been reported to occur in 5% to 14% of SOT recipients, typically occurring several weeks after initiation of antifungal therapy. IRIS in this cohort may result in the loss of graft function.[28] For these patients, cessation of calcineurin inhibitors has been identified as a risk factor. The manifestations of *Cryptococcus*-associated IRIS include a paradoxical worsening of CNS symptoms (i.e., new brain lesions, recurrent meningitis) and the unmasking of disease in organs not previously recognized to be affected (i.e., adenitis). Cryptococcal IRIS also occurs in SOT recipients and can result in the loss of allograft function. IRIS must be distinguished from failure of antifungal therapy. Both entities result in a recrudescence of symptoms, although treatment failure is associated with microbiologic failure, whereas with IRIS cultures are generally sterile. Some manifestations of CME-associated IRIS may resolve on their own. For more severe symptoms (including increased ICP and persistent symptoms), the addition of corticosteroids to antifungal therapy is recommended with a 2- to 6-week taper.[24]

Disease Prophylaxis/Prevention

Owing to the relatively low incidence of cryptococcosis in transplant recipients and children with malignancies, neither primary antifungal prophylaxis based on CD4 cell count nor screening with serum antigen testing is recommended to prevent disease.[18] Given the ubiquitous nature of the pathogen, it is difficult to prevent exposure; nonetheless, owning and/or breeding birds (e.g., pigeons, canaries, parakeets) may pose additional risk.

OTHER INVASIVE YEAST INFECTIONS

In addition to *Candida* and *Cryptococcus* spp., a variety of other yeasts have been found to cause serious, invasive disease in immunocompromised individuals. Because of their rarity, the precise incidence of these infections is difficult to define, but it is generally considered to

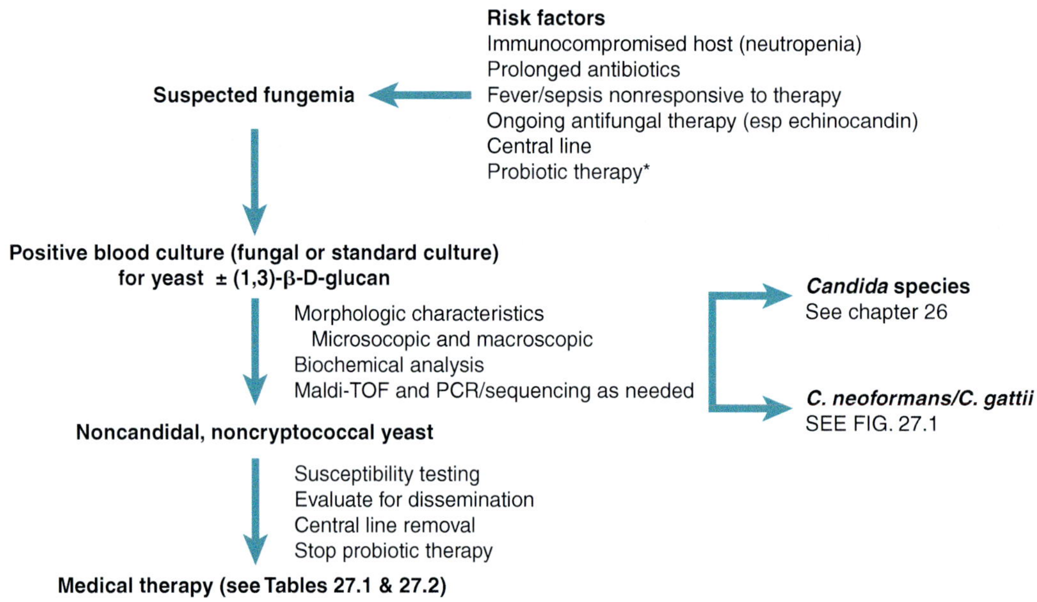

*Associated with *saccharomyces* infection

Fig. 27.3 Approach to the patient with fungemia. *esp*, especially; *MALDI-TOF*, matrix-assisted laser desorption/ionization time-of-flight mass spectrometry; *PCR*, polymerase chain reaction.

represent less than 5% of fungemias.[29] Likewise, the description of these infections (especially for children) is limited, consisting of case reports, case series, and systematic reviews of these series. Thus many of the features and treatment recommendations for these infections represent extrapolations from adult literature. These yeasts and the disease they cause tend to share several important epidemiologic and clinical characteristics (Fig. 27.3). These organisms are commonly found in the environment but also colonize humans, causing disease in the appropriate clinical context. Risk factors for these infections tend to be similar to those for invasive candidiasis including underlying immunosuppression, neutropenia, and the presence of a central line. Because of these epidemiologic similarities and their shared morphologic appearance, initial misidentification of these yeasts is common. The mortality from these invasive infections is generally high. Importantly, these infections often occur in the context of ongoing antifungal therapy (especially echinocandins), which should alert clinicians to the possibility of a noncandidal infection and antifungal resistance. Owing to the rarity of these infections, there are no randomized, controlled treatment studies. Removal of potentially infected central lines should be considered early in the course of disease. Initial therapeutic recommendations (Tables 27.1 and 27.2) are generally based on reports in the literature and historic patterns of susceptibility. Therapy is further complicated by the absence of standardized susceptibility cutoff values, and the observation that in vitro susceptibilities may not correlate with clinical response.

TABLE 27.1 Pathogen and Preferred Therapy

	ANTIFUNGAL SUSCEPTIBILITIES[37,a]			
Pathogen	**AMB**	**VCZ**	**5-FC**	**FLU**
Trichosporon spp.	+	++	[b]	–
Rhodotorula spp.	++	–	[b]	+
Saccharomyces spp.	++	+	[b]	++
Geotrichum spp.	++	++	–	–

[a]Based on extrapolation of breakpoints of fermentative yeast established by either the Clinical and Laboratory Standards Institute (CLSI)[42] or the European Committee on Antimicrobial Susceptibility Testing to determine susceptibilities.
[b]Consider in combination with amphotericn B.
5-FC, flucytosine; *AMB*, amphotericin B; *FLU*, fluconazole; *VCZ*, voriconazole; –, limited or no data available; + and ++, relative activity.

TRICHOSPORON SPECIES INFECTION

Epidemiology and Risk Factors

Trichosporon spp. belong to the phylum Basidiomycota and are commonly found in the environment but are also known to colonize humans. This fungus causes hair shaft infections (known as white piedra) and summer hypersensitivity pneumonitis in immunocompetent individuals. Although 50 trichosporon species have been identified, invasive disease is caused by a limited number of species. *T. asahii* (formerly known as *T. beigleii*) is the most common cause of invasive disease. Less commonly *T. mucoides*, *T. inkin*, and *T. asteroides* also cause invasive disease. *Trichosporon* spp. exhibit a variety of traits that contribute to its pathogenicity, including biofilm formation, protease secretion, and the production of glucuronoxylomannan, a polysaccharide that has been linked to cryptococcal virulence (reviewed in Colombo and colleagues[30]).

Case series and systematic reviews of adults suggest that hematologic malignancies (especially AML) are disproportionately associated with trichosporonosis, but disease may also occur in solid organ and stem cell transplant recipients as well as in patients with solid tumors.[31] In a recent review of pediatric trichosporonosis, ALL was the most common underlying diagnosis (47% of patients).[32] Affected patients have risk factors that are typical for invasive fungal diseases. This includes neutropenia, the presence of a central venous catheter, and recent antibiotic therapy. Peritonitis in patients receiving dialysis has also been described as has endocarditis in patients with prosthetic valves (reviewed in Colombo and colleagues[30]).

TABLE 27.2 Antifungal Considerations

Antifungal	Formulation	Interactions	Renal Impairment	Caution
Voriconazole	IV PO: Tablets and oral suspension	Substrate: • CYP2C19 • CYP2C9 • CYP3A4 Inhibits: • CYP2C19 • CYP2C9 • CYP3A4	None necessary unless <50 mL/min for the IV formulation	Patients with impaired renal function with a creatinine clearance <50 mL/min may have accumulation of cyclodextrin for the IV formulation; the manufacturer recommends to change to the oral formulation; • Goal trough: 1-5 mg/L
Fluconazole	IV PO: Tablets and oral suspension	Inhibits: • CYP2C19 • CYP2C9 • CYP3A4	• CrCl 10-50 mL/min per 1.73 m^2: Administer 50% of recommended dose at the normal interval. • CrCl ≤10 mL/min per 1.73 m^2: Administer 50% of recommended dose every 48 hours • Intermittent HD: 12 mg/kg per dose after HD • PD: 6 mg/kg per dose every 48 hours • Continuous renal replacement: 6 mg/kg per dose every 24 hours	
Amphotericin	IV		No renal adjustment issued by the manufacturer; however, patients with preexisting renal conditions	Premedicate with acetaminophen and diphenhydramine 30 to 60 min before the administration of the amphotericin. Use meperidine when necessary for rigors. Providers can use saline solution boluses to reduce the nephrotoxic affects.
Flucytosine	PO		• CrCl 30-50 mL/min per 1.73 m^2: 25-37.5 mg/kg per dose every 8 hours • CrCl 10-29 mL/min/1.73 m^2: 25-37.5 mg/kg per dose every 12 hours • CrCl <10 mL/min per 1.73 m^2: 25-37.5 mg/kg per dose every 24 hours • HD or PD: mL/min per 1.73 m^2: 25-37.5 mg/kg per dose every 24 hours • Continuous renal replacement therapy: mL/min per 1.73 m^2: 25-37.5 mg/kg per dose every 24 hours	

CrCl, creatine clearance; *HD*, hemodialysis*: IV*, intravenous; *PD*, peritoneal dialysis, *PO*, oral.
Data from Lexi-Drugs. Lexicomp. Wolters Kluwer Health, Inc. Riverwoods, IL. Available at: http://online.lexi.com. Accessed January 24, 2019.

Clinical Manifestations

Invasive trichosporonosis usually presents as fever with or without sepsis that is nonresponsive to antibiotics. As the organism is resistant to echinocandins, disease is often described in patients receiving echinocandin therapy. The initial detection may be as fungemia, but trichosporonosis can also be recognized because of dissemination to a specific organ system, including the skin, lungs, liver, and spleen. Urinary tract infections also occur. The mortality rate of invasive disease is extremely high, up to 58% in children.[32] Within the lung, trichosporon infection appears as a nodule(s), masses, or infiltrates.[33] The rash of invasive trichosporonosis is polymorphic and can be maculopapular, nodular, or vesicular. More recently, an inflammatory-mediated disease similar to hepatosplenic candidiasis has been described in association with *T. pullulans* infection.[34] With this syndrome, fungal dissemination is believed to occur while the patient is neutropenic, with symptoms occurring in association with neutrophil count recovery. Patients may have persistent fever and develop lesions in the liver or spleen.

Diagnosis

The gold standard for the diagnosis of trichosporonosis is a positive culture result from the infected site. The significance of positive culture results from nonsterile areas must be interpreted with caution because *Trichosporon* spp. are known colonizers. The most common source for a positive culture result is the blood. On standard solid culture media, the organism grows to produce cream to white yeastlike colonies. The organism produces hyphae, pseudohyphae, and barrel-shaped arthroconidia. This latter feature distinguishes it from *Candida* spp. These histopathologic elements and (occasionally blastoconidia) can be seen on microscopic examination of colonies and histopathologic examination of tissues. Unlike cryptococcosis, there are no reliable fungal serum antigen tests for diagnosing invasive trichosporonosis. Because of shared antigens with *Aspergillus* spp. and *Cryptococcus* spp., affected patients may at times have positive serum galactomannan and glucuronoxylomannan assays.[30] Furthermore, the organism does produce β-D-glucan, but at relatively low concentrations and elevated serum β-D-glucan levels are not a good marker of disease.[35] *Trichosporon* isolates can be identified by standard biochemical testing; however, species identification may not be possible using this technique. MALDI-TOF has been successfully used to rapidly identify and speciate trichosporon but is not available in all clinical microbiology laboratories.[18] In addition, PCR identification techniques in conjunction with sequencing (which is available through select reference laboratories) have been increasingly studied for the identification of *Trichosporon* spp. from both fixed and nonfixed tissues.[36]

Treatment

There are no breakpoints for the 17 medically relevant species of trichosporon. Most studies use the breakpoints of fermentative yeast established by either the Clinical & Laboratory Standards Institute or the European Committee on Antimicrobial Susceptibility Testing to determine susceptibilities.[37] As a class, these yeasts should be considered resistant to echinocandins. Furthermore, amphotericin susceptibility is variable. Among the antifungals, triazoles generally have the lowest minimum inhibitory concentrations with voriconazole being the most active agent and fluconazole and intraconazole being the least active. Furthermore, animal and human case reports have also shown the most favorable data in regard to clearance and survival with voriconazole.[38] Based on these findings, voriconazole is generally considered the drug of choice for invasive trichosporon. However, clinicians should be aware that variation in susceptibility to voriconazole exists across *Trichosporon* spp. and resistance to voriconazole by previously susceptible species is emerging. Furthermore, even with appropriate antifungal therapy, the mortality of invasive trichosporon disease is extremely high. In patients in whom the central line is considered the source of infection, strong consideration should be given to removing it.

RHODOTORULA SPECIES INFECTIONS

Epidemiology and Risk Factors

Rhodotorula spp. belong to the phylum Basidiomycota and produce a distinctive orange to salmon-colored colony when grown in culture. These organisms are found throughout the environment but can also colonize the skin, respiratory, gastrointestinal, and genitourinary tracts. *R. mucilaginosa* (formerly known *R. rubra*) is the most commonly implicated species, but *R. glutinis* and *R. minuta* also cause disease.[39] *Rhodotorula* spp. have been reported to be responsible for 0.5 % to 2.3 % of fungemias (reviewed in Wirth and Goldani[40]).

Clinical Manifestations

Fungemia is the most common form of rhodotorula disease and may be associated with sepsis and end-organ involvement. Dissemination to other organs, including the skin, liver, and urinary tract, may also occur.[39] *Rhodotorula* spp. may also cause an acute, subacute, or chronic meningoencephalitis in immunocompromised patients. The primary risk factor for infection appears to be the presence of a central venous catheter in patients with malignancy or recipients of a solid organ or hematopoietic stem cell transplant. Specific risk factors within this population include include broad-spectrum antibiotic exposure, neutropenia, receipt of parenteral nutrition, or exposure to immunosuppressive agents such as corticosteroids. The organism is typically resistant to echinocandins and fluconazole; therefore infection may occur in the context of ongoing antifungal prophylaxis with these agents.

Similar to *Trichosoporon* spp., *Rhodotorula* spp. can also cause localized infections (i.e., keratitis, peritonitis, and prosthetic joint infections) in the absence of underlying immunosuppression, likely related to direct inoculation of the organism and/or the presence of a foreign body.

Diagnosis

Growth on solid media remains the gold standard for the diagnosis of rhodotorula infections. The salmon-orange coloring of the colony is distinctive and assists in establishing a tentative diagnosis. The organism is most commonly isolated from blood cultures but can also be isolated from other sterile and nonsterile sites. Microscopic examination of the colony and affected tissues reveals round or oval yeasts without pseudohyphae or hyphae. Because the organism is commensal, determining the significance of growth from a nonsterile site must be done in the context of clinical symptoms. The utility of serum β-D-glucan testing in the diagnosis of rhodotorula infections has not been studied and false-negative results have been reported.[41] The genus can be distinguished from other yeasts using routine biochemical testing; however, species identification requires MALDI-TOF or PCR with sequencing.[18]

Treatment

Like the other yeasts described in this section, breakpoints for *Rhodotorula* spp. have not been defined, and thus most studies extrapolate from *Candida* and *Cryptococcus* spp. testing to define susceptibility. As a class this yeast should be considered resistant to echinocandins. Furthermore, susceptibility to azoles is variable with isavuconazole reported to be the most active agent.[42] Currently an amphotericin formulation with or without flucytosine is considered the therapy of choice for invasive rhodotorula infections. However, resistance to amphotericin has been described.[38] The best outcomes are often associated with source control such as removal of the central line in the setting of a central line–associated bloodstream infection.

SACCHAROMYCES SPECIES INFECTIONS

Epidemiology and Risk Factors

Saccharomyces species belong to the Ascomycota phylum and are genetically related to *Candida*. This organism is used in the food industry for fermentation and as a probiotic. They are also used to make recombinant proteins. *Saccharomyces* are known to colonize the respiratory, gastrointestinal, and genitourinary tracts. The species most commonly implicated in human disease is *S. cerevisiae*, also known as baker's or brewer's yeast. *S. boulardii*, a species frequently used in probiotic products, is considered a subtype of *S. cerevisiae*.[43] Although exposure to *Saccharomyces* through food products is common, disease is rare and is generally limited to high-inoculum exposures as with probiotics in the context of an impaired gastrointestinal or skin barrier in immunosuppressed patients. Infection after abdominal surgery or in patients with a central venous catheter has been reported, even in the absence of an exogeneous exposure. In addition, hospital outbreaks of saccharomyces infection infection have been described.[44] These reports support the fact that the organism can colonize patients and become opportunistic in the right clinical setting.

Clinical Manifestations

In a review of SOT and stem cell transplant recipients, the most common form of saccharomyces disease was fungemia with sepsis, but other forms of the disease have been reported, including pneumonia, endocarditis and liver abscess.[45] When compared with *S. cerevisiae* infections, *S. boulardii* infections are more closely linked to digestive tract disease, the presence of a central venous catheter, and intensive care unit admission. However, impaired immunity is more common among patients with *S. cerevisiae* infections.[43] In contrast to the other yeasts described in this section, *Saccharomyces* spp. are generally not resistant to echinocandins.

Diagnosis

The diagnosis of saccharomyces infection is made by isolation of the organism by culture from the affected site. The organism is most commonly isolated from blood but can also be grown from other infected tissue. When grown on solid media, the organism produces smooth, cream- to tan-colored colonies. Microscopically, the organism demonstrates several features that help distinguish it from other yeasts, including, multipolar budding, blastoconidia, and ascospores. The organism can be identified biochemically, but molecular techniques are needed to distinguish the subtype boulardii from other types.

Treatment

An amphotericin formulation is generally considered the drug of choice for *Saccharomyces* spp. Infections,[38] Flucytosine has been added in some patients with severe disease.[46] Removal of a central venous catheter should be considered and probiotics therapy should be discontinued. There are currently no standards for breakpoints for *Saccharomyces* spp. from the Clinical & Laboratory Standards Institute and the European Committee on Antimicrobial Susceptibility Testing. Variable susceptibility to the azoles has been reported.[46] Although echinocandins generally have good activity against *Saccharomyces* spp., resistance mutations can occur.

GEOTRICHUM SPP. INFECTIONS

Epidemiology and Risk Factors

Geotrichum spp. belong to the Ascomycota phylum, and like the other yeasts discussed in this section, are widely distributed in the environment. Humans can be colonized and invasive disease occurs in individuals with risk factors for invasive yeast infections. The taxonomy of *Geotrichum* has been revised so that 2 clinically relevant species previously classified as *Geotrichum* (*G. capitatum* and *G. clavatum*) are now classified as *Magnusiomyces capitatus* and *Saprochaete clavata,* respectively.[47] The third clinically relevant organism is *G. candidum*. Reports of invasive disease are mainly from Europe.[31] Prolonged neutropenia is an important risk factor for disease, and invasive infection has been reported in a range of diseases, including AML, ALL, hematopoietic stem cell transplantation, SOT, high-dose steroids, chronic granulomatous disease, and diabetes mellitus.

Clinical Presentation

Infections with these yeasts generally present with fever and sepsis with multiorgan involvement, including lung, liver, kidney, skin, or the CNS. The mortality from these infections is typically reported to exceed 60% of affected patients.[48]

Diagnosis

Culture (usually blood) is the gold standard in making a diagnosis of geotrichum infection. Results of serum β-D-glucan and galactomannan assays have been reported to be positive in individual case reports, but the overall utility of tests in the diagnosis of these infections is unknown.[49] Furthermore, biochemical profiles may not be reliable in distinguishing these yeasts from each other and from other yeasts. However, both MALDI-TOF and DNA sequencing have been reported as helpful in this regard.[18]

Treatment

An amphotericin formulation with or without flucytosine is the recommended empiric therapy for these infections.[38] Voriconazole and isavuconazole generally have good activity in vitro and may also be useful in therapy. There have also been case reports describing, with varying degrees of success, combination therapy with voriconazole and caspofungin, as well as sequential use of liposomal amphotericin and an azole.[50]

28

Histoplasmosis, Blastomycosis, and Coccidioidomycosis

John C. Christenson, MD and Thomas G. Fox, MD

Histoplasmosis, blastomycosis, and coccidioidomycosis are the most common endemic mycoses in North America. Their geographic distribution encompasses close to two-thirds of the United States and parts of Canada, Mexico, Central and South America, and Africa. *Histoplasma capsulatum*, *Blastomyces dermatitidis*, *Coccidioides immitis*, and *C. posadasii* are dimorphic fungi that grow as yeast in the human body and as a mycelial form in the environment. Infections occur as a result of exposures to contaminated environments. Although most infections result in a subclinical process, higher-inoculum exposures and infections in immunocompromised hosts can result in severe life-threatening conditions. Most immunocompromised patients affected by these pathogens are adults. Limited pediatric data are available for various aspects of the epidemiology, risk factors, clinical manifestations, and treatment. Recommendations have been mostly extrapolated from adult studies and anecdotal clinical experiences.

EPIDEMIOLOGY OF ENDEMIC MYCOSES

Most infections involve the respiratory tract. Symptomatic extrapulmonary disease is more likely in immunocompromised individuals, which is more likely to lead to hospitalization. A retrospective cohort using a nationwide database of hospital admissions for 2002 estimated that 332 pediatric patients with symptomatic endemic mycoses were hospitalized in the United States, at a rate of 4.6 cases per 1 million with a mortality rate of 5%, compared with 6003 adults at a rate of 28.7 cases per million population and a mortality rate of 7%. Hospitalized children with histoplasmosis were more likely to have an immunodeficiency than adults: 32% versus 14%, respectively. The database provided geographic information confirming prior observations that coccidioidomycosis is most likely to be observed in the West, whereas blastomycosis and histoplasmosis usually occurs in the Midwest and southern states. Although distinctive geographic regions are associated with specific endemic mycoses, in recent years many cases have appeared in areas outside their usual regions, such as blastomycosis in Oregon and Colorado; histoplasmosis in Idaho, California, and New Mexico; and coccidioidomycosis in Washington State. Clinicians will need a greater index of suspicion when evaluating patients with signs and symptoms compatible with endemic mycoses, even in the absence of travel to or residence in traditional endemic regions. When considering a diagnosis of endemic mycoses in a patient with pulmonary disease, several factors need to considered, such as residence or travel to an endemic region, occupation, hobbies and leisure activities, the presence of birds and bats in dwellings, demolition of old structures, excavation or soil tilling, and animal exposures.

A retrospective study of 30 transplant patients with histoplasmosis or blastomycosis at 3 midwestern medical centers between 1996 and 2008 demonstrated a cumulative incidence of infection of 0.5%.[1] A majority (73%) had undergone renal transplantation and were receiving multiple immunosuppressive agents, including corticosteroids. The median time from transplant to infection was approximately 10 months. As expected, the lungs were the most common site of infection. Sixty percent of patients had disseminated disease. A mortality rate of 13% was attributable to infection. Among the 22 patients with histoplasmosis, the median time from onset of symptoms to diagnosis was 30 days (range 4 to 42 days), whereas for blastomycosis it was 14 days (range 3 to 90 days). Graft loss was reported in 27% of patients.

Endemic mycoses are often overlooked as a cause of community-acquired pneumonia. A delay in diagnosis and treatment may result in severe disease in an immunocompromised host such as those affected by human immunodeficiency virus (HIV)/AIDS. In the case of blastomycosis, pulmonary findings on chest radiographs may resemble a bacterial etiology because lobar consolidation is a common feature. Nodular infiltrates may be seen in severe cases. Mediastinal or hilar adenopathy and pleural effusions are less common in blastomycosis. Diffuse reticulonodular or miliary infiltrates along with mediastinal and hilar adenopathies and eventual calcifications are seen in disseminated or severe histoplasmosis, as well as in tuberculosis.

An increased risk of fungal and mycobacterial infections is reported in patients receiving tumor necrosis factor (TNF) inhibitors.[2] Histoplasmosis represents 60% of reported fungal infections in this group, and coccidioidomycosis and blastomycosis 10% and 4%, respectively.

Endemic mycoses are rare in solid organ transplant (SOT) patients. In one study, infection developed in only 33 patients among 16,806 patients who had undergone an SOT; the most common infection was histoplasmosis.[3] However, invasive endemic mycoses can be a major cause of morbidity and mortality in kidney transplant patients, resulting in 41% graft failures and a fatality rate of 19%.[4] Coccidioidomycosis was responsible for graft failures in 67% of patients. The use of antithymocyte globulin, diabetes mellitus, and age were also risk factors for infection. The risk of infection may persist for years after transplantation.

HISTOPLASMOSIS

Epidemiology and Risk Factors

Histoplasmosis is the most common pulmonary and systemic mycosis in humans and affects millions of people.[5] The highest incidence was found in residents of the Ohio-Mississippi-Missouri, the St. Lawrence, and the Rio Grande river valleys. From 2001 to 2012, histoplasmosis-associated hospitalizations in the United States were estimated to be 50,778.[6] Infection rates were lowest in persons younger than18 years. The significance of *H. capsulatum* as a cause of opportunistic infection has escalated in proportion to the increasing numbers of individuals who are immunosuppressed. An increase in hospitalizations has been observed in transplant recipients and in those receiving biologic agents.

The optimal conditions for *H. capsulatum* var. *capsulatum* to survive in the environment are moist, nitrogen-rich soils at temperatures of 37°C or higher. *H. duboisii,* the cause of African histoplasmosis, is a variant of *H. capsulatum.* Infections caused by *H. capsulatum* var. *duboisii* have been described across central and western Africa.

The majority of illnesses occur sporadically and are not associated with exposure to a specific site or specific activity. Infection rates are higher in summer months when persons are more likely to be outdoors in conditions that favor the aerosolization of spores. Asymptomatic infections are common in children and are usually clinically unrecognized. Regions with high rates of infection are considered endemic. Implicated sites have included blackbird and pigeon roosting areas, chicken houses, bat-infested caves, attics, chimneys, old structures, and decaying woodpiles and trees. Activities that disturb these areas have been implicated in localized outbreaks. Infections in children have been associated with exploring caves, playing in barns or hollow trees, silos, cleaning abandoned buildings, cutting firewood or decayed tree stumps, renovation of older homes, and digging in contaminated sites. Contact with these areas must be avoided by the immunocompromised person.

In a large outbreak in Indianapolis, Indiana, affecting an estimated 100,000 individuals, illnesses were identified in 435 individuals (including 49 children <15 years of age), and disseminated disease developed in 46.[7] In reported outbreaks, 51% of cases occurred among children with a majority associated with common source exposures in schools. Rarely, infections occur in nonendemic areas and may result from reactivation of quiescent infection in patients who become immunosuppressed.

Mother-infant transmission with resulting dissemination has been documented after exposure to TNF-α blocker therapy. Transmission has been confirmed in the recipients of 2 cadaveric organs from a donor who had resided in an endemic area.

Antibodies against the organism are measurable approximately 1 month after infection, but these play no major role in controlling infection. Cell-mediated immune response is key in controlling fungal growth and provides a degree of protection against reinfection. *H. capsulatum* replicates within macrophages until T lymphocytes are activated. Granuloma formation occurs in response to infection of macrophages. The release of proinflammatory cytokines and chemokines is required for the development of a protective immune response. Reinfection usually results from reexposure; recurrences have shorter incubation periods and are generally milder than primary infections. Recrudescence of latent infection has been documented in recipients of transplanted organs from infected donors, and in people receiving corticosteroids or TNF-α inhibitors.

The length of the incubation period of histoplasmosis varies inversely with the size of the inoculum, the integrity of the host immune response, and the presence of immunity from previous infection. The range of incubation periods is reported to be 1 to 3 weeks in nonimmune hosts. Because most infections occur sporadically and are either asymptomatic or result in nonspecific and self-limited flu-like illnesses that are not diagnosed, the upper range may be longer. In patients who retain specific protective T-cell immunity from previous infection, reexposure results in milder symptoms and shorter incubation periods. A proportion of individuals with primary or acquired cellular immune dysfunction are more likely to experience symptomatic illness after exposure.

Granulomas appear after the development of an effective acquired immune response. Inflammation ultimately progresses to fibrosis and often is accompanied by calcification. The rate of calcification is age dependent, and it may occur within months in children and over several years in adults. Exuberant granulomatous inflammation or fibrosis or both can result in obstruction or dysfunction of adjacent mediastinal or, less commonly, abdominal structures. In areas endemic for histoplasmosis, old granulomas in the lung, bone marrow, or other sites may be seen as incidental findings. In patients with disseminated histoplasmosis, especially those with preexisting cellular immune dysfunction, or in otherwise healthy infants, the inflammatory response is impaired and granuloma formation is poor, leading to extensive parasitization of macrophages by yeasts. Many organ systems are often involved.

The use of antithymocyte globulin as part of a rejection prevention regimen is associated with severe histoplasmosis in kidney transplant patients.

Clinical Manifestations

Histoplasmosis begins as an acute inflammatory pneumonitis and undergoes self-limited or progressive dissemination. Aside from patients with known preexisting conditions or those receiving therapy that impairs immune function, all patients with serious disseminated disease, persistent antigenuria after completion of therapy, relapse, or recurrent infections should undergo comprehensive assessment of immune function. Most symptoms of acute primary histoplasmosis are mild, self-limited, and undifferentiated resembling a flu-like illness with cough, myalgia, headache, and variable low-grade fever, with a resolution in 3 to 5 days. After a more significant fungal exposure, fever, myalgia, chills, persistent cough, and nonpleuritic chest pain may last as long as 2 weeks. Fatigue and weight loss improve slowly after the fever resolves. In about 5% of children, symptoms are subacute, persisting longer than 2 weeks.

Pericardial effusion, hypercalcemia, and mediastinal and abdominal manifestations resulting from irritation, compression, or destruction of structures adjacent to infected lymph nodes and granulomas are well described. Osteomyelitis and central nervous system (CNS) infections are unusual manifestations of histoplasmosis in healthy, older children. Hepatosplenomegaly occasionally is present, although its occurrence should raise suspicion of the early onset of progressive dissemination. Rheumatologic manifestations, including erythema nodosum, erythema multiforme, and polyarthropathy, can occur.

Acute primary infections after a high-inoculum exposure results in a diffuse pneumonitis associated with severe symptoms, particularly dyspnea or adult respiratory distress syndrome (ARDS) early in the infection. This may lead to dissemination with a high risk of progression. This presentation resembles the clinical picture observed in immunocompromised hosts with severe disease.

The appearance of intrathoracic and, less commonly intraabdominal, lymphadenitis can mimic malignant tumors. These are mostly seen when acute primary infections are accompanied by fever, weight loss, and masses visible on chest radiograph (mediastinal adenitis) or computed tomographic (CT) scans. The presence of mediastinal lymphadenopathy in the absence of any recognized clinical symptoms often requires definitive diagnosis to exclude a neoplasm, especially lymphoma. Complications of acute primary histoplasmosis are mostly seen when granulomatous lymphadenitis results in inflammation, compression, or obstruction of contiguous structures within the thorax, such as trachea, bronchi, pulmonary vasculature, vena cava, nerves, and lymphatics (mediastinal granuloma). In rare instances, this granulomatous inflammation may progress to the formation of a dense irreversible fibrosis, resulting in stenosis, obstruction, or malfunction of contiguous critical mediastinal structures. Fibrosing mediastinitis does not respond to antifungal therapy or antiinflammatory agents. This condition is rare in children. Constrictive pericarditis and cavitary histoplasmosis are also rarely observed in children.

Disseminated Histoplasmosis

Fungal dissemination that occurs early in infection is almost always self-limited in normal individuals. The term "progressive disseminated histoplasmosis" is applied to instances of continued and overwhelming reticuloendothelial infection and is fatal if untreated. The clinical entity is defined as an illness that is accompanied by active replication of *H. capsulatum* in multiple organ systems. This manifestation often suppresses cellular immune function in previously immunocompetent hosts and is a common opportunistic infection in individuals with acquired or congenital cellular immune dysfunction.[8]

Disseminated histoplasmosis may result from exogenous exposure of a susceptible or immune-impaired host or from reactivation of endogenous quiescent foci of infection. Although reactivation of infection may occur in an immunosuppressed host, epidemiologic data in immunosuppressed individuals who reside in areas highly endemic for histoplasmosis favor a new episode of exogenous exposure as the most common mechanism. Rates of disseminated histoplasmosis in immunocompromised patients increase only during periods in which infection rates increase in the general population and do not increase in interepidemic periods.[9]

In a single-center retrospective analysis of pediatric patients with histoplasmosis, 16 patients (22%) were immunocompromised, with 5 affected by malignancy receiving chemotherapy, whereas others were receiving TNF-α inhibitors and corticosteroids.[10] Disseminated and pulmonary disease affected 56% and 44% of patients, respectively. Cough, fever, fatigue, shortness of breath, and weight loss were common complaints. Immunocompromised patients had longer hospitalizations when compared with non-immunocompromised patients. Children with disseminated disease were also more likely to have antigenemia and antigenuria. Pneumonia with a rapid progression to marked hypoxemia and an ARDS-like picture is not uncommon in the immunosuppressed host with severe histoplasmosis. Fevers, chills, fatigue, anorexia, weight loss, and hepatosplenomegaly are features suggestive of disseminated disease.[11]

CNS involvement is well recognized in patients with disseminated histoplasmosis. Clinical manifestations are varied and include chronic meningitis and arachnoiditis, hydrocephalus, focal parenchymal lesions, cerebellar ataxia, cranial nerve neuropathy, vasculitis, stroke, and/or diffuse encephalitis.

Unusual manifestations of histoplasmosis, especially in patients with disseminated disease, include skin and oral lesions, terminal ileitis, colonic ulcerations, adrenal involvement with insufficiency, endocarditis, genitourinary ulcerations, arthritis, osteomyelitis, sepsis-like syndrome, and superior vena cava syndrome.

Histoplasmosis-induced hemophagocytic syndrome is a well-recognized complication. It is a lethal complication of histoplasmosis observed in immunocompromised patients. Cytopenias, splenomegaly, and hyperferritinemia are clinical markers of the disease. Response to therapy can be measured by a reduction in ferritin levels.[12]

Histoplasmosis in Oncology Patients

A retrospective review of 57 children with acute histoplasmosis at a pediatric oncology center provides a comprehensive view of the clinical spectrum of disease in children with cancer. A majority of patients had acute lymphocytic leukemia (64%). Ten patients were identified with acute pulmonary disease, and 23 (with 26 episodes) with disseminated disease. Most of the children with acute pulmonary histoplasmosis were not neutropenic at the onset of symptoms. Fever was the most common clinical feature with acute pulmonary and disseminated histoplasmosis, present in 60% and 96% of patients, respectively. Bilateral lung disease was observed in 9 of 13 patients. Nodular infiltrates were present in one-half of the patients with chest radiographs, whereas isolated hilar adenopathy or masses were observed in only two patients. Chest CT demonstrated parenchymal lung disease in 8 and hilar adenopathy in 5. Findings were not suggestive of invasive aspergillosis. The diagnosis of histoplasmosis was based on clinical findings and histopathologic features of lung biopsies in 60% of patients. Liver enzyme and serum lactate dehydrogenase levels were elevated in one-third of patients. No deaths were attributable to histoplasmosis. However, cancer therapy had to be delayed in several of the patients.

In the children with disseminated disease, clinical features, epidemiology, and laboratory findings were similar to those with acute pulmonary disease. Most patients were not neutropenic at the time of the diagnosis. One-third of patients had mediastinal adenopathy and masses compatible with granulomatous disease. Fifteen of 26 patients had positive blood culture results for *H. capsulatum* using lysis centrifugation tubes. In addition, detection of antigen in urine and histopathologic findings in bone marrow and tissue helped support the diagnosis. Of interest, in only 8 of 26 patients was histoplasmosis suspected before diagnosis. The mean time between onset of symptoms and diagnosis was 18.6 ± 8.2 days. The overall mortality for patients with disseminated disease was 26%. Inactive histoplasmosis was found in a group of children with solid tumors. In a cohort of patients with newly diagnosed solid tumors, inactive histoplasmosis was found in 48% of them at the time of diagnosis.

Histoplasmosis in Transplant Patients

Infections with endemic mycoses are rare in children who have undergone SOT; no histoplasmosis infections were documented among 584 children with SOTs during a 13 year-study period. Histoplasmosis usually occurs in the first 18 months after transplant.[13] In organ transplant patients, the most common clinical feature of histoplasmosis is prolonged fevers.

In a study at three medical centers in the midwestern United States, 22 adult transplant patients were affected by histoplasmosis.[1] Sixty-four percent of patients had a renal transplant, whereas 36% had liver transplant, and 14% had pancreas transplant. Some patients had multiple organs transplanted with some receiving more than one organ. Ninety-five percent of patients were receiving two or more immunosuppressive agents. Corticosteroids were administered to 73% of patients. The majority of patients (77%) had pulmonary disease, with disseminated disease developing in 64%; a majority (95%) had positive culture result, most often from bronchoalveolar lavage (BAL) or blood. Urine antigen assays were positive in 91% of patients. Two patients (9%) died from the infection, whereas 5 (23%) had graft loss.

Between 2001 and 2006, the Transplant-Associated Infection Surveillance Network identified 52 transplant patients with histoplasmosis.[3] A majority had an SOT, mostly kidney or liver. Disseminated disease was recognized in one-third of patients, whereas pulmonary plus dissemination was documented in another one-third. Disease limited to the lungs was noted in 36% of patients. A majority of patients were receiving 2 or more immunosuppressive agents, including corticosteroids. Fifty-three percent of patients had positive blood culture results, whereas 35% of BAL/sputum specimens were positive. Of interest, serum and urine antigen assays were used to make the diagnosis in 25% and 57% of patients, respectively.

Histoplasmosis is a serious complication of kidney transplantation. Among infected patients documented between 1994 and 2014, graft failure was documented in 21% of patients.

In another study, moderate-to-severe disease was documented in 96% of transplant patients.[14] Fever, cough, and diarrhea were present in 87%, 39%, and 35% of patients, respectively. Urine *Histoplasma* antigen assay results were positive in 95% of patients. Interstitial and alveolar infiltrates were documented in 63% of patients, with a miliary pattern was observed in only 6% of transplant patients, in contrast to recipients of TNF-α inhibitors, in whom a miliary pattern was documented in 44% of patients. The overall mortality rate in transplant was 9%.

A study of SOT patients from 24 institutions determined that 81% of recipients had disseminated disease, with 28% requiring admission to intensive care units.[15] Of 152 patients with histoplasmosis, 10% died, with 72% of deaths occurring in the first month of diagnosis. The median time from transplant to diagnosis was 27 months, with disease diagnosed in 34% of patients in the first year after transplant.

At another institution, disseminated histoplasmosis was documented in six children with kidney transplants, with one-third of patients presenting in the first year after transplantation. No deaths resulted from these infections. In five of the patients, cytopenia was evidence of dissemination. Five of the patients had received induction with thymoglobulin and steroids.[8]

Diagnosis

The early diagnosis of histoplasmosis in an immunosuppressed host can be achieved only if there is high clinical suspicion of the condition. A thorough consideration of the epidemiology preceding the onset of symptoms and key clinical features are essential in making a diagnosis. Distinguishing histoplasmosis from other fungal infections can be challenging. In patients with disseminated disease, elevated lactate dehydrogenase levels, liver enzymes, especially alkaline phosphatase, and erythrocyte sedimentation rate are commonly present. An elevated aspartate aminotransferase/alanine aminotransferase ratio is suggestive of disseminated histoplasmosis. A markedly elevated ferritin level and pancytopenia are frequently present in disseminated disease.

Medical Imaging

The radiographic findings seen most commonly in children with histoplasmosis are not pathognomonic and may mimic the findings seen in tuberculosis or other granulomatous processes and, in some instances, neoplastic conditions, especially lymphoma. CT is highly sensitive and likely to reveal parenchymal infiltrates that are not visualized in plain radiographs. The most common pulmonary parenchymal changes are "soft" single or multiple, poorly defined areas of airspace consolidation often found in the basilar portions of the lungs. Immunocompromised hosts with evidence of dissemination are likely to have a diffuse pneumonitis pattern (Fig. 28.1).

The appearance of enlarged hilar/mediastinal nodes, either in association with pulmonary infiltrates or as isolated findings, also is a common radiographic finding of acute pulmonary histoplasmosis. Low signal intensity within nodes is often observed. Infected nodes may enlarge and compress or obstruct adjacent structures. Isolated calcifications may be seen in the spleen or liver months to years after infection.

Histopathology

In clinical and epidemiologic settings compatible with histoplasmosis, observation of 2- to 4-μm typical yeast forms (Fig. 28.2) in histopathologic specimens demonstrating granulomatous inflammation is strong supportive evidence of histoplasmosis. Caution is merited because intracellular pathogens such as *Toxoplasma gondii*, *B. dermatitidis*, yeast forms of *Cryptococcus neoformans*, and spherules of *C. immitis* may resemble the yeast forms of *H. capsulatum*. Both Giemsa- and hematoxylin-eosin–stained specimens may reveal intracellular yeasts in sputum, blood smears, bone marrow aspirates, and biopsy specimens. The Gomori methenamine silver stain is the most sensitive reagent.

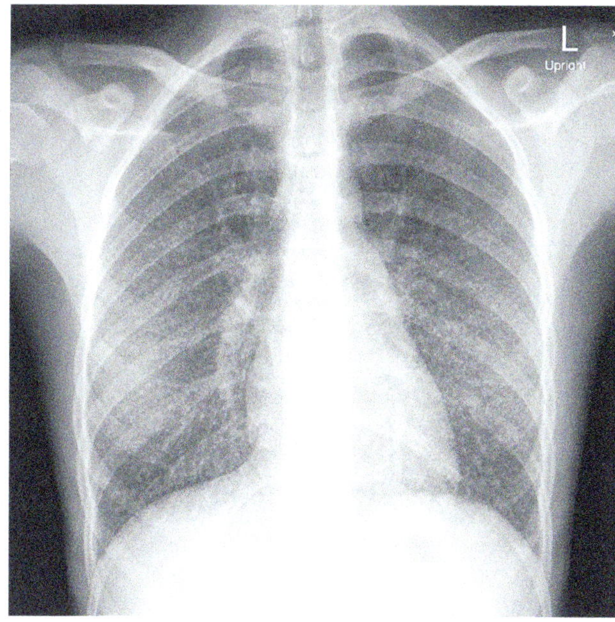

Fig. 28.1 Diffuse pneumonitis in an adolescent with disseminated histoplasmosis

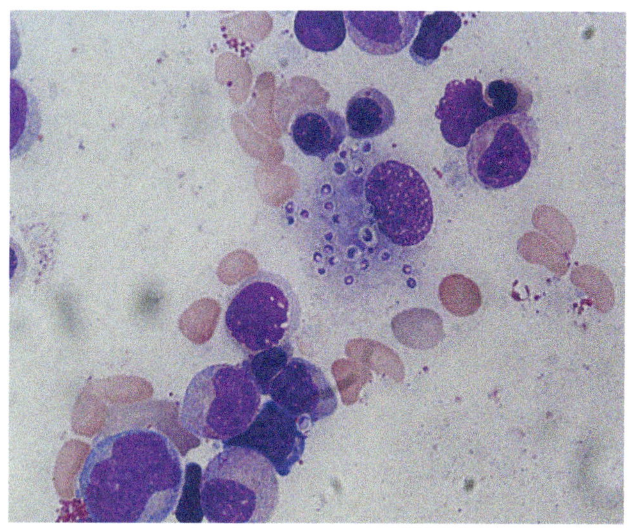

Fig. 28.2 Yeast forms of *Histoplasma capsulatum* in bone marrow of patient with disseminated histoplasmosis. Hematoxylin-eosin stain.

Culture

Recovery of *H. capsulatum* from a clinical specimen obtained from a symptomatic patient with a compatible illness confirms the diagnosis of active histoplasmosis. Normally, sterile specimens and minced or homogenized tissue can be inoculated onto suitable media, usually Sabouraud glucose (dextrose) agar. Mycelial growth of a white-to-tan mold has the highest specificity, with confirmation by use of DNA probe. Along with cultures, histologic examination of infected tissue can be a complementary test in the diagnosis of histoplasmosis. The optimal method for recovery of *H. capsulatum* from blood is the lysis-centrifugation technique. Culture results are positive in 75% to 85% of patients with disseminated disease. In the latter patients, sites from which *H. capsulatum* commonly is recovered include the lower respiratory tract, blood, bone marrow, cerebrospinal fluid (CSF), liver, spleen, skin lesions, and synovium of affected joints. The highest yield is from bone marrow. In adults with disseminated histoplasmosis, rates of positive lysis-centrifugation cultures of peripheral blood are 90% to 100% in acute dissemination.

In children, culture plus staining of BAL fluid has been rewarding in diagnosing high–fungal burden infections in patients with HIV, but it is less sensitive than lung biopsy in other immunocompromised patients, especially those receiving chemotherapy for reticuloendothelial malignancy.

Serology

Serologic methods are frequently used to make the diagnosis of histoplasmosis. The detection of antibodies by immunodiffusion (ID) and complement fixation (CF) have equal sensitivity (75% to 85%); however, ID is slightly more specific (>95% vs. 85% to 90%).[16] In immunocompetent patients, either or both test results are positive in 95% of patients with acute primary pulmonary infection. CF titers often become positive 2 to 4 weeks earlier, usually within 4 to 6 weeks after exposure.[17] When the ID test is reactive, however, it remains so for a longer period of time. In addition to the 4- to 6-week lag in developing elevated titers, an important limitation of both serologic assays is their reduced sensitivity in immunosuppressed patients. Only 50% of immunosuppressed children and adults with disseminated histoplasmosis are seropositive.[18]

A 4-fold increase between acute and convalescent sera provides the best serologic evidence of recent infection. The individual yeast (CF-Y) and mycelial (CF-M) phases are measured. The CF-Y phase is more sensitive than the CF-M phase when performed in a patient with a recent or active infection. In highly endemic areas, background low-titer CF serologic reactions may be present. The titer of antibody by the complement fixation test is directly proportional to severity of illness and degree of exposure.[19]

The ID method detects precipitins (reported as bands) against the H and M glycoprotein antigens of *H. capsulatum.* The H band is present infrequently in patients with histoplasmosis; when seen, it is transient and its presence suggests active infection. In patients with active pulmonary histoplasmosis, one-half to three-fourths have an M band alone. The H band is present in only 10% to 20% of acute infections, and only 10% of individuals have both M and H bands present. The presence of both is highly suggestive of active histoplasmosis. Only approximately 50% of patients with disseminated disease have a positive M band.

A newer enzyme immunoassay that measures *Histoplasma* immunoglobulin (Ig) M and IgG antibodies appears to have demonstrably higher sensitivity than CF and ID.[20]

Cross-reactivity with other fungal antigens affects CF and ID assays. CF cross-reactivity occurs most commonly with *B. dermatitidis* (40%) and *C. immitis* (16%). Cross-reactions also occur, albeit rarely, with candidiasis, tuberculosis, aspergillosis, and cryptococcosis. Single titers of 1: 32 or higher performed by an experienced laboratory are strong supportive evidence of acute or recent infection, especially when the accompanying clinical symptoms are compatible. However, patients with non-*Histoplasma* febrile pneumonia may have false-positive CF titers. However, other laboratory and clinical data should be considered when making the diagnosis of histoplasmosis. A low CF titer of a person living in an endemic region is not diagnostic.

The serologic diagnosis of patients with isolated meningitis caused by *H. capsulatum* often is problematic because no single test exhibits high sensitivity. CF and ID results can be positive in CSF, but one-half of patients with other chronic fungal meningeal infections may show false-positive results. CF-M antibody appeared to be the most sensitive and specific test for the diagnosis of meningitis caused by histoplasmosis. However, a recent study demonstrated that the combined use of *Histoplasma* antigen assay and anti-*Histoplasma* IgG or IgM antibody assay detected 98% of cases of *Histoplasma* meningitis.[21]

Antigen Detection

Antigen detection is most sensitive in infections accompanied by high fungal burdens. Antigen detection assays on serum, urine, or other selected body fluids provide a rapid, accurate, noninvasive diagnostic result for the most serious manifestations of disease. It is especially useful for the evaluation of infections in immunocompromised hosts, in whom serologic method results often are negative. In immunocompromised hosts and patients with primary pulmonary infection, the detection of antigen reflects the early hematogenous dissemination that occurs before being aborted by an effective cellular immune response.

The sensitivity of urine antigen detection in patients with acute primary pulmonary infection surpasses 75%, with the highest rates seen in patients tested within a few weeks of exposure, in those with large inoculum exposure, and in patients with extensive pulmonary involvement. The sensitivity of antigen detection is very high in patients with disseminated disease, where antigen is detected in 91% of immunosuppressed patients. In children with disseminated disease, urinary antigen testing was positive in 100 percent. Although *Histoplasma* antigen can be detected in serum, the sensitivity is substantially less than that of urine. Antigen often is found in BAL fluid of patients after high-inoculum exposure to histoplasmal spores and in immunocompromised patients with hematogenous dissemination and lung involvement.[22] Inactive histoplasmosis consisting of calcified hilar nodes or liver granulomas universally have negative antigen assay results, whereas patients with untreated severe disseminated disease always have positive urine and serum antigen assay results. In a group of immunocompromised children, higher rates of antigenemia and antigenuria were observed compared with non-immunocompromised children, along with longer durations.[9]

A multicenter study of an *H. capsulatum* antigen detection assay demonstrated a higher sensitivity in immunocompromised hosts compared with immunocompetent patients. Antigenuria was detected in approximately 92% of patients with disseminate histoplasmosis, approximately 84% of patients with acute histoplasmosis, and approximately 30% of patients with subacute histoplasmosis.[23] Antigenemia was present in 100% of patients with disseminated histoplasmosis. Cross-reactivity was observed in 90% of patients with blastomycosis. Specificity of the assay was 90%.

Variations in sensitivity have been reported between commercially available antigen detection assays. These are not considered interchangeable as they are not comparable.[24]

Cross-reactivity between the various endemic mycoses is well recognized; therefore epidemiology, clinical features, and geographic exposures should be factors in determining which mycosis is most likely.

In addition to its usefulness in diagnosis, an antigen assay provides a quantitative parameter with which to assess the pace and adequacy of response to therapy and, thereafter, a sensitive monitor that promptly detects relapse in patients who are at high risk for recurrence. Antigen concentration decreases during effective therapy. Failure of the antigen concentration to decline or documentation of progressive increase may indicate treatment failure. Persistent but decreasing concentrations of antigenuria may be present after completion of an appropriate and effective course of antifungal therapy. Patients who have completed appropriate courses of therapy for serious infections and have had resolution of their clinical symptoms yet demonstrated persistent but decreasing concentrations of antigenuria have fared well after the completion of the planned course of antifungal therapy. Residual excretion of urine antigen after adequate treatment continues to decrease and eventually ceases; monitoring is recommended to confirm resolution of antigenuria.[25] The persistence of moderate antigenuria has been associated with a risk for recrudescence.

If urine concentration is too high and unable to quantitate, monitoring is more informative if antigen concentrations of serum are initially followed because concomitant serum concentrations are lower than those of concomitant urine samples and more likely to be within the range in which differences in concentration could be measured accurately. Thereafter, when antigenemia is resolved, urine concentrations can be followed with the quantitative assay. Testing should be performed routinely at 3- to 4-month intervals during treatment, at the end of therapy, if symptoms recur, and periodically for another year to monitor for relapse.

Molecular Testing

Polymerase chain reaction (PCR) methodology has been evaluated for identifying *H. capsulatum* in tissue and body fluids, but false-negative results were encountered in one-third of specimens. PCR methodology used with clinical specimens (urine, serum, BAL, CSF) containing urine antigen showed specificities of 80% to 100% but sensitivities of only 0 to 22%. In situ hydridization of tissue appears to be a valuable tool in evaluating cutaneous lesions in patients with endemic mycoses. Real-time PCR can detect the presence of *B. dermatitidis* and *H. capsulatum* in cultures and clinical specimens with high specificities, 99% and 100%, respectively. Sensitivities are somewhat lower: 73% for *H capsulatum*, and 86% for *B. dermatitidis*.

Other Assays

In cancer patients undergoing stem cell transplantation and found with pulmonary nodular opacities, false-positive galactomannan assay results may result in delays in initiating effective therapy for disseminated histoplasmosis. Clinicians must be aware of this problem, especially if caring for patients in endemic regions.

Testing of patients with histoplasmosis and blastomycosis may result in a positive (1,3)-β-D-glucan assay. However, caution is merited if this assay is used as a screening test because many patients with blastomycosis are likely to have a negative assay result. However, even though the assay appears to reliably detect individuals with disseminated histoplasmosis, *H. capsulatum*–specific antigen assays are more sensitive and specific and can be used reliably to assess response to therapy. (1,3)-β-D-Glucan was measured in the CSF of patients with CNS histoplasmosis. The sensitivity of the assay was found to be approximately 53% with a specificity of approximately 87%. Compared with other CNS fungal infections, the specificity was just 46%.

Treatment

Immunocompromised patients with histoplasmosis require antifungal therapy. They are more likely to have symptomatic and disseminated disease. Incidental findings of calcified granulomas in lungs, mediastinum, and/or liver-spleen represent inactive ("old") histoplasmosis and will not benefit from antifungal therapy. Evidence-based, consensus practice guidelines for treatment of histoplasmosis have been published and include recommendations for treatment of children (Table 28.1).[26]

TABLE 28.1 Treatment of Histoplasmosis

Disease Manifestation	Treatment	Comments
Acute pulmonary histoplasmosis Moderately severe or severe	LAB[a]: 3-5 mg/kg per day IV for 1-2 wk,followed by ITR 5-10 mg/kg per day orally divided twice daily (maximum adult dose, 200 mg twice daily) for 12 wk[b,c,d] Methylprednisolone: 0.5-1.0 mg/kg daily IV for 1-2 wk	Higher dosing is recommended in patients with suspected CNS infection, where liposomal amphotericin B is the preferred agent. Severe pulmonary disease usually follows high-inoculum exposure, or if patient is immunocompromised. Corticosteroids appear to be beneficial in patients with severe respiratory disease requiring mechanical ventilation.
Acute pulmonary histoplasmosis Mild to moderate	No treatment if symptoms <4 wk Symptoms >4 wk (fever, cough): ITR: for 6-12 wk (same dose as above)[b]¶	
Progressive disseminated histoplasmosis Moderately severe or severe	LAB[a]: 3-5 mg/kg per day for 1-2 wk,followed by ITR 5-10 mg/kg per day PO divided twice daily (maximum adult dose, 200 mg twice daily) for at least 12 mo[b,c,d]	Because the incidence of CNS involvement is high in immunocompromised hosts with disseminated disease, liposomal amphotericin B is the preferred agent.
Progressive disseminated histoplasmosis Mild to moderate	ITR: 5-10 mg/kg per day (maximum adult dose, 200 mg twice daily) for at least 12 mo	
CNS histoplasmosis	LAB: 5 mg/kg per day for 4-6 wk followed by ITR for at least 12 mo[b,c]	Liposomal amphotericin B is the preferred agent. Combination therapy with azoles is not recommended.
Mediastinal lymphadenitis	Symptoms <4 weeks: No therapy Symptoms >4 weeks: ITR 5-10 mg/kg per day PO divided twice daily (maximum adult dose, 200 mg twice daily) for 6-12 weeks[b,c]	Patients with symptoms of airway or esophageal obstruction may benefit from corticosteroid therapy. Prednisone, 0.5-1.0 mg/kg daily with tapering dosing over 1-2 wk is the recommended regimen.
Mediastinal granuloma	Asymptomatic: No treatment necessary Symptomatic: ITR 5-10 mg/kg per day orally divided twice daily (maximum adult dose, 200 mg twice daily)[b]¶	Surgery may be required for patients with airway or esophageal obstruction.

Continued

TABLE 28.1 Treatment of Histoplasmosis—cont'd

Disease Manifestation	Treatment	Comments
Pericarditis Moderately severe or severe	ITR: 5-10 mg/kg per day PO divided twice daily (maximum adult dose, 200 mg twice daily) for 6-12 weeks only if prednisone is used.[b,c,d] Prednisone: 0.5-1.0 mg/kg daily with tapering dosing over 1-2 wk	Antifungal therapy is given in patients receiving corticosteroids. Cardiac tamponade requires prompt drainage.
Mediastinal fibrosis	Antifungal therapy has not been shown to be effective. However, most experts would give a single course of ITR for 6-12 wk because at initial evaluation it is difficult to differentiate from mediastinal granuloma. Stenting of obstructed vessels is warranted.	Debulking surgery should be avoided.
Salvage antifungal agents	Fluconazole: 5-6 mg/kg per dose twice daily (usual adult dose, 600 mg/day) Voriconazole: Loading dose 6 mg/kg per dose q12h for 2 doses, then 4 mg/kg per dose q12h for 3 days, then 200 twice daily (usual adult dose 400-600 mg/day divided q12h) Posaconazole: (≥13 years): 400 mg twice daily Isavuconazole: (adult dosing): Loading dose 372 mg (200 mg isavuconazole) q8h for 6 doses, then 372 mg (200 mg isavuconazole) daily starting 12-24 h after last loading dose.	Large randomized trials are not available in children. Anecdotal reports support their use in special circumstances. Echinocandins are not effective against *Histoplasma capsulatum*. With the exception of fluconazole and isavuconazole, therapeutic drug monitoring is needed for all azoles used in the treatment of histoplasmosis.

[a]Liposomal amphotericin B or amphotericin B lipid complex. Amphotericin B deoxycholate is generally not recommended because lipid formulations appear to be more effective in immunocompromised hosts.
[b]Itraconazole suspension is the recommended formulation because it has higher bioavailability compared with capsules. Therapeutic drug monitoring is indicated. A random serum concentration of more than 1.0 μg/mL is desirable.
[c]A loading dose should be administered. The usual loading dose is 5 mg/kg per dose (maximum adult dose, 200 mg per dose) 3 times daily for the first 3 days, followed by 10 mg/kg per day divided twice daily (maximum adult dose, 200 mg twice daily).
[d]Immunocompromised persons may require longer courses of therapy.
CNS, central nervous system; *h,* hour; *ITR,* itraconazole; *IV,* intravenous; *LAB,* lipid amphotericin B; *mo,* months; *PO,* oral; *q,* every; *wk,* weeks.
Adapted from Wheat LJ, Freifeld AG, Kleiman MB, et al. Clinical practice guidelines for the management of patients with histoplasmosis: 2007 update by the Infectious Diseases Society of America. *Clin Infect Dis.* 2007;45:807-825.

Lipid formulations of amphotericin B have been shown to be more effective in reducing fungal burden in immunocompromised hosts. Higher response rates and resulting lower mortality have been reported. Amphotericin B deoxycholate has been shown to be effective and well tolerated in children. However, many experts recommend a lipid formulation, such as liposomal amphotericin B, because of its lower incidence of infusion-related side effects and less potential for nephrotoxicity. No controlled therapeutic trials have been conducted in children.

Amphotericin B preparations are fungicidal for *H. capsulatum*, whereas itraconazole is fungistatic. Combined use of the 2 agents does not result in synergy. Amphotericin B is used most commonly as "induction" therapy. After substantial clinical improvement has occurred, it is stopped and itraconazole is used to complete treatment. Monotherapy with itraconazole is effective for treating patients who have mild or only moderately severe symptoms.

Itraconazole is generally well tolerated by children and, in adults, is more effective and less likely to induce resistance than the other azoles. Although formal trials using itraconazole have not been conducted in children, clinical experience has confirmed its effectiveness as the oral azole of choice. The erratic bioavailability of the capsule form can be improved when it is taken with liquids with low pH and caloric content (concomitant food, preferably fatty in composition, and a cola drink are recommended). Serum levels should be monitored, particularly if symptoms persist. Itraconazole oral solution is the recommended preparation used for children with blastomycosis and histoplasmosis. Its bioavailability is superior to the capsule form and can be taken with an empty stomach. However, its adverse gastrointestinal effects affect compliance. Most children complain of gastric discomfort with this preparation. Itraconazole serum concentration should be determined once the agent has reached steady state. With its long half-life, serum concentrations vary little after steady state is achieved (usually within 2 weeks of starting the agent). When used as monotherapy or as step-down treatment after amphotericin B induction, a loading dose consisting of 150% of the total daily dose is recommended for the initial 3 days of therapy. Random serum concentrations of itraconazole above 1.0 μg/mL are considered therapeutic, whereas levels above 10.0 μg/mL are considered toxic. Laboratories generally report itraconazole and its metabolite hydroxyitraconazole. Because both are bioactive, the sum of both determines your concentration. Clinicians are cautioned to be aware of potential drug interactions frequently observed in immunosuppressed patients, especially those receiving antirejection agents.

Electrolytes and renal function needs to be monitored in patients receiving amphotericin B, including lipid formulations. Azole therapy may lead to hepatitis. Liver enzymes need to be monitored during therapy, every 2 weeks for the first month, followed by testing every 3 months if the patient continues therapy. Azoles may also cause electrolyte imbalances such as hypokalemia, so electrolytes also need to be monitored. Caution is merited if voriconazole is used as therapy.

Ocular disturbances, hallucinations, and paresthesias have been reported with this agent, especially at high serum concentrations. Drug interactions with antirejection agents used in transplant patients merits caution and close monitoring.

Fluconazole was less effective than itraconazole in treating disseminated histoplasmosis. It also has been associated with relapse in disseminated infection, and is less effective than itraconazole for secondary prophylaxis in adults with disseminated infection. It clears fungemia more slowly in adults with disseminated infection than does itraconazole.

Both voriconazole and posaconazole have in vitro activity against *H. capsulatum*. Posaconazole has shown greater activity and seems to be more active in experimental models and several case reports. Patients with severe forms of histoplasmosis received salvage treatment with posaconazole, all with favorable outcomes. Resistance that seems to have been induced by fluconazole when used in patients with AIDS also was accompanied by an increase in minimum inhibitory concentration values for voriconazole, suggesting that resistance may emerge during treatment with voriconazole. Voriconazole and posaconazole have been effective in isolated reports describing differing manifestations of infection. These agents and fluconazole remain second-line alternatives to itraconazole. If these agents are elected for use, therapeutic drug and antigen monitoring is essential. Preliminary data suggest isavuconazole as an alternative agent for the treatment of histoplasmosis, especially in patients intolerant of amphotericin B and itraconazole. Isavuconazole has demonstrated favorable clinical activity against endemic fungi, with an overall 63% success rate. Voriconazole has been used as salvage therapy with favorable outcomes in patients with histoplasmosis, coccidioidomycosis, and blastomycosis.

Echinocandins such as caspofungin and micafungin lack adequate activity against *H. capsulatum*.

Concomitant use of corticosteroids is beneficial in treating patients with severe lung disease and ARDS. Disseminated infections in children require treatment with antifungal agents.

If untreated, patients with acute progressive disseminated histoplasmosis have a mortality rate approaching 100%. Treatment with amphotericin B results in survival of more than 90% of infants with the condition. Initial monotherapy with itraconazole is not recommended for children with disseminated histoplasmosis. Itraconazole is recommended for step-down therapy after induction and clinical improvement with amphotericin B. If amphotericin B is elected as monotherapy, a course of 4 to 6 weeks is recommended.

Amphotericin B preparations enter the CSF poorly; however, liposomal amphotericin B concentrations are higher in brain parenchyma.

Disease Prophylaxis and Prevention

Complete prevention of histoplasmosis is currently impossible, but reasonable precautions can substantially decrease the exposure to individuals with risk factors that predispose them to serious complications should they acquire the infection. Individuals with impaired cellular immunity who reside in, or plan travel to, endemic regions should be counseled about the potentially serious consequences of infection. This should include education about areas that are endemic for histoplasmosis, sites likely to be heavily contaminated with *H. capsulatum*, and the circumstances, activities, and events that may aerosolize spores and result in inhalation and infection.

Screening for antibodies to *H. capsulatum* before transplant or chemotherapy is not recommended, even in endemic areas. Only 5% of individuals living in endemic areas will have a weakly positive titer. A group of seropositive individuals undergoing transplantation did not develop histoplasmosis up to a year after initiation of immunosuppression. The presence of mediastinal or pulmonary calcifications indicates old infection and do not merit treatment in immunocompromised hosts. An active infection would indicate a new infection rather than reactivation.

Primary prophylactic regimens using itraconazole may be considered for immunocompromised hosts with exposure to soil mixed with bird or bat droppings. If such activities are unavoidable, the use of high-efficiency mask filtration devices should be encouraged. When potentially contaminated sites, such as old or unused structures in which birds or bats have roosted, dampening the areas with water is likely to reduce aerosolization of spores.

Although educating and counseling high-risk patients affords some protection against acquiring infection from microfoci, some of which can result in intense exposure, this is not helpful in protecting against "sporadic" exposure to contaminated aerosols. Prophylaxis for patients residing in a hyperendemic area and who are undergoing immunosuppression for management of neoplasms, inflammatory syndromes, or transplantation of allogeneic bone marrow, or solid organs is not routinely done, even in individuals with evidence of past infection.

Vaccines directed against any of the endemic mycoses have not yet been developed.

BLASTOMYCOSIS

Epidemiology and Risk Factors

Blastomycosis is caused by the dimorphic fungi *B. dermatitidis* and *B. gilchristii*. Persons affected by this infection mostly reside in the midwestern, southeastern, and south-central United States and in Canadian provinces bordering the Great Lakes. In a recent study, an increase in the incidence of blastomycosis was documented in the province of Ontario, Canada. From 1990 to 2015, 1,092 cases were diagnosed at an incidence rate of 0.41 cases per 100,000 population. Between 1995 and 2001 a significant increase in disease activity was observed in the Northwest region of the province with an incidence rate of 10.9 cases per 100,000 population. This represented a rate more than 12 times higher than other regions in the province.[27]

Canine cases have been often recognized as sentinels for human infection as their incidence of disease is more than 8 times higher than those seen in humans. Outdoor activities near rivers, stream, irrigation or drainage ditches, and construction sites with moist, decaying vegetation have been implicated in outbreaks of the disease. Like most fungal infections, inhalation of infective conidia leads to an infection in the respiratory tract. Inoculation through the skin has also been reported.

Between 2001 and 2006, the Transplant-Associated Infection Surveillance Network identified 9 SOT patients with blastomycosis.[3] Disseminated disease was recognized in 22% of patients, whereas pulmonary plus dissemination was documented in 11%. A majority of patients had disease limited to their lungs. A majority of patients were taking 2 or more immunosuppressive agents, including corticosteroids.

Invasive fungal infections are a serious complication of kidney transplantation. In a study from the University of Wisconsin, graft failure was documented in 40% of adult patients with blastomycosis. The mean interval from transplant to infection was 1.8 ± 2.2 years.[4]

Clinical Manifestations

Similar to other endemic mycoses, the clinical spectrum of blastomycosis ranges from subclinical infection to fulminant multilobar pneumonias and ARDS. Focal disease resembling bacterial pneumonia is not uncommon, and in many cases is self-limiting, requiring no antifungal therapy. Necrotizing pneumonia with cavitation has also been reported. Chronic lung disease may resemble lung cancer and tuberculosis. It is estimated that children represent 5% or more of all cases of blastomycosis but 50% to 100% of the extrapulmonary disease. Extrapulmonary disease involving the skin appears to be very common. In patients with any type of cell-mediated immune system impairment, disease tends to be more disseminated and associated with a greater mortality. Cutaneous, osteoarticular, and CNS disease and involvement of the genitourinary tract have been reported. CNS blastomycosis is reported in 1% to 15% of patients. Symptoms of chronic meningitis or focal neurological deficits are commonly observed. Magnetic resonance imaging findings include leptomeningeal enhancement, epidural abscesses, ocular involvement, and enhancing mass lesions. The clinical presentation of CNS blastomycosis is nonspecific with patients reporting headache, altered mental status, fever, vision changes, and seizures. Approximately 80% of patients with disseminated disease have cutaneous involvement. Crusted verrucous lesions (Fig. 28.3), plaquelike lesions, tender subcutaneous nodules, and painful ulcers with raised borders are commonly described with cutaneous blastomycosis. Some of the lesions may resemble pyoderma gangrenosum or types of skin cancer. Erythema nodosum can be observed; however, it is more common in patients with histoplasmosis and coccidioidomycosis.

Pulmonary disease was reported in 86% of a cohort of 14 children with active blastomycosis.[28] None of the patients were immunocompromised, but 21% had an underlying cardiac disorder. This retrospective study from Chicago documented extrapulmonary dissemination in 46% of the cohort, with skin and bone involvement in 31% of patients. Median age was 11.5 years. Fever, cough, and weight loss were the most common clinical features. The majority of patients (86%) were hospitalized and one-third required mechanical ventilation. Three patients died; 2 had ARDS and another had hypotension and respiratory failure.

In a multicenter study in the midwestern United States, 8 adult renal transplant patients had blastomycosis. All were receiving immunosuppressive therapy consisting of tacrolimus, with 75% receiving corticosteroids and 63% receiving mycophenolate mofetil. All patients had pulmonary disease, with disseminated disease developing in 50%. The majority (88%) had positive culture results, either from BAL or from skin biopsy. Three patients had positive urine antigen assay results. Two patients (25%) died from the infection, whereas 3 (38%) had graft loss.[1] Pneumonia was also common in another cohort of adult renal, liver, and lung transplant patients. Mortality was much higher in those patients with ARDS.

Diagnosis

The most common radiographic finding in patients with pulmonary blastomycosis is acute airspace consolidation that resembles a bacterial process (25% to 75%) (Fig. 28.4). It may be patchy, confluent, and segmental. Cavitation in the consolidated lung can be observed in approximately 48% of patients. A nodule or mass is observed in one-third of patients. Similar to histoplasmosis, a diffuse interstitial or miliary pattern is generally observed in patients with disseminated disease. The organism can be isolated from the sputum and bronchoalveolar washings in persons with lung disease. In addition, histopathologic findings and cultures help document extrapulmonary involvement. Blastomycosis is known to result in a pyogranulomatous histologic appearance on infected tissue.

The detection of antibodies to make a diagnosis of blastomycosis is problematic because assays are insensitive and nonspecific. The specificity of antigen assays is low because they frequently cross-react with other endemic mycosis such as histoplasmosis. Cultures remain the confirmatory test for diagnosis.

In a retrospective study of 14 children with blastomycosis, serologic results were positive in 1 patient of 7 tested, whereas urine antigens for either histoplasmosis or blastomycosis were positive in all patients tested.[28] An enzyme immunoassay using *B. dermatitidis* surface protein BAD1 performed well compared with ID. A specificity of 99.2% was observed in patients with nonfungal infections and 94% in patients with histoplasmosis. When combined with antigen testing, diagnostic sensitivity was 97.6%.

Antigen detection for blastomycosis in urine, serum, and BAL has high sensitivity (~90%) in patients with disseminated disease.[29] The use of antigen detection assays in bronchoalveolar lavage fluid is a valuable tool in the diagnosis of pulmonary blastomycosis. The use of a second-generation assay had a demonstrable sensitivity of approximately 83%. Antigen can also be detected in CSF in patients with CNS involvement. An immunoassay for *B. dermatitidis* antigen in the urine demonstrated a sensitivity of 92.9% and a specificity of 79.3%. Cross-reactions with other causes of endemic mycoses were observed,

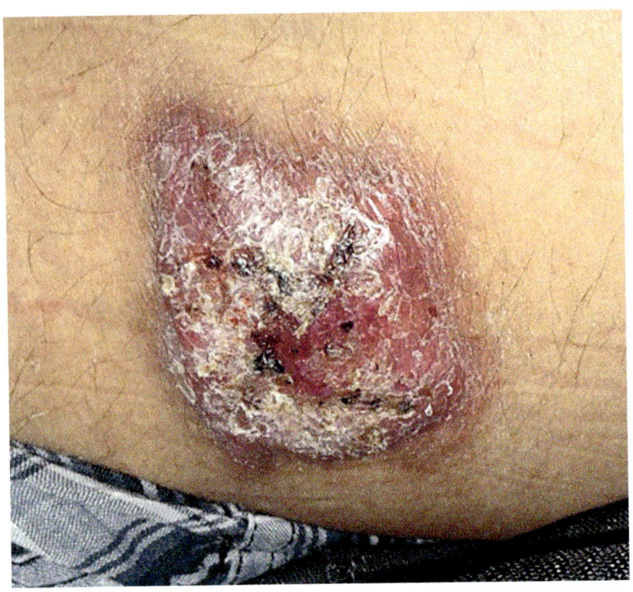

Fig. 28.3 Culture-positive skin lesion in adolescent with blastomycosis.

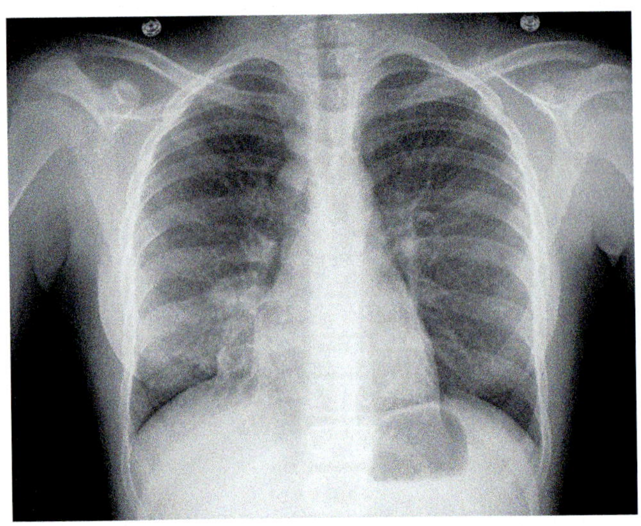

Fig. 28.4 Pneumonia secondary to *Blastomyces dermatitidis*.

specifically 96.3% with histoplasmosis. As with *H. capsulatum* antigen detection assays, cross-reactivity also occurs with other endemic mycoses. Further development of antigen detection assays are focused on improving the detection of serum antigen. Pretreatment of serum with ethylenediamine tetraacetic acid (EDTA) that dissociates immune complexes has been shown to increase the test's sensitivity, from approximately 35% to approximately 57%.

CSF analysis usually demonstrates elevated protein, low glucose concentration, and pleocytosis consisting early with a predominance of neutrophils followed by a predominance of lymphocytes. *B. dermatitidis* grows in culture in two-thirds of specimens.

Treatment

Treatment guidelines have been published (Table 28.2).[30] Liposomal amphotericin B is the preferred agent for disseminated disease. Most of the existing literature on the antifungal treatment of blastomycosis has involved the use the amphotericin B deoxycholate. Although there is a lack of controlled trials, all amphotericin B preparations appear to be effective. Irrespective of agent used, all patients receive additional therapy with an azole such as itraconazole. Studies have demonstrated the efficacy of ketoconazole in the treatment of types of blastomycosis, but because safer and more effective agents are available (with lower relapse rates), ketoconazole is no longer used.

Immunosuppressed individuals are at an increased risk of severe and disseminated disease. The severity of the disease is greatly influenced by the magnitude of the immunosuppression. Patients with cancer, solid organ, and stem cell transplants, and HIV/AIDS appear to be at the highest risk. Immunosuppressed persons should continue azole suppressive or prophylactic therapy once initial and step-down therapy has been completed.

Echinocandins such as caspofungin, micafungin, and anidulafungin have limited activity against *B. dermatitidis* and should not be used as therapy.

Relapses after completion of therapy is not uncommon in immunocompromised patients. Long-term observation for signs of disease plus serial monitoring with antigen detection assays are imperative.

Limited data in children suggest that itraconazole is an effective agent for the treatment of mild-to-moderate blastomycosis. In addition, previously healthy children receiving itraconazole solution for uncomplicated disease may not require therapeutic drug monitoring. Similar to most severe disease, azoles should not be used as the sole agent in the treatment of CNS disease.

Immunosuppressed patients with ARDS secondary to blastomycosis can benefit from the administration of corticosteroids. Anecdotal clinical observations have documented their clinical utility.

Disease Prophylaxis and Prevention

In endemic regions, patients with cellular immunodeficiencies or HIV infection or people who receive immunosuppressive drugs should be counseled concerning high-risk activities. If such activities are unavoidable, protective masks should be used.

Chronic suppressive therapy is critical in immunocompromised patients with endemic fungal infections. Azoles are the most commonly used agents. They have been shown to be safe and effective in preventing relapses.

COCCIDIOIDOMYCOSIS

C. immitis and *C. posadasii* are thermally dimorphic fungi responsible for coccidioidomycosis. Coccidioidomycosis affects humans and animals in distinct geographic areas in the Western Hemisphere where hot, arid climates exist. Coccidioidomycosis in SOT recipients is uncommon, even in highly endemic areas, especially in the modern era of antifungal prophylaxis. The incidence in hematopoietic stem cell transplant (HCT) recipients appears to be rare, with only a few cases reported in the literature. Severe, disseminated, life-threatening infections are more common in transplant patients due primarily to the T-cell inhibitory effects of immunosuppressants such as calcineurin inhibitors and corticosteroids. *Coccidioides* infection in the transplant

TABLE 28.2 Treatment of Blastomycosis in Immunocompromised Patients

Disease Manifestation	Treatment	Comments
Disseminated blastomycosis		
Moderately severe to severe	LAB[a]: 3-5 mg/kg per day for 1-2 wk followed by ITR 10 mg/kg per day divided bid (maximum adult dose, 200 mg bid) for 12 mo[b,c,d]	
Disseminated	ITR: 10 mg/kg per day divided bid (200 mg bid) for 6-12 mo[b,c,d]	Osteoarticular infections are treated for 12 mo.
Mild-to-moderate		
CNS disease	Liposomal amphotericin B: 5 mg/kg per day for 4-6 wk followed by an azole for at least 1 year[b,c,d]	Fluconazole, itraconazole, or voriconazole has been used.
Additional antifungal agents	Fluconazole: 5-6 mg/kg per dose twice daily (usual adult dose, 600 mg/day)	High doses of fluconazole (400-800 mg) may be useful in patients with CNS disease.
	Voriconazole: Loading dose 6 mg/kg per dose q12h for 2 doses, then 4 mg/kg per dose q12h (usual adult dose 400–600 mg/day divided q12h).	Voriconazole can also be used to treat CNS disease. Because these alternative agents have been shown to be less effective than itraconazole, they should not be used in immunosuppressed hosts.
	Posaconazole (≥13 years of age): 400 mg twice daily	

[a]Liposomal amphotericin B or amphotericin B lipid complex. Amphotericin B deoxycholate is generally not recommended because lipid formulations appear to be more effective in immunocompromised hosts.
[b]Itraconazole suspension is the recommended formulation because it has higher bioavailability compared with capsules. Therapeutic drug monitoring is indicated. A random serum concentration of more than 1.0 μg/mL is desirable.
[c]A loading dose should be administered. The usual loading dose is 5 mg/kg per dose (maximum adult dose, 200 mg per dose) 3 times daily for the first 3 days, followed by 10 mg/kg per day divided twice daily (maximum adult dose, 200 mg twice daily).
[d]Immunocompromised persons may require longer courses of therapy.
bid, twice a day; *CNS,* central nervous system; *h,* hour; *ITR,* itraconazole; *LAB,* lipid amphotericin B; *mo,* months; *q,* every.
Chapman SW, Dismukes WE, Proia LA, et al. Clinical practice guidelines for the management of blastomycosis: 2008 update by the Infectious Diseases Society of America. *Clin Infect Dis.* 2008;46:1801-1812.

recipient portends the poorest prognosis among the endemic mycoses, but prophylaxis is effective in preventing primary and recrudescent disease. Unfortunately, the existing literature regarding *Coccidioides* infection specific to the pediatric transplant patient is scarce; therefore the information presented here is primarily from the adult experience. Additionally, most of the literature on infections in transplant patients is in SOT. Because coccidioidomycosis in HCT recipients appears to be such a rare event, accurate data on infection rates and treatment recommendations are not available; therefore this section focuses mainly on the SOT recipient unless otherwise specified. The recommendations provided are in congruence with available current guidelines from the American Society of Transplantation[31] and the Infectious Diseases Society of America.[32]

Epidemiology and Risk Factors

Coccidioidomycosis is endemic in certain desert regions of Arizona, California, and northern Mexico as well as parts of Central and South America. Infection is acquired through inhalation of fungal spores and in most individuals leads to a self-limited, often asymptomatic pulmonary infection, but severe pulmonary disease and dissemination occur in a minority of cases. Of the cases in the United States, 95% are reported from Arizona and California, but occasional cases have been reported in states not recognized to be endemic either because patients have previously traveled to or resided in *Coccidioides*-endemic areas or, rarely, because *Coccidioides* was acquired from infected fomites. Coccidioidomycosis is a common infection in endemic regions, responsible for approximately 150,000 infections annually in the United States, but extrapulmonary disease occurs in less than 1% and death is rare.[33] A 10-fold increase in cases was reported from endemic states from 1998 to 2011 owing to multiple factors.[34] The incidence of infection can vary widely from year to year as a result of differing climate and environmental conditions.

Although most cases of disseminated infection occur in otherwise healthy individuals, certain immunocompromising conditions substantially increase the likelihood of severe and disseminated disease. Cellular immunity is critical in controlling the spread of infection; therefore any genetic or acquired impairment of T-cell function can be a risk factor for severe disease. Because SOT and HCT recipients require anti–T-cell medications to prevent graft rejection and graft-versus-host disease, respectively, they are at substantially higher risk for severe infection compared with the general population. Before the widespread use of antifungal chemoprophylaxis, coccidioidomycosis affected 7% to 9% of SOT recipients in endemic areas. Most infected patients had disseminated infection and mortality was as high as 72%. More recent data indicate infection rates of 1% to 2% but mortality remains high at approximately 25%. Risk factors for infection in SOT recipients include receipt of high-dose corticosteroids, treatment of rejection, and a pretransplant history of *Coccidioides* infection or positive serology. Only a few cases of *Coccidioides* infection have been reported in HCT recipients but the mortality in this population appears high. Mendoza and colleagues reviewed all cases of active coccidioidomycosis in HCT recipients from 2003 to 2013 at the Mayo Clinic Hospital in Phoenix, Arizona. Eleven of 426 (2.6%) HCT recipients experienced active infection a median of 14 months after HCT, of whom 5 (45%) died.[35] Most of these patients were receiving immunosuppression at the time of diagnosis with either tacrolimus or corticosteroids and the majority were not receiving antifungal prophylaxis.

Coccidioidomycosis in SOT and HCT patients most often results from environmental exposure to spores near the time of transplant or after transplant or recrudescence of past infection. However, several reports of donor-derived infection (i.e., acquired from an infected graft) in SOT recipients exist, and one infected donor has the potential to spread infection to multiple recipients through the various organs, and infection can be spread from organs other than lungs.[36] SOT recipients who acquire infection from the graft present sooner (typically within 1 month of transplant) and have more severe disease compared with environmentally acquired infection. Donor-derived coccidioidomycosis in the SOT recipient highlights the importance of the epidemiologic history of the donor; when *Coccidioides* infection is not suspected, empiric antifungal therapy is not always begun and the diagnosis is often made only at autopsy.[37]

Clinical Manifestations

Most cases of coccidioidomycosis in SOT occur in the first year after transplant surgery. The clinical presentation of coccidioidomycosis in transplant patients is protean and can range from asymptomatic seroconversion to fulminant disseminated disease and death. Pulmonary disease is often nondescript and can mimic community-acquired pneumonia. Symptoms of pulmonary infection common to both healthy patients and transplant recipients include fever, cough, rash, weight loss, myalgias, chest pain, and fatigue. Consolidative pneumonia is common and pleural effusion can be seen. Transplant patients are more likely to have severe pneumonia that can progress to multilobar involvement, ARDS, and respiratory failure. Extrapulmonary (i.e., disseminated) disease is more common in SOT and HCT recipients, occurring in up to 75% of transplant patients,[38] and typical sites of involvement include the skin, bones and joints, and the meninges. Multiorgan involvement is not uncommon in this population. Involvement of other organs, including the implanted graft, can occur. In a recent review of pediatric patients with coccidioidomycosis at a clinic in Madera, California, 18 of 108 (17%) had disseminated infection that mostly involved bones.[39] Patients with musculoskeletal infection present with local swelling and pain; most commonly affected sites include the tibia, vertebrae, skull, and metatarsals/metacarpals.[40] Patients with coccidioidal meningitis can present with headache, altered mental status, and focal neurologic defects; fever is not always present and meningismus is often absent. Headache may be due to hydrocephalus. CNS coccidioidomycosis can occur in the absence of detectable pulmonary disease. Fungal dissemination can result in cutaneous seeding manifesting as a variety of skin findings such as papules, nodules, and plaques. Verrucous granuloma at the nasolabial fold is the most common presentation of disseminated cutaneous disease. Skin rashes such as erythema nodosum and erythema multiforme can be seen early in the disease course and are most commonly seen in healthy individuals. As opposed to the dermatologic manifestations mentioned previously, these skin findings do not represent fungal dissemination.

Diagnosis

A multifaceted approach should be used in the diagnosis of coccidioidomycosis in the transplant patient that includes serology, fungal culture, and histopathologic examination of body fluids and tissues, and potentially antigen and molecular testing. Using multiple methods of serologic testing and performing repeated testing can substantially improve the sensitivity in transplant patients.[41] The diagnosis of coccidioidomycosis is challenging even in previously healthy hosts because there are no pathognomonic clinical findings and the sensitivity of any one diagnostic assay is not high. Growth of *Coccidioides* in culture or identification of classic histopathology in biopsy specimens provides definitive evidence of infection. Respiratory cultures often grow the organism in adults with pulmonary infection and the organism grows readily on fungal culture media within 5 days. Common but nonspecific hematologic findings seen in infection include leukocytosis, eosinophilia, and elevated erythrocyte sedimentation rate.[40] Patients with coccidioidal meningitis can show CSF with hypoglycorrhachia, elevated protein, and mononuclear pleocytosis. CSF stains are usually negative, and the yield of CSF culture is low. CSF serology is the most reliable method of diagnosis for meningeal disease with the enzyme immunoassay (EIA) results positive in 82% of cases,[40] but negative test results do not rule out CNS infection.

Radiographic imaging can be helpful in the workup of suspected coccidioidomycosis, but the findings are not specific. In a recent study of coccidioidomycosis diagnostics in adult SOT recipients, chest CT findings were abnormal in 19 of 22 (86%) with findings including multifocal nodules (n = 7), consolidation (n = 4), consolidation and multifocal nodules (n = 4), and pleural effusion and multifocal nodules (n = 1).[41] In this study, chest radiography was abnormal in 16 of 25 (64%) but repeat examinations increased the probability of finding abnormalities to 84%.

Most patients with coccidioidomycosis are diagnosed by serologic testing. A variety of options are available in local and reference laboratories. EIAs are commercially available and are often used as initial screening because of their enhanced sensitivity compared with antibody measurements by ID, tube precipitin, and CF.[32] However, the sensitivity of the EIA can vary, depending on manufacturer and performing laboratory. Additionally, the EIA may have reduced specificity compared with other methods, so repeated testing that includes other methods is recommended when the EIA is the only positive result.[32] Measurement of IgG by CF provides a quantitative measurement that can be used to monitor treatment response. Higher CF titers at diagnosis are associated with an increased risk of disseminated disease. Controversy exists as to whether the serologic response to *Coccidioides* infection is impaired in transplant patients. Earlier studies reported a depressed antibody response in SOT recipients,[38] but more recent investigations show that serologic testing may be reliable in these patients and comparable to immunocompetent individuals.[42] It is important to recognize that in contrast to many other pathogens—including the other endemic mycoses—the serum IgG antibody after *Coccidioides* infection wanes rapidly (within months). Therefore any transplant patient with positive *Coccidioides* serology results should be presumed to have recent infection, and prompt workup for disseminated disease and initiation of treatment should begin.[32]

Newer diagnostic methods include antigen quantification and molecular assays. A research group previously reported that cross-reactivity occurred in patients with severe coccidioidomycosis in whom 58% had a positive *Histoplasma* urine antigen EIA result.[43] They developed a *Coccidioides* EIA assay that was 71% sensitive in severe coccidioidomycosis. Of the patients in this study, 79% were immunocompromised, including 2 SOT recipients[44]. PCR-based molecular assays are commercially available at certain reference laboratories and may provide a more rapid means of diagnosis, especially for coccidioidal meningitis. How these tests should best be used in the diagnostic workup remains to be determined, but they show promise, especially in the immunocompromised patient who may have an impaired serologic response.

Treatment

Although antifungal therapy is often not required in normal hosts with coccidioidomycosis, it should always be provided to transplant patients with suspected or confirmed infection because of the high risk of mortality from severe/disseminated disease.[32] There are no randomized controlled trials for the treatment of coccidioidomycosis in SOT or HCT recipients. Interpreting existing case reports and case series is problematic owing to differences in reported disease severity, immunosuppression, and comorbidities that could affect outcome. Additionally, pediatric-specific studies are lacking, so the recommendations for treatment of *Coccidioides* infections in children are extrapolated from existing data and guidelines in adults. Table 28.3 provides a visual representation of the treatment recommendations.

Azoles are the mainstay of therapy for coccidioidomycosis in all patients. They are safe, well tolerated, and effective. For the treatment of mild-to-moderate (nonsevere) *Coccidioides* infection in adults, fluconazole is recommended.[32] Similar to histoplasmosis and blastomycosis, amphotericin B is recommended as initial therapy for all patients with nonmeningeal severe pulmonary and disseminated disease because of its superiority over azoles in the rapidity of treatment response. Although there is no evidence that liposomal amphotericin B is superior to amphotericin B deoxycholate, the lipid formulations are preferred owing to their better tolerance and side effect profile.[32] Some experts recommend initial treatment of severe infection with amphotericin B in combination with an azole, but data for this practice are lacking. Patients can be transitioned from intravenous amphotericin B to an oral azole after 2 weeks as long as significant response to initial therapy is documented.[31]

Meningeal/CNS coccidioidomycosis is best treated with fluconazole. This recommendation differs from CNS histoplasmosis and blastomycosis in which amphotericin B is preferred. The recommended adult dose of fluconazole is 400 mg/day but some experts recommend 800 to 1200 mg/day.[32] The recommended dose for children is 12 mg/kg per day, although some advocate for doses up to 23 mg/kg per day.[40] Intrathecal amphotericin B deoxycholate was the

TABLE 28.3 Primary and Alternate Treatment Recommendations for Pediatric Coccidioidomycosis in Transplant Patients

Disease Manifestation	Primary Therapy	Alternatives
Nonsevere, nonmeningeal	Fluconazole 6-12 mg/kg once daily IV/PO (maximum dose 400 mg).	Itraconazole 2-5 mg/kg per dose 3 times daily for 3 days, then 2-5 mg/kg per dose twice daily thereafter (maximum dose 200 mg) Liposomal amphotericin B: 5 mg/kg IV once daily
Severe, nonmeningeal	Liposomal amphotericin B 5 mg/kg IV once daily. Some experts would escalate dose to 10 mg/kg in cases of treatment nonresponse.	Amphotericin B deoxycholate: 0.5-1 mg/kg IV once daily Fluconazole: 12 mg/kg once daily IV/PO (maximum dose 800mg)
Meningeal	Fluconazole 12 mg/kg once daily IV/PO (maximum dose 800-1200 mg). Some experts recommend doses up to 23 mg/kg.	Liposomal amphotericin B: 5 mg/kg IV once daily with possible dose escalation Amphotericin B deoxycholate: 0.5-1 mg/kg IV once daily Other azoles (itraconazole, voriconazole, posaconazole) have been successfully used

IV, intravenous; *PO*, oral.

gold standard for coccidioidal meningitis in the pre-azole era, but its use via this route affords additional toxicity without proven benefit above systemic azole therapy and is therefore not recommended.[32] Lipid formulations of amphotericin B have improved CNS penetration compared with deoxycholate and have been used in azole-refractory cases.

Besides fluconazole, other azoles are active against *Coccidioides* and have proven successful in treating disease. Itraconazole was found to be equivalent to fluconazole in an adult study of nonmeningeal coccidioidomycosis, with itraconazole showing a trend for better activity in a subgroup analysis of patients with skeletal infection.[45] Itraconazole may be superior to fluconazole in pediatric skeletal disease as well, but caution should be taken in its use given the erratic enteric absorption, difficulty with tolerance, and need for therapeutic drug monitoring compared to fluconazole.[40] Serum itraconazole levels should be monitored during therapy. Voriconazole and posaconazole have been used as alternative therapy in cases of disseminated, including meningeal coccidioidomycosis.[46] As with the other endemic mycoses, the echinocandins have variable in vitro activity and are not recommended as therapeutic agents for coccidioidomycosis.[31]

In transplant patients with coccidioidomycosis, consideration should be made for reduction of immunosuppression when possible. Additionally, clinicians should use caution when administering azoles to patients receiving calcineurin inhibitors (cyclosporine and tacrolimus) and sirolimus because azoles inhibit cytochrome P450 3A4, the enzyme that metabolizes these immunosuppressants. The addition of azole therapy frequently leads to elevated levels of the antirejection medications; therefore their levels should be monitored closely when starting, changing dosage, and discontinuing azoles. Preemptive dose reduction of the antirejection drug is advised.[32]

Transplant patients with coccidioidomycosis should be monitored closely for treatment response. With effective therapy, improvements in objective measures such as oxygenation requirements and temperature should be observed. As discussed earlier, the CF titer should decline with effective therapy and can be used as a marker of response. It is unclear if the *Coccidioides* antigen can be used in a similar manner to *Histoplasma* antigen to monitor treatment. Therapeutic drug monitoring is advised in patients receiving itraconazole (and potentially the other azoles except fluconazole). Transplant recipients who acquire coccidioidomycosis require azole therapy for life. Long-term fluconazole use in SOT appears to be safe.[47]

Disease Prophylaxis and Prevention

All patients should undergo a thorough epidemiologic history and appropriate laboratory and radiographic testing for coccidioidomycosis before SOT or HCT. Suspected active coccidioidomycosis at the time of evaluation requires a thorough workup and initiation of empiric antifungal therapy. Transplantation should be delayed if possible in this case. Epidemiologic history and testing should similarly be obtained in the donor because infection in the recipient can occur from donors with active coccidioidomycosis at the time of organ procurement or in those with a prior history of infection based on serology. History of living in or travel to *Coccidioides* endemic areas is important, even if it occurred in the distant past, because reactivation of disease can occur years later.[31] Patients with any risk factors for *Coccidioides* infection should have screening serologic testing before transplant and afterward if risk factors persist (e.g., living in an endemic area). A reasonable approach is to perform serologic testing (including EIA, CF, and ID antibodies) at (1) the pretransplant evaluation; (2) the time of SOT/HCT; (3) every 4 months for the first year after transplantation; and (4) yearly or twice-yearly thereafter.[31,48] After their introduction, azoles were found to be effective in the prevention of *Coccidioides* disease in SOT recipients. Given the clear risk of recrudescent disease in SOT recipients with a previous history of *Coccidioides* infection and/or positive serology results,[48] targeted prophylaxis with oral fluconazole was recommended in this patient group. De novo coccidioidomycosis in SOT recipients—*Coccidioides* infection acquired after transplant in patients with no prior history of infection and with negative serology findings at the time of transplant—was previously thought to be uncommon: 1.4% in a study from 2003.[49] However, further studies revealed the rate of infection in SOT recipients naïve to *Coccidioides* to be higher.[50] Risk factors for infection in these patients were not identified; therefore the Infectious Diseases Society of America currently recommends that universal azole prophylaxis be provided to all patients without evidence of active coccidioidomycosis undergoing SOT in *Coccidioides*-endemic areas.[32] Prophylaxis is provided for a duration of 6 to 12 months based on studies, demonstrating that the majority of cases of de novo or recrudescent disease occur in the first year after transplantation. Patients who receive organs from donors with active coccidioidomycosis or positive serologic resting results should receive lifelong antifungal prophylaxis.[31]

The recommended dose of fluconazole dose for primary prophylaxis in adult patients is 200 mg by mouth once daily. The optimal dosage in pediatric patients is unclear.

Because the risk of recrudescent disease is high and potential consequences are severe, transplant patients treated for coccidioidomycosis should receive secondary prophylaxis with an oral azole for the duration of immunosuppression (i.e., indefinitely for SOT recipients).[32] The term "secondary prophylaxis" is slightly misleading, however, because the recommended fluconazole secondary prophylaxis dose in adults is 400 mg once daily, identical to the treatment dose, although some experts would transition to the lower dose of 200 mg once daily (the same dose as recommended for primary prophylaxis).[32] The optimal dose of fluconazole to be used in pediatric patients for secondary prophylaxis is unknown, but it seems prudent to continue the treatment dosage.

Patients should be counseled before and after transplantation about the avoidance of activities or situations in which they may be more likely to be exposed to *Coccidioides* spores, which are found in high concentrations in aerosolized dust. Complete elimination of risk is impossible in endemic areas, but patients should avoid areas or activities that are likely to have large amounts of dust such as construction/excavation sites and home remodeling.[31] Wearing a protective mask to prevent dust inhalation may be helpful if exposure is unavoidable.

Standard precautions should be followed in hospitalized patients with coccidioidomycosis. Patients with active *Coccidioides* infection pose no risk for human-to-human transmission. However, contamination of materials such as dressings and casts occurs, so care should be taken in the handling and disposal of these items.

Although human-to-human transmission of *Coccidioides* does not occur, *Coccidioides* growing on culture media poses a significant risk to laboratory personnel. Clinicians should alert the laboratory before submission of specimens for culture in cases of suspected coccidioidomycosis so that appropriate precautions can be followed, which includes opening cultures only inside a biological safety cabinet appropriate for containing spore-forming fungi.[32] Detailed guidance in cases of laboratory exposure is available.[32]

Endemic mycoses such as histoplasmosis, blastomycosis, and coccidioidomycosis are known to cause significant morbidity and mortality in immunocompromised individuals who are frequently affected by severe pulmonary and disseminated disease. Clinicians must have knowledge of the epidemiology, risk factors, and clinical manifestations of these conditions and institute prompt therapy while awaiting diagnostic test results. Patients also need to be counseled on behaviors that minimize the risks of acquiring such an infection.

29

Toxoplasma gondii

Sharon F. Chen, MD, MS and Hayley A. Gans, MD

EPIDEMIOLOGY AND RISK FACTORS

Toxoplasma gondii is a protozoan parasite in the phylum Apicomplexa. It infects humans and almost all warm-blooded animals, including mammals and birds.

Transmission of *T. gondii* is linked to its biological life cycle and occurs most frequently with the ingestion of oocysts in soil and water or with the ingestion of tissue cysts from infected animals and, less frequently, with transplacental dissemination to a fetus[1] (Fig. 29.1). Tissue cysts can be found in any organ, so organ transplantation is also a potential source of transmission[2] (Table 29.1). The Felidae family, domestic and stray cats and wild felids (e.g., cougars, bobcats, lions), are the definitive host in which *T. gondii* undergoes sexual reproduction (see Fig. 29.1). Infected cats can shed more than 100 million oocysts in their stool. Unsporulated oocysts in the environment are not infectious until matured, which takes 1 to 5 days; therefore direct contact with cats is not considered a transmission risk. Sporulated oocysts remain viable for more than a year in moist environments because they can resist chemical and mechanical damage and detergents.

Oocysts house a protozoan stage of *T. gondii* called sporozoites. If a human or animal ingests oocysts, the gastric enzymes destroy the cyst wall and sporozoites penetrate the intestinal epithelium and differentiate into another stage (rapidly dividing tachyzoites). Tachyzoites can invade almost all nucleated cells and remain intracellular, evading the immune response within a parasitophorous vacuole.

Tachyzoites disseminate throughout the body via the blood or lymph circulation, transported within a monocyte, dendritic cell, or other nucleated cells, and can lodge in any tissue, including a fetus via a transplacental route. Tachyzoite replication is generally thought to be controlled by the host immune response within a few weeks after initial infection.[3] Outside the host cell, tachyzoites are fragile and are usually killed rapidly.[4] Theoretically, during the acute dissemination phase, tachyzoites could be transmitted to a patient if the bone marrow or blood was collected during this transient phase. Reports have suggested this scenario but have not been confirmed.[5-8]

Within the tissue, asexually replicating tachyzoites can differentiate into bradyzoites, a slowly dividing stage that eventually forms a tissue cyst. The signals for differentiation between the stages are not completely defined.[9] Tissue cysts can develop as early as 7 to 10 days after initial infection[1] and can form in any organ. More often, tissue cysts are found in neural tissues, such as the brain and the eye, and in muscular tissues such as skeletal muscles and the heart. Tissue cysts can remain in the host for years.[10]

Protective immunity may be sustained throughout the lifetime because of antigenic stimulation from intermittent asymptomatic reactivation of persistent tissue cysts.[10] The host immune response is protective but does not eradicate the protozoa, resulting in a balance that allows survival of the host by limiting *T. gondii* replication and allows persistence of the protozoa by subverting the host immune response.[10] If tissue cysts rupture in an immunocompromised individual, bradyzoites transform into tachyzoites that can disseminate to any tissue, transforming back into bradyzoites and forming new tissue cysts. "Reactivation" of persistent tissue cysts can lead to uncontrolled tachyzoite replication and dissemination, leading to the clinical signs and symptoms observed in severely immunosuppressed patients. Interferon-gamma–secreting CD4 and CD8 T cells and natural killer (NK) cells are important for controlling bradyzoite reactivation within a cyst,[11] because interferon-gamma is key for controlling acute *T. gondii* infection.[12] Therefore immune suppression medications that interfere with cell-mediated immunity or myeloablative conditioning can increase the risk of *T. gondii* infection and disease.[13] The level of immune suppression also contributes to the clinical severity of *T. gondii* disease.[13]

Another means of transmission is by ingestion of tissue cysts in raw or undercooked meat (see Fig. 29.1). When the cysts rupture within the intestinal tract, bradyzoites are released, enter the intestinal epithelial cells, and differentiate into tachyzoites, which disseminate throughout the body in the intermediate and definitive hosts. To complete the life cycle, bradyzoites can also differentiate into gametocytes in the definitive host cat, leading to development of oocysts, which are shed in feces.[1]

Since the 1980s, it has been recognized that tissue cysts can also be transmitted within a transplanted organ. This scenario occurs more often with heart organs because there is a predilection of *T. gondii* for muscle.[2] However, tachyzoites can disseminate to all tissues and thus other organs may harbor tissue cysts but at a lower frequency.[1,]

On a population level, seroprevalence is dependent on the climate and culture of a country. Approximately 20% to 30% of the world's population is infected with *T. gondii.*[15] North America has a low seroprevalence (10% to 30%), south and central Europe, including France, has intermediate prevalence (30% to 50%), whereas South America, especially Brazil, has high prevalence (up to 80%).[13,16] However, decreasing seroprevalence is being reported in Paris.[17] The incidence of *T. gondii* disease is dependent on seroprevalence of the population, immunosuppression level, and administration of prophylaxis to an individual.[18,19] In transplant recipients, the estimated incidence of *T. gondii* infection or disease is highest in seropositive allogeneic hematopoietic stem cell transplant (HSCT) recipients, ranging from 2.1% to 19.6%, varying geographically[13] (see Table 29.1). This supports reactivation as the strongest risk factor for *T. gondii* disease in the HSCT population. The incidence is lower for solid organ transplant (SOT) recipients and much lower for oncology and autologous HSCT patients.[20] For the SOT population, donor-recipient mismatch (D^+/R^-) is a risk factor for acquiring *T. gondii.*[2] Within all SOT recipients, D^+/R^- heart ($\pm$lung) transplant recipients have the highest incidence of

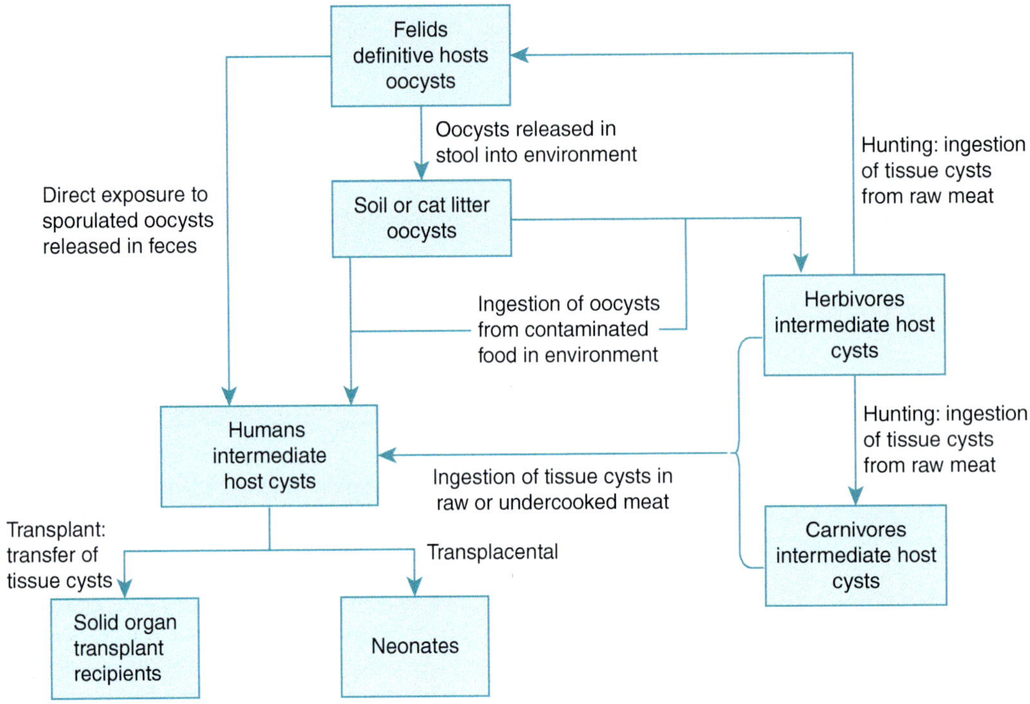

Fig. 29.1 Sources, parasitic stage, and mechanisms of transmission of *Toxoplasma gondii*.

TABLE 29.1 Risk of *Toxoplasma gondii* Disease

Risk Level	Type of Patient (Mode of Transmission) (Incidence)
High	HSCT (reactivation) (2.1%-19.6%)
	D^+/R^- Heart transplant (graft transmission) (0.6%-25%)
Intermediate	D^+/R^- Liver, kidney, lung, small intestine, pancreas (graft transmission) (0.08%-0.2%)
	Enhanced immunosuppression in HSCT, SOT, oncology patients (e.g., with treatment for GVHD or allograft rejection)
Low	Seropositive R^+ SOT recipients (reactivation)
	Seropositive oncology patients (reactivation)
	Autologous HSCT (reactivation)
None	Eye, bone, artery transplant

D, donor; *GVHD*, graft versus heart disease; *HSCT*, hematopoietic stem cell transplant; *R*, recipient; *SOT*, solid organ transplant.

TABLE 29.2 Clinical Manifestations of *Toxoplasmosis gondii* Infection

Clinical Manifestations by Transplant Type	Percent
Allo-Hematopoietic Stem Cell Transplant	
Disseminated disease	25
Cerebral toxoplasmosis	10
Isolated fever	4
Ocular toxoplasmosis	4
Solid Organ Transplant	
Bone marrow suppression	63
Central nervous system	56
Liver	26
Heart	23

T. gondii, up to 25% in patients with no prophylaxis.[13] Incidence for noncardiac organ transplant recipients is lower, estimated at 0.08% to 0.2%.[13] There is no risk of transmission with eye, bone, or artery transplants.[21] Although data on vascularized composite allotransplantation are sparse, it would be anticipated that those containing skeletal muscle will be at risk. Mortality rates from the largest study of SOT recipients was shown to be 13%,[2] which is lower than the approximately 38% observed in HCST recipients.[1]

Clinical Manifestations

The severity of clinical manifestations of *T. gondii* disease is dependent on the level of the individual's immune suppression (Table 29.2). Clinical findings do not distinguish between primary or reactivated *T. gondii* disease. Fever is common and should prompt the inclusion of *T. gondii* disease in the differential diagnosis.[13,22] Delayed diagnosis is a common theme for fatal cases.

In HSCT recipients, reactivation of persistent tissue cysts is the predominant mechanism leading to clinical disease, manifesting typically in the first 6 months after transplant.[23-25] In a severely immunosuppressed individual, dissemination of tachyzoites can present as a rapidly progressive infection and can clinically manifest as fever with multiple organ involvement, most commonly the lungs.[26,27] For those less immunosuppressed, the brain is the most affected organ clinically and in autopsy.[24] Clinical symptoms of brain involvement include somnolence or obtundation and seizures. Brain abscesses can be detected on imaging.[24] After the brain, lung involvement can be prominent and manifest as a pneumonitis and, in severe cases, evolve to acute respiratory distress syndrome.[13] Computed tomography chest imaging may reveal a reticulonodular or interstitial pattern.[28] The heart and eyes can be affected, manifesting as myocarditis and retinochoriditis, respectively.[24] Cutaneous involvement is rare, presenting as multiple erythematous macules or papules.[13] In some reports, up to 36% of HSCT patients have no symptoms because transient, self-resolving positive *T. gondii* polymerase chain reaction (PCR) findings have been detected in asymptomatic patients.[25,28,29]

Depending on the level of immune suppression, SOT recipients manifest signs and symptoms generally within 3 months after transplant. A broad spectrum of disease can be observed (see Table 29.2), including dissemination similar to that seen in severely immunosuppressed HSCT patients as well as isolated organ involvement[2,22,30-32] or no symptoms.[33]

The relationship between genotype of *T. gondii* and clinical findings in immunocompromised patients is controversial. Case reports suggest more severe disease associated with non–type II after allogeneic HSCT,[34] but another study of 88 *T. gondii* strains showed no differences in clinical outcomes.[35]

DISEASE PROPHYLAXIS AND PREVENTION

Pretransplant Monitoring

The serologic status of the donor and recipient is helpful in stratifying risk for *T. gondii* infection and disease. Patients with the highest risk of *T. gondii* infection and disease are seropositive HSCT recipients and seronegative recipients of a seropositive donor organ (D^+/R^-). The benefit of serology screening for organ transplantation may be debatable in low-seroprevalence countries such as the United States, especially with suppressive trimethoprim-sulfamethoxazole (TMP/SMX) therapy.[36] In the United States, serology screening for HSCT and SOT patients varies by institution. In contrast, pretransplant serology screening in France and many European countries is mandatory.[13] Since 2017 all deceased organ donors in the United States are routinely screened for *T. gondii*,[37] and this additional information may drive the desire to know the recipient's serostatus, especially with a seropositive donor heart organ. In the United States, routine pretransplant screening for allogeneic HSCT recipients, heart transplant recipients, and selected SOT and oncology patients seems prudent to strategize prevention of *T. gondii* disease.

Posttransplant Monitoring

Serology screening after transplant is not as useful, especially in HSCT recipients.[19] Transient increases of *T. gondii*–specific immunoglobulin (Ig) G may be due to passive antibody via blood transfusions. In addition, with immunosuppression, the antibody response may be altered or difficult to interpret. In these situations, *T. gondii* quantitative PCR assays are available and can be helpful.[38,39] Routine monitoring of peripheral blood with PCR assays in high-risk situations can detect circulating DNA, sometimes before manifestation of clinical signs and symptoms. A preemptive strategy, with routine serial PCR testing and initiation of treatment if test results are positive, may be useful for a HSCT patient before engraftment when routine suppressive TMP/SMX therapy is not favorable owing to myelosuppressive side effects.[40] In SOT patients, posttransplant serology testing can detect seroconversion with primary *T. gondii* infection, manifested as a positive *T. gondii*–specific IgM followed by a positive *T. gondii*–specific IgG. In a mismatched D^+/R^- scenario, seroconversion early after transplant suggests graft transmission.

Chemoprophylaxis

TMP/SMX is the most widely used therapy for prophylaxis, although no definitive clinical trial has been conducted to show efficacy (Table 29.3). Despite this, studies have shown that TMP/SMX

TABLE 29.3 Chemoprophylaxis for Prevention of *Toxoplasma gondii*

	Medication	Dose Infants/ Children	Dose Adults	Formulations	Notes
Preferred choice	TMP-sulfamethoxazole	75 mg/m²/dose twice a day 3 times per week on alternate days (2.5 mg/kg/dose twice a day 3 times per week on alternate days) OR 150 mg/m²/day once a day for 3 consecutive days per week (5 mg/kg/day once a day for 3 consecutive days per week) OR 150 mg/m²/day once a day[14] (dosing based on TMP)	1 single strength tablet (80 mg) once a day[45] OR 1 double strength tablet (160 mg) once a day 3 times weekly OR 1 double-strength tablet (160 mg) once a day [14] (dosing based on TMP)	Suspension 8 mg/mL (TMP) Tablets Single strength 80 mg (TMP) Double strength 160 mg (TMP)	These doses are also effective as prophylaxis for *Pneumocystis jirovecii.* If given daily, there is added benefit for preventing infection from bacteria, e.g. *Listeria, Nocardia, Salmonella, Haemophilus, Staphylococcus*[14]
Alternative	Atovaquone	*1-3 months old:* 30 mg/kg/day once a day *4-24 months old:* 45 mg/kg/day once a day WITH or WITHOUT pyrimethamine 1 mg/kg/day once a day AND leucovorin (folinic acid) 5mg once a day every 3 days[14] *>24 months:* 30 mg/kg/day once a day *Adolescents:* 1500 mg once a day Maximum: 1500 mg/day	1500 mg once a day	Suspension only Mepron 750 mg/5mL (5 mL, 210 mL) Generic 750 mg/5 mL (5 mL, 210 mL)	Administer with food, especially high-fat meal Expensive Mepron contains benzyl alcohol; citrus flavor

Continued

TABLE 29.3 Chemoprophylaxis for Prevention of *Toxoplasma gondii*—cont'd

	Medication	Dose Infants/ Children	Dose Adults	Formulations	Notes
Alternative	Dapsone (in combination with pyrimethamine and leucovorin)	*≥1 month old:* 2 mg/kg/dose once a day (15 mg/m^2/day once a day) AND pyrimethamine 1 mg/kg/day once a day AND leucovorin 5 mg once a day every 3 days.	50 mg once a day (AND pyrimethamine 75 mg once a week AND leucovorin 25 mg once a week) OR 200 mg once a week (AND pyrimethamine 75 mg once a week AND leucovorin 25 mg once a week)	Tablet (scored) 25 mg	Need to test for G6PD deficiency Do not use if severe TMP allergy Use in combination with pyrimethamine because of breakthrough. For HIV-infected patients, dapsone/pyrimethamine is preferred alternative compared to atovaquone based on more data

G6PD, Glucose-6-phosphate dehydrogenase deficiency; *mo*, month; *TMP*, trimethoprim.

prevented graft-transmitted *T. gondii* in D$^+$/R$^-$ mismatched scenarios when TMP/SMX was used for *Pneumocystis jirovecii* pneumonia prophylaxis.[2,36] In HSCT recipients, TMP/SMX seems to protect against *T. gondii* reactivation.[23] In one study, the absence of prophylaxis increased the odds of *T. gondii* disease and infection approximately 12-fold.[41] TMP/SMX has the added benefit of activity against several other pathogens. Other potential drugs are available for prophylaxis, but their efficacy is not definitively known.[23] In heart transplant recipients, one small study showed that no *T. gondii* infections occurred after starting pyrimethamine for routine prophylaxis.[42] For HSCT recipients intolerant of TMP/SMX, small studies show protection with weekly pyrimethamine-sulfadoxine and with atovaquone.[43,44] None of the current drugs eradicate tissue cysts, but TMP/SMX and atovaquone rapidly kill tachyzoites.[21] Prophylaxis can fail because of impaired absorption or drug interruption from intolerance.[40] Although it is used for prophylaxis against *Pneumocystis jirovecii* pneumonia, pentamidine has no activity against *T. gondii.*[23] Prophylaxis should continue for about 6 months in SOT[45] and HSCT patients.[23]

DIAGNOSIS

Diagnostic methods for *T. gondii* include serologic assays, molecular-based techniques (such as PCR), and histopathology (Table 29.4). Diagnosis of *T. gondii* infection is defined by detection of a positive PCR assay result in peripheral blood or primary seroconversion without organ involvement, with or without fever. Definitive diagnosis of *T. gondii*

TABLE 29.4 Diagnostic Testing for *Toxoplasma gondii*

Clinical Scenario	Laboratory Tests	Sample Source
Toxoplasma infection	PCR assay	Peripheral blood
	Toxoplasma IgM and IgG (in seronegative patient)	Peripheral blood
Toxoplasma disease	Sampling depends on organ involvement and/or dissemination	
	PCR assay	Peripheral blood, bone marrow, BAL, CSF, tissue biopsies, aqueous humor, vitreous fluid
	Giemsa-staining for tachyzoites	Peripheral blood, bone marrow, BAL, CSF
	Giemsa-staining and immunohistochemistry for tachyzoites	Tissue
	Intrathecal IgG (Western blot)	CSF (IgG production may be altered owing to immunosuppression)
	Intraocular IgG (Goldmann-Witmer coefficient [GWC] and Western blot)	Aqueous humor (AH) and serum in parallel GWC = *T. gondii* IgG (AH)/*T. gondii* IgG (serum) × Total IgG (serum)/Total IgG (AH) (IgG production may be altered owing to immunosuppression)
Pretransplant testing	*Toxoplasma* IgG • In SOT recipients with seropositive donor organs. • In all allogeneic HSCT recipients • Strongly consider in all SOT recipients	Peripheral blood
Posttransplant monitoring	PCR assay (e.g., weekly testing) • In HSCT when TMP/SMX prophylaxis is not provided during pre-engraftment period (preemptive strategy).	Peripheral blood
	Toxoplasma IgM and IgG • In mismatched D$^+$/R$^-$ SOT recipient	Peripheral blood

BAL, bronchoalveolar lavage; *CSF*, cerebral spinal fluid; *D*, donor; *HSCT*, hematopoietic stem cell transplant; *Ig*, immunoglobulin; *PCR*, polymerase chain reaction; *R*, recipient; *SOT*, solid organ transplant; *TMP/SMX*, trimethoprim-sulfamethoxazole.

TABLE 29.5 Treatment Options for *Toxoplasma gondii*

Preferred Regimen	Alternative Regimens	Notes
Adults: Pyrimethamine: loading dose: 200 mg by mouth once, then 50-100 mg/day orally *plus* Sulfadiazine: 4-6 g/daily by mouth or intravenously divided 4 times daily *plus* Leucovorin: 10-25 mg by mouth once daily *Pediatrics:* Pyrimethamine: loading dose: 2 mg/kg body weight (maximum 50 mg) by mouth once daily for 3 days, then 1 mg/kg body weight (maximum 25 mg) by mouth once daily, *plus* Sulfadiazine 25-50 mg/kg body weight (maximum 1- 1.5 g/dose) by mouth per dose 4 times daily *plus* Leucovorin 10-25 mg by mouth once daily *Treatment duration:* 4-6 weeks or longer depending on clinical response	*For sulfonamide-intolerant patients:* *Adults:* Clindamycin (maximum 600 mg/dose) by mouth or IV per dose given 4 times a day *plus* pyrimethamine *plus* Leucovorin *Pediatrics:* Clindamycin 5-7.5 mg/kg body weight (maximum 600 mg/dose) by mouth or IV per dose given 4 times a day *plus* Pyrimethamine *plus* leucovorin The following regimens have been used in adults but not studied in children: 1. TMP-SMX: TMP 5 mg/kg body weight *plus* SMX 25 mg/kg body weight per dose IV or by mouth given twice daily has been used as an alternative to pyrimethamine-sulfadiazine in adults 2. Azithromycin: 900-1,200 mg/day, *plus* pyrimethaminesulfadiazine, (has not been studied with sulfadiazine alone, or as a single agent in patients intolerant to both pyrimethamine and sulfadiazine) 3. In patients intolerant to both pyrimethamine and sulfadiazine: Atovaquone 1.5 g by mouth twice daily as a single age or *plus* pyrimethamine/leucovorin *OR plus* sulfadiazine	Pyrimethamine use requires CBC monitoring at least weekly while using daily dosing and at least monthly while using less than daily dosing. Corticosteroids (e.g., prednisone, dexamethasone) have been used in children with CNS disease when CSF protein is very elevated (>1000 mg/dL) or there are focal lesions with significant mass effects, with discontinuation as soon as clinically feasible.

CBC, complete blood cell count; *CNS*, central nervous system; *CSF*, cerebral spinal fluid; *IV*, intravenous; *TMP/SMX*, trimethoprim-sulfamethoxazole.

disease (*T. gondii* infection and organ involvement)[13] is based on detecting tachyzoites in blood, body fluids, or tissues. With microscopy, Giemsa stain can detect tachyzoites in bone marrow aspirates and in bronchoalveolar lavage (BAL) fluid. Giemsa stain and immunohistochemistry can detect tachyzoites and cysts in tissue.[46,47] Compared with microscopy, PCR may be more sensitive and specific,[38] but it has limitations. For example, although PCR assays can detect parasite DNA in blood, cerebrospinal fluid, aqueous humor, and BAL fluid with high specificity, its findings can be negative with localized disease.[29] Conversely, PCR assay findings can be transiently positive in HSCT and SOT patients who are asymptomatic.[28,29,33] Serology assays include *T. gondii*–specific IgM, IgG, and IgA. These test results may be negative in both primary and reactivation disease in immunocompromised individuals and therefore are not recommended for diagnosis of *T. gondii* disease.[19,37] In addition, for seropositive individuals, rising *T. gondii*–specific IgG titers should not be used to diagnose *T. gondii* disease because rising titers have been detected in asymptomatic patients.[19,32]

TREATMENT

Although not well studied, the most common first-line therapy for *T. gondii* disease is pyrimethamine with sulfadiazine as a synergistic combination, inhibiting tachyzoite proliferation[15,48] (Table 29.5). Because of hematologic adverse effects of pyrimethamine, folinic acid or leucovorin is administered simultaneously.[13] For patients with sulfadiazine allergy, clindamycin or azithromycin have been used in combination with pyrimethamine.[49] However, macrolides and clindamycin have a delayed effect against tachyzoites.[21] Atovaquone, doxycycline, and dapsone are potential alternatives.[13] Prognosis is dependent on the level of immunosuppression; therefore reduction of immune suppression may help. The benefit of adjuvant corticosteroids for central nervous system and ocular disease is not clear.[50] the duration of therapy is at least 4 to 6 weeks.[13]

INFECTION PREVENTION AND ANTICIPATORY GUIDANCE

Mitigating against exposure to *T. gondii* before and after transplantation will decrease the risk of environmental infection and disease. Transmission occurs with ingestion of oocysts in soil or water and ingestion of tissue cysts from infected animals (detailed in the "Epidemiology and Risk Factors" section); thus prevention against infection is based on avoiding these transmission mechanisms. Guidance for prevention measures is outlined in Table 29.6. Preventing donor transmission relies on screening donors and instituting prophylaxis strategies.

TABLE 29.6 Infection Prevention Measures

Transmission Route	Prevention Measure	Notes
Oocysts in the environment	• Wash hands and brush nails after gardening or any outdoor activities. • Wear gloves for gardening. • Avoid ingestion of water from lakes, rivers, reservoirs, wells, and raw surface water. • Avoid ingestion of raw oysters, clams, and mussels. • Thoroughly wash vegetables, fruits, and herbs that are eaten raw.	• Oocysts are killed within 1-2 minutes by heating to 55°C-60°C. • Oocysts are resistant to chemical disinfectants such as sodium hypochlorite. • Oocysts can survive for long periods in fresh water, in seawater, and in various species of shellfish
Oocysts in cat feces	• Wash hands after touching cats. • Avoid changing cat litter or wear gloves. • Change cat litter frequently and wash tray with >60°C hot water.	• Oocysts become infectious 2-3 days after shedding, so frequent changing of cat litter will mitigate exposure. • Oocyst shedding is about 2 weeks.
Tissues cysts in meat	• Cook meat well done or stew meat. • Avoid microwave cooking. • Freeze meat at −20°C or colder for at least 15 days before cooking and eating.	• Any type of meat may harbor tissue cysts, but sheep, goats, and pigs (raised in organic outdoor systems) and wild game are highest risk. • Cysts are immediately killed at 67°C • Cysts are killed if frozen for ≥3 days at −12°C or colder.

Adapted from Robert-Gangneux F, Darde M-L. Epidemiology of and diagnostic strategies for toxoplasmosis. *Clin Micro Rev.* 2012;25:264-296.

30

Nocardia and *Actinomyces*

Grant C. Paulsen, MD and Paul K. Sue, MD

NOCARDIA

Epidemiology and Risk Factors

Nocardia species are a heterogeneous group of ubiquitous aerobic, gram-positive filamentous organisms that reside in soil and decaying organic matter and are associated with an array of infections in both immunocompetent and immunocompromised hosts. First described by Edmond Nocard in 1888, *Nocardia* infections are associated with a range of illnesses, from localized suppurative skin lesions and chronic mycetomas, to invasive pulmonary infections, bacteremia and central nervous system (CNS) infection. Although nocardiosis remains a relatively rare infection overall, with an estimated 500 to 1000 cases diagnosed annually in the United States; immunocompromised hosts, particularly those with impaired T-cell immunity, are at significant risk for infection, with prevalence rates as high as 2.0% to 3.5% in select populations.[1,2] Geographically, *Nocardia* infections occur throughout the world, with variations in local incidence and *Nocardia* subspecies attributable to differences in climate and geography.[3] Within the United States, dry, warmer climates (such as in the Southwest) are associated with higher rates of *Nocardia* infection, potentially caused by increased aerosolization of pathogens with dust, or contamination of wounds with dirt.[4] Among children, 60% to 70% of cases occur in the setting of underlying immune deficiency (e.g., systemic lupus erythematosus, solid organ transplant [SOT], bone marrow transplant (BMT), chronic granulomatous disease, or cancer), with pulmonary infection the most common manifestation, followed by central nervous system (CNS) infection, disseminated bacteremia, and skin and soft tissue disease.[4] In contrast, approximately 30% of pediatric cases occur in otherwise immunocompetent children and typically present as lymphocutaneous disease, orbital cellulitis, arthritis, or pneumonia. Outcomes in this setting are almost uniformly good and rarely fatal.[5-7] In the largest single-center study of pediatric nocardiosis to date, 31 cases of *Nocardia brasiliensis* infection were identified among healthy children in south Texas over a 5-year period; all presented with lymphocutaneous disease, with no noted episodes of dissemination and no reported deaths.[8] In contrast, mortality rates among SOT and BMT recipients have been reported to be as high as 60% to 70%.[9]

Microbiology of *Nocardia*

The recent advent of molecular diagnostic tools such as gene sequencing and matrix-assisted laser desorption ionization/time-of-flight mass spectrometry has led to significant changes in the classification of *Nocardia* species. Although classic methods of identification previously relegated most pathogenic species to a relatively limited number of *Nocardia* groups or complexes, (*N. asteroides* complex, *N. brasiliensis* and *N. otitidiscaviarium*), the use of molecular diagnostics has led to the discovery of more than 50 distinct pathogenic *Nocardia* species previously classified within these groups. As a result, the complex previously known as *N. asteroides* complex, once considered the most pathogenic of *Nocardia* complexes, has in recent years been reclassified into six distinct taxa, each of which demonstrates unique antimicrobial susceptibility patterns; these include *N. nova, N. abscessus, N. transvallensis, N. brevicatena/N. paucivorans, N. cyriacigeorgica, and N. farcinica complexes.*[3] Other important pathogenic *Nocardia* species include *N. brasiliensis, N. otitidiscaviarium,* and *N. pseudobrasiliensis*. As a result of these classification changes, in recent years, the majority of Nocardia infections in the U.S. have been attributable to these species, specifically *N. nova*, *N. abscessus*, *N. farcinica*, and *N. cyriacigeorgica*.[2]

Given the unique pathogenic characteristics and antimicrobial susceptibility patterns of various *Nocardia* species, identification of *Nocardia* infections to the species level is recommended. Given the recognized limits of classic phenotypic testing, current guidelines recommend the use of molecular methods to identify Nocardia isolates in cases of suspected infection.[2,3]

Nocardiosis in Solid Organ Transplant Recipients

SOT recipients are at increased risk for nocardiosis, with high rates of associated morbidity and mortality.[11] Although estimates vary based on the type of organ transplanted, immunosuppressive regimen, and geographic region, the frequency of *Nocardia* infection among kidney, heart, and lung transplant recipients has been reported to be between 0.6% and 3.5%, with incidence estimates in transplant recipients suggesting a 100- to 3000-fold greater risk for *Nocardia* infection than in the general population.[12,13] As can be expected from an environmental pathogen that primarily enters the host via inhalation, lung transplant recipients are likely to be uniquely susceptible to nocardiosis. Among North American SOT recipients, lung transplant recipients are at greatest risk for *Nocardia* infection (3.5%), followed by heart transplant recipients (2.5%) and multivisceral transplant recipients (1.3%). Infection risk among liver and kidney transplant recipients is low, with less than 1% diagnosed with nocardiosis in most studies.[13] Potential donor-derived *Nocardia* transmission is another consideration in the SOT population. Although there are no published reports of donor-derived nocardiosis in pediatrics, it is listed a single time as a potential donor-derived transmission from the ad hoc Disease Transmission Advisory Committee based on the 2005-2009 Organ Procurement and Transplant Network reports.[14,15] Geography and environment are also likely to affect risk of infection among SOT recipients, with individuals residing in warm dry climates at increased risk of nocardiosis. In a study of more than 2000 SOT recipients in the American Southwest, the risk of infection was noted to be between 2 and 3 times higher across all SOT groups, compared with other regions. In this setting, lung transplant recipients remained at greatest risk (9.28%), with heart transplant (4.57%), kidney transplant (1.13%), and liver transplant recipients (0.45%) following, respectively.[16]

Nocardia infection is associated with significant morbidity and mortality among SOT recipients, with an overall estimated 10-fold increase in 1-year mortality risk over noninfected individuals.[17] Risk factors for infection among SOT recipients include receipt of high-dose steroids, cytomegalovirus disease in the preceding 6 months, use of tacrolimus, and high median calcineurin inhibitor levels in the preceding 30 days.[11,13] The majority of infections occur between 1 month and 1 year after, with a range of clinical presentations from predominately isolated pulmonary infections (~70%) in North American studies to higher rates of disseminated disease (~40%) and CNS infection (25%) in European studies.[11]

Nocardiosis in Hematologic Malignancy and Stem Cell Transplant

Hematology/oncology patients and recipients of hematopoietic stem cell transplant (HSCT) are also at increased risk for morbidity and mortality owing to nocardiosis. Incidence estimates from a systematic review between 1966 and 2004 reported 13 cases/1000 person-years among BMT recipients, 300 times greater than the estimated risk in the general population.[12] Other more recent (2008 to 2013) retrospective studies in HSCT recipients found an incidence rate of 2.4 cases/1000 patients.[18] Depending on the type of HSCT, such as autologous versus allogeneic, other reported incidence rates vary from 0.4% to 3.6%. Predisposing risk factors for nocardiosis in the HSCT population include high prednisone doses (≥20 mg of prednisone per day), lymphopenia, concurrent opportunistic infections (e.g., cytomegalovirus), $CD4^+$ T cells <100 cells/μL and active graft-versus-host disease.[18,19] Sites of infection in adult HSCT and oncology patients are similar to those seen in SOT with pulmonary infection the most common (70% to 87%), followed by CNS/disseminated infection (47% to 50%), and skin (6% to 8%). *Nocardia* infection-related mortality in HSCT and oncology patients remains high with reports ranging from 60% to 70% mortality and one report of approximately 25% survival at 300 days after diagnosis of *Nocardia*.[18-20]

Clinical Presentation

Because of its ubiquitous presence in the environment, *Nocardia* often gains entry via the respiratory tract into the lungs. From there, *Nocardia* species can cause localized pulmonary disease or continue to spread to other sites, resulting in a diverse spectrum of infection. In general, the clinical presentation of nocardiosis tends to be similar across SOT, HSCT, and oncology patients.

Pulmonary nocardiosis is the most frequent manifestation of infection in immunocompetent and immunocompromised patients. Symptoms in both groups and across SOT, HSCT, and oncology patients most commonly consist of fever (80%) and productive cough (60%) with or without shortness of breath/dyspnea, chills, pleuritic chest pain, and/or weight loss; hemoptysis is less frequently reported (<10%).[20] Generally, pulmonary nocardiosis presents as a subacute process with symptoms present for up to several weeks and abnormal thoracic imaging is a common finding (see "Diagnosis" section). Reports of presenting symptoms in pediatric SOT patients include fever and chest pain.[21]

Extrapulmonary nocardiosis is common in immunocompromised patients and is often due to hematogenous dissemination to other sites or contiguous spread from a pulmonary focus into the nearby structures. Although estimates of disseminated nocardiosis vary, approximately 30% to 50% of immunocompromised patients with *Nocardia* infections are found to have disseminated disease, with the CNS as the most common secondary site.

The clinical presentation of patients with CNS or disseminated nocardiosis has been documented in adults and can be quite variable and nonspecific. Although CNS infection can present as classic meningismus, *Nocardia* infections of the CNS tend to occur as one or more focal abscesses, and symptoms may also be more indolent than other more common bacterial etiologies. Clinical presentation of CNS nocardiosis covers a spectrum of symptoms from silent with no focal neurologic findings to altered mental status and unresponsiveness.[22] Signs and symptoms at the time of clinical presentation can be those seen with any space-occupying lesion, including headaches, seizures, motor and sensory deficits, personality changes, fevers, nausea, emesis, visual changes, weight loss, and other nonspecific generalized symptoms. One case reported presenting symptoms in immunocompromised children including fever, diarrhea, lethargy, nausea, and meningismus.[23]

Skin and soft tissue infections can occur after direct inoculation, including minor trauma, or as a manifestation of hematogenous spread. Initially, in most immunocompromised patients, it is often not readily apparent which route is responsible for the lesions seen on examination; therefore a broad workup is often necessary. Cutaneous manifestations are variable and include cellulitis, subcutaneous nodules/pustules, lymphocutaneous disease (sporotrichoid nocardiosis), abscesses, pyomyositis, and/or mycetomas. Erythema may also be present in addition to spontaneous drainage of lesions. Cutaneous nocardiosis also more frequently involves the face and lower extremities as opposed to the upper extremities or torso. Soft tissue nocardiosis as the result of disseminated infection tends to more commonly manifest as a deeper abscess or nodules rather than more superficial lesions. Localized, nondisseminated cutaneous infections are most often seen in immunocompetent patients, including otherwise healthy children.[10]

Although localized cutaneous nocardiosis remains relatively uncommon in the SOT, HSCT, and oncology patient populations, skin and soft tissue nocardiosis is more commonly a sign of disseminated disease. In an analysis of adult SOT recipients with nocardiosis, localized skin and soft tissue infection as the only site of infection was seen in only 7% of patients, whereas skin and soft tissue infection as part of disseminated infection was seen in 32%.[11]

Other less common manifestations include bone or joint, endocarditis/pericarditis, renal, and ocular infections. Although *Nocardia* bacteremia is generally regarded as a relatively uncommon finding, it has been reported in approximately 8% of adult SOT and 27% of adult HSCT recipients with nocardiosis.[17,19] Central venous catheter (CVC)-associated *Nocardia* has been reported in immunocompromised pediatric and adult patients, either as disseminated (or secondary) bacteremia or as central line–associated bloodstream infection alone.[24] Symptoms include fever, chills, malaise, pain, and/or erythema at the CVC insertion site.

Prevention and Prophylaxis

There is no proven intervention that has been shown to be clearly effective in preventing nocardiosis in SOT, HSCT, or oncology patients. Despite what would appear to be an appealing biologically plausible link, and historic reports on the benefit of trimethoprim-sulfamethoxazole (TMP/SMX) prophylaxis, evidence of clear efficacy of TMP/SMX prophylaxis for nocardiosis remains elusive. One case-control study in adult SOT recipients with nocardiosis reported up to 18% of cases occurring in the setting of TMP/SMX prophylaxis given for *Pneumocystis jirovecii* pneumonia (PJP), and although there was a slight reduction in risk (odds ratio 0.36, 95% confidence interval 0.14 to 0.93, $P = 0.03$), this was not present in multivariable analysis.[11]

Other studies in immunocompromised patients have reported similar, and even greater, rates of breakthrough nocardiosis—up to 69% in some cases.[13] Of the *Nocardia* isolates from those patients with breakthrough infection treated with TMP/SMX, the majority of isolates (79% to 100%) are typically found to be susceptible to TMP/SMX, leaving resistance to TMP/SMX as an unlikely explanation for the failure.

The most commonly proposed explanation for this somewhat confounding result is that the efficacy of TMP/SMX for the prevention of nocardiosis may be dependent on dose and frequency, and routine prophylaxis (often given 2 to 3 times per week for PJP) is not sufficient. Data are similar in the HSCT population in that TMP/SMX does not reliably prevent nocardiosis. Although some report a potential benefit of TMP/SMX prophylaxis in preventing disseminated nocardiosis, this is also not a reproducible finding.[25] Additionally, there are reports of breakthrough nocardiosis in HSCT recipients receiving daily (single-strength) TMP/SMX.[25] While the data on efficacy of TMP/SMX for prevention of nocardiosis remain mixed, fortunately there is little evidence that prophylaxis given for other reasons (i.e., PJP or toxoplasmosis) will select for TMP/SMX-resistant *Nocardia* isolates.[18]

Diagnosis

The diagnosis of *Nocardia* infection typically relies on culture and identification of the organism from the appropriate clinical site. Because of the broad variability in clinical manifestations of nocardiosis as well as the other potential pathogens on the differential for most immunocompromised patients, the time to definitive diagnosis of *Nocardia* can be prolonged, with interval from symptom development to diagnosis of 20 to 30 days in both SOT and HSCT. Rarely, patients in both groups can have symptoms for more than 3 months before diagnosis. Culture of *Nocardia* species requires special consideration, as opposed to simply obtaining routine aerobic and anaerobic bacterial cultures. Because of their relatively slow growth, isolation of *Nocardia* can require extended incubation periods.[26] In some cases, *Nocardia* species may grow after a minimum of 2 to 5 days, whereas in other cases up to 4 weeks can be necessary; therefore the microbiology laboratory should be made aware of the clinical suspicion for *Nocardia* and samples should also be set up on media optimized for fungi and/or mycobacteria to allow for longer incubation times. Although standard fungal and mycobacterial cultures readily grow *Nocardia*, in some cases the digestion and decontamination procedures used for mycobacterial culture may render *Nocardia* nonviable. Therefore mycobacterial culture media should not be the sole method used for testing, and culture for fungi may be preferred.[10]

Direct examination of gram-stained specimens can demonstrate filamentous, beaded, and/or branching rods that stain weakly gram-positive and are partially acid-fast.[9] In the appropriate clinical setting, microscopic visualization of the organism can allow for an early, presumptive diagnosis while complete culture results are still in process.

In clinical practice, the approach to diagnosing nocardiosis often requires a combination of clinical suspicion, examination findings, and radiographic studies, which in turn leads to site selection for sampling of material for culture (i.e., blood, spinal fluid, respiratory fluid, and/or biopsy specimen). See Fig. 30.1 for a proposed diagnostic workup schema for *Nocardia*; other/additional diagnostic studies may be indicated to evaluate alternative etiologies and/or disseminated nocardiosis to less common sites, such as musculoskeletal, ocular, cardiac, or other sites. As with many infections in immunocompromised hosts, a low threshold for broad diagnostic testing and imaging is often warranted.

Although some findings indicative of pulmonary nocardiosis can be seen on a chest radiograph, computed tomography (CT) is preferred to evaluate and characterize any lesions (Fig. 30.2). Common findings in SOT recipients include airspace consolidation (64%), nodules (57%), masses (21%), pleural effusions (28%), and mediastinal/hilar lymphadenopathy (15%).[27] Nodules can be variable in distribution and appearance, with either ill-defined or well-defined borders, smooth or spiculate margins; lesions may be solitary or in clusters and may also be cavitary (40%). In one series of adult SOT recipients, 43% of those ultimately found to have CNS nocardiosis had no neurologic abnormalities on examination.[11] Therefore, CNS imaging should be performed in any immunocompromised host with nocardiosis, once the diagnoses is established. Contrast-enhanced magnetic resonance imaging is the modality of choice, as CT imaging may not be sensitive enough to detect subtle findings and small lesions.[27] Imaging in CNS nocardiosis is variable, with up to 80% of imaging in SOT recipients showing multiple lesions made up of a combination of 53% bihemispheric, 93% supratentorial, and 30% infratentorial locations.[11] Ring-enhancing lesions, sometimes with surrounding edema (Fig. 30.3), in an immunocompromised patient should place *Nocardia* firmly in the differential diagnosis in addition to other etiologies, such as toxoplasmosis.

In addition to microbiologic culture and histopathology, molecular methods are used extensively in the identification of *Nocardia* and have been used for diagnosis as well. Historically, phenotypic characterization methods were used to identify *Nocardia* to the species level, but these steps are laborious, time-consuming, and require expert interpretation. Currently available molecular methods are sensitive and less time-consuming; therefore a combination of phenotypic and molecular methods is now essentially required for full identification of any *Nocardia* species.[10] Molecular techniques for initial diagnosis of *Nocardia* infection, using 16S ribosomal ribonucleic acid/DNA polymerase chain reaction testing, have also been used in a few reported cases and are an additional consideration for diagnostic testing.[28,29]

Treatment

Treatment of nocardiosis typically consists of an initial, presumptive phase followed by a more tailored course of antimicrobials based on susceptibility testing. Since the 1940s, the mainstay of treatment for nocardiosis has been the sulfonamide class of antibiotics, and they have remained the cornerstone of treatment ever since. Aside from the generally reliable utility of sulfonamides, most often TMP/SMX, a number of questions still remain regarding the optimal management of nocardiosis in transplant patients, including choice and number of agents, duration of therapy, and need for secondary prophylaxis.

The choice of initial treatment regimen, before the availability of susceptibility results, largely depends on the site, or sites, of infection (Fig. 30.4).[2,9] If the *Nocardia* species has been identified based on molecular methods before antibiotic susceptibility testing, then species-specific antibiograms should be weighed into the decision regarding initial antimicrobial therapy.[10] In addition, Brown-Elliott and colleagues identified six characteristic antimicrobial susceptibility testing patterns and grouped the known *Nocardia* species into each of these groups. In the absence of definitive susceptibility results, these pattern types (I-VI) can be used, in addition to TMP/SMX, to guide initial therapy decisions before the return of organism-specific susceptibility testing results (Table 30.1).[3,10]

Given the relatively high mortality of CNS and/or disseminated nocardiosis and the different antibiotic resistance patterns among *Nocardia* species, most recommendations include initial combination therapy for these infections.[9,10] Synergy and/or an additive effect have been shown for imipenem combined with TMP/SMX, cefotaxime or amikacin, as well as for amikacin combined with TMP/SMX or

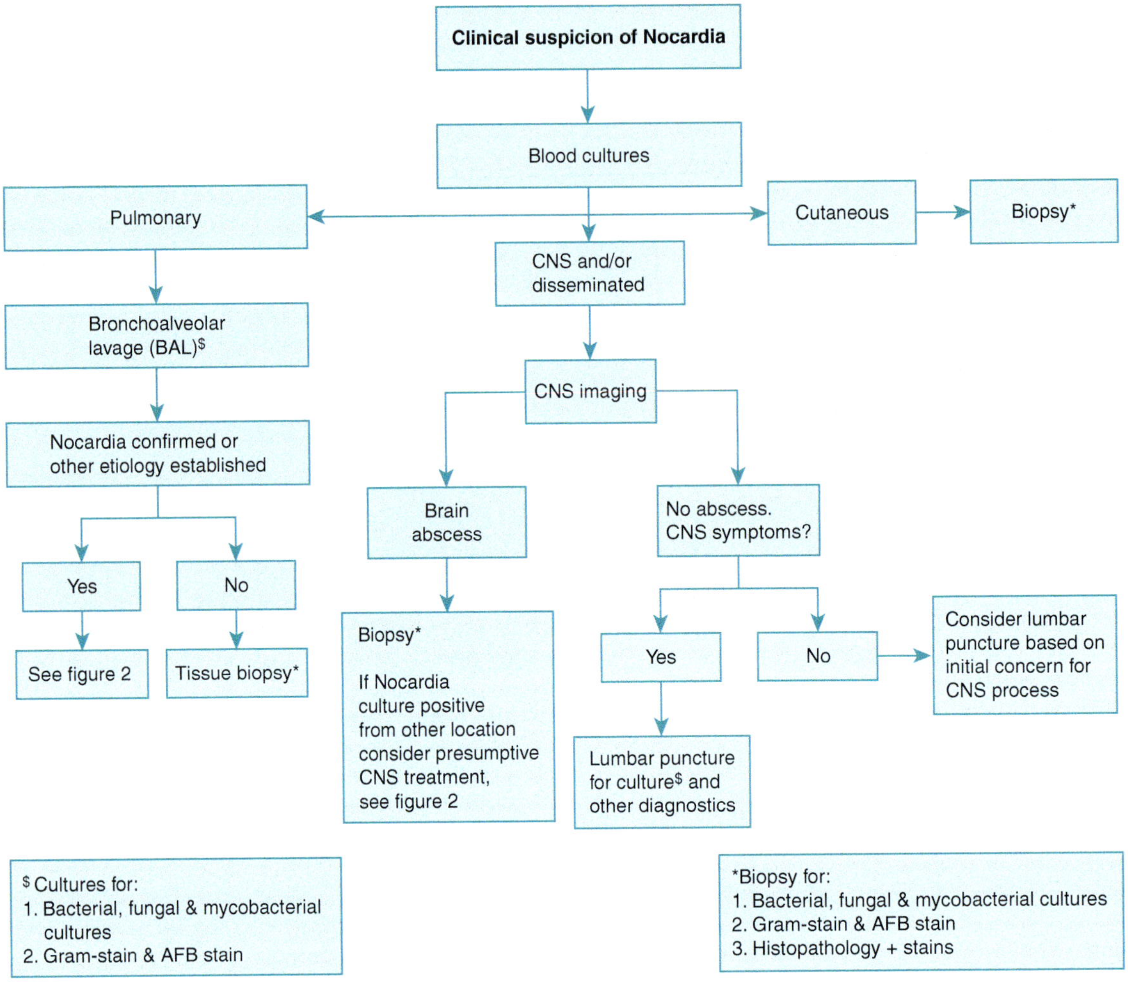

Fig. 30.1 Diagnostic algorithm for *Nocardia* infection. *AFB,* acid-fast bacillus; *BAL,* bronchoalveoler lavage; *CNS,* central nervous system. (Adapted from Restrepo A, Clark NM. Nocardia infections in solid organ transplantation: Guidelines from the Infectious Diseases Community of Practice of the American Society of Transplantation. *Clin Transplant.* 2019:e13509; and Lebeaux D, Freund R, van Delden C, et al. Outcome and treatment of nocardiosis after solid organ transplantation: new insights from a European study. *Clin Infect Dis.* 2017;64[10]:1396-1405.)

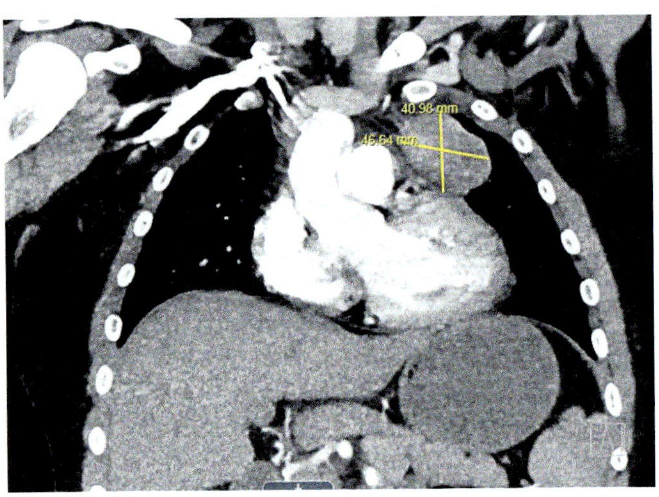

Fig. 30.2 A 20-year-old man with *Nocardia farcinica* pulmonary infection after second renal transplant.

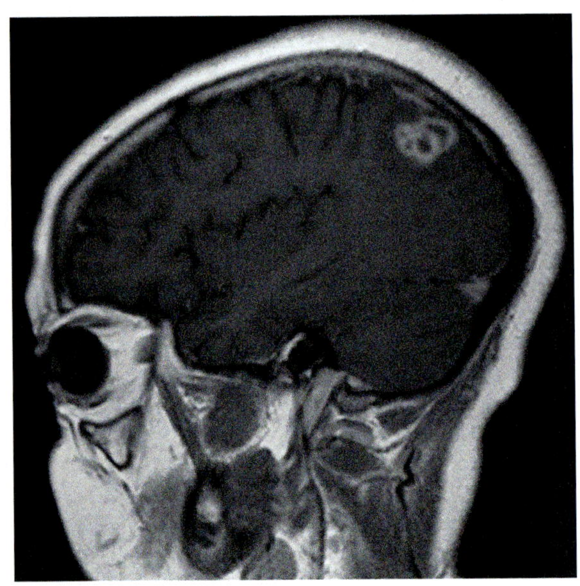

Fig. 30.3 A 21-year-old woman with a history of liver and kidney transplant with disseminated (pulmonary and central nervous system) *Nocardia otitidiscaviarum.*

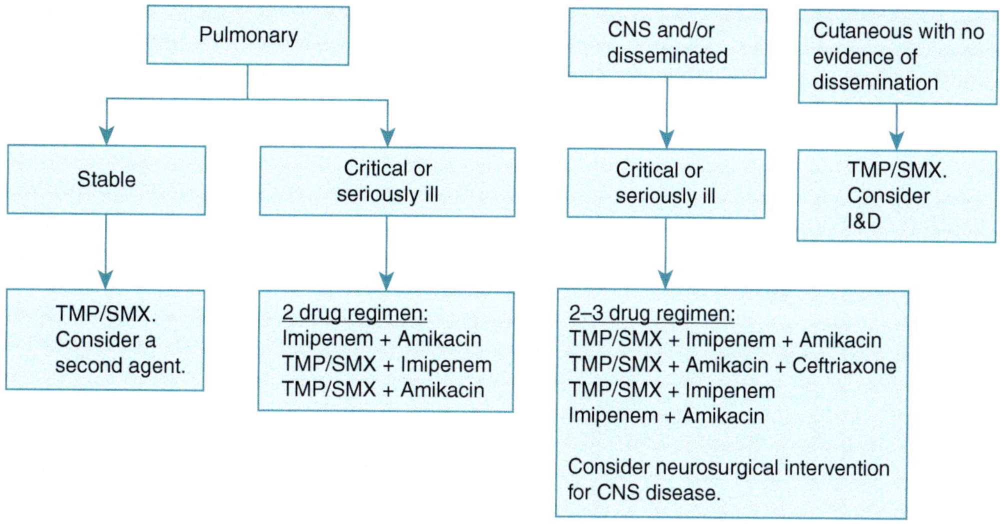

Fig. 30.4 Treatment algorithm for *Nocardia* infection. *CNS,* central nervous system; *I&D,* incision and drainage; *TMP/SMX,* trimethoprim-sulfamethoxazole. (Adapted from Restrepo A, Clark NM. Nocardia infections in solid organ transplantation: guidelines from the Infectious Diseases Community of Practice of the American Society of Transplantation. *Clin Transplant.* 2019:e13509; and Lebeaux D, Freund R, van Delden C, et al. Outcome and treatment of nocardiosis after solid organ transplantation: new insights from a European study. *Clin Infect Dis.* 2017;64[10]:1396-1405.)

TABLE 30.1 Antimicrobial Susceptibility Patterns: Nocardia

Complex or Species	Drug Pattern Type	Major Drug Pattern Characteristics
Nocardia abscessus complex	I	Susceptible to ampicillin, amoxicillin-clavulanic acid, ceftriaxone, linezolid, sulfamethoxazole and amikacin; most have resistant MICs for imipenem; resistant to ciprofloxacin and clarithromycin
N. brevicatena/paucivorans complex	II	Same as type I but kanamycin MICs low (1 μg/mL) and susceptible to ciprofloxacin; usually resistant to gentamicin; resistant to clarithromycin
N. nova complex	III	Susceptible to ampicillin but resistant to amoxicillin-clavulanic acid; susceptible to erythromycin, clarithromycin, linezolid, and ceftriaxone; very low MICs to imipenem and amikacin
N. transvalensis complex	IV	Resistant to all aminoglycosides, including amikacin; susceptible to ciprofloxacin, ceftriaxone, linezolid, and imipenem; resistant to erythromycin and clarithromycin
N. farcinica complex	V	Resistant to ampicillin, broad-spectrum cephalosporins, and clarithromycin; resistant to aminoglycosides except amikacin; susceptible to ciprofloxacin, linezolid, and imipenem
N. cyriacigeorgica complex	VI	Resistant to amoxicillin-clavulanic acid, clarithromycin, and ciprofloxacin; susceptible to ampicillin, ceftriaxone, amikacin, linezolid, and imipenem
N. brasiliensis	N/A	Susceptible to minocycline, amoxicillin-clavulanic acid, carbenicillin and sulfamethoxazole; resistant to kanamycin, cefamandole, ampicillin, ciprofloxacin, and clarithromycin
N. pseudobrasiliensis	N/A	Susceptible to carbenicillin, ciprofloxacin, clarithromycin and sulfamethoxazole; resistant to kanamycin, cefamandole, ampicillin, minocycline, and amoxicillin-clavulanic acid
N. otitidiscaviarum complex	N/A	Susceptible to kanamycin, gentamicin, amikacin, sulfamethoxazole, and ciprofloxacin; resistant to ceftriaxone, ampicillin, amoxicillin-clavulanic acid, carbenicillin, and imipenem (often resistant to all β-lactam antibiotics)

MIC, minimum inhibitory concentration; *N/A,* not applicable.
Adapted from Brown-Elliott BA, Brown JM, Conville PS, Wallace RJ Jr. Clinical and laboratory features of the *Nocardia* spp. based on current molecular taxonomy. *Clin Microbiol Rev.* 2006;19(2):259-282; and Conville PS, Brown-Elliott BA, Smith T, Zelazny AM. The complexities of *Nocardia* taxonomy and identification. *J Clin Microbiol.* 2018;56(1).

cefotaxime.[30] Pulmonary nocardiosis in a critical or seriously ill patient should also be treated with combination therapy. Although single-agent TMP/SMX treatment may be considered for stable pulmonary nocardiosis, given reports of treatment failures of single-agent TMP/SMX therapy in SOT recipients, consideration of a second agent may be reasonable, at least until clinical improvement is seen.

Susceptibility testing, as opposed to reliance on published species-level susceptibility reports, should be performed on isolates from any *Nocardia* infection in an immunocompromised host. Clinical and Laboratory Standards Institute guidelines for antimicrobial susceptibility testing were first published in 2003, recommending broth microdilution as the preferred method. Owing to the complexities in performance and interpretation of susceptibility testing, referral for testing to a qualified and experienced laboratory is reasonable, especially for those microbiology laboratories that do not frequently culture and test *Nocardia*. One illustration of the complexity and difficulty in susceptibility testing for

Nocardia is the issue of TMP/SMX resistance. A number of studies in 2010 and 2011 reported a surprisingly high degree of TMP/SMX resistance—up to 43% of some cases. A subsequent study of 552 isolates from six major centers experienced in *Nocardia* susceptibility testing found only 2.5% of isolates were resistant to TMP/SMX (0.5%) and/or sulfamethoxazole (2.0%).[31] The authors emphasized the need for careful training and close scrutiny of laboratory proficiency with respect to accurate *Nocardia* susceptibility testing.

Although TMP/SMX is generally the preferred agent in the treatment of nocardiosis, there are a number of other agents with potential activity. As previously stated, the activity of different antimicrobials varies across the different species of *Nocardia*. In addition to TMP/SMX, both linezolid and amikacin typically have the highest reliability against almost all species of *Nocardia*, with 100% and 99% susceptibility reported, respectively.[32] Other agents with potential activity include imipenem, meropenem, ceftriaxone, cefotaxime, clarithromycin, fluoroquinolones, amoxicillin-clavulanate, tigecycline, tobramycin, and minocycline. Tedizolid has also shown excellent in vitro activity against all *Nocardia* species tested. While there is currently little experience with its use in nocardiosis or pediatrics, it is a potentially attractive future therapeutic option owing to its reportedly improved side effect profile compared with linezolid. Although tigecycline, minocycline, and some fluoroquinolones do have activity against some strains, their use in pediatrics, especially children younger than 8 years, should be undertaken with caution.

Full susceptibility testing of the specific *Nocardia* isolate is generally recommended, as susceptibility to one agent does not always predict the same degree of activity to other agents, even within the same class of antimicrobials. One example is that imipenem susceptibility does not always equate to meropenem susceptibility for the same isolate; therefore meropenem for definitive treatment should only be used after specific susceptibility testing.[9] Along the same lines, ertapenem is significantly less active against *Nocardia* than either imipenem or meropenem. Although While linezolid has 100% in vitro activity against all clinically significant *Nocardia* species, there are in vitro reports of antagonism with both amikacin and imipenem, although without clear clinical impact.[9] Therefore even though linezolid is a potential option in place of imipenem or amikacin, combination therapy should be undertaken cautiously.

As combination therapy is often necessary and often for a prolonged period of time, comprehensive susceptibility testing can also provide information on treatment options that may be necessary during the treatment course. Changes to the initial treatment regimen are common, with one series reporting more than 50% of treated adult SOT or HSCT patients required between two and five different regimens, most commonly because of either intolerance or progression of disease.[18]

In addition to antimicrobial therapy, aspiration or drainage of any abscess or similar collection should be considered. Although this can be a relatively low-risk procedure for a soft tissue abscess, the risks involved in drainage of a CNS abscess warrant careful attention. Retrospective mortality in an adult cohort with CNS nocardiosis found those treated with both targeted antimicrobial therapy and neurosurgery (evacuation or aspiration) had decreased mortality (7%) compared with those treated with antimicrobial therapy alone (mortality 22%) or neurosurgery alone (mortality 36%).[22] Despite the paucity of data in pediatrics to supplement the consideration for surgical intervention versus antibiotics alone, there are successful reports of pediatric transplant recipients with CNS nocardiosis treated with medical therapy alone.[33]

The recommended duration of therapy in immunocompromised hosts is typically is 6 to 12 months for pulmonary nocardiosis, 9 to 12 months for CNS and disseminated infections, with 3 to 6 weeks parenteral therapy followed by oral therapy to complete the course.[2] Optimal timing on changing from an initial intravenous (IV) regimen to an oral/enteral regimen is not well defined. It is reasonable to consider a change from IV to oral once good clinical response has been demonstrated, and identification and susceptibility testing has been completed with susceptibility data of at least one oral antimicrobial option with good bioavailability.

Although many experts would recommend 12 months of treatment for nocardiosis in any immunocompromised patient, there are reports of successful treatment in adult SOT recipients receiving shorter courses of therapy, with good outcomes in pulmonary and cutaneous infections treated with median courses of 56 (23 to 120) days, as well as pulmonary nocardiosis after adult heart transplant treated for less than 120 days.[17] Reports of treatment regimens and outcomes in pediatric SOT and HSCT remain scarce, with successful cases reporting durations of approximately 1 year in CNS nocardiosis after renal and liver transplant, and approximately 24 months for CNS disease in a pediatric oncology patient.[21,23,33] Treatment regimens included TMP/SMX monotherapy in one case, TMP/SMX plus a second agent in one case, and monotherapy with sequential linezolid, then meropenem followed by amoxicillin-clavulanate in one case. Duration of treatment for CVC-associated *Nocardia* bacteremia is not well defined. There are reports of relapsed infection in a pediatric oncology patient treated with line retention and ceftriaxone for 28 days, as opposed to successful treatment with removal of the CVC and antibiotic courses of 14 to 90 days.[34]

After completion of therapy for all *Nocardia* infections, patients should be monitored closely for any sign of relapse. For patients with CNS disease, repeat imaging of the brain is also suggested.[2] Similar to primary prophylaxis for nocardiosis, there are few data to guide the use of secondary prophylaxis after the completion of therapy. Although primary prophylaxis with TMP/SMX for PJP does not reliably prevent nocardiosis, some providers believe there may be benefit with respect to prevention of relapse and choose to use TMP/SMX for long-term secondary prophylaxis.[18,35] The most commonly reported regimen is 3 times a week, up to daily, TMP/SMX, and there are also (fewer) reports of azithromycin used as secondary prophylaxis.

Infection Prevention and Anticipatory Guidance

Because the primary route of transmission for *Nocardia* is likely inhalation from the environment, there have been reports of presumed nosocomial spread via contact with a health care worker and/or nearby construction, as well as clusters of infection from a common environmental source. Standard transmission-based isolation precautions for nocardiosis are appropriate in most cases, with additional precautions potentially used if the isolate is considered multidrug resistant based on local criteria. To prevent direct inoculation, immunocompromised patients should cover their skin when working in soil or similar settings.[26]

ACTINOMYCES

Epidemiology

Actinomyces species are slow-growing, microaerophilic to facultative anaerobic, gram-positive, filamentous branching bacilli that are known to cause infection in three distinct anatomic sites: cervicofacial, thoracic, and abdominal.[26] They belong to the order Actinomycetales, along with *Mycobacteria* and *Nocardia*. There are more than 40 known species of *Actinomyces*, and infections have commonly been reported owing to *A. israelii*, *A. odontolyticus*, *A. mayeri*, *A. naeslundii*, *A. neuii*, *A. turensis*, and *A. graerenitzii*.[36]

In general, pediatric actinomycosis is uncommon, representing less than 3% of reported *Actinomyces* cases.[37] *Actinomyces* species are generally opportunistic pathogens, with disease reported after penetrating or nonpenetrating trauma as well as any breach of the mucosal barrier. The pathogens are also notorious for their ability to directly cross tissue planes and extend into bone to cause soft tissue abscesses and chronic suppurative granulomatous infections.

Actinomycosis in pediatric SOT and HSCT recipients remains a rare infection, with reported cases in the literature occurring only in adults. An adult center reporting on 16 years of actinomycosis found 2 of 36 (6%) proven infections occurred in SOT recipients and 6 (17%) occurred in patients with concurrent malignancy. Alcohol abuse and foreign bodies/devices are commonly reported factors associated with actinomycosis in adults, whereas breaks in the mucosal barrier, including trauma, perforation, or surgery, are often risks in pediatrics.[38] In another analysis of 366 surveillance and clinically triggered bronchoscopy specimens after adult lung transplantation, only a single culture (0.3%) was positive for *Actinomyces*.[39] Although there are reports of actinomycosis in patients with human immunodeficiency virus as well as patients with other immune-compromising conditions, such as autoimmune disorders and certain primary immunodeficiencies, the degree of association between SOT and/or HSCT and the risk of *Actinomyces* infection remains elusive. A national study of actinomycosis after renal transplantation found an estimated prevalence of 0.02% (7 cases of 34,268 renal transplant recipients).[36] All cases were in adult SOT recipients, and the median time between transplant and diagnosis was 104 months. Based on population data in the same region, the authors estimated that actinomycosis prevalence may be increased up to 10-fold in adult kidney transplant recipients. As there are no similar data for pediatric SOT, HSCT, or oncology patients, the associated risk in these populations remains unknown. Although overall treatment outcomes are generally good, as with many other opportunistic infections, an infection with invasive actinomycosis is potentially a marker of poor overall prognosis.[40]

Clinical Presentation

The most commonly reported sites of actinomycosis in SOT and HSCT patients remain the same as for nontransplant recipients: cervicofacial (50% to 60%), thoracic (15% to 20%), and abdominal (20%).[37] Less commonly reported infections include skin and soft tissue, musculoskeletal, bacteremia, endocarditis/pericarditis, and infection of the CNS. In general, polymicrobial infections are common, with up to 80% of invasive *Actinomycosis* infections reported as polymicrobial. Common copathogens include *Actinobacillus actinomycetemcomitans, Fusobacterium, Clostridia, Klebsiella, Bacteroides, Eikenella, Enterococccus,* and *Peptostreptococcus*. Although rare, there are cases reported of actinomycosis occurring after adult renal, liver, heart ,and heart-lung SOT as well as HSCT and peripheral blood stem cell transplant.[36,41-44] No similar case series or reports of pediatric actinomycosis in SOT, HSCT, or oncology patients are in the current literature. *Actinomyces* organisms are routinely included in the category of infections labeled "great masqueraders" and are often misdiagnosed initially, frequently as a malignancy. In the adult SOT and HSCT population, this is a commonly reported scenario.

Clinical presentations in adult SOT and HSCT recipients are not significantly different than those reported in immunocompetent patients. The reported clinical presentation of cervicofacial actinomycoses in adult SOT or HSCT recipients includes oropharyngeal, glottis, and esophageal abscess or ulceration, as well as sinusitis with or without symptoms of pneumonia.[41,44-46] In a review of immunocompetent pediatric cases of cervicofacial actinomycosis, all patients presented with mandibular or neck masses and associated pain (47%), fever (29%), dysphagia (6%), and/or draining sinus (6%).[47] Lesions often develop along one of two lines: slowly over weeks to months, often without pain, or more rapidly with associated constitutional symptoms often culminating in a suppurative infection/abscess.

Thoracic actinomycosis in children often presents with cough, chest pain, hemoptysis, fever, and weight loss.[48] Chest imaging can vary from parenchymal opacity/consolidation with or without pleural thickening and hilar lymphadenopathy to frank abscess formation with lung destruction and extension into the mediastinum or through the diaphragm.

Abdominal actinomycosis in children typically presents as abdominal pain (79%), palpable abdominal mass (68%), fever (53%), and/or sinus tract/drainage (37%).[37] Abdominal imaging may demonstrate a mass with an invasive pattern that mimics malignancy, bowel wall inflammation/thickening, fistulae, or complete obstruction.[43]

Prevention and Prophylaxis

Although pediatric SOT, HSCT and oncology patients routinely receive a variety of antimicrobial prophylaxis before, during, and after transplant or chemotherapy, prevention of *Actinomyces* is typically not a specified goal of these regimens. It is also unclear if prophylaxis is effective for prevention, as two of the five cases reported after adult SCT occurred in patients receiving penicillin prophylaxis, although adherence was uncertain in one of those two patients. In a series of adult renal transplant recipients with actinomycosis, the suspected portal of entry was dental in 57%, raising the consideration for comprehensive treatment of any dental caries or other oral disease before transplant and the importance of dental hygiene after transplant.

Diagnosis

Although the gold standard for diagnosis of *Actinomyces* is a positive culture result from a normally sterile site, however, growing the organism requires special considerations. Culture material should be freshly obtained, using specific anaerobic media and maintained for a longer duration than typical aerobic and anaerobic cultures, often requiring 14 to 21 days to grow. Communication with the microbiology laboratory is an important step if there is clinical suspicion of actinomycosis. Microscopically, *Actinomyces* species appear as beaded, branched, gram-positive bacilli and are often described as filamentous. As opposed to *Nocardia, Actinomyces* species are acid-fast negative. Yellow "sulfur granules" seen microscopically or macroscopically are also highly suggestive of *Actinomyces* species, but they are not specific, since similar lesions can also be seen in infections caused by *Nocardia* and *Streptomcyes* species. Conversely, not all species of *Actinomyces* form sulfur granules, including *A. odontolyticus*. Sulfur granules are 1- to 3-mm aggregates of *Actinomcyes* surrounded by neutrophils, often seen within purulent collections and can give the collection a yellow, sulfur-like appearance.[26] There is no actual sulfur in the granules. Owing to their fastidious nature and generally slow growth, *Actinomyces* species can be difficult to accurately identify and both matrix-assisted laser desorption ionization–time-of-flight mass spectrometry and 16S ribosomal ribonucleic acid gene sequencing have been used for reliable species-level identification.[49] Histopathology is also frequently used in the diagnosis, most often in those cases when malignancy is highest on the differential diagnosis and a specimen is not sent for culture. Histopathology in patients with actinomycosis routinely demonstrates sulfur granules with or without surrounding fibrotic granulation tissue.

Treatment

Appropriate management of actinomycosis often requires both surgical and medical management. Surgical drainage may also allow for a shorter duration of antibiotic therapy. In thoracic actinomycosis surgical intervention is often indicated for empyema drainage, fistula repair, and resection of necrotic lung tissue. Surgical intervention is also important in the management of abdominal actinomycosis, often for both diagnosis and treatment.

The generally recommended initial antibiotic therapy for *Actinomyces* in pediatrics includes IV penicillin G or ampicillin for 4 to 6 weeks, followed by high doses of oral penicillin for a total of 6 to 12 months.[26] This extended duration of therapy is based on previously reported risk of relapsed infection, but some authors have reported success in adults with shorter courses, with median duration of therapy ranging from 82 to 167 days.[40] *Actinomyces* species are uniformly susceptible to penicillin and amoxicillin and are also typically susceptible to doxycycline, erythromycin-clarithromycin, amoxicillin-clavulanate, piperacillin-tazobactam, ceftriaxone, linezolid, vancomycin, and meropenem. *Actinomyces* species are unusual compared with other anaerobic bacteria in that metronidazole has no activity and clindamycin has variable activity.[50]

Infection Prevention and Anticipatory Guidance

Standard transmission-based isolation precautions for actinomycosis are appropriate in most cases; there is no person-to-person spread. As stated previously, comprehensive oral hygiene and treatment of any dental caries or disease may prevent infection.

31

Pneumocystis Pneumonia

Catherine Burton, MD, MSc, FRCPC and Benjamin Hanisch, MD

EPIDEMIOLOGY AND RISK FACTORS

Pneumocystis jirovecii (formerly *Pneumocystis carinii*) is an infrequent though potentially deadly cause of fungal pneumonia (*P. jirovecii* pneumonia [PJP]) in immunocompromised patients. *P. jirovecii* is a ubiquitous unicellular organism found around the world with an affinity for the respiratory tract. Most individuals are exposed in childhood and many are colonized,[1] but disease occurs almost exclusively in immunocompromised hosts. Individuals with impaired cellular immunity, which is common in the setting of malignancy, primary immunodeficiencies, or a history of solid organ or bone marrow transplant, are vulnerable and repeat exposure can lead to fatal infection if untreated.[2]

Aside from human immunodeficiency virus (HIV), the most robust studies of PJP have been in hematopoietic stem cell transplant (HSCT) patients. PJP was a common cause of nonbacterial pneumonia and was associated with substantial morbidity and mortality[3] before the implementation of prophylaxis with trimethoprim-sulfamethoxazole (TMP-SMX) in the late 1970s. PJP infections in HSCT patients are no longer common (incidence of 0.63% for allogeneic and 0.28% for autologous transplants), although infections are still associated with high mortality in breakthrough cases with a 6.9-fold increased risk of death.[4] HSCT patients at highest risk are those with graft-versus-host disease and poor immune reconstitution.

In patients with hematologic malignancy, PJP risk is related to the underlying disease as well as the treatment regimen. The most significant risk factors include acute lymphoblastic leukemia, corticosteroids (particularly 2 mg/kg per day or more of prednisone or equivalent), and use of T-cell–depleting agents, such as alemtuzumab. High-intensity chemotherapy and prolonged CD4 lymphopenia also appear to be associated with an increased risk of PJP. The risk of PJP in children with acute myelogenous leukemias and solid tumors is not well defined, with a wide range of incidences reported (0.5 to 25 %) in children with solid tumors. Steroid use is a key factor in determining PJP risk in these populations.

Reported rates of PJP in patients receiving solid organ transplants (SOTs) are between 5% and 15%. The risk correlates with increased immunosuppression, temporal proximity to transplant, corticosteroid use, therapies to treat rejection, as well as low CD4 counts, and lymphopenia.[5]

CLINICAL MANIFESTATIONS

Classically, *Pneumocystis* pneumonia has an acute presentation in non-HIV immunocompromised individuals with symptoms of fever, cough, and dyspnea evolving over a few days, although symptoms can progress more gradually over the course of 1 to 2 weeks.[6-8] Tachypnea, tachycardia, and evidence of increased work of breathing, with nasal flaring and intercostal retractions, are common in children, whereas lung auscultation is often normal. Illness can progress rapidly, and many children require intensive care unit admission and mechanical ventilation. As the clinical presentation is nonspecific, it is critical to maintain a high index of suspicion in at-risk patients to facilitate early diagnosis and treatment. Co-infection with other pathogens, including cytomegalovirus as well as bacteria, fungi, and respiratory viruses, occurs frequently in patients with PJP and may influence the clinical presentation.[7,9]

Impaired oxygenation is common in PJP and can be severe. The degree of hypoxemia at presentation, as measured by the arterial blood oxygen tension (Pao_2), is commonly used to evaluate disease severity. Contrary to conventional teaching, PJP may present without hypoxemia in non-HIV immunocompromised individuals. A recent small retrospective study in adult SOT recipients found that less than half of SOT patients with PJP were hypoxemic on admission.[5] However, the lack of hypoxemia could reflect earlier diagnosis and therefore less severe disease, because of the high index of suspicion for PJP in the SOT population, rather than an actual difference in how the disease presents.

Imaging

Chest radiographic findings in PJP are nonspecific, most commonly showing bilateral perihilar interstitial infiltrates that spread peripherally. Chest radiographic findings can be normal early in the disease.[5,8,9] High-resolution computed tomography is much more sensitive than chest radiography and typically shows bilateral patchy ground-glass opacities, concentrated in the perihilar regions, with or without consolidation.[10] Cystic lesions and nodules can also be seen, although less commonly.[9-11] Patients receiving inhaled pentamidine prophylaxis more commonly have upper lobe infiltrates, likely because of decreased deposition of pentamidine in this area.[12] Pneumothorax is a recognized complication of PJP and may be more common in HSCT patients.[9]

DISEASE PROPHYLAXIS AND PREVENTION

Administration of PJP prophylaxis significantly reduces the risk of PJP in high-risk individuals. The generally accepted threshold for starting prophylaxis is greater than 3.5% risk of developing PCP to justify the potential toxicities. Indications for PJP prophylaxis in pediatric oncology and transplant populations are listed in Table 31.1 and suggested dosing in Table 31.2.

Trimethoprim-Sulfamethoxazole

TMP-SMX is the most studied agent for PJP prophylaxis and is considered the agent of choice to prevent disease. A 2014 Cochrane

TABLE 31.1 Indications for Prophylaxis

Condition/Indication	Duration/Notes
Oncology	
Acute lymphoblastic leukemia	Continue from induction to end of maintenance
Acute myeloid leukemia	
Solid tumors	When treatment is likely to result in lymphopenia for the duration of chemotherapy
Hematopoietic Stem Cell Transplant	
Allogeneic	Continue from engraftment through at least 6 months and until discontinuation of immunosuppression
Autologous	Generally given for 3-6 months after transplant
Solid Organ Transplant[a]	
Heart, liver, kidney	6-12 months after transplant
Lung, small bowel	Often lifelong
Treatment of rejection	For 3-6 months after treatment (depending on treatment)[b]
Other	
Steroids (>0.4 mg/kg per day or >16 mg/day for >1 month)	For the duration of therapy
Rituximab	For ≥6 months after treatment
Alemtuzumab	

[a]Some experts recommend lifelong prophylaxis for all solid organ transplant recipients.
[b]Prophylaxis for 3 months with pulse steroids, 6 months with antithymocyte globulin.

meta-analysis evaluating the effectiveness of TMP-SMX for prophylaxis of PJP in hematologic malignancy, stem cell transplant, and SOT patients found that the risk of PJP was 85% lower in patients receiving TMP-SMX compared with those receiving no PJP prophylaxis.[13] Multiple guidelines, including those of the American Society for Blood and Marrow Transplantation, the American Transplant Society, the American Society of Clinical Oncology, and the Infectious Diseases Society of America, support the use of TMP-SMX as the first-line agent for PJP prophylaxis.[14-16] In addition to its activity against *Pneumocystis,* TMP-SMX is protective against toxoplasmosis, listeriosis, and nocardiosis if given at sufficient doses.

Side effects of TMP-SMX include rash, fever, neutropenia, pancytopenia, hepatitis, and anaphylaxis. The Cochrane review of TMP-SMX prophylaxis in non-HIV immunocompromised patients reported that adverse events leading to permanent discontinuation of TMP-SMX occurred in approximately 3.1% of adult patients, but no serious adverse events were reported in children.[13] TMP-SMX should be used with caution in patients who are glucose 6-phophate dehydrogenase (G6PD) deficient as hemolysis may occur. Mutations leading to resistance to TMP-SMX have been reported,[17] though fortunately, they have been uncommon.

Multiple TMP-SMX prophylactic dosing regimens have been used and for PJP, and there is no clear difference in efficacy between twice-weekly and other more frequent dosing schedules.[18] There may be beneficial effects of more frequent dosing for prophylaxis against non-PJP infections in some high-risk populations. TMP-SMX needs to be dose adjusted in patients with creatinine clearance less than 30 mL/min.

Alternative Agents

Alternatives to TMP-SMX include intravenous (IV) and inhaled pentamidine, dapsone, and atovaquone; however, there have been few prospective comparison studies and thus there is no clear consensus with respect to the preferred alternative agent.

Pentamidine is the most studied second-line prophylaxis option. A retrospective study in adult HSCT patients found that patients receiving inhaled pentamidine had a higher probability of developing PJP (9.1%) than those receiving TMP-SMX (0%).[19] There is some concern that the IV form of pentamidine may not result in sufficient intra-alveolar concentrations to be protective[20]; however, recent retrospective studies in pediatric oncology, HSCT and SOT patients report good outcomes with inhaled and IV pentamidine.[21,22] The dosing interval for pentamidine is traditionally every 4 weeks, although a higher frequency has been used in young children, particularly those younger than 2 years, safely.[23] Pentamidine does not have activity against toxoplasmosis.

The inhaled form of pentamidine can be associated with coughing and wheezing that can be reduced with pretreatment with β-adrenergic agonists. Bronchospasm may be more common or severe in patients with chronic respiratory conditions.[24] Inhaled pentamidine therapy requires a specific nebulizer capable of producing particles smaller than 1 μm, as larger particles may be unable to reach the alveoli and would be less effective. The use of inhaled pentamidine in young children may be limited by their ability to coordinate and cooperate with medication inhalation. There have been reports of extrapulmonary infections with *Pneumocystis* in patients using inhaled pentamidine. The American Society of Transplantation recommends that inhaled pentamidine be considered a third-line

TABLE 31.2 Prophylaxis Options and Dosing

Agent	Dose and Frequency	
Trimethoprim-sulfamethoxazole	5-10 mg/kg per day of trimethoprim component divided into twice daily dosing. Given every day or 2-3 days per week.	Maximum dose of trimethoprim 320 mg/day
Dapsone	2 mg/kg once daily if >1 month of age	Maximum 100 mg daily
Atovaquone	30 mg/kg once daily if >2 years 45 mg/kg once daily if 4 months to 2 years	Maximum 1500 mg daily
Pentamadine	9 mg/kg every 4 weeks (age <5 years)	Maximum 300 mg/day
aerosolized	300 mg every 4 weeks (age >5 years)	
Intravenously	4 mg/kg every 2-4 weeks (age >2 years)	

agent, as there are more breakthrough infections than with atovaquone and dapsone.[25]

Atovaquone is another second-line agent that is available only in oral solution form. In HIV-infected individuals, atovaquone has been compared with once-daily dapsone and aerosolized monthly pentamidine with no significant differences in mortality or PJP infections,[26,27] but data for non-HIV-immunocompromised children are scarce. A small prospective study comparing atovaquone and TMP-SMX in adult autologous transplant patients did not identify any cases of PJP with either drug but found that TMP-SMX was discontinued significantly more frequently because of intolerance.[28] Atovaquone is generally well tolerated with minimal side effects, including rash, gastrointestinal symptoms, and headache. It also has the advantage of having activity against toxoplasma. High cost and poor palatability are the most common limitations in the use of atovaquone. There have also been reports of development of PJP resistance in a transplant center with widespread use.[29]

The final prophylactic option is dapsone. There has been limited study of dapsone prophylaxis outside the HIV-infected population, where dapsone appears to have efficacy similar to atovaquone in patients who could not tolerate TMP-SMX.[29] A retrospective study in HSCT recipients who could not tolerate TMP-SMX reported a 7.2% incidence of PJP in the dapsone group, using 3 times weekly dosing, compared with 0.37% in the TMP-SMX group ($P < .001$).[27] The same group reported a 1.3% incidence of PJP in HSCT recipients taking daily dapsone prophylaxis, suggesting that daily prophylaxis may be more effective.[30]

Dapsone can induce neutropenia, rash, and gastrointestinal upset. It can also cause methemoglobinemia. It should be avoided in those with severe TMP-SMX reactions as there may be cross-reactivity between the two drugs. Children should be screened for G6PD deficiency before initiation of dapsone treatment, as it can cause hemolytic anemia in children with G6PD deficiency and should be avoided in this population. Dapsone may have some activity against toxoplasma but is not recommended as monotherapy for toxoplasma prophylaxis.

Duration of Prophylaxis

PJP prophylaxis should be continued throughout the periods of most intense immunosuppression, but the optimal duration of PJP prophylaxis is unknown. In SOT recipients, PJP prophylaxis is generally provided for at least 6 to 12 months after transplant. Some experts recommend lifelong prophylaxis for all SOT recipients. PJP prophylaxis should be extended or restarted in patients receiving high-dose steroids or treatments for rejection. Given their intense immunosuppression, lifelong prophylaxis is often provided for lung and small bowel transplant recipients. Lifelong secondary prophylaxis is recommended in patients with a history of PJP.

In HSCT patients, TMP-SMX is usually held until engraftment because of concern for potential marrow suppression, although it is unclear if this is necessary.[31] Prophylaxis should continue for at least 6 months after allogeneic transplant. Longer prophylaxis is required for those with graft-versus-host-disease and/or ongoing immunosuppression. In autologous transplants, prophylaxis is often provided for 3 to 6 months after transplant. Although good-quality evidence for PJP prophylaxis in children with solid tumors and acute myeloid leukemia is lacking, it is common practice to prescribe prophylaxis throughout the course of chemotherapy.

DIAGNOSIS

PJP diagnosis can be quite difficult because of wide variations in presentation. Even when suspected, the diagnosis can be difficult to confirm as *P. jirovecii* cannot be cultured through traditional methods. Bronchoalveolar (BAL) fluid is the preferred specimen to diagnose PJP. If BAL fluid is not available, multiple induced sputum samples are often required to establish the diagnosis, as there are fewer cysts in the upper respiratory airways. Specific staining techniques of respiratory specimens, including Giemsa, can be used establish the diagnosis and to identify trophic forms, and toluidine blue or calcofluor white can be used to detect cysts. Immunofluorescent monoclonal antibodies to PJP that can identify both trophic forms and cysts are commonly used to establish the diagnosis. Staining and immunofluorescent assays may have sensitivities of 90% or better in BAL specimens, but sensitivity is lower in sputum specimens.[32]

Polymerase chain reaction (PCR) is the most sensitive method to establish the diagnosis of PJP; however, PCR diagnosis is complicated by the possibility of detecting *Penumocystis* colonization in the absence of clinical disease.[33] There are a variety of PJP PCR assays with differing targets and performance characteristics. Quantitative PJP PCR assays appear to be more promising than qualitative assays, but there is no currently established threshold to distinguish colonization from clinical PJP disease.

Serum (1,3)-β-D-glucan can be used as a screening tool for PJP, especially when bronchoscopy is not feasible or immediately available. A negative (1,3)-β-D-glucan test result has a high negative predictive value and can be used to exclude PJP.[34] It should not be used in isolation to diagnose PJP as it is a nonspecific marker positive in many fungal infections, including infections with *Candida* and *Aspergillus* species. Lactate dehydrogenase is commonly obtained but is not particularly helpful because of its low sensitivity and specificity.[35]

Diagnostic algorithms using multiple diagnostic methods are recommended to establish the diagnosis of PJP[33,36] (Fig. 31.1).

TREATMENT

Prompt administration of PJP-specific treatment is critical in patients at risk of PJP with consistent clinical features, as delay in treatment administration is associated with increased mortality.[8] Although obtaining a definitive diagnosis is of utmost importance, PJP-specific treatment should be empirically started in high-risk patients with consistent clinical findings and should not be delayed awaiting diagnostic procedures. Definitive diagnosis should still be pursued after empiric treatment has been initiated, as *Pneumocystis* remains detectable in bronchial secretions for days after treatment initiation.

Grading of PJP disease severity should take into account Pao_2 as well as other clinical signs and symptoms. Generally, a Pao_2 less than 70 mmHg while breathing room air is considered to indicate moderate to severe disease.

Recommendations regarding optimal treatment of PJP in non-HIV immunocompromised children are largely based on studies in HIV-positive children and observational data from non-HIV immunocompromised adults.[37-39] Therapeutic options for treatment of PJP in children are summarized in Table 31.3 and a treatment algorithm is presented in Fig. 31.2.

TMP-SMX is the preferred therapy for PJP of any severity. It is readily accessible, cost-effective, and has proven to be a highly effective therapy for PJP that is relatively well tolerated in non-HIV immunocompromised children. In patients with moderate or severe disease, treatment should be initiated parenterally, whereas oral therapy may be considered in mild cases if there are no concerns with enteral absorption or adherence to therapy. Standard duration of PJP treatment in HIV-positive children is 3 weeks, but optimal treatment duration is not well defined in non-HIV immunocompromised children.

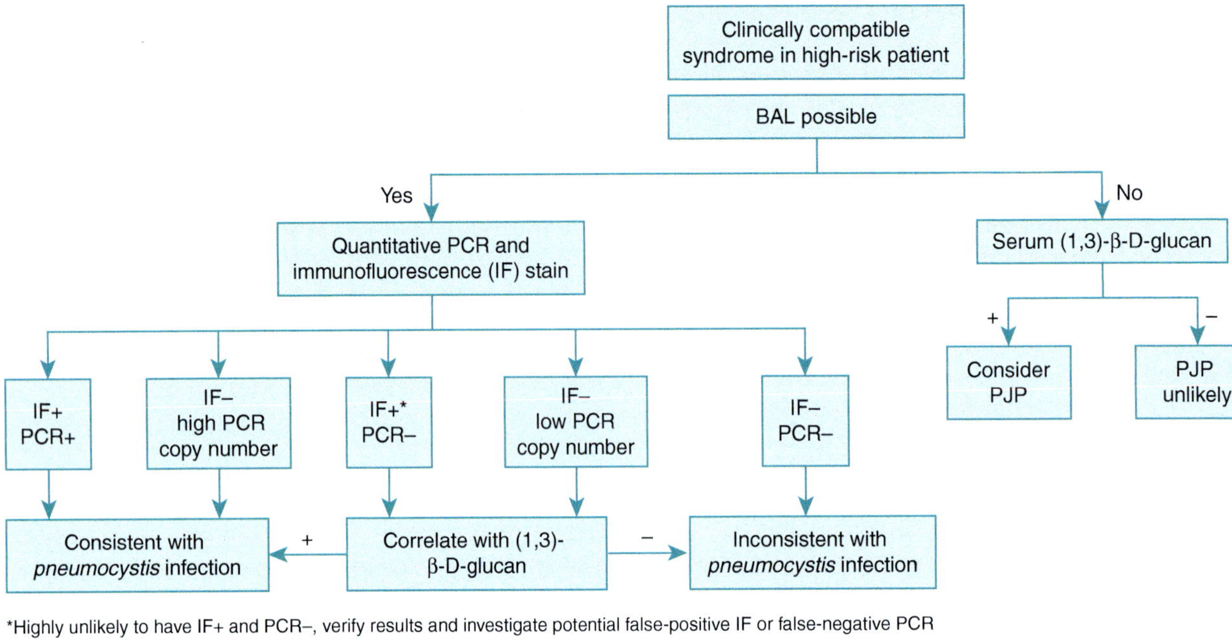

Fig. 31.1 Diagnosis of *Pneumocystis jirovecii* pneumonia. *BAL*, bronchoalveolar lavage; *IF*, immunofluorescence; *PCR*, polymerase chain reaction; *PJP*, *Pneumocystis jirovecii*.

TABLE 31.3 Therapeutic Options for Treatment of *Pneumocystis jirovecii* Pneumonia in Children

Agent	Dose	Monitoring/Precautions[a]
First-Line Therapy		
Trimethoprim-sulfamethoxazole (TMP-SMX) drug of Choice all severities of PJP	• TMP 15-20 mg/kg per day, IV or PO, divided q6h • SMX 75-100 mg/kg per day, PO or IV, divided q6h	• Regular monitoring of blood cell counts, potassium, creatinine, liver enzymes
Alternative Therapies		
Pentamidine	4 mg/kg per day, IV, once daily infused over ≥60 min	Regular monitoring of creatinine, blood cell counts, potassium, calcium, glucose, liver enzymes Hypotension (with rapid infusion) Cardiac arrhythmias and pancreatitis reported
Clindamycin plus primaquine	• Clindamycin 40 mg/kg per day, IV, divided q6h • Primaquine 0.3 mg/kg per day (maximum 30 mg/day), PO, once daily	• Avoid primaquine with G6PD deficiency (test for G6PD before use) • Monitor blood cell counts • Increased risk of *Clostridium difficile*–associated diarrhea
Atovaquone Not recommended for severe PJP	• *1-3 months and >24 months of age:* 30 mg/kg per day PO, divided bid (maximum 1500 mg/day) • *3-24 months of age:* 45 mg/kg per day, PO, divided BID	• Administer with food (increase bioavailability)
Dapsone plus trimethoprim Not recommended for severe PJP	• Dapsone 2 mg/kg per day (maximum 100 mg), PO, once daily • Trimethoprim 15 mg/kg per day, PO, divided q8h	• Avoid dapsone in children with a history of a severe reaction to TMP-SMX[b] • Monitor blood cell counts, liver enzymes • Dapsone can cause methemoglobinemia
Adjunctive Agents		
• Corticosteroids • Consider for moderate-to-severe PJP	• Prednisone 1 mg/kg per dose bid on days 1-5, 0.5 mg/kg per dose bid on days 6-10, and 0.5 mg/kg per dose once daily on days 11-21	

[a]Always check for drug interactions before administration.
[b]Severe TMP-SMX reactions: severe cutaneous adverse reactions, hepatitis, acute interstitial nephritis, agranulocytosis.
bid, twice a day; *G6PD*, glucose 6-phophate dehydrogenase; *h*, hour; *IV*, intravenous; *min*, minutes; *PJP*, *Pneumocystis jirovecii* pneumonia; *PO*, oral; *q*, every; *SMX*, sulfamethoxazole; *TMP*, trimethoprim.

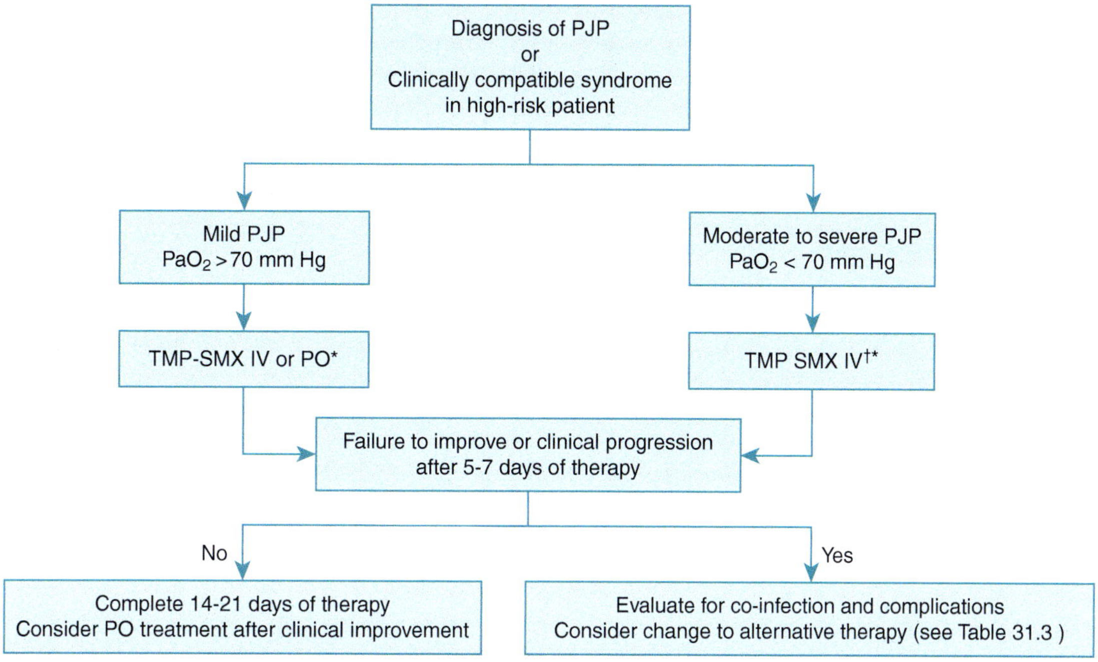

†Some experts recommend use of steroids in moderate to severe PJP, as is recommended in HIV-infected individuals
*If documented history of severe reaction to TMP SMX or if severe reaction develops during therapy, choose alternative therapy (see Table 31.3)

Fig. 31.2 Treatment of *Pneumocystis jirovecii* pneumonia. *IV*, intravenous; *Pao_2*, arterial blood oxygen tension; *PJP*, *Pneumocystis jirovecii* pneumonia; *PO*, oral; *TMP-SMX*, trimethoprim-sulfamethoxazole.

Treatment should be continued for at least 2 weeks and should be extended to 3 weeks in moderate and severe cases.[25,37,38]

The most common adverse reaction to TMP-SMX in children is maculopapular rash. Nausea, vomiting, and diarrhea can occur but are not generally treatment limiting. Hematologic abnormalities, including neutropenia and anemia, occur but are often multifactorial in these populations. Other more rare side effects include hyperkalemia, hepatitis, renal dysfunction and acute interstitial nephritis, and anaphylaxis. Severe cutaneous adverse reactions, including Stevens-Johnson syndrome, toxic epidermal necrolysis (TEN), and drug reaction with eosinophilia and systemic symptoms are rare but well-recognized complications of TMP-SMX therapy.

Desensitization to TMP-SMX can be considered in children who have had mild reactions to TMP-SMX, including isolated rash without mucous membrane involvement.[40] For children who have had a serious adverse reaction to TMP-SMX (anaphylaxis, severe cutaneous adverse reaction, aplastic anemia, hepatitis, acute interstitial nephritis), alternative agents should be used.

For treatment of severe PJP, IV pentamidine has generally been the preferred alternative in patients who cannot tolerate TMP-SMX, as well as the preferred second-line therapy for children in whom TMP-SMX treatment has failed.[38] However, recent European guidelines for treatment of PJP in hematology patients recommend clindamycin plus primaquine over pentamidine for second-line therapy of PJP, based on observational studies in HIV-infected and uninfected adults.[37,39] Dapsone plus trimethoprim and atovaquone are alternative oral options for mild-to-moderate PJP in children who cannot tolerate TMP-SMX. As there is no clear evidence of superiority in clinical outcomes in children, the choice of alternative and second-line therapy should take into consideration patient-specific factors, severity of PJP, as well as the risk and impact of potential drug-related side effects (see Table 31.3).

Caspofungin, a broad-spectrum antifungal agent, may have a role in the treatment of PJP. It has activity against *Pneumocystis* in animal models, and there are several case series and reports supporting its use in treatment of PJP in combination with other agents, most often TMP-SMX.[25,37]

Detection of drug resistance in *Pneumocystis* is very challenging as the organism cannot be cultured in vitro. Evaluation of *P. jirovecii* dihydropteroate synthase, an enzyme involved in folic acid synthesis that is targeted by TMP-SMX, has led to the discovery of mutations associated with an increased risk of failure of TMP-SMX prophylaxis, but the effect of these mutations on clinical treatment failure is unclear.[41,42]

Although studies in HIV-infected children have shown benefits of early administration of corticosteroids in moderate-to-severe PJP, including decreased mortality and decreased need for mechanical ventilation, the role of adjunctive steroids is much less clear in non-HIV infected individuals with PJP. Although steroids are commonly administered to non-HIV immunocompromised patients with PJP, the available evidence is limited and contradictory in adults and is essentially nonexistent in children. The most recent and largest study, a retrospective propensity-matched cohort study including 323 non-HIV immunocompromised adults with PJP, failed to find any benefit of early corticosteroid administration.[43] The use of adjunctive steroids should be considered on an individual basis, weighing the potential benefits and the recognized side effects of steroids. If steroids are used, prednisone dosing recommended for PJP in HIV-positive children is as follows: 1 mg/kg per dose twice daily on days 1 through 5, 0.5 mg/kg per dose twice daily on days 6 through 10, and 0.5 mg/kg per dose once daily on days 11 through 21.[38]

Clinical deterioration is common in the first 5 days after treatment initiation, but improvement should be expected by the end of the first week of PJP-specific therapy. If clinical status has not improved or is deteriorating by day 7 of therapy, then patients should be investigated for the presence of co-infections and complications. If no alternative explanation is identified, a switch to second-line therapy should be considered. Studies in adults with hematologic malignancies have identified long-term steroid use, longer time from symptom onset to treatment initiation, and co-infection with cytomegalovirus or herpes simplex virus as poor prognostic factors in PJP.[8,37] Other factors associated with worse prognosis include ongoing clinical deterioration by day 8, need for mechanical ventilation, shock, and acute respiratory distress syndrome.[8,37]

PJP is associated with significant morbidity and mortality in non-HIV immunocompromised adults, but outcomes of PJP pneumonia in non-HIV immunocompromised children are not well characterized. A recent retrospective review of PJP in children in the United States found that in-hospital all-cause mortality was highest in HSCT recipients (32.4%) and lowest in SOT recipients (9.8%), which is consistent with previous adult studies.[8,9,44] In-hospital mortality for children with hematologic malignancy and malignant solid tumors was 13.9% and 19.5%, respectively.[44]

INFECTION PREVENTION AND ANTICIPATORY GUIDANCE

Pneumocystis is most likely transmitted through airborne spread and can be passed from person to person. Clusters of infections have been reported in transplant units,[45] although it remains unclear what isolation precautions are needed in patients with PJP. Some centers use respiratory isolation for patients with PJP pneumonia, although at a minimum, it would seem prudent to have immunocompromised patients avoid other patients with known PJP.

32

Strongyloides, *Cryptosporidium*, and Other Parasitic Infections

Ivan A. Gonzalez, MD, MSc and Terri Stillwell, MD, MPH

Parasitic infections are an uncommon but potentially important cause of morbidity and mortality in children undergoing solid organ transplantation (SOT). Although few data have been published relating to parasitic infections in children undergoing hematopoietic stem cell transplantation (HSCT) or being treated for cancer, the high degree of immunodeficiency relating to treatment with chemotherapy and ablation therapy early after HSCT transplant, as well as the potential presence of ongoing immunosuppression treatment to prevent or treat graft-versus-host disease (GVHD), also places these children at increased risk for serious disease if they are exposed to these parasitic pathogens. This chapter reviews several important parasitic pathogens and their impact on these immunosuppressed children.

STRONGYLOIDIASIS

Epidemiology and Risk Factors

There are more than 40 species within the genus of Strongyloides; however, the main species that infects humans is *S. stercoralis*. It is an intestinal nematode predominantly present in the subtropics and tropical areas as well as in the Appalachian area and southeastern United States.[1-3] It is estimated that between 30 million and 100 million people worldwide are infected with *Strongyloides* spp.[2,4-7] *S. rhabditiform* larvae are excreted in stool of infected individuals and either develop into free-living adult worms or into the filariform larvae.[7] During the free-living adult worm stage, they can produce fertilized eggs that can then develop into the rhabditiform larvae.[2,3] Transmission often occurs when the filariform larvae penetrate the skin of a person walking barefoot on soil in endemic areas.[7] Larvae then travel to the intestines and mature into adult worms.[3] It is the only nematode that can cause autoinfection once it completes the life cycle within a human host.[2,7] In autoinfection, adult female worm lay eggs within the intestinal mucosa that become rhabditiform larvae. Subsequently, these larvae develop into the filariform larvae and can penetrate the intestinal mucosa or perianal skin and migrate to the intestines via the lungs to restart the cycle.[2]

Possible outcomes to an initial infection are eradication of the infection, autoinfection, and hyperinfection or disseminated disease, which is rare in immunocompetent hosts. Transmission from human to human is extremely rare. Transmission can occur as part of SOT seen as donor-derived infections,* which is most often associated with kidney transplantation (KTx) with an increased number of hyperinfections related to corticosteroid use.[1,7,9] Infections in bone marrow transplant recipients have been rarely reported.[10] Hyperinfection occurs during autoinfection, with an increase larval migration into the pulmonary system. In disseminated disease, larvae migrate within the venous system to reach other organs.[7] In disseminated disease, there is an increased risk of enteric gram-negative bacteremia and meningitis. Data on *Strongyloides* in children being treated for cancer are not available.

The main epidemiologic risk factor for developing strongyloidiasis is living or visiting endemic areas, such as Central and South America, the Caribbean, Puerto Rico, Mexico, sub-Saharan Africa, Asia, India, and Oceania.[9] The highest seropositivity in these areas can exceed 80% as opposed to only 3.8% in the United States,[6] yet 6.7% of pretransplant evaluations reveal positive serology results in asymptomatic Hispanic transplant candidates.[4]

Clinical Manifestations

Most infections are asymptomatic, but strongyloidiasis can present with abdominal pain, diarrhea, bloating, anorexia, cough, sore throat, or rash in the immunocompetent patient.[3,9] Owing to the use of immunosuppression, including corticosteroids, SOT recipients can present with gastrointestinal symptoms, respiratory distress, sepsis-like picture, bacteremia, and/or meningitis.[6,7] The pathogenesis stems from autoinfection through intestinal mucosa allowing for bacterial seeding. In disseminated disease, end-organ dysfunction specific to the larval migration is seen. Eosinophilia can be present in up to 30% of patients with hyperinfection syndrome.[1,5,6] Mortality associated with hyperinfection can range from 25% to 87%, with better outcomes depending on early detection.[1,7,8] Patients have also developed acute respiratory distress syndrome as a complication of hyperinfection.[1]

Disease Prophylaxis and Prevention

There are few existing guidelines suggesting the use of universal screening as it pertains to KTx programs.[4,6,9,11] However, reports based on surveys show that only 10% of organ procurement organizations actually screen for *Strongyloides* infection.[9] Screening is based on the presence of epidemiologic risk factors, such as traveling to or having lived in an endemic area, unexplained eosinophilia, or a history of previous *Strongyloides* infection.[6] However, geographic risk is not reliable enough to serve as the primary screening tool as adult worms can live up to 5 years. More robust screening algorithms are warranted to reduce the risk of donor-derived infections along with increased screening from organ procurement organizations. Depending on geographic location, transplant programs should perform *Strongyloides* screening universally. The Miami Transplant Institute has recently adopted a universal prophylaxis protocol given it experience with adults in whom donor-derived *Strongyloides* infections developed—one with a positive serologic test result and another with a false-negative serologic test result. If a screening test result is positive, the recipient should receive prophylaxis with ivermectin to reduce the risk after transplantation.[6] Considerations to timing for prophylaxis must include assurance of ivermectin absorption. Therefore prophylaxis can

*References 1, 2, 4, 6, 8, 9.

occur during the pretransplant period or soon after transplantation, depending on recipient or donor seropositivity.

Diagnosis

The gold standard for diagnosis is isolation of larvae from stool specimens. However, the sensitivity of this method remains low, ranging from 15% to 30%.[7] Serial stool examinations can be submitted to increase the sensitivity. Based on the life cycle of this organism, larvae may not be present during the time of stool examinations. Additionally, the gastrointestinal function of the individual needs to be considered. Recently serologic testing has become more popular and has become the method of choice for screening.[4,6,7] Sensitivity varies depending on the assay performed; indirect immunofluorescence assays having the highest sensitivity. However, these are not commercially available. Sensitivity ranges from 80% up to 96% and specificity ranges from 90% up to 96%.[1-5,9] Serologic test results may remain positive even after appropriate treatment for *Strongyloides* infection. Experimentally, investigators have attempted to use immunoglobulin Ig A levels in saliva as an alternative, but serologic testing has higher sensitivity.[3] Polymerase chain reaction (PCR) has been investigated as well and demonstrates potential, but it is not commercially available and the reliability needs to be evaluated in larger clinical trials.[11] Eosinophilia may only be present in 30% of cases, but if present and unexplained, it should prompt screening immediately. An approach to risk-based screening and symptom-based diagnostic testing for *Strongyloides* in organ donors and organ recipients is shown in Fig. 32.1.

Treatment

The drug of choice is ivermectin for the treatment of asymptomatic disease, hyperinfection, and disseminated disease. Treatment may be prolonged in immunocompromised patients. Prophylactic dosing is 200 μg/kg once daily for 2 days; some experts recommend repeating the dose 2 weeks apart. Albendazole is an alternative treatment for *Strongyloidiasis* infection for 3 to 7 days. However, some experts recommend the combination of ivermectin and albendazole in hyperinfection and disseminated disease in the SOT population.[4,12] Parenteral formulations are not approved and may not be available; however, the veterinary formulation may be used subcutaneously.[13] The pediatric and adult dosing for ivermectin and albendazole is shown in Table 32.1.

TABLE 32.1 Medications and Dosing Regimens for the Treatment of Strongyloidiasis

Treatment Drug	Adult Dosing	Pediatric Dosing
Ivermectin	200 μg/kg daily once a day for 1 to 2 days	*<15 kg:* No dosing available *≥15 kg:* 200 μg/kg daily once a day for 2 days
Albendazole	400 mg twice a day	*≤10 kg:* 200 mg a day *>10 kg:* 400 mg twice a day

Infection Prevention and Anticipatory Guidance

The best preventative effort to avoid infection is to wear shoes while walking on soil in endemic areas. Human-to-human transmission is extremely rare except in donor-derived infections in SOT recipients. Standard precautions such as hand hygiene after stool contact are recommended in hospitalized patients. Screening for *Strongyloides* infection should be performed in patients who will receive immunosuppressive therapy.

CRYPTOSPORIDIUM SPECIES

Epidemiology and Risk Factors

Cryptosporidium is an intracellular parasite that has become one of the leading causes of diarrheal disease worldwide. The first human *Cryptosporidium* infection was noted in 1976. Since that time, it has increasingly become recognized as a common cause for diarrheal disease, with

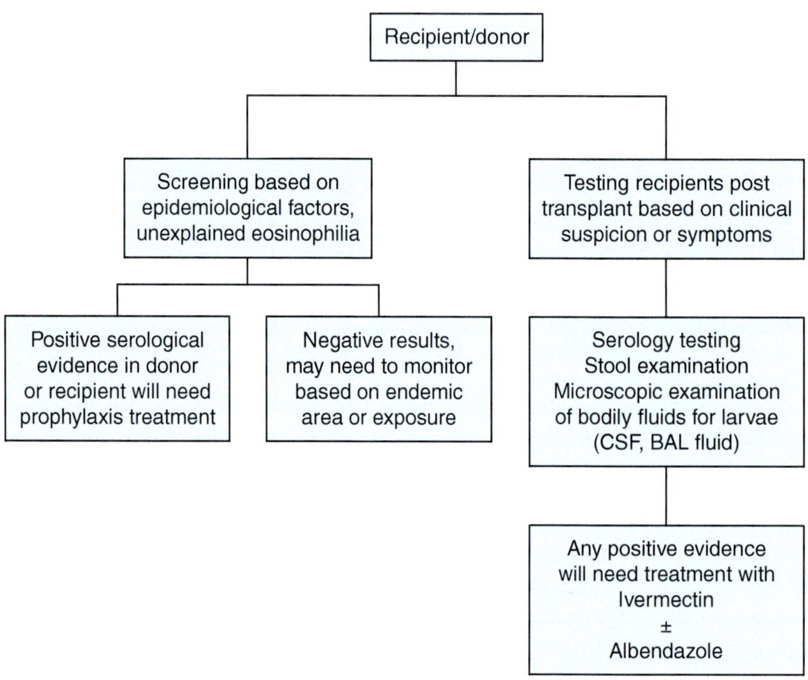

Fig. 32.1 Risk-based screening and symptom based diagnostic testing algorithm for *Strongyloides* in organ donors and organ recipients. *CSF,* cerebral spinal fluid; *BAL,* bronchoalveolar lavage.

the Centers for Disease Control and Prevention (CDC) estimating approximately 750,000 cases occur annually, only a fraction of which are reported.[14-16] From 2001 to 2010, *Cryptosporidium* was the leading cause of all waterborne outbreaks of diarrheal disease in the United States. Per the CDC, *Cryptosporidium*-related disease hospitalizations cost $45.8 million dollars per year.[16] Estimated *Cryptosporidium* seroprevalence in North America ranges from 25% to 35%.[17,18]

Although there are many species of *Cryptosporidium*, the species that most commonly infect humans are *C. parvum* and *C. hominis*, with some studies noting that *C. parvum* causes nearly 97% of *Cryptosporidium* infections[18,19] *C. hominis* primarily causes human-to-human infection, whereas *C. parvum* can cause both human-to-human disease and animal-to-human infection.[16] Cattle and sheep seem to serve as the primary animal reservoirs for human disease, with animal waste contaminating ground water.[14,15,18]

Fecal-to-oral transmission occurs via contaminated drinking water, food, recreational water, and indirectly via fomites.[14,18,19] In the United States, *Cryptosporidium* oocysts are estimated to be in 55% to 87% of surface water tested. Individuals participating in recreational water activities are at increased risk for *Cryptosporidium* infection, with 90% of recreational outbreaks from 1991 to 2000 linked to swimming pools and water parks. Some studies report a seasonal increase from June to September, thought to be due to increased exposures to contaminated water via recreational activities.[15] Exposure to contaminated drinking water has also led to many *Cryptosporidium*-related outbreaks; one of the largest was the 1993 Milwaukee outbreak, the in which nearly 400,000 individuals were affected.[14,15,20]As an intracellular parasite, once *Cryptosporidium* oocysts are ingested, they infect intestinal epithelial cells. *Cryptosporidium* undergoes both asexual replication, resulting in merozoites that infect neighboring epithelial cells, and sexual replication, which results in oocysts. Once excreted, oocysts are immediately infectious and can lead to autoinfection and contamination of the immediate environment. Oocysts do not reproduce outside the host. Infection can result from a very small number of oocysts; some studies note as few as 10 oocysts result in infection. With an infected individual shedding up to 10^8 oocysts per day, outbreaks occur easily.[16,19]

Although *Cryptosporidium* infections affect all people, both immunocompetent and immunocompromised, children and immunosuppressed individuals are at higher risk for disease. Children 2 to 11 years old are at increased risk for person-to-person transmission, with the highest number of cases in children younger than 5 years.[15,16,21] Immunosuppressed individuals are also at increased risk for disease; one study showed *Cryptosporidium* spp. as the cause for 21% of diarrheal cases in SOT patients compared with only 3% of cases in the control group.[22]

Clinical Manifestations

The pathophysiology of *Cryptosporidium* infection is still unknown. The inflammatory response to intracellular infection leads to villous blunting and atrophy and increased cell permeability, which causes significant watery diarrhea and can contribute to malabsorption.[14,17] Rarely does bloody diarrhea occur and stool is often without fecal leukocytes. It is believed to be a secretory diarrhea process; however, no enterotoxin has been found.[14,20] Although the mechanism of infection remains unknown, it seems that the immune system's ability to control *Cryptosporidium* infection is reliant on cell-mediated immunity. Given this information, transplant and oncologic patients are at significant risk for disease.[14,17,18] The incubation period for *Cryptosporidium* is up to 2 weeks. Most infections in immunocompetent individuals are either asymptomatic or self-limited.[14,15]

Clinical syndromes from *Cryptosporidium* infection can include acute infection, chronic infection, and fulminant disease. Acute infection often occurs in immunocompetent individuals, presenting primarily with watery diarrhea. About 90% of acute symptoms last 2 weeks, although symptoms can last up to 5 weeks. Chronic disease is classified as diarrheal symptoms lasting more than 2 months. Both acute and chronic infections can also be associated with abdominal pain, bloating, nausea, vomiting, and occasionally fever. Fulminant disease is most often seen in immunocompromised individuals and results in profuse, watery, cholera-like stool output, with liters of output per day, leading to significant concerns for hypovolemia.[14,17]

Extra-intestinal symptoms can also occur with *Cryptosporidium* infection; these symptoms are mostly biliary and respiratory. Biliary disease, manifesting as right upper quadrant pain, nausea, and vomiting, was seen in up to 26% of patients with AIDS.[14] Studies have shown that upper respiratory tract symptoms occur in 15% of pediatric cases. Symptoms manifest as bronchitis, cough, dyspnea, chest pain, and increased secretions.[18] Studies from developing nations have linked cryptosporidiosis to decreased growth and physical development, as well as diminished cognitive development.[18]

Disease Prophylaxis and Prevention

At present, there are no recommendations for screening of *Cryptosporidium* infection in immunocompromised patients. Testing is suggested only for patients with prolonged diarrheal symptoms. Prevention focuses on good hygiene and decreasing exposures to potential environmental contamination.

Diagnosis

Cryptosporidium oocysts are not generally found on routine ova and parasite testing; if there is concern for infection with *Cryptosporidium*, the laboratory should be notified of this concern. Often a modified acid-fast stain can be used to detect the oocysts in the stool sample.[14,17,18,20] Given that oocysts are only shed intermittently, a single stool sample has an estimated sensitivity of about 30%; therefore multiple stools samples on multiple days are suggested to increase sensitivity of testing.[16,20] Most sources would recommend a minimum of three stool samples. Direct fluorescent antibody testing, enzyme immunoassays, and PCR testing are now more commonly used for diagnosis because they have increased sensitivity compared with microscopic testing; some studies report near 100% sensitivity and specificity with these newer methods.[14,17] Point-of-care rapid antigen testing is also available.

Treatment

Currently there are very few effective treatments for *Cryptosporidium* infection. For immunocompetent individuals, supportive care alone is often sufficient. In 2005, the U.S. Food and Drug Administration (FDA) approved nitazoxanide as a treatment for *Cryptosporidium* infection; it is the only FDA-approved treatment currently available.[16] Even with this as approved treatment, efficacy is still in question, particularly in immunocompromised patients.

An Egyptian study compared 3 days of nitazoxanide treatment versus placebo in immunocompetent individuals with *C. parvum* infection. Treatment with nitazoxanide significantly reduced symptoms; 80% of the patients had resolution of symptoms at the 7-day follow-up compared with only 20% in the placebo group. Additionally, 67% of patients in the treatment arm had no oocysts present in the posttreatment stool samples compared with only 22% in the placebo group.[18,23] Another study comparing nitazoxanide treatment versus placebo in Zambian HIV-infected and HIV-uninfected children showed improved symptoms and improved parasitologic findings in the HIV-uninfected children treated with nitazoxanide versus those who received placebo; however, this significance was not seen in the HIV-infected children treated with nitazoxanide.[18,19,21,24]

Current recommendations suggest a 3-day course of nitazoxanide for immunocompetent individuals, with a minimum of 14 days of treatment for those who are immunosuppressed.[17,24] If nitazoxanide is not available, paromomycin is an alternative treatment option, although the limited data available show mixed results regarding efficacy.[17-19,21] Additionally, there is scant literature on combination therapy—paromomycin plus azithromycin—in the treatment of *Cryptosporidium* infection in HIV populations, showing some success, particularly for chronic cryptosporidiosis.[18,19] Other case studies of treatment in immunosuppressed patients suggest that decreased immunosuppression and combination therapy resulted in improvement in clinical course.[17]

Adjunct treatment with oral human immunoglobulin and immune bovine colostrum have also been evaluated in various case reports, showing that these treatments may attenuate clinical infection, but there are no trials evaluating these treatment options.[17,21] Additional studies on effective treatments for *Cryptosporidium* infections are needed.

Infection Prevention and Anticipatory Guidance

Cryptosporidium oocysts are hardy organisms and are able to survive in the environment for long periods of time.[18] Most standard disinfectants and cleaners are not effective against *Cryptosporidium* spp.; therefore hydrogen peroxide and bleach are the preferred disinfectants for *Cryptosporidium* in the health care setting.[14] Additionally, alcohol-based hand sanitizers are ineffective and soap and water is the preferred hand hygiene method. In the health care setting, standard precautions should be used for all patients with *Cryptosporidium* infections. For those who are diapered or incontinent of stool, contact precautions should also be implemented.

Outside the healthcare setting, good hygiene is the best method of prevention. Both foodborne-related outbreaks and animal-to-human transmission can be lessened by practicing good hand hygiene. Given the link between *Cryptosporidium* and waterborne outbreaks from various water sources, participation in recreational water activities should be done with caution. For those recovering from infection with *Cryptosporidium*, participation in recreational water activities should be avoided until at least 2 weeks after diarrheal symptoms resolve to help prevent contaminating the water. Individuals should also avoid ingestion of recreational water or water from any untreated water source. If an individual is in an area with unsafe water, boiling and filtration can help mitigate risk. International travel has also been associated with increased risk for infection, particularly when traveling to locations without safe water sources. Immunocompromised individuals should be aware of this risk and take precautionary steps where appropriate.[14,16]

CHAGAS DISEASE

Epidemiology and Risk Factors

Human trypanosomiasis in the Americas, also known as Chagas disease (CD), is caused by *Trypanosoma cruzi*.[25-28] It is endemic to the regions of Mexico and Central and South America.[4,26-29] It is estimated that 65 million people are at risk and 7 to 8 million people are infected in Latin America.[4,28] Because of immigration and international travel, it is estimated that more than 300,000 people living in the United States are infected with *T. cruzi*.[26,27] Therefore Chagas disease is becoming an emerging infectious disease in the United States. Triatomine bugs are responsible for vector-related transmissions. After initial infection, individuals enter the acute phase of infection characterized by mild febrile illness or nonspecific signs and symptoms.[30] Most infected people are asymptomatic. In endemic areas, there is a high level of parasitemia during the acute phase. After a few months, infected people progress to the chronic phase without symptoms.[31] However, 20% to 40% of people in the chronic phase develop cardiac, gastrointestinal, and rarely, peripheral nervous system disease.[26,29,32] Cardiomyopathy is the most recognized complications during the chronic phase, necessitating heart transplantation (HTx).[33] During the chronic phase, approximately 60% to 80% of patients enter a clinical latency, which is referred to as the indeterminate form.[30,32] During the acute phase, blood smear or buffy coat testing can be used to look for parasites.[26] However, during the chronic phase, in particular during the indeterminate form, diagnoses can only be made through serologic testing.[4,26]

Vector-related, oral, and vertical transmission are the most common routes of infection in endemic areas, whereas blood transfusion and SOT are most commonly associated with transmission in nonendemic areas.[30,34,35] The increasing number of people traveling to and from endemic areas has increased the pool of donors who are infected with CD.[4,26,28] The rate of seropositivity in the United States approaches 0.9%; however. the rate can be affected by geographic location and population demographics.[25,27] Studies in transplant candidates from Central America have demonstrated seropositivity rates of 4.5%.[28] In the United States, Florida and California account for more than 50% of seropositive cases for CD.[28]

As of 2016, 14 cases of donor-derived infections were documented in United States with a 13% to 18% rate of transmission reported.[4,26] However, in HTx the rate of donor-derived CD owing to reactivation of the parasite within the cardiac allograft may be as high as 61% within the first 24 months after transplantation.[26] The rate of transmission in KTx is between 8% and 22%; the rate in liver transplant is between 20% and 22%; and in HTx the rate is approximately 75%.[4,25,29-31] Recipient-negative and donor-positive (R^-/D^+) patients have a low risk of donor derived infection whereas R^+/D^- patients may have a 33% risk of reactivation of prior infection within the recipient. Few cases have been reported in bone marrow transplant recipients.[36-38] Risk factors leading to a positive serologic test result are being born in Latin America, born to a mother from Latin America, living in mud houses, receipt of unscreened blood transfusion, or residence in an endemic area from 3 to 6 months.[4,30,33,39] Demographics for patients treated under an investigation new drug program from the CDC showed a few pediatric cases including a congenital infection.[40] These data suggest that pediatric screening may also be warranted and that clinicians caring for pediatric organ candidates and recipients should likely follow adult guidelines. Most guidelines suggest against accepting heart or intestine allografts from a positive donor but support acceptance of kidney, pancreas, liver, and lung allografts. Risk/benefit analysis must be performed to accept organs from positive donors as transmission is not extremely high.[4]

Clinical Manifestations

During the chronic stage of CD, immunocompetent hosts can present with cardiac arrhythmias, progressive heart failure, and/or segmental dilatation of the gastrointestinal tract with megaesophagus or megacolon.[26,28] CD can manifest as myocarditis leading to allograft dysfunction, with rapid onset of congestive heart failure in HTx recipients.[28] Other symptoms may include fever, inflammatory panniculitis, and skin nodules. In other organs, CD may present with fever, atypical skin lesions, myocarditis, or meningoencephalitis.[30] In some cases, the skin lesions resemble erythema nodosum.[32] In CD, mortality has been reported as low as 0.7%, with other studies suggesting early detection and treatment leading to favorable outcomes.[41]

Disease Prophylaxis and Prevention

There are few guidelines suggesting universal screening in endemic areas with serologic laboratory tests. In the United States, only 19% of organ procurement organizations screen for CD, either universally or based on epidemiologic risk factors, such as being born in Latin America, born to a mother from Latin America, living in mud houses, receipt of unscreened blood transfusion, or residence in an endemic area from 3 to 6 months.[4,26,28,30] There are no randomized controlled trials to evaluate the efficacy of prophylaxis in the prevention of CD.[30] Case reports on the use of prophylaxis to prevent transmission in living related transplant programs as well posttransplant prophylaxis do not provide sufficient evidence to inform recommendations either way.[30,41,42] Some programs suggest screening after transplant to inform treatment instead of providing prophylaxis.[30] In Brazil, an endemic area, transplant programs do not routinely provide prophylaxis.[43] Additionally, there are reports that use of mycophenolate mofetil and corticosteroids increases the risk of CD.[27,30,31,33] However, there is no consensus on which immunosuppressive regimens should be used in a transplant recipient with a positive donor.[33,41] Current guidelines are hindered by a lack of widespread data collection.[4] Therefore there is little consensus relating to screening recipients and donors, prophylaxis questions, and immunosuppressive regimens.

Diagnosis

During the acute phase of CD, the use of microscopic examination for parasites using blood smear or buffy coat is the optimal laboratory examination.[26] Biopsy specimens can be submitted for histopathology and PCR-based testing. However, for screening purposes one serologic test is sufficient to diagnose the chronic phase of CD. For a clinical diagnosis, two separate antigen and/or techniques are needed.[28] There are three distinct methodologies that can be performed: enzyme-linked immunosorbent assay, immunofluorescence assay, and radioimmunoprecipitation assay. Currently two companies have FDA approval for donor screening using enzyme-linked immunosorbent assay kits.[4] Overall sensitivity is 99% to 100% and specificity is 98% to 100%.[4,44] PCR is not routinely used for screening donors as it would miss patients in the chronic phase.[4,30] PCR is the preferred methodology for posttransplantation screening for CD.[4] Blood PCR may lead to early detection before the onset of clinical symptoms as it is interpreted as parasitemia.[25,26] However, there are some studies suggesting specificity may be lower and some experts would recommend to wait for clinical symptoms.[45] In postmortem organs examined by PCR, *T. cruzi* was detected by PCR and may explain transmission to the recipient. PCR may not be readily available commercially; however, it is reliably available from the CDC. For patients screened based on epidemiologic risk factors with a positive serologic screening result before transplant, follow-up after transplant should include PCR and microscopic examination every week for the first 2 months, then every 2 weeks during the third month, and monthly until 6 months after transplant.[26,28] However, recently programs have adopted a modified posttransplant screening process based on specific organs. For HTx patients, the process is weekly PCR and microscopic examination weekly during the first 2 months, then every other week for months 3 through 12, every 3 weeks for months 13 through 24, and every 6 months thereafter. For non-HTx patients, the process is weekly during the first 2 months, then every other week for months 3 through 6, and then annually thereafter.[30]

Treatment

The drug of choice is benznidazole for the treatment of CD.[25,26,28,29] Benznidazole is available commercially and is approved by the FDA for children as young as 2 years.[26] Treatment is prolonged in immunocompromised patients up to 60 days with negative test results documented for clearance.[30] Nifurtimox is an alternative treatment for CD and is only available through an investigational new drug program from the CDC.[26,28] Nifurtimox is not FDA approved for the treatment of CD and the length of therapy is approximately 90 days with a negative test result indicating cure.[30] Patients should be monitored annually post treatment to assess for potential reactivation. The pediatric and adult dosages of the medications are shown in Table 32.2.

TABLE 32.2 Medications and Dosing Regimen for the Treatment of Chagas Disease

Treatment Drug	Adult Dosing	Pediatric Dosing
Benznidazole	5-7 mg/kg per day divided twice (or thrice) daily	*Ages <12 years:* 5-7.5 mg/kg per day divided twice (or thrice) daily *Ages ≥12 years:* 5-7 mg/kg per day divided twice (or thrice) daily
Nifurtimox	8-10 mg/kg per day divided 3 or 4 times a day	*Ages <10 years:* 15-20 mg/kg divided in 3 or 4 doses *Ages 11-16 years:* 12.5-15 mg/kg divided in 3 or 4 doses

Infection Prevention and Anticipatory Guidance

The best preventative effort in endemic areas is improving sanitation and the quality of housing to limit vector exposure and using insecticides to decrease vector presence. Travelers to endemic areas should avoid contact with triatomine bugs; the use of insecticide-impregnated netting is useful along with avoidance of buildings constructed with mud or adobe brick. In nonendemic areas, transmission is mainly through blood transfusion and donor-derived infections in SOT recipients. Standard precautions should be followed in hospitalized patients. Screening for CD should be performed in patients who will receive immunosuppressive therapy with epidemiologic risk factors.

OTHER INTESTINAL PARASITES

Epidemiology and Risk Factors

Diarrheal disease in transplant and oncologic patients can be due to various causes, both infectious and noninfectious. Although noninfectious etiologies, such as medication-related, mucositis, and even GVHD, are more common, infectious causes should remain in the differential diagnosis, particularly if diarrheal disease is prolonged. Intestinal parasites, such as *Giardia*, *Cyclospora*, *Cystoisospora belli*, and *Entamoeba histolytica* have all been associated with disease in immunocompromised host, often leading to prolonged diarrheal episodes.[46-50]

Although billions of people have parasitic infections worldwide, only 5% of known parasites have been found in transplant patients.[47] Infections are more frequently seen in those with links to developing nations or those in contact with contaminated food and drinking water. A study of primarily adult renal transplant patients found a symptomatic parasitic infection prevalence of 2.2%.[47] An Iranian study of renal transplant patients revealed a 33.3% prevalence of intestinal parasitic infection, compared with a prevalence of only 20% in the control group.[50] Another study, from Turkey, evaluating the causes of diarrhea in SOT patients found a comparable prevalence of *Giardia* in the transplant patient group compared with the control group: 27.2% versus

21.2%, respectively, with a much lower prevalence of *E. histolytica* in transplant patients compared with controls, 3.0% versus 21.2%.[49] As noted earlier, cellular-mediated immunity seems to play a large role in controlling parasitic infection, placing transplant and oncologic patients at greater risk for morbidity related to these types of infections.[50]

Clinical Manifestations

Intestinal parasites can be asymptomatic but are more often known to cause gastroenteritis, leading to either acute or chronic infection. Some cases of enteritis can mimic GVHD. Diarrhea, nausea, vomiting, and abdominal bloating are associated symptoms. Depending on the degree of disease, significant stooling can be accompanied by weight loss and malabsorption, particularly with *Giardia* infection.[48] *Cyclospora* and *Cystoisopora* can cause profound watery diarrhea, leading to significant dehydration, prompting the need for electrolyte replacement. Grossly bloody stools are the hallmark of *E. histolytica* infection, which can also lead to liver abscess formation.

Disease Prophylaxis and Prevention

Although there are no specific recommendations regarding pretransplant screening for these organisms, if an individual has significant epidemiologic risk, including a positive travel history to endemic areas and comparable clinical symptoms, an infectious workup to rule out these intestinal parasites should be performed. Treatment should be in accordance with the pathogen found.

Diagnosis

Most intestinal parasites can be seen on conventional ova and parasite examinations. Often it is difficult to differentiate *E. histolytica* from nonpathogenic *Entamoeba* spp. by microscopy; therefore additional testing may be needed to make the diagnosis. For *Cyclospora* and *Cystoisospora*, modified acid-fast staining may be required. Direct fluorescent antibody assays, enzyme immunoassays, and antigen detection assays are available depending on the parasite. For some, PCR testing on the newer multiplex PCR platforms can aid in diagnosis of intestinal parasites, offering greater sensitivity than standard microscopy.

Treatment

Metronidazole is the mainstay of treatment for *Giardia* infections. Tinidazole and nitazoxanide have also been found to be effective. For *Cyclospora* and *Cystoisopora*, TMP-SMX is the treatment of choice. When treating invasive amebiasis (*Entamoeba*), treatment consists of both metronidazole and a luminal agent, such as paromomycin or iodoquinol. Tinidazole can also be used in the place of metronidazole. In addition to antimicrobial treatments, all of these infections types require supportive management with electrolyte and nutritional replacements.

Infection Prevention and Anticipatory Guidance

Transmission of intestinal parasites occurs via the fecal-oral route, primarily from contaminated food and water supply. Good hand hygiene practices are key to prevention of these infections. Additionally, individuals should avoid contaminated water supplies whenever possible, with particular attention when traveling to endemic areas. Recreational water activities in endemic areas should also be undertaken with caution by avoidance of ingesting untreated water. Additionally, precautions should be taken with all food preparations to avoid potential contamination.

33

Gastrointestinal Viruses

Inci Yildirim, MD, PhD, MSc and
Elizabeth Doby Knackstedt, MD

Diarrheal disease is the second most common cause of death in children younger than 5 years worldwide, according to the World Health Organization (WHO). In the United States, viruses are the major cause of acute gastroenteritis in children; norovirus, rotavirus, adenovirus, astrovirus, and sapovirus are the most commonly detected.[1] Viral gastroenteritis also affects immunocompromised children, in whom it causes more morbidity and mortality, including longer duration of illness, increased hospitalization rates, renal injury, and graft rejection.[2,3]

With increasing availability and use of molecular diagnostic testing, especially multipathogen platforms, etiologic diagnosis of viral gastroenteritis is increasing and improved epidemiologic data are becoming available.[4] No U.S. Food and Drug Administration (FDA)-approved medications exist for the treatment of viral gastroenteritis (except for cytomegalovirus [CMV]. For a complete discussion of CMV disease in immunocompromised children, see Chapter 17). Therapeutics for viral gastroenteritis are an area of active research, especially among immunocompromised patients, where disease is more severe and prolonged.[5] Although an effective vaccination against rotavirus is now being used worldwide, vaccines for the other major viral causes of gastroenteritis do not exist. This too is an area of active research.[6]

NOROVIRUS

Norovirus infection is the most common cause of acute gastroenteritis worldwide, accounting for approximately 20% of all cases.[7] Noroviruses are part of the family *Caliciviridae* and are 27- to 40-nm, nonenveloped, single-stranded ribonucleic acid (RNA) viruses. Owing to genetic drift, the genus norovirus is genetically diverse and divided into seven genogroups, which are further subdivided into more 40 genotypes. Three of the genogroups (GI, GII, and GIV) have been isolated in humans, with GII.4 causing the majority of illness.[7]

Epidemiology and Risk Factors

Norovirus is transmitted through the fecal-oral route by close person-to-person contact. It can also be transmitted through contaminated food or water, and environmental contamination has been implicated in outbreaks.[8] In addition, because norovirus is present in the vomitus of infected individuals, it can be spread by droplets to those who are in close contact with or caring for individuals who are vomiting.[9] Norovirus is very infectious and a low inoculum is needed to cause disease. Norovirus virions are quite stable in the environment and can remain infectious on fomites for at least 7 days.[8] Norovirus can be detected in the stool of asymptomatic individuals; one meta-analysis found norovirus in the stools of 7% of healthy controls (3% to 10%).[10] This is likely a consequence of asymptomatic infection and/or convalescent excretion after illness has resolved. The role of asymptomatic shedding in transmission is unknown.

Noroviruses are a leading cause of both sporadic cases and outbreaks of acute gastroenteritis in the community worldwide.[10] Community outbreaks occur year-round but the majority occur in the winter. They are also important causes of institutional and nosocomial infection and outbreaks. A recent survey of U.S. hospitals revealed that noroviruses were among the most commonly detected nosocomial pathogens and caused the highest rate of hospital unit closures.[11]

Norovirus affects all age groups. Globally, norovirus prevalence in acute gastroenteritis cases in children younger than 5 years was 18% (15% to 20%) and 19% (7% to 21%) in all age groups.[10] In the United States, norovirus is associated with 19 million to 21 million episodes of gastroenteritis and up to 71,000 hospitalizations annually.[12] Nearly 800 deaths are caused by norovirus each year, which is the second most common cause of gastroenteritis-related death in the United States. Deaths occur disproportionately among individuals with chronic and/or immunocompromising conditions, such as transplantation and/or chemotherapy.[13] Norovirus has been detected in 22% to 32% of immunocompromised children with diarrhea.[4,13,14]

Clinical Manifestations

Symptoms of norovirus infection are similar to other causes of acute viral gastroenteritis and include vomiting, abdominal pain, watery, nonbloody diarrhea, and low-grade fever after an incubation period of about 24 hours. Vomiting is common and may be the only symptom. Symptoms usually last 12 to 60 hours in immunocompetent individuals. In contrast, the immunocompromised can have more severe and prolonged symptoms. A study of pediatric oncology patients with diarrheal illness found that 44% of these patients with norovirus required hospitalization. The median duration of diarrhea was 6 days (interquartile range 3 to 10 days).[4] Another study of immunocompromised pediatric patients found that the mean duration of symptoms was 10 days; the majority (70%) had symptoms for 4 days or longer and more than 20% had symptoms for longer than 14 days. In addition, nearly half of these children had seven or more diarrheal episodes daily.[14]

Chronic norovirus diarrhea (lasting ≥4 weeks) has been well described, especially in solid organ transplant (SOT) recipients and other immunocompromised individuals.[15-17] Illness can be associated with significant weight loss, failure to thrive, dehydration requiring hospitalization, renal dysfunction, and relapsing diarrhea.[16-18] One study found that the strongest association with duration of diarrhea was having received induction immunosuppression with antithymocyte globulin and having received plasmapheresis, in addition to human antigen leukocyte– and/or ABO-incompatible kidney transplant status, suggesting that more significant immunosuppression could be associated with a more severe course.[18] Another study of norovirus in SOT patients also found that CMV infection in the 90 days preceding norovirus diagnosis and nausea at presentation were two significant risk factors for diarrhea persisting more than 2 weeks.[15]

Disease Prophylaxis and Prevention

No licensed norovirus vaccines exist. Five different norovirus vaccines are currently being developed. Two vaccines have been studied in humans with promising results. One safety and immunogenicity trial in children is ongoing (NCT02153112).[6] All of these are virus-like particle vaccines targeting the major capsid protein.[6] It is unclear whether candidate vaccines would be effective in patients with significant immunosuppression. However, an effective vaccine might still protect immunocompromised patients via herd effects.

Diagnosis

The genetic (and antigenic) diversity of noroviruses has led to low sensitivity for antigen detection tests, whereas polymerase chain reaction (PCR)-based detection has proven very sensitive. Multiple single-plex PCR-based tests that have high sensitivity are commercially available. Recently sensitive multiplex PCR-based tests for multiple gastrointestinal pathogens (including norovirus) have become increasingly available and used.[19] None of the three commercially available multipathogen gastrointestinal panels can distinguish between norovirus GI and GII.[6] Because norovirus can be shed by healthy and/or asymptomatic individuals and given the high sensitivity of many of the PCR-based assays, clinicians must interpret a positive test result in the context of the clinical situation and symptoms.

Treatment

Clinical management of norovirus is supportive and targeted at maintaining adequate hydration, nutrition, and electrolyte balance. The WHO recommends low-osmolarity oral rehydration solution as opposed to traditional oral rehydration solution, and it has been shown to decrease vomiting and stool output in children with acute gastroenteritis. Ondansetron reduces vomiting in children with acute gastroenteritis and decreases need for intravenous hydration.[20]

Multiple potential therapies have been tried, with limited success in immunocompromised patients, to manage the more severe manifestations. Reduction of immunosuppression, when possible, often is helpful in immunocompromised patients with prolonged and/or severe symptoms but may be associated with the risk of graft rejection. One small study in kidney transplant patients described decreased immunosuppression associated with clinical improvement, but continued viral shedding in two-thirds of the patients.[21]

No medications are currently approved for treatment of norovirus infection. Nitazoxanide is an antiparasitic drug licensed in the United States for treatment of *Cryptosporidium parvum* and *Giardia lamblia* in adults and children older than 12 months. However, nitazoxanide has been reported to have broad-spectrum antiviral activity as well through a variety of poorly understood mechanisms.[22] A recent systematic review of five studies of nitazoxanide for the treatment of acute gastroenteritis caused by norovirus, rotavirus, or adenovirus showed use of this agent shortened duration of diarrhea by approximately 24 hours compared with placebo.[5] Multiple published case reports describe the use of nitazoxanide for norovirus gastroenteritis in immunocompromised individuals with variable effect on clinical symptoms and/or viral shedding.[16,23] A multicenter, randomized, placebo-controlled trial of nitazoxanide for treatment of symptomatic norovirus infection in SOT and hematopoietic stem cell transplantation (HSCT) recipients is ongoing and will hopefully provide definitive evidence regarding the efficacy of this agent for norovirus disease (NCT03395405).

Both intravenous and enteral administration of immunoglobulin have been used in immunocompromised patients with norovirus, but published experience is limited to case reports. Two single case reports in heart and pancreas transplant recipients cited no difference in symptoms after intravenous immunoglobulin administration.[24] Enteral administration of immunoglobulin has been described in case reports as well, with mixed results.[24] Concern exists about protein degradation by the acidic environment, so jejunal administration has been used. A case-control study of pediatric oncology and transplant patients (primarily SOT) evaluated enteral immunoglobulin in 12 patients and found a trend toward resolution of diarrhea and stool output 7 days after treatment.[25] However, the study did not find a difference in length of stay, hospitalization cost, or time to resolution of diarrhea. Because of the possible antiviral effects of mammalian target of rapamycin inhibitors, substituting rapamycin for other immunosuppressants is a theoretical strategy whose use has been reported in a few cases of chronic norovirus.[24] Additional studies of potential therapeutics are clearly needed for immunocompromised pediatric patients.

Infection Prevention and Anticipatory Guidance

Norovirus is relatively resistant to many available disinfectants, including alcohol-based hand sanitizers. It is also relatively resistant to many commonly used hospital disinfectants based on phenolic compounds (triclosan and quaternary ammonium). Bleach-based solutions are recommended for environmental cleaning. Handwashing with soap and water is effective at preventing transmission, including in institutional settings. Guidelines recommend standard precautions for viral gastroenteritis, including norovirus, with the use of contact precautions for diapered or incontinent patients for the duration of illness.[9] Owing to the description of nosocomial outbreaks[6] and the potential for serious consequences among transplant patients, we recommend contact precautions for all transplant patients with viral gastroenteritis, In addition, transmission has been described through aerosolized vomitus or fecal material[9]; thus droplet precautions are appropriate if a patient is actively vomiting. Ideally, these patients should be in private rooms. Given the infectiousness of symptomatic individuals, infected health care workers should be excluded from work for at least 48 hours after resolution of symptoms.[26]

ROTAVIRUS

Rotavirus is the leading cause of severe gastroenteritis among children worldwide. Despite the success of rotavirus vaccines, more than 90 million infants still lack access to a rotavirus vaccine, and rotavirus infections are still responsible for 180,000 to 450,000 deaths each year in children younger than five years globally.[27] Rotaviruses are non-enveloped, double-shelled RNA viruses in the family Reoviridae. The genome is composed of 11 segments of double-stranded RNA, coding for six structural and five nonstructural proteins. One of these non-structural proteins, NSP4, is an intracellular receptor and has been shown to have direct toxic effects on the gastrointestinal mucosa.

Epidemiology and Risk Factors

Young children 6 months to 2 years of age who are immunologically naïve are at highest risk for rotavirus infection.[27] Most children have experienced an initial rotavirus infection by age 5. Older children and adults who are immunocompetent are usually asymptomatic or have mild disease with subsequent episodes of infection. Transmission occurs via a fecal-oral route, usually through direct contact between people, and a small inoculum, such as 100 virions per gram of stool can be contagious. Transmission also can occur via ingestion of contaminated water or food and contact with contaminated surfaces or objects. Family outbreaks are common, and up to 50% of exposed immunocompetent children within a household develop rotavirus gastroenteritis.[25] Rotavirus is present in the stools of infected children several days before and after the onset of clinical symptoms. Asymptomatic excretion of rotavirus in stool is relatively common and likely plays a role in transmission. The virus is stable in the environment and can be found on toys or hard surfaces. The incubation period is short, usually less than 2 days. In the United States, incidence peaks during late winter and early spring with annual epidemics occurring from December through June.[25]

Clinical Manifestations

Rotavirus infections are characterized by watery nonbloody diarrhea, vomiting, fever, or abdominal pain. Vomiting usually lasts for 2 to 3 days and other symptoms resolve within a week.[27] Gastroenteritis caused by rotavirus cannot be clinically distinguished from that caused by other viral enteric pathogens. Severe cases can result in dehydration with shock, electrolyte imbalance, and death.[25] Central nervous system involvement with seizures and encephalopathy has been described and rotavirus has been detected in cerebrospinal fluid on occasion.[28] Necrotizing enterocolitis, intussusception, biliary atresia, and diabetes mellitus have also been described in association with rotavirus infection.[29-31] However, it is uncertain whether rotavirus is an etiologic factor for these clinical syndromes.

Among immunocompromised children, particularly those with T-cell immunodeficiency or those who have undergone HSCT, rotavirus infections can cause severe disease with prolonged diarrhea fever, dehydration, electrolyte imbalances, acidosis, and mortality. Among 183 pediatric patients who received an allogeneic HSCT at St. Jude Children's Research Hospital, 36 (19.7%) had at least one episode of rotavirus infection over the first 3 years after transplant and the median duration of diarrhea was 17.5 days (range 4 to 122 days).[32] In a retrospective case-control study among pediatric oncology patients, the median duration of rotavirus-related symptoms was 7 days (range 4 to 34 days) and the median duration of viral shedding was 17 days (range 4 to 73 days).[33] Children with SOT usually have more severe disease compared with healthy children and may experience prolonged hospitalization; however, the infection usually resolves without treatment. In addition, rotavirus may promote acute cellular rejection, particularly among intestinal transplant patients.[34]

In addition, rotavirus infection can lead to increased serum levels of particular immunosuppressive agents in organ transplant recipients, particularly in liver transplant recipients. Fruhwirth and colleagues described three pediatric SOT recipients in whom rotavirus infection caused increased trough levels of tacrolimus.[35] Although exact mechanisms are uncertain, as tacrolimus is significantly metabolized in the intestine, increased intestinal permeability and decreased gastrointestinal transit time, which would enhance drug availability in areas with lower intestinal metabolism such as the colon, have been proposed as potential mechanisms for increasing trough levels of tacrolimus.

Disease Prophylaxis and Prevention:

The most effective way to prevent rotavirus infections is through the use of the rotavirus vaccine.[25] The WHO, the American Academy of Pediatrics, and other institutions recommend universal infant immunization against rotavirus. Two live attenuated oral rotavirus vaccines are licensed for use in the United States: pentavalent human-bovine rotavirus reassortant vaccine (RV5, PRV, RotaTeq [Merck, Kenilworth, NJ]) and attenuated human rotavirus vaccine (RV1, HRV, Rotarix [GlaxoSmithKline Biologicals, Rixensart, Belgium). RV5 is administered in three oral doses at 2, 4, and 6 months of age, whereas RV1 is administered in two oral doses at 2 and 4 months. Both vaccines may be started as early as 6 weeks of age and the first dose of both vaccines should be given before 14 weeks 6 days of age. No rotavirus vaccine should be administered to infants older than 8 months 0 days. The minimum interval between doses is 4 weeks. Vaccine effectiveness against severe gastroenteritis caused by vaccine genotypes is reported as 98% (95% confidence interval 88% to 100%) for RV5, and 85 % (95% confidence interval 72% to 92%) for RV1. Children with severe combined immunodeficiency and history of intussusception cannot receive this vaccine.[25] Further studies are needed to evaluate the safety and effectiveness of rotavirus vaccines among transplant recipients; however, to date, there are no known vaccine-derived rotavirus infections in either SOT or HSCT recipients. However, family and household member of these patients can and should be vaccinated. Highly immunocompromised individuals should avoid handling diapers of infants for 4 weeks after rotavirus vaccination.[25]

Diagnosis

Rotavirus can be detected in stool samples using enzyme immunoassay, latex agglutination, and nucleic acid testing, such as PCR. Enzyme immunoassays are widely used and have high sensitivity and specificity. PCR-based tests are rapid, specific, and highly sensitive and can detect viral shedding for a longer period than enzyme immunoassay.[36] Immunocompromised children with unexplained diarrhea should be tested for viral agents of gastroenteritis including rotavirus. Multiplex PCR assays may be preferred for their increased sensitivity and ability to detect multiple viral agents.

Treatment

Similar to other causes of viral gastroenteritis, supportive measures remain the primary treatment for rotavirus infection. Currently there are no FDA-approved antiviral agents for the treatment of rotavirus infections. Enteral administration of immunoglobulin has been used. Nitozoxanide has some in vitro activity for rotavirus. The clinical efficacy of both therapies remains unclear and data are limited. In a retrospective study of 41 episodes of rotavirus infection in pediatric HSCT recipients, the median duration of clinical symptoms after initiation of nitazoxanide was shorter (11 days [range 2 to 85 days]) compared with those who received enterally administered immunoglobulins (23 days [range 10 to 107 days]) or a combination of both treatments (26 days [range 6 to 90 days]), but was similar to those who received no treatment ($P = .1$). No adverse effects of either treatment were documented.[32] In a single-center study including four pediatric HSCT patients with confirmed rotavirus infections, median time from initiation of enteral immunoglobulin to symptom resolution was 3 days, and stool frequency and consistency were improved compared with historical controls.[37] Additional studies are necessary before any of these can be considered for routine use.

Infection Prevention and Anticipatory Guidance

Contact precautions are indicated for children with rotavirus during the duration of diarrhea. Soap, water, and bleach solutions can be used to prevent transmission through environmental surfaces.

ASTROVIRUS

Astrovirus infections are among the most common causes of gastroenteritis in children.[38] Astroviruses are small, non-enveloped, positive-sense single-stranded RNA viruses in the family Astroviridae. Astroviruses have a distinctive surface star-like appearance under electron microscope. The family is divided into two genera; the genus *Mamastrovirus* infects mammals and the genus *Avastrovirus* infects poultry. There are at least eight distinct serotypes of human astroviruses, with serotype 1 viruses detected most commonly.

Epidemiology and Risk Factors

Human astrovirus infections affect predominantly children, particularly those younger than 2 years. Elderly and immunocompromised hosts are also at risk for astrovirus infection. Astrovirus is transmitted predominantly through the fecal-oral route, although ingestion of contaminated food and water and contamination of surfaces may play a role. Fresh produce washed with contaminated water has been implicated in outbreaks. Most of the published outbreaks have occurred in closed populations of younger children and elderly, such as in child care centers or hospitals. Globally, human astroviruses are estimated to cause 2 to 9% of cases of acute, nonbacterial diarrhea requiring hospitalization in children.[39] Mendez-Toss and colleagues reported that 4.6% of stool samples collected from Mexican children younger than 5 years with diarrhea had positive findings for human astroviruses.[40] Astrovirus circulates year-round but the incidence peaks in cold weather periods in temperate regions. Viral shedding lasts a median of 5 days after onset of symptoms; however, it can be prolonged to several weeks in healthy children and persistent shedding may occur in immunocompromised patients.[41,42]

Clinical Manifestations

Human astrovirus infections often cause self-limiting diarrhea in immunocompetent individuals, but they can also disseminate to organs beyond intestines and cause severe infections in immunocompromised patients. The mean incubation period is 3 to 4 days. In immunocompetent children, astrovirus infections usually present with a mild, watery diarrhea that lasts 2 to 3 days, associated with vomiting, anorexia, abdominal pain, and sometimes fever. Vomiting and diarrhea are usually milder in astrovirus infection than rotavirus infection. Asymptomatic infections are common. In a recent study from Mexico, 2.6% of stool samples collected from children younger than 5 years without diarrhea were positive for human astrovirus using an enzyme-linked immunosorbent assay.[40] Severe disseminated lethal infection and prolonged viral shedding have been described in immunocompromised patients.[41,42] Wunderli and colleagues described three pediatric recipients of HSCT with disseminated astrovirus infection with meningoencephalitis and chronic diarrhea; one infant died.[43] Astrovirus RNA was detected in the respiratory tract, blood, bone marrow, skin, and brain. Astrovirus RNA has been detected in premature infants with necrotizing enterocolitis, but the causal association is uncertain.[44]

Disease Prophylaxis and Prevention

No vaccine for astroviruses currently exists and, to our knowledge, none is under investigation.

Diagnosis

It is not possible to distinguish gastroenteritis caused by astrovirus infection from cases caused by other viral pathogens based on clinical presentation. Enzyme immunoassays have been used in epidemiologic studies to detect human astroviruses in stool specimens, and although they cannot identify the serotypes, they are helpful for rapid detection. Several FDA-cleared multiplex nucleic acid–based assays can detect astrovirus and have good sensitivity.

Treatment

Supportive treatments, including maintaining adequate hydration, nutrition, and electrolyte balance, are the mainstays of therapy. Currently there are no specific antiviral medications with FDA-approved labeling for the treatment of astrovirus and few data on potential strategies.

Infection Prevention and Anticipatory Guidance

General measures for control of diarrheal infections, such as training care providers on general sanitation measures, hand hygiene practices, keeping food preparation areas separate from child care activities, and maintaining cleanliness of environmental surfaces using soap, water, and bleach solutions, can be used to prevent transmission. Symptomatic patients should have contact and standard precautions. Sick health care workers should be excluded from work until they are asymptomatic.

SAPOVIRUS

Sapoviruses cause acute gastroenteritis in both humans and animals. Sapovirus is in the family Caliciviridae but is a separate genus from norovirus. Sapoviruses are genetically and antigenically diverse. They are small (30 to 38 nm), non-enveloped, single-stranded RNA virus. Five genogroups exist, and nine additional genogroups have been proposed. To date, only four genogroups (GI, GII, GIV, and GV) have been found to cause disease in humans.[45]

Epidemiology and Risk Factors

The initial human outbreak of sapovirus was described at an orphanage in Sapporo, Japan, in 1977.[46] Commercially available testing has only recently been available. Sapoviruses, like noroviruses and other human caliciviruses, are transmitted via fecal-oral route. Sapoviruses have been isolated from animals and contaminated water and food, including shellfish; foodborne and environmental transmission has been reported.[45] Sapoviruses infect all age groups worldwide. Most cases are probably sporadic, but outbreaks have been reported associated with child care centers, hospitals, schools, and other group care settings.[47]

Globally, sapoviruses cause a substantial proportion of pediatric diarrhea. A recent reanalysis of a multisite, international study (MAL-ED [Malnutrition and Enteric Disease Study]) using molecular diagnostic methods found that sapoviruses had the second and third greatest attributable incidence for diarrhea in children 12 to 24 months and younger than 12 months, respectively.[48] In recent studies in the United States, sapovirus was isolated from the stools of approximately 5% to 10% of children with gastroenteritis[1,49] and 3% to 6 % of healthy, asymptomatic children.[1,49] Although sapovirus disease occurs year-round, the highest prevalence of sapovirus has been found in cold months, although studies have shown differences in seasonality.[45]

Sapovirus also causes problematic infections in immunocompromised patients, although data are limited. A study among pediatric oncology patients with diarrhea isolated sapoviruses in 5% of the study population.[4] Another study of immunocompromised patients found sapoviruses in 2% of symptomatic patients, although this study included adults and a large percentage of primary immunodeficiency patients.[2]

Clinical Manifestations

The clinical symptoms of acute gastroenteritis caused by sapoviruses are similar to those of other viral causes of gastroenteritis and include low-grade fevers, vomiting, nonbloody diarrhea, abdominal pain, and cramping. Sapovirus gastroenteritis may cause milder symptoms compared with norovirus[50] and may cause more vomiting than diarrhea.[1] Among immunocompromised patients, disease may be more severe. One study of immunocompromised patients with gastroenteritis cited a similar percentage requiring hospitalization (56%) compared with other viral causes, although numbers were small.[2] Prolonged fecal excretion and diarrhea have been described in a renal transplant patient with sapovirus.[3] A larger, more recent study of sapovirus infection in immunocompromised patients did not find any with chronic excretion.[2]

Disease Prophylaxis and Prevention

No vaccine for sapoviruses currently exists and none is known to be under investigation.

Diagnosis

Antigen detection methods exist, but as for norovirus, these tests generally have low sensitivity owing to antigenic diversity. Reverse-transcription PCR is the diagnostic method of choice because of its excellent sensitivity and specificity and is available in both single-pathogen and one multipathogen testing platform.[45] Of the three commercially available multipathogen testing platforms, only one includes sapoviruses. Therefore published data regarding sapovirus are somewhat limited compared with other viral causes of gastroenteritis. Because sapovirus is found in the stools of asymptomatic individuals and the PCR-based diagnostic testing has high sensitivity, a positive test result must be interpreted in the context of the clinical scenario.

Treatment

Supportive treatments, including maintaining adequate hydration, nutrition, and electrolyte balance, are the mainstays of therapy. No approved medications for sapovirus currently exist, and no published data exist regarding potential treatment in immunocompromised children. Nitazoxanide might have theoretical activity as for norovirus,[5] but no data exist.

Infection Prevention and Anticipatory Guidance

Prevention consists of general sanitation measures, including handwashing with soap and water and use of bleach-based disinfectants. Because of the similarity of sapoviruses and noroviruses, approaches to prevention and infection control are based on data for norovirus. Guidelines recommend standard precautions for all viral gastroenteritis with the use of contact precautions for diapered or incontinent patients for the duration of illness.[9] Owing to the description of nosocomial outbreaks[45] and the potential for serious consequences among transplant patients, we recommend contact precautions for all transplant patients with viral gastroenteritis and droplet precautions if vomiting. Sick health care workers should be excluded from work until they are asymptomatic.

ADENOVIRUS

Human adenoviruses are a large group of double-stranded DNA viruses, which cause a broad spectrum of clinical disease in both healthy and immunocompromised individuals. In one study of children younger than 5 years in the United States with viral gastroenteritis, adenovirus was the third most common cause.[1] Similarly, it is an important cause of gastrointestinal illness in immunocompromised children as well, isolated from 15% of pediatric oncology patients with diarrhea.[4] Although adenovirus gastroenteritis is generally a self-limited disease in healthy children, it can be associated with more prolonged illness and disseminated disease in children who have undergone HSCT or SOT. For a complete discussion of adenovirus disease in immunocompromised children, please see Chapter 22.

CONCLUSION

Diarrhea is a frequent and potentially debilitating condition in immunocompromised pediatric patients. The pathogens causing infectious diarrhea in immunocompromised children are similar to those causing disease in healthy children; however, symptoms can be prolonged and systemic and/or disseminated disease may occur. With increasing availability and use of molecular diagnostic testing, especially multiplex PCR-based tests, diagnosis of specific pathogens in viral gastroenteritis is increasing, leading to improved epidemiologic data on the viral causes of gastrointestinal illness in immunocompromised children. Because of the severity, multiplex PCR-based tests may be an important tool for immunocompromised children with diarrhea. Although the mainstay of therapy is supportive care and immunosuppression reduction when feasible, antiviral medications are being studied in this population, but more data are needed. Vaccine has been successful for prevention of rotavirus, and vaccines targeted against norovirus are under investigation, but additional vaccines for other viral causes of gastroenteritis are needed.

34

Clostridioides difficile Infection

Erick F. Mayer Arispe, MD, MSc and Andi L. Shane, MD, MPH, MSc

Clostridioides difficile, formerly knowns as *Clostridium difficile*, is a Gram-positive, anaerobic bacillus, with a spore phase that prolongs survival in the environment. Ingestion of spores that are resistant to gastric acid results in maturation into the bacillus stage. *C. difficile* replicates disproportionally to other colonic flora when the balance is affected by another pathogen, absence of enteral feeds, exposure to antimicrobials, or chemotherapeutics. *C. difficile* produces two different toxins. Toxin A is an enterotoxin that attaches to the basal membrane damaging the villi. Toxin B is an extremely potent cytotoxin that induces apoptosis. Toxin-mediated damage, with progressive neutrophilic infiltration and fluid secretion by the intestine, results in many of the symptoms that are a sequelae *C. difficile* activity.

The presence of *C. difficile* in the gastrointestinal tract is the normal, baseline state. Newborns have sterile gastrointestinal tracts and *C. difficile* colonization is highest by 1 month of life, then declines in the following months until there are very low rates of colonization by 2 years of age.[1] Most infants do not develop clinical disease, probably secondary to lack of toxin-binding receptors in their immature intestinal mucosa and/or by protection from secretory immunoglobulin A and oligosaccharides in human milk.[2] Differentiating colonization from active infection in immunocompromised children is challenging, as dysbiosis is the common baseline state. Diarrhea, abdominal pain, and other nonspecific gastrointestinal symptoms are the result of numerous factors, including medications, chemotherapy, and frequent courses of antimicrobials.

Despite shared risk factors for *C. difficile*, there are differences in the epidemiology of *C. difficile* colonization and disease between children and adults that are essential to understand in order to interpret results and manage disease. Most of the limited evidence for the diagnosis and treatment of *C. difficile* is derived from studies in immunocompetent adults, with few studies in children. The focus of this chapter is to outline the differences between immunocompetent and immunocompromised *C. difficile* colonization and disease in children, focusing on pediatric solid organ (SOT), hematopoietic stem cell transplant (HSCT) recipients, and pediatric oncology patients.

EPIDEMIOLOGY AND RISK FACTORS

Definitions of *C. difficile* Disease and Colonization

C. difficile disease is defined as new-onset of diarrhea (at least three unformed stools in less than a 24-hour period) and a positive diagnostic test result for *C. difficile* in stool, or colonoscopic or histopathologic evidence of pseudomembranous colitis.[3] Because the probability of colonization is higher in younger children (usually those younger than 2 years), it is important to consider other common infectious and noninfectious etiologies of diarrhea even when *C. difficile* testing results are positive. There is no accepted definition for severe *C. difficile* disease. The presence of a complication of *C. difficile* disease or at least two abnormal laboratory findings (Table 34.1) has been used in previous research studies,[4,5] but validation of this proposed scoring system is still required.

Several studies noted an increase in the rates of *C. difficile* disease among children.[6,7] A retrospective study of more than 20 children's hospitals in the United States reported that the rates of pediatric *C. difficile* disease doubled between 2001 and 2006.[6] Another study analyzing secondary data from more than 30,000 pediatric patients noted an increase in the rates of *C. difficile* disease diagnosed by toxin assay between 1999 and 2006, and a decrease in rates of *C. difficile* disease between 2006 and 2010.[7] Molecular diagnostics have altered surveillance. The increased sensitivity of molecular assays has limited the ability to make comparisons between rates of colonization and disease calculated using toxin assays with those calculated using molecular diagnostics.

A retrospective study of 200 children with *C. difficile* disease reported that 38 (19%) had underlying conditions that increased their risk of infection, and 149 (75%) had received antibiotics in the 2 months before the episode.[8] Risk factors for the development of *C. difficile* disease in children include younger age (1 to 4 years), prolonged hospitalization, feeding via gastrostomy or jejunostomy, use of broad-spectrum antibiotics, HSCT, SOT, cancer, immunodeficiency, and human immunodeficiency virus (HIV) infection, fungal infections, viral gastroenteritis, cystic fibrosis, and inflammatory bowel disease.[9] A nested case-control study in children identified the following risk factors for CDI: SOT, lack of hospitalization, presence of gastrostomy or jejunostomy, and receipt of fluoroquinolones or nonquinolone antibiotics in the 4 weeks before *C. difficile* disease.[10]

C. difficile Infection in Pediatric SOT Recipients

The estimated prevalence of *C. difficile* disease among pediatric SOT recipients is 12%,[11] varying by transplanted organ. The rates of *C. difficile* disease among pediatric SOT recipients ranges between 5% and 16% for kidney recipients; between 11% and 12.9% for heart recipients; between 11% and 18% for liver recipients; between 11.5% and 9% for lung recipients[13]; between 3% and 7% for pancreas recipients[14,15]; and 20% for small bowel transplant recipients.[16] A study that evaluated secondary data from more than 50,000 hospitalized adult SOT recipients reported that those with *C. difficile* disease had higher mortality rates, longer hospital stays, higher costs, more colectomies, and higher rates of complications associated with the transplanted organ compared with those patients without *C. difficile* disease.[17]

Among pediatric kidney transplant recipients, young age (younger than 5 years), female gender, treatment with monoclonal antibodies, antibiotic use, and intraabdominal placement of the graft were associated with the development of *C. difficile* disease.[12] Other risks factors

TABLE 34.1 Clinical and Laboratory Criteria of Severe *Clostridioides difficile* Disease

Clinical Criteria (At Least One)
• Pseudomembranous colitis (endoscopy or histopathology)
• Required surgical intervention because of CDI
• Gastrointestinal perforation
• Toxic megacolon
• Pneumatosis intestinalis
• Admission to the ICU on the date of diagnosis or readmitted within 2 days of the diagnosis
Laboratory Criteria (2 or More)
• WBC > 15 × 10^3 cells/mL
• Albumin <2.5 g/dL
• Elevated age-adjusted creatinine level
• Bloody stools
• Fever >38.5°C for 1 or more days within 7 days before diagnosis or the day after the diagnosis

CDI, Clostridioides difficile infection; *ICU,* intensive care unit; *WBC,* white blood cell count.
Adapted from Zar FA, Bakkanagari SR, Moorthi KM, Davis MB. A comparison of vancomycin and metronidazole for the treatment of *Clostridium difficile*-associated diarrhea, stratified by disease severity. *Clin Infect Dis.* 2007;45(3):302-307; and Kim J, Shaklee JF, Smathers S, et al. Risk factors and outcomes associated with severe *Clostridium difficile* infection in children. *Pediatr Infect Dis J.* 2012;31(2):134-138.

for the development of *C. difficile* disease described for adult SOT recipients include recent hospitalization, augmentation of steroid dose, use of steroids before transplant, ganciclovir prophylaxis, the use of antithymocyte globulin, and transplant other that kidney alone.

C. difficile Infection in Pediatric HSCT Recipients

The rates of *C. difficile* disease are similar in pediatric and adult HSCT patients, although some studies have found even higher rates in children compared with adults. The rate of *C. difficile* disease among pediatric allogeneic HSCT recipients was 17% compared with 11% among adult patients in the same institution.[18] Infection with *C. difficile* is more common in adult patients undergoing allogeneic (9% to 27%) than autologous (7% to 9%) transplants, respectively.[19-21] Differing rates of posttransplant *C. difficile* disease has been noted in several observational studies. Recipients of allogenic HSCTs are subject to prolonged use of broad-spectrum antibiotics, a higher immunosuppressive state, and an increased risk for graft-versus-host disease (GVHD), all of which are risk factors for *C. difficile* disease. Another contributing factor may be higher colonization rates with *C. difficile* before allogenic transplantation, a factor that has been reported among adult[22] and pediatric allogenic HSCT recipients.[23]

A nested case-control study with a multivariate analysis comparing 62 adult allogeneic HSCT recipients with 123 controls matched by graft type demonstrated that receipt of chemotherapy before conditioning, exposure to broad-spectrum antibiotics after transplant, and vancomycin-resistant enterococci colonization were associated with the development of *C. difficile* disease. Cord blood as the source of the stem cells, acute GVHD, and total body irradiation were associated with *C. difficile* disease among adult allogenic HSCT recipients.[19]

C. difficile Disease in Pediatric Oncologic Patients

One-third of children younger than 3 years and one-fifth who are 3 years and older are colonized with *C. difficile* at the time of their first admission to the pediatric oncology ward. After 2 weeks of inpatient hospitalization, colonization rates increase to 90% for children younger than 3 years and 50% for those older than 3 years.[24] Another surveillance study that used polymerase chain reaction (PCR) testing and culture, reported that 29% of asymptomatic pediatric oncology patients were colonized with *C. difficile* at the time of admission to an inpatient unit. Slightly more than half (55%) of those who had a history of *C. difficile* disease had positive results for stool sampling by molecular testing or culture noted intermittently for over 20 weeks, sometimes with different *C. difficile* strains.[25] The high prevalence of colonization, gut dysbiosis, gastrointestinal effects of chemotherapy regimens, antibiotic exposure, other infections, and underlying conditions make the diagnosis of *C. difficile* disease challenging in pediatric oncologic patients.

Cancer has been reported as the most common comorbidity in pediatric *C. difficile* disease, with 25% of infections reported among children whose data was collected in administrative databases.[6,7] According to these databases, the rate of *C. difficile* disease is 10 times higher in pediatric patients with cancer compared with children without cancer. A multicenter retrospective cohort study evaluating children with acute myeloid leukemia reported that 37 (11%) developed diarrhea and had positive test results for *C. difficile* toxin while receiving chemotherapy.[26]

A study that evaluated the risk factors associated with *C. difficile* disease among children with cancer reported that exposure to aminoglycosides, third- and fourth-generation cephalosporins, and proton pump inhibitors in the week before admission, and chemotherapy in the 8 to 14 days before admission were associated with the development of *C. difficile* disease.[7] Another retrospective cohort study in children with acute myeloid leukemia reported that the duration of broad-spectrum antibiotics and infection of a sterile site were independently associated with *C. difficile* disease.[26]

CLINICAL MANIFESTATIONS

Toxin Detection and Clinicopathologic Correlation

Diarrhea or other gastrointestinal symptoms frequently develop in pediatric immunocompromised patients as the result of infections, as an adverse effect of antibiotics or chemotherapeutic agents, or as the result of an underlying disease. The detection of *C. difficile* toxin in stool samples does not necessarily correlate with organism activity. One of 11 children from whom *C. difficile* toxin was detected in their stools had postmortem histologic evidence of clostridial infection and abundant pseudomembranes. The other 10 children had negative clostridial immunohistochemistry and PCR results, and the macroscopic findings varied significantly, from normal to the presence of pseudomembranes.[27]

C. difficile Disease

C. difficile disease may be considered in children with new-onset diarrhea, with three or more episodes of unformed stools in less than 24 hours.[3] The median time for development of *C. difficile* disease after SOT was 57 days (interquartile range [IQR] 14 to 227 days) varying by transplanted organ.[11] In pediatric kidney transplant recipients *C. difficile* disease developed significantly earlier than in adults (mean time of onset of symptoms was 33 days for children, compared with 15 months in adults).[12] *C. difficile* disease has been reported in four children who underwent a lung transplant for cystic fibrosis; two had disease within the first 4 months after transplant, whereas in the other two infection developed during the first 3 years of follow-up.[13] The median time for detection of *C. difficile* disease was 204 days after the procedure (range 77 to 339 days) in small bowel transplant recipients.[16]

Reports of the time of onset of gastrointestinal symptoms in patients with *C. difficile* disease after HSCT vary from center to center, likely related to differences in colonization rates, criteria for diagnostic testing, and differences in patient populations. The highest risk for *C. difficile* disease among HSCT recipients spans the duration of conditioning through 3 months post-transplant. *C. difficile* disease tends to develop earlier in recipients of autologous HSCT than in allogeneic HSCT recipients, with a median time of onset of 6.5 versus 33 days, respectively.[19] When compared with adult allogeneic HSCT recipients, *C. difficile* disease developed in pediatric allogeneic HSCT recipients later, at a median of 51 days (IQR 5 to 72 days) compared with 16 days (IQR 5 to 49 days).[18]

Severe *C. difficile* Disease

The definition of severe *C. difficile* disease in immunocompromised hosts is challenging. Severe *C. difficile* disease with leukocytosis or fulminant colitis with pseudomembranes has been reported in pediatric SOT recipients.[28] Nevertheless, most patients are neutropenic during and after chemotherapy or cytoreduction. Because the development of pseudomembranous colitis requires neutrophilic infiltration of the intestinal mucosa, this severity marker is not a common occurrence in patients with neutropenia.[29]

Pseudomembranous colitis has been reported after both autologous and allogeneic bone marrow transplants, but patients were not neutropenic at the time of diagnosis of *C. difficile* disease.[30] Another case series reported four allogeneic HSCT patients with *C. difficile* disease in whom nonspecific inflammatory changes developed within their colonic mucosa, without evidence of pseudomembranous colitis.[29]

There are two sets of proposed criteria for the definition of severe *C. difficile* disease. The Society for Healthcare Epidemiology/Infectious Diseases Society of America (SHEA/IDSA) guidelines include the presence of white blood cell count higher that 15,000 cells/mL or a serum creatinine level greater than 1.5 mg/dL.[3] The European Society of Clinical Microbiology and Infectious Diseases (ESCMID) guidelines require the presence of any of the following: fever; rigors; hemodynamic instability; signs or peritonitis or ileus; marked leukocytosis or marked left shift; elevated creatinine; reduced serum albumin; elevated lactate level; evidence of pseudomembranous colitis on endoscopy; distention of large bowel, colonic wall thickening, pericolonic fat stranding, or ascites on imaging.[31] Given the differences between immunocompromised children and adults, it is reasonable to assume that classic clinical, pathologic, or diagnostic criteria for severe *C. difficile* disease may not be adequate for pediatric oncology patients and transplant recipients. When these criteria were applied to immunocompetent pediatric patients, half of the children with severe infections were not detected using the SHEA/IDSA criteria, whereas all children with severe infections were detected by the ESCMID criteria.[32] Previous studies, one in adults and one in children, have used the presence of a complication of *C. difficile* disease or at least two abnormal laboratory findings (see Table 34.1) as indicators of severe *C. difficile* disease,[4,5] but this scoring system has not been validated.

Clinical Outcomes

A large cohort study from Canada reported that 90% of children with *C. difficile* disease had resolution of symptoms by 30 days after onset, and 2% experienced severe outcomes (five required intensive care and one patient's *C. difficile* disease was associated with mortality).[33]

A large retrospective cohort study using secondary data from 41 free-standing children's hospitals in the United States reported that children with a *C. difficile* diagnosis had a significantly higher mortality than those without a *C. difficile* diagnosis (1.4% vs. 0.7%).[34] When subgroups were analyzed based on time of onset of disease, those who had *C. difficile* detected before the third day of hospitalization had mortality similar to *C. difficile*–negative children. Children with *C. difficile* detected after the third inpatient day had higher mortality rates than *C. difficile*–negative children, longer hospital stays, and higher costs.[34] Other risk factors associated with higher mortality rates included older age (>13 years), underlying malignancy, cardiovascular disease, hematologic or immunologic conditions, gastric acid suppression, and the presence of more than one severity illness marker in the previous 48 hours (admission to intensive care unit, receipt of vasopressors, or need for respiratory support).[35] A study of 200 children in Canada reported a *C. difficile*–associated mortality rate of 1%. The cohort included 38 children with underlying conditions that increased their risk of *C. difficile* disease. Both children who died were immunocompromised.[8] A small cohort of pediatric lung transplant recipients in whom *C. difficile* disease developed had poor outcomes. Of four lung transplant recipients with *C. difficile* disease, one required an ileostomy, another died after developing renal insufficiency, and two had subsequent episodes of *C. difficile* disease that eventually resolved.[13] Although it is challenging to separate *C. difficile* infection from disease and even more difficult to separate comorbidities of immunocompromised children from the clinical presentation of *C. difficile* disease, clinicians should be aware of the poorer clinical outcomes of children with *C. difficile* infection and disease that have been demonstrated both on the individual and population levels.

Recurrence of *C. difficile* Disease

The rate of recurrence of *C. difficile* disease in children has been reported as between 20% and 30%.[8,36] In comparison, 10 (40%) of pediatric SOT recipients had a recurrent episode of *C. difficile*. Two (20%) of the SOT recipients had a recurrent *C. difficile* in the 8 weeks after the initial episode.[11] Factors associated with recurrence included malignancy, recent surgery, and the number of antibiotic classes to which the patient was exposed.[36] The mean time to recurrence was 34 days after the onset of the first episode.[32] A case-control study comparing 48 children with severe *C. difficile* disease with 34 children with nonsevere *C. difficile* disease found no difference between these groups in terms of recurrence or treatment failure.[4]

Children who received an HSCT had higher rates of recurrence *C. difficile* disease compared with those who did not receive a transplant, but the difference in rates was not statistically significant.[36,37] Patients in whom gastrointestinal GVHD (GI GVHD) developed had a 5-fold higher odds of recurrent *C. difficile* disease. GI GVHD remained significant after adjusting for recognized risk factors for *C. difficile* recurrence, including receipt of systemic steroids.[19] In a case-control study, adults in whom *difficile* disease developed were more likely to have GI GVHD disease in the year after transplantation. In a subgroup of 12 (85%) patients, the diagnosis of *C. difficile* disease preceded the diagnosis of GI GVHD. The median time to development of GI GVHD was 21 days after the diagnosis of *C. difficile* disease.[19] A retrospective cohort of adult and pediatric T-cell–depleted allogeneic HSCT recipients did not find an association between the development of GI GVHD and *C. difficile* disease.[21]

Diagnosis

The diagnosis of *C. difficile* disease may be considered in high-risk patients with new onset of diarrhea. Current guidelines recommend consideration of *C. difficile* testing when a patient has more than three episodes of unformed stools in less than 24 hours.[3] Clinicians should consider how they will interpret the results of diagnostic testing in the context of risk factors of the host. In immunocompromised pediatric hosts, the clinician should consider the likelihood of infection versus colonization, underlying conditions, recent antimicrobial, administration, radiation, and chemotherapy, as well as non–*C. difficile* etiologies for the symptoms.

Toxigenic culture and cell cytotoxicity neutralization assays in stools have been largely replaced by the detection of glutamate dehydrogenase (GDH, an enzyme present in all isolates of *C. difficile*), and *C. difficile* toxins using enzyme immunoassays; and by nucleic acid amplification tests (NAAT) that can target *C. difficile*–specific genes, including *tcdA*, *tcdB*, and 16S ribosomal RNA.

Selection of a diagnostic assay should consider the sensitivity, specificity, and positive and negative predictive values. of the tests used. Enzyme immunoassay has a sensitivity of 35% compared with 95% with a PCR when pediatric samples are analyzed. Both tests have a specificity of 100%.[38] PCR increases the yield of detection of *C. difficile* by toxin 2-fold compared with cytotoxin assays.[39]

Diagnostic algorithms that include a multistep process (i.e., GDH plus toxin; GDH plus toxin, with NAAT; or NAAT plus toxin) to adjudicate inconclusive results have the optimal positive predictive value. The use of NAAT alone has a high sensitivity, which may lead to overdiagnosis of *C. difficile*. Currently NAAT alone or a multistep process is recommended as the preferred diagnostic method.[3]

Clinicians caring for both immunocompetent and immunocompromised infants must carefully interpret of *C. difficile* diagnostic results, given the high rates of colonization and clinical insensitivity to *C. difficile* toxin in this age group. Although rare, *C. difficile* disease has been reported and the diagnosis should be considered, especially when an infant has manifestations of pseudomembranous colitis, toxic megacolon, or significant diarrhea when other etiologies have been excluded. Children between 1 and 2 years of age are also likely to have high *C. difficile* colonization rates, making diagnosis of active disease in a symptomatic host with clinical symptoms challenging. Children older than 2 years have similar colonization rates as older children and adults.

Increased reporting of severe gastrointestinal infections after transplantation, including *C. difficile* infection,[40] have been affected by the use of molecular panels with increased sensitivity and multiple targets. The detection of co-infections with *C. difficile*, including rotavirus, norovirus, and sapovirus, has been noted. Comparisons of different commercial multiplex PCR platforms for enteropathogens have yielded equivalent results from stools of immunocompromised children.[41]

Diagnostic tests of cure are not beneficial, as toxin may continue to be detected in up to 60% of asymptomatic children. Guidelines emphasize that repetitive diagnostics within 7 days of the initial test are not beneficial. Children with recurrence of symptoms after treatment and initial resolution may be evaluated with repeat diagnostics[3] considering non–*C. difficile* etiologies.

The evidence to support the use of stool inflammatory markers to diagnose *C. difficile* disease is limited.[3] A study evaluating *C. difficile*–positive and *C. difficile*–negative diarrheal stool samples found higher stool levels of lactoferrin, calprotectin, interleukin (IL)-8 and IL-23 in *C. difficile*–positive stool samples Other markers present included C5a, CD40L, granulocyte colony-stimulating factor, I-309, IL-13, IL-16, IL-27, monocyte chemoattractant protein-1, tumor necrosis factor alpha, and IL-8.[42] The diagnostic utility of stool inflammatory markers in the management of children with diarrhea is undergoing assessment.

TREATMENT

The mainstay of treatment of *C. difficile* disease is to restore normal flora and reduce dysbiosis. Optimally this is accomplished by discontinuing antimicrobials, if this is feasible. The 2017 IDSA/SHEA *C. difficile* guidelines recommend that either metronidazole or vancomycin may be considered for the treatment of a nonsevere, first episode of *C. difficile* disease in children.[3] An Emerging Infectious Disease Network survey of 285 pediatric infectious disease specialists noted that all respondents use oral metronidazole for a mild, first episode of *C. difficile* disease. In this survey, 41% to 79% of physicians would still use metronidazole for a mild, first episode of *C. difficile* disease when the patient had an underlying co-morbidity, including SOT.[43]

In children with an initial, severe *C. difficile* disease episode, the treatment of choice is oral vancomycin.[3] Either vancomycin or fidaxomicin is recommended for the treatment of an initial, severe episode of *C. difficile* disease in adults. These antibiotics have similar rates of cure, including resolution of symptoms, although adult fidaxomicin recipients had lower recurrence rates (71% vs. 57%) compared with oral vancomycin recipients.[44] Fidaxomicin has been administered to adult oncology patients who have recurrent *C. difficile* disease, with resolution of clinical symptoms in 20 of 22 patients.[45] Fidaxomicin has not been approved by the FDA for use in children younger than 18 years, although it has been tolerated in children with a pharmacokinetic profile similar to adults.[46] A 10-year old boy, who was gastrostomy tube dependent, had five episodes of *C. difficile* disease after being treated for recurrent pneumonia. He received crushed fidaxomicin at a dose of 200 mg twice daily administered via his gastrostomy tube. His diarrhea resolved in less than 24 hours. *C. difficile* disease recurred after a subsequent course of antibiotics, and fidaxomicin receipt was accompanied by quick symptom resolution.[47]

Oral vancomycin is the antimicrobial of choice for children with two or more episodes of recurrent *C. difficile* disease. If the antimicrobial used previously was vancomycin, an extended course of oral vancomycin (tapered and pulsed regimen) or oral vancomycin followed by rifaximin or fidaxomicin could be considered for treatment, extrapolated from adult studies.[3] A survey of pediatric infectious diseases specialists reported that 23 (18%) would recommend fecal microbiota transplantation (FMT) and 20 (16%) would recommend off-label use of fidaxomicin for recurrent or severe *C. difficile* disease in children.[43]

A review article summarized the experience of FMT in children with refractory *C. difficile* disease; 23 patients aged 16 months to 19 years (8 were immunocompromised) had cure rates between 50% and 100%.[48] In a case series of 10 children with recurrent *C. difficile* disease, four immunocompromised (three with inflammatory bowel disease, one received chemotherapy for Wilms tumor), concluded that FMT administered via nasogastric tube was safe and effective. Nine (90%) had symptom resolution. One child had recurrence of symptoms 2 months after FMT while he was receiving chemotherapy, and *C. difficile* recurred after a second FMT[49] (Table 34.2).

Primary and Secondary Prevention

Children, both immunocompetent and immunocompromised, with diarrhea, including that attributed to *C. difficile*, should be cared for in a single-occupancy room, when feasible. Staff should wear gowns and gloves, and dedicated equipment should remain in the single-occupancy room to be used only to care for the patient. These contact precautions should be maintained for at least 48 hours after resolution of diarrhea. Hand hygiene practices of staff, family members, and the patient are the mainstay of prevention of reinfection and transmission to others. Handwashing with soap and water is preferable to the use of alcohol-based sanitizers owing to the *in vitro* observation that handwashing with soap and water is more effective for spore removal.[3] However, use of an alcohol-based sanitizer is acceptable if handwashing with soap and water cannot be performed.

There is moderate evidence to support the use of probiotics for the primary prevention of *C. difficile* disease among immunocompetent

TABLE 34.2 Suggested Treatment Regimens for Immunocompromised Children with CDI

Clinical Presentation	Recommended Treatment	Dose	Maximum Dose
Initial episode, non-severe	Metronidazole × 10 days (PO)[a]	7.5 mg/kg/dose tid or qid	500 mg tid or qid
	or		
	Vancomycin × 10 days (PO)[a]	10 mg/kg/dose qid	125 mg qid
Initial episode, severe/fulminant[b]	Vancomycin × 10 days (PO or PR)[a]	10 mg/kg/dose qid	500 mg qid
	with or without		
	Metronidazole × 10 days (IV)[a]	10 mg/kg/dose tid	500 mg tid
First recurrence, non-severe	Vancomycin × 10 days (PO)[a]	10 mg/kg/dose qid	125 mg qid
	or		
	Vancomycin tapered and pulsed regimen[c]		
Second or subsequent recurrence	Vancomycin tapered and pulsed regimen[c]	10 mg/kg/dose qid	125 mg qid
	or		
	Vancomycin × 10 days, followed by rifaximin for 20 days[d]		Vancomycin: 125 mg qid Rifaximin: 400 mg tid
	or		
	Fidaxomicin × 10 days[e]	200 mg bid (>6 years of age) 16 mg/kg bid (6 months to <6 years of age)	400 mg/day

[a]The duration of treatment used by most of the clinical trials was 10 days, but if symptoms have not subsided, extension of treatment to 14 days should be considered.
[b]In case of fulminant CDI disease, consider the addition of intravenous metronidazole to oral or rectal vancomycin.
[c]Tapered and pulsed regimen: vancomycin 10 mg/kg with max of 125 mg 4 times per day for 10-14 days, followed by 10 mg/kg with max of 125 mg two times per day for a week, followed by 10 mg/kg max of 125 mg once a day for a week, and then 10 mg/kg max of 125 mg every 2 or 3 days for 2-8 weeks.
[d]No pediatric dose for rifaximin. FDA approved for the use only in children >12 years of age.
[e]No pediatric dose for fidaxomicin. FDA approved for the use >18 years of age.
IV, intravenous; *PO*, oral; *PE*, rectal; *tid*, three times per day; *qid*, four times per day.

hosts.[50] The potential risk of bacteremia and fungemia in the immunocompromised host, who may be more likely to translocate probiotic organisms into the bloodstream, must be considered. The risks and benefits of probiotic supplementation in pediatric transplant recipients and oncology patients in need of evidence-based recommendations.

There is no supportive evidence for screening people for asymptomatic colonization of *C. difficile* in a non-outbreak setting.[3] There are no data to support routine screening of immunocompromised hosts, despite recognition of high rates of *C. difficile* infection among previously colonized immunocompromised patients. Diseases developed in 11 of 18 adults colonized with toxigenic *C. difficile* strains a median of 12 days after HSCT. In contrast, disease developed in only one patient of 26 colonized with non-toxigenic strains of *C. difficile*.[22] Further research is needed to determine if interventions, such as prophylactic metronidazole, vancomycin, or fidaxomin, are warranted for prevention of disease before and during profound immunosuppression.

Antibiotic stewardship programs have an active role in educating clinicians about strategies to reduce the risk of *C. difficile* disease. Balancing the use of broad-spectrum antimicrobials for empiric therapy in immunocompromised hosts and limiting duration are strategies that can be jointly promoted by clinicians. Additional guidance from antibiotic stewardship programs can inform interventions based on local practices and the epidemiology of *C. difficile*.[3]

CONCLUSION

C. difficile can be both a commensal and a pathogenic member of the gastrointestinal flora, with high rates of asymptomatic colonization in neonates and infants. When the balance of the gut microbiome homeostasis is perturbed, *C. difficile* has the potential to cause disease. Among immunocompromised children with diarrhea, abdominal pain, and other nonspecific gastrointestinal symptoms, *C. difficile* disease, along with other infectious and noninfectious etiologies, should be considered. The interpretation of diagnostics for *C. difficile* in an immunocompromised child requires differentiating *C. difficile* colonization from disease. The objective of *C. difficile* treatment is the restoration of the normal flora and reduction of dysbiosis. The mainstay of management is to discontinue or narrow antimicrobial therapy, if feasible, while optimizing enteral nutrition. Selection of *C. difficile*–therapeutics should be done based on severity of infection, number of recurrences, and host immunocompromise. Infection prevention, antimicrobial and diagnostic stewardship should be incorporated into the management of immunocompromised children with *C. difficile* to optimize care.

INDEX

A

Abdominal actinomycosis, 239
Actinomyces, 238–240
  epidemiology of, 238–239
Actinomycosis, pediatric, 239
Active immunization, for herpes simplex virus, 138
Active immunoprophylaxis, for Epstein-Barr virus, 128
Acute cellular rejection, after solid organ transplant, 4
Acute gastroenteritis, norovirus in, 253
Acute lymphoblastic leukemia (ALL), 22, 23–24t, 26–27
Acute myelogenous leukemia (AML), 23–24t, 27
  candidiasis with, 196
Acute primary histoplasmosis, complications of, 215
Acute rejection, after solid organ transplant, 4
Acyclovir, for herpes simplex virus, 136
Adaptive cellular immune recovery, after HSCT, 13–14
Adaptive humoral immune recovery, after HSCT, 14
Adaptive immunotherapy, for PTLD treatment, 132
Adenoviruses, 155, 257
  anticipatory guidance for, 161
  clinical manifestations of, 156–157
  common disease association with, 156t
  diagnosis of, 158–159
  disease prophylaxis/prevention for, 157–158, 158f
  epidemiology and risk factors of, 155–156
  hematopoietic cell transplantation and, 156
  immunotherapy for, 161
  infection prevention for, 161
  solid organ transplantation and, 155–156, 156t
  treatment for, 159–161
Adolescent, CMV in, 125
AIDS, cryptococcosis with, 206
Air quality, good practice recommendations and, 86
Albendazole, for strongyloidiasis, 248, 248t
Alcohol-based hand sanitizers, for norovirus, 254
Alemtuzumab (Campath), 6
  for herpes simplex virus, 136
Alkylating agents, 25–26t, 29
ALL. *see* Acute lymphoblastic leukemia
Allograft rejection, 76
AML. *see* Acute myelogenous leukemia
Amphotericin
  for cryptococcosis, 209
  for *Geotrichum* spp. infections, 213
  for *Rhodotorula* species infections, 212
  for *Saccharomyces* species infections, 213
Amphotericin B, for histoplasmosis, 220
Amphotericin B-based monotherapy, for mucormycosis, 185–186
Amphotericin B deoxycholate
  for blastomycosis, 223
  for histoplasmosis, 220
Animal contact, after transplantation and chemotherapy, 94–95
Animal safety, 85
Antibacterial prophylaxis, role of, 78
Antibiotic therapy, for actinomycosis, 240
Antibiotics, microbiome implications and, 74
Anti-CD20 monoclonal antibody, for PTLD treatment, 132
Anticipated donor-derived infections, 40–41
Antifungal prophylaxis, breakthrough invasive mold infections reported on, 182t
Antifungal therapy
  for fusariosis, 191
  for invasive aspergillosis, 177–179
  for invasive mold diseases, 193–194, 194t
  for *L. prolificans,* 191
  for mucormycosis, 185–187
  for *S. apiospermum* species complex, 191
Antigen detection
  assays, for cryptococcosis, 208–209
  for histoplasmosis, 218–219
  methods, for sapovirus, 257
Antigenemia, 218
Antigen-presenting cell (APC), 2–3
Antigenuria, 218
Antimetabolites, 8, 25–26t, 29
Antimicrobial resistance, rates of, 81
Antimicrobial stewardship programs (ASPs), 78, 80
  basic goals of, 78
  immunocompromised children, barriers to in, 79–80
Antineoplastic therapies, cancer and, 22
Anti-thymocyte globulin (ATG), 4
Antiviral agents, for adenoviruses, 159–161
Antiviral resistance, of cytomegalovirus, 123
Antiviral treatment, for respiratory virus, 151–153, 152t, 153t
APC. *see* Antigen-presenting cell
Arabinitol, 201
Aspergillosis, 170
  anticipatory guidance for, 180
  cerebral, 172
  clinical manifestations of, 172
  cutaneous, 172
  diagnosis of, 173–176, 174f
    (1, 3)-β-D-glucan for, 176
    culture for, 173
    galactomannan antigen for, 175–176
    polymerase chain reaction for, 176
    radiology for, 173–175
  disease prophylaxis/prevention for, 172–173
  epidemiology of, 170–172
  in hematopoietic stem cell transplant, 170–171
  infection prevention for, 180
  invasive pulmonary, 172
  in oncology, 171
  pediatric-specific invasive, 171–172
  risk factors for, 170–172
  in solid organ transplant, 171
  treatment of, 176–180, 177f
    adjunctive therapies for, 180
    alternative antifungal therapy for, 179
Aspergillosis *(Continued)*
    combination antifungal therapy for, 180
    primary antifungal therapy for, 177–179
    salvage antifungal therapy for, 179–180
Aspergillus, 170
Aspergillus serum galactomannan assay, for fusariosis, 190
ASPs. *see* Antimicrobial stewardship programs
Astrovirus, 255–256
Asymptomatic candiduria, 197
ATG. *see* Anti-thymocyte globulin
Atovaquone, for *Pneumocystis* pneumonia, 243
Attenuated human rotavirus vaccine, 255
Atypical pneumonia, *Mycoplasma* and, 108
Autologous hematopoietic stem cells, 14–15
Autologous stem cell transplant, 30
Avastrovirus, 255
Azathioprine (Imuran), 8
Azithromycin
  for *Bartonella,* 105
  for *Legionella,* 106
Azole therapy
  for blastomycosis, 223
  for coccidioidomycosis, 225
  for histoplasmosis, 220–221

B

BA. *see* Bacillary angiomatosis
Bacillary angiomatosis (BA), 103
Bacillary peliosis (BP), 103
Bacteremia, candidemia and, 197
Bacterial infections
  management of, 59–61
    empiric antibacterial therapy for, 60
    with high-risk fever and neutropenia, 59–60
    initial antibiotic therapy for, 59
    with low-risk fever and neutropenia, 60
  prevention of, 49–50
    active, 49
    early disease, 49
    exposure, 49
    late disease, 49
Bacterial pathogens, 56–57, 57t
Bartonella, 103–105
  anticipatory guidance for children with, 105
  clinical manifestations of, 103–104
  diagnosis of, 104
  disease prophylaxis/prevention, 104
  epidemiology of, 103
  infection prevention for children with, 105
  risk factors of, 103
  treatment of, 104–105
Basiliximab (Simulect), 6
Belatacept (Nulojix), 8
Benznidazole, for Chagas disease, 251
Biologic agents
  cryptococcosis associated with, 207
  as induction therapy, 6
  as maintenance immunosuppressive therapy, 8
  for pediatric cancers, 30–32
  as rejection therapies, 8–9

BK polyomavirus (BKPyV), 162
Blastomycosis, 221–223
  clinical manifestations of, 221–222, 222f
  diagnosis of, 222–223, 222f
  disease prophylaxis and prevention of, 223
  epidemiology and risk factors of, 221
  treatment of, 223, 223t
Bleach-based solutions, for norovirus, 254
Blood culture
  for candidiasis, 200
  for *Geotrichum* spp. infections, 213
Blood products, window of time between, 63
Bloodstream infection (BSI), 22
  proposed pathogenesis of, 73f
Bone marrow, 16
  laboratory screening of, 41, 42–43t
Bortezomib, 8
BP. *see* Bacillary peliosis
Brain abscesses, *T. gondii* infection and, 228–229
Brain imaging, for aspergillosis, 175
Brincidofovir, for adenoviruses, 160
Bronchoalveolar (BAL) fluid, for *Pneumocystis* pneumonia, 243
Bronchoalveolar lavage, for aspergillosis, 175–176
BSI. *see* Bloodstream infection

C

Calcineurin inhibitors, as maintenance immunosuppressive therapy, 7–8
Caliciviridae, 253
Cancer
  candidiasis and, 196
  Epstein-Barr virus in, 127
  histoplasmosis in, 216
Candida albicans, 195
Candida endophthalmitis, 198
Candida genus, 195
Candida glabrata, 195
Candida parapsilosis, 195
Candidal esophagitis, 196
Candidemia, 195, 197
  definitive therapy for, 202–203, 203f
Candidiasis, 195
  central nervous system, 198
  clinical manifestations of, 196
  definitive therapy for
    based on *Candida* species, 201–202, 202t
    based on location of infection, 202–205
  diagnosis of, 199–201
  disease prophylaxis and prevention of, 198–199
  endovascular, 197
  epidemiology and risk factors of, 195–197
  genitourinary and renal, 197
  hepatosplenic (chronic disseminated), 197
  infection prevention and anticipatory guidance for, 205
  intraabdominal, 197
  invasive, 197–198
  laboratory findings of, 200
  non-culture detection methods for, 200
  non-culture DNA-based diagnostic tests for, 200–201
  non-DNA and non-culture diagnostic tests for, 201
  ocular, 198
  osteoarticular, 197
  pulmonary, 198
  treatment of, 201–205
Carbapenem-resistant Enterobacteriaceae, 99–101, 100t
  infection, 84
Carbapenem-resistant *Klebsiella pneumoniae,* 84
Carbapenem-resistant *Pseudomonas aeruginosa,* 101
Caspofungin, for *Pneumocystis* pneumonia, 245
Cat-scratch disease (CSD), 103
CD. *see* Chagas disease
CDC. *see* Centers for Disease Control and Prevention
CDI. *see Clostridium difficile* infection
Cell-mediated immune response, histoplasmosis and, 215
Cell-mediated rejection, after solid organ transplant, 4
Cellular treatment, for cytomegalovirus, 123–124, 124f
Cellular-based immunotherapy, 32
Centers for Disease Control and Prevention (CDC), 82
  surveillance studies, 91
Central line associated bloodstream infections (CLABSIs), 82–83
Central nervous system candidiasis, 198
Central nervous system tumors, 23–24t, 28
Central venous catheter (CVC)-associated *Nocardia,* 234
Central venous catheters, presence of, 88
Cerebral aspergillosis, 172
Cerebrospinal fluid (CSF) exam, for cryptococcosis, 208
Chagas disease (CD), 250–251, 251t
Chemoprophylaxis
  for Epstein-Barr virus, 128
  for *T. gondii* infection, 229–230t, 229–230
Chemotherapy
  for PTLD treatment, 132
  safe living after, 90
    animal contact and pet safety, 94–95
    food safety, 93
    prevention of infections by direct contact, 90
    recreational activities including travel, 95–96
    returning to school, 95
    water safety/exposure to *Cryptosporidium,* 91–93
  vaccination issues for, 63
Chemotherapy-induced mucositis, 75
Chest radiograph, for *Nocardia,* 235
CHG. *see* Chlorhexidine gluconate
Chickenpox, pretransplantation vaccination for, 64
Children
  with histoplasmosis, 214
  microbiome to, 72, 73f
  Nocardia in, 233
Chlorhexidine gluconate (CHG), 85
Chromoblastomycosis, 192
Chronic lymphocytic leukemia, cryptococcosis with, 207
Chronic myeloid leukemia (CML), 23–24t, 27
Chronic norovirus diarrhea, 253–254
Chronic rejection, after solid organ transplant, 4–5
Cidofovir
  for adenoviruses, 159–160
  for cytomegalovirus, 121t
Ciprofloxacin, for *Bartonella,* 105
CLABSIs. *see* Central line associated bloodstream infections
Clindamycin, for *Mycoplasma,* 108
Clostridioides difficile infection, 258
  clinical manifestations of, 259–260
  clinical outcomes of, 260
  clinicopathologic correlation, 259
  colonization, 258
  definition of, 258
  diagnosis of, 260–261
  epidemiology of, 258–259
  in pediatric HSCT recipients, 259
  in pediatric oncologic patients, 259
  in pediatric SOT recipients, 258–259
  primary and secondary prevention for, 261–262
  recurrence of, 260
  risk factors of, 258–259
  severe, 260
  toxin detection in, 259
  treatment for, 259t, 261–262
Clostridium difficile, 84
Clostridium difficile colitis, 71
Clostridium difficile infection (CDI), 78
CML. *see* Chronic myeloid leukemia
CMV. *see* Cytomegalovirus
CNS nocardiosis, 234
Coccidioidomycosis, 223–226
  clinical manifestations of, 224
  diagnosis of, 224–225
  disease prophylaxis and prevention of, 226
  epidemiology and risk factors of, 224
  treatment of, 225–226, 225t
Colonization resistance, 71
  mechanism of, 72f
Combination antifungal therapy, for mucormycosis, 187
Commensal microbes, 71, 75
Complex microbial communities, 71
Computed tomography (CT)
  chest imaging, for *T. gondii* infection, 228–229
  for histoplasmosis, 217
  for *Nocardia,* 235
Computed tomography (CT)-guided lung biopsy, for mucormycosis, 184–185
Conventional chemotherapeutic agents, 29–30, 31t
Corticosteroids
  for histoplasmosis, 221
  for induction therapy, 6–7
  in oncology, aspergillosis and, 171
Cough, legionellosis and, 105
Crusted verrucous lesions, with blastomycosis, 221–222, 222f
Cryptococcal meningoencephalitis, 207, 207f
Cryptococcal pneumonia, 208f
Cryptococcal polymerase chain reaction (PCR) assays, for cryptococcosis, 208–209
Cryptococcosis, 206–210
  clinical manifestations of, 207–208
  diagnosis of, 208–209
  disease prophylaxis/prevention of, 209
  epidemiology and risk factors of, 206
  pulmonary, 207–208, 208f
  skin involvement in, 208
  treatment of, 209
Cryptococcus, polysaccharide capsule of, 206
Cryptococcus gattii, 206
Cryptococcus neoformans, 206

Cryptococcus neoformans-Cryptococcus gattii complex, 206
Cryptococcus-associated IRIS, 209
Cryptosporidium hominis, 91–92, 249
Cryptosporidium infection, water safety/ exposure to, 91–93
Cryptosporidium parvum, 91–92, 249
Cryptosporidium species, 248–250
clinical manifestations of, 249
diagnosis of, 249
disease prophylaxis and prevention of, 249
epidemiology and risk factors of, 248–249
fecal-to-oral transmission of, 249
infection prevention and anticipatory guidance for, 250
treatment of, 249–250
CSD. *see* Cat-scratch disease
CTLA-4. *see* Cytotoxic T-lymphocyte antigen-4
Culture
for aspergillosis, 173
for candidiasis, 200
for histoplasmosis, 217–218
of *Nocardia* species, 235
Cutaneous aspergillosis, 172
Cutaneous mucormycosis, 182
Cutaneous nocardiosis, 234
Cystitis
CMV, 120t
hemorrhagic, polyomavirus and, 166
Cytomegalovirus (CMV), 4, 40, 118
antiviral resistance of, 123
clinical manifestations of, 119
diagnosis of, 122–123
disease, definitions of, 120t
disease prophylaxis and prevention for, 120–122, 121t
emerging prevention therapies and strategies, 121–122
HSCT-specific strategies, 121
oncology-specific strategies, 121
solid organ transplant-specific strategies, 120, 121t
epidemiology and risk factors for, 118–119, 119t
infection prevention and anticipatory guidance for, 124–125
primary, 119
specific immunity, 123
testing modalities, 122t
treatment for, 123–124
Cytomegalovirus infection, posttransplant lymphoproliferative disorders, 126
Cytomegalovirus status, HSCT and, 17–18
Cytotoxic T-lymphocyte antigen-4 (CTLA-4), 8

D

Dapsone, for *Pneumocystis* pneumonia, 243
Deep surgical site infections, 2
Deficient immune mechanisms, children with, 82
Dematiaceous molds, 191–192
Dermatitis, candidiasis and, 196
β-D-glucan (BDG), 201
Diagnostic stewardship, 79
Diarrhea
Clostridioides difficile infection and, 259
legionellosis and, 105
Diarrheal disease, 253
Diphtheria toxoid vaccine, for hematopoietic stem cell transplantation, 68
Disease Transmission Advisory Committee (DTAC), 41
Disseminated disease, herpes simplex virus and, 135
Disseminated histoplasmosis, 216
Disseminated mucormycosis, 182
Donor age, HSCT and, 17
Donor evaluation, of hematopoietic stem cell transplantation, 47–49, 47b
active infections in, 48
donation, special considerations and contraindications to, 48–49, 49b
history in, 47
imaging in, 49
pathogen-specific testing in, 47–48, 48t
Donor Patient Safety Monitoring Advisory Group (DPSM), 41
Donor screening, 40
regulatory oversite of, 41–43, 42–43t
Donor-derived infections, 40, 88
ad hoc disease transmission advisory committee, lessons from, 43–44
anticipated, 40–41
in HSCT and SOT recipients, lessons from, 43
importance of recognizing, 44
reporting of, 41–43, 42–43t
before transplant, educating candidates about, 44
unanticipated, 40–41
Down syndrome (DS), 27
Doxycycline, for *Bartonella,* 105
DPSM. *see* Donor Patient Safety Monitoring Advisory Group
Drinking water, 92t
DS. *see* Down syndrome
DTAC. *see* Disease Transmission Advisory Committee

E

Early postengraftment period, after HSCT, 11
EBV. *see* Epstein-Barr virus
Echinocandins
for blastomycosis, 223
for candidiasis, 198
for histoplasmosis, 221
Eculizumab, 8–9
Elevated aspartate aminotransferase/ alanine aminotransferase ratio, for histoplasmosis, 217
ELISA. *see* Enzyme-linked immunosorbent assay
Empiric antibacterial therapy
cessation of, 60–61
for IFD, 61
modification of, 60
Encephalitis, CMV, 120t
Endemic mycoses, epidemiology of, 214
End-of-Life care, 80
Endogenous endophthalmitis, 198
Endovascular candidiasis, 197
Enzyme immunoassays
for astrovirus, 256
for rotavirus, 255
Enzyme-linked immunosorbent assay (ELISA), for aspergillosis, 175
Eosinophilia, strongyloidiasis in, 247
Epstein-Barr virus (EBV), 4, 40–41, 126
in cancer, 127
clinical manifestations of, 127, 127t
diagnosis of, 129–130, 129f, 130t
Epstein-Barr virus *(Continued)*
epidemiology and risk factors for, 126–127
in hematopoietic stem cell transplantation, 126–127
immunoprophylaxis for, 128–129
prevention of, 128
in solid organ transplant recipient, 126
viral load monitoring and preemptive prevention strategies for, 128–129
Ertapenem, for nocardiosis, 238
Esophagitis, herpes simplex virus and, 135
Extended-spectrum β–lactamase-producing enterobacteriaceae, 99

F

Fastidious gram-negative bacillus, *Legionella* and, 105
Fecal microbiome transplantation (FMT), 74–75
Felidae family, 227
Fever, histoplasmosis with, 216
Fever and neutropenia (FN), 56
high-risk, 59–60
low-risk, 60
FK778 (manitimus), 9
Fluconazole
for candidiasis, 201
for histoplasmosis, 221
Flucytosine
for cryptococcosis, 209
for *Saccharomyces* species infections, 213
Fluoroquinolone prophylaxis, 78
Fluoroquinolones
for *Legionella,* 106
for polyomavirus, 169
FMT. *see* Fecal microbiome transplantation
FN. *see* Fever and neutropenia
Focal disease, definitive therapy for, 203–205, 204–205t, 204t
Food safety, after transplantation and chemotherapy, 93
Foscarnet
for cytomegalovirus, 121t
for HHV-6, 147t
FTY720 (fingolimod), 9
Fungal biomarkers, for candidiasis, 201
Fungal dissemination, 216
Fungal pathogens, 57
Fungemia, 209–210, 210f, 212
Fungitell BGD assay, for candidiasis, 201
Fusariosis, 188–191
adjunctive therapy of, 191
clinical manifestations of, 189, 190f
diagnosis of, 190
disease prophylaxis for, 190
epidemiology and risk factors of, 188–189
infection prevention and anticipatory guidance for, 191
prognosis and modifying factors of, 189
surgical management of, 191
treatment of, 191
Fusarium, 188

G

Galactomannan antigen, 175–176
Ganciclovir
for adenoviruses, 161
for cytomegalovirus, 121t
for HHV-6, 147t

Gastroenteritis, caused by rotavirus, 255
Gastrointestinal disease, CMV, 120t
Gastrointestinal viruses, 253
G-CSF. *see* Granulocyte colony-stimulating factor
Genitourinary candidiasis, 197
Geotrichum spp. infections, 213
Gingivostomatitis, herpes simplex virus and, 134–135
(1, 3)-β-D-Glucan
for aspergillosis, 176
for histoplasmosis, 219
Gomori methenamine silver stain, for histoplasmosis, 217
Good bathing practices: showers and wipes, 85
Graft failure, blastomycosis in, 221
Graft-versus-host disease (GVHD), 18–19, 73–74, 73f
acute, 10
on immune reconstitution, 18–19
prophylaxis, 18
Graft-versus-leukemia effect, 19
Gram-negative infections
common mechanism of, 97
multidrug-resistant, in transplant and oncology patients, 97
anticipatory guidance, 102
clinical manifestations of, 98–102
diagnosis of, 99, 100f
epidemiology of, 97–98
infection prevention of, 102
risk factors of, 97–98
treatment of, 99–101
Granulocyte colony-stimulating factor (G-CSF), 56
Granulomas, histoplasmosis and, 215
Gut bacteria, taxonomic classification of, 72t
GVHD. *see* Graft-versus-host disease

H

HAIs. *see* Health care-associated infections
Handwashing, for norovirus, 254
HAV. *see* Hepatitis A virus
Health care epidemiologist, close collaboration with, 82
Health care worker attire, care of linens and, 87
Health care-associated infections (HAIs), 82
importance of, 82–83
Health care-associated mold infection, surveillance for, 86–87
Heart transplant recipients, 97–98
T. gondii infection in, 229–230
Heart transplantation, deep space infection after, 2
Hematologic malignancies, 26–28
acute lymphoblastic leukemia, 26–27
acute myelogenous leukemia, 27
chronic myeloid leukemia, 27
down syndrome, 27
fusariosis with, 189
infant leukemia, 27
lymphoma, 27–28
mucormycosis with, 181
nocardiosis in, 234
in *Pneumocystis* pneumonia, 241
Hematopoietic cell transplant (HCT) recipients, respiratory viruses in
clinical manifestations of, 149–150
diagnosis of, 151
disease prophylaxis/prevention for, 150
Hematopoietic cell transplant (HCT) recipients *(Continued)*
epidemiology and risk factors for, 148
infection prevention in, 154
treatment for, 151–153, 152t, 153t
Hematopoietic cell transplantation
adenoviruses and, 156, 157
polyomavirus and, 165
Hematopoietic stem cell transplant (HSCT)
actinomycosis in, 239
aspergillosis in, 170–171
candidiasis in, 195, 198
fusariosis and scedosporiasis in, 189
human herpesvirus and, 143
infectious disease evaluation of infants and children awaiting, 34
additional screening measures for, 37–38, 37b
approach to, 36–37
extremes of age, considerations for, 38–39
future directions of, 38–39
herpesvirus screening in, 36, 36t
HIV and hepatitis screening in, 35–36
immunization, pretransplant, 38
pretransplant, principles of, 34–38
tuberculosis screening in, 37
invasive mold diseases in, 192
mucormycosis in, 181, 183t
nocardiosis in, 234
patients, oncology and, 99
in *Pneumocystis* pneumonia, 241
recipients, 97
donor-derived infections in, 43
T. gondii infection in, 228–229, 228t
Hematopoietic stem cell transplant (HSCT) recipient, pediatric, immunologic recovery and basis for infections in, 10, 11f
adaptive cellular immune recovery after, 13–14
adaptive humoral immune recovery after, 14
alloreactivity, factors affecting, 15–19
autoreactivity, factors affecting, 15–19
fixed time periods after, infection risk by, 10–12
early postengraftment, 11
late postengraftment, 11–12
pre-engraftment, 10
prophylaxis relative to, 12
immune reconstitution after
assessment of, 19–20
autologous for, 14–15
factors affecting, 15–19
improving, 20, 20t
timing of, 12–14, 13t
pretransplant conditioning, 16–17
recipient- and donor-specific factors, 17–18
cytomegalovirus status, 17–18
donor age, 17
graft-versus-host disease, 18–19
recipient age, 17
sex and parity, 17
Hematopoietic stem cell transplantation (HSCT), 68–70, 72
cytomegalovirus and, 121
Epstein-Barr virus in, 126–127
graft-versus-host disease, 73–74, 73f
in immunocompromised pediatric populations, 88
infections, 74
Hematopoietic stem cell transplantation *(Continued)*
microbiome and, 73–75
PTLD therapy in, 133
therapeutics, 74–75
Hematopoietic stem cell transplantation (HSCT) recipient, prevention of infections in, 46
bacterial, 49–50
invasive fungal disease, 50
other infections, 52–53
Pneumocystis jirovecii pneumonia, 52
Strongyloides Stercoralis, 53
Toxoplasma Gondii, 53
tuberculosis, 52–53
pretransplant evaluation of, 46–49, 47b
donor, 47–49
recipient, 46–47
vaccination for, 49
viral, 50–52
Hematopoietic stem cells (HSCs), 14
autologous, 14–15
Hemophagocytic lymphohistiocytosis (HLH), 142
Hemorrhagic cystitis, polyomavirus and, 166
diagnosis of, 168–169, 168t
Hepatitis, CMV, 120t
Hepatitis A vaccines
for oncology patients, 67
for solid organ transplantation, 66
Hepatitis A virus (HAV), 93
Hepatitis B vaccines
for oncology patients, 67
for solid organ transplantation, 65–66
Hepatitis screening, in infectious disease evaluation, 35–36
Hepatoblastoma, 29
Hepatosplenic (chronic disseminated) candidiasis, 197
Hepatosplenomegaly, histoplasmosis and, 215
Herpes simplex virus (HSV), 4, 134
active or passive immunization for, 138
clinical manifestations of, 134–135
diagnosis of, 135
epidemiology and risk factors of, 134
future directions for, 141
infection prevention for, 137–138
in oncology, 134–138
suppressive therapy for, 135–137
in transplant, 134–138
treatment of, 136–137, 137t
Herpesvirus screening, in infectious disease evaluation, 36, 36t
Herpesviruses, 118
Heterologous immunity, with CMV, 118
High-resolution computed tomography, for *Pneumocystis* pneumonia, 241
High-risk neuroblastoma, 23–24t
Histoplasma capsulatum, 214–215
Histoplasmosis, 214–221
antigen detection of, 218–219
clinical manifestations of, 215
culture for, 217–218
diagnosis of, 217
disease prophylaxis and prevention of, 221
disseminated, 216
epidemiology and risk factors of, 214–215
histopathology of, 217, 217f
medical imaging for, 217, 217f
molecular testing for, 219
mother-infant transmission with, 215

Histoplasmosis *(Continued)*
in oncology patients, 216
other assays for, 219
progressive disseminated, 216
serology for, 218
in transplant patients, 216–217
treatment of, 219–220t, 219–221
Histoplasmosis-induced hemophagocytic syndrome, 216
HIV screening, in infectious disease evaluation, 35–36
HL. *see* Hodgkin lymphoma
HLA. *see* Human leukocyte antigen
HLA matching, HSCT and, 15–16
HLH. *see* Hemophagocytic lymphohistiocytosis
Hodgkin lymphoma (HL), 23–24t, 27–28
Hospital infection prevention, for pediatric transplant recipients and oncology patients, 82
good practice recommendations, 85–88
air quality, 86
animal safety, 85
care of linens and health care worker attire, 87
cleaning and disinfecting environmental surfaces within hospital units, 87–88
construction and renovation, 86–87
environmental impact on medical care of immunocompromised patients, 86
food safety, 86
furnishings, 87
good bathing practices: showers and wipes, 85
mask use in patients during ambulation/transportation within hospitals, 86
plants, 87
policies for ill providers, 85
toys, 86
vaccinations of health care workers and close contacts, 85
visitation policies, 85
water damage, 87
water quality, 87
infection prevention practices in specific immunocompromised pediatric populations, 88–89
pathogen-specific infection prevention strategies, 83–85, 83t
HSCs. *see* Hematopoietic stem cells
HSCT. *see* Hematopoietic stem cell transplant
HSV. *see* Herpes simplex virus
Human astrovirus infections, 256
Human herpesvirus, 142
anticipatory guidance for, 146
clinical manifestations of, 143–144
diagnosis of, 144–145, 145f, 146f, 147f
disease prophylaxis/prevention for, 144
epidemiology and risk factors of, 142–143
infection prevention for, 146
in oncology, 144
solid organ transplant and, 143–144
treatment for, 145–146, 147t
Human herpesvirus 6
clinical manifestations of, 143–144
diagnosis of, 144, 145f, 146f
epidemiology and risk factors for, 142–143
in hematopoietic stem cell transplant, 143
in solid organ transplant, 143
treatment for, 145
Human herpesvirus 7
diagnosis of, 144
epidemiology and risk factors for, 143
in hematopoietic stem cell transplant, 143
in solid organ transplant, 144
treatment for, 145
Human herpesvirus 8
diagnosis of, 144–145, 147f
epidemiology and risk factors for, 143
in hematopoietic stem cell transplant, 143
in solid organ transplant, 144
treatment for, 146, 147t
Human immunodeficiency virus (HIV), in *Pneumocystis* pneumonia, 241
Human leukocyte antigen (HLA), 3
Human papilloma virus, for hematopoietic stem cell transplantation, 68
Human papillomavirus vaccines
for oncology patients, 67
for solid organ transplantation, 66
Human polyomaviruses (HPyVs), 162, 163t
Human trypanosomiasis, 250
Hyperacute rejection, after solid organ transplant, 4
Hyperbaric oxygen therapy, for mucormycosis, 188
Hyperinfection, strongyloidiasis in, 247

I

Ibrutinib, cryptococcosis associated with, 207
IC. *see* Invasive candidiasis
IFDs. *see* Invasive fungal diseases
Ill providers, policies for, 85
Imaging, of *Pneumocystis* pneumonia, 241
IMDs. *see* Invasive mold diseases
Immune bovine colostrum, for *Cryptosporidium* species, 250
Immune reconstitution, after HSCT
assessment of, 19–20
autologous for, 14–15
factors affecting, 15–19
improving, 20, 20t
timing of, 12–14, 13t
Immune reconstitution inflammatory syndrome (IRIS), 209
Immune recovery, after HSCT
adaptive cellular, 13–14
adaptive humoral, 14
Immune system
components of, 2–4, 3f
evolution of, 3–4, 5f
Immunity, CMV-specific, cellular assays for, 123
Immunization
in immunocompromised hosts, 63
pretransplant, 38
Immunocompetent children, *Mycoplasma* spp. infections and, 107
Immunocompromised children
CMV in, 125
microbiome on, 73f
rotavirus in, 255
Immunocompromised hosts
antimicrobial stewardship in, 78
barriers to antimicrobial stewardship programs in, 79–80
donors and contacts of, 63–64
goals of stewardship in, 78–79
osteoarticular candidiasis in, 197
strategies and tactics for stewardship in, 80
Immunocompromised patients, environmental impact on medical care of, 86
Immunocompromised pediatric populations, specific, infection prevention practices in, 88–89
Immunodiffusion (ID) test, for histoplasmosis, 218
Immunologic disorders, children with, 82
Immunoprophylaxis, for Epstein-Barr virus, 128–129
Immunosuppressed host, histoplasmosis in, 217
Immunosuppression, reduction of, in PTLD treatment, 130–131
Immunosuppressive medications, for solid organ transplant
induction therapies, 6–7
maintenance therapies, 7–8
standard approach to, 8
rejection therapies, 8–9
standard approach to, 9
Immunosuppressive regimens, cryptococcosis associated with, 207
Immunosuppressive therapy, children with, 82
Immunotherapy
adaptive, for PTLD treatment, 132
for adenoviruses, 161
for pediatric cancers, 30–32
Impaired oxygenation, in *P. jirovecii* pneumonia, 241
Inactivated vaccines
for oncology patients, 67
for solid organ transplantation, 64, 65t
Increased intracranial pressure (ICP)
in cryptococcal meningoencephalitis, 207
management of, 209
Infant leukemia, 27
Infants, rotavirus vaccination of, 64
Infection prevention, hospital, for pediatric transplant recipients and oncology patients, 82
Infections
Clostridioides difficile, 258
clinical manifestations of, 259–260
clinical outcomes of, 260
clinicopathologic correlation, 259
colonization, 258
definition of, 258
diagnosis of, 260–261
epidemiology of, 258–259
in pediatric HSCT recipients, 259
in pediatric oncologic patients, 259
in pediatric SOT recipients, 258–259
primary and secondary prevention for, 261–262
recurrence of, 260
risk factors of, 258–259
severe, 260
toxin detection in, 259
treatment for, 259t, 261–262
diagnostic uncertainty of, 79
by direct contact, prevention of, 90
donor-derived, 40
ad hoc disease transmission advisory committee, lessons from, 43–44
anticipated, 40–41
in HSCT and SOT recipients, lessons from, 43
importance of recognizing, 44
reporting of, 41–43, 42–43t
before transplant, educating candidates about, 44
unanticipated, 40–41

Infections *(Continued)*
hematopoietic stem cell transplantation and, 74
organisms transmitted from animals, 94t
paucity of evidence for prevention and management of, 79
polymicrobial or multiple, concerns for, 79
prevention of, in solid organ transplantation recipient, 54
perioperative antimicrobial prophylaxis for, 54–55
posttransplant prophylaxis and monitoring of, 55
pretransplant evaluation of, 54
vaccination for, 54
respiratory, prevention of, 90–91
risk by fixed time periods after transplantation, 10–12
early postengraftment, 11
late postengraftment, 11–12
pre-engraftment, 10
prophylaxis relative to, 12
Infectious disease evaluation, of infants and children awaiting solid organ or hematopoietic stem cell transplant, 34
additional screening measures for, 37–38, 37b
approach to, 36–37
candidate, screening of, 35, 35b
extremes of age, considerations for, 38–39
future directions of, 38–39
herpesvirus screening in, 36, 36t
HIV and hepatitis screening in, 35–36
pretransplant
immunization, 38
principles of, 34–38
tuberculosis screening in, 37
Influenza
antiviral treatment for, 152–153
vaccination, for hematopoietic stem cell transplantation, 68
vaccines
for oncology patients, 67
for solid organ transplantation, 65
Innate immune recovery, after HSCT, 12–13
Intervention without disease transmission (IWDT), 43–44
Intestinal parasites, 251–252
Intestinal transplant recipients, 98
Intraabdominal candidiasis, 197
Intravenous immunoglobulin (IVIG), 4
window of time between, 63
Invasive aspergillosis
antifungal therapy for
adjunctive, 180
alternative, 179
combination, 180
primary, 177–179
salvage, 179–180
pulmonary, 172
sinusitis, 172
Invasive *Aspergillus* sinusitis, 172
primary antifungal therapy for, 177–179
Invasive candidiasis (IC), 197–198
Invasive fungal diseases (IFDs), 57, 61
empiric antifungal therapy for, 61
evaluation of, 61
prevention of, 50
active infections, 50
exposure, 50
Invasive fungal infections, 88
Invasive mold diseases (IMDs), 191–194
adjunctive therapy of, 194
clinical manifestations of, 192, 193t
diagnosis of, 192
disease prophylaxis for, 192
epidemiology and risk factors of, 192
infection prevention and anticipatory guidance for, 194
surgical management and other source control measures of, 194
treatment of, 192–194
Invasive pulmonary aspergillosis, 172
Invasive trichosporonosis, 211
Invasive yeast infections, 209–210, 210f, 210t, 211t
Irinotecan-induced mucositis, 75
IRIS. *see* Immune reconstitution inflammatory syndrome
Isavuconazole
for histoplasmosis, 221
for mucormycosis, 186–187
Isolation precautions, for nonrespiratory viruses, 85
Itraconazole, for histoplasmosis, 220
Ivermectin, for strongyloidiasis, 248, 248t
IVIG. *see* Intravenous immunoglobulin
IWDT. *see* Intervention without disease transmission

K

Kaposi sarcoma (KS)-associated herpesvirus, 142
Kidney transplantation (KTx)
deep space infection after, 2
histoplasmosis in, 216
polyomavirus and, 163–165, 164f
strongyloidiasis in, 247

L

Lactobacillus rhamnosus GG, 74
Late postengraftment period, after HSCT, 11–12
Lavage, bronchoalveolar, for aspergillosis, 175–176
LD. *see* Legionnaires' disease
Legionella, 83, 105–106
anticipatory guidance for children with, 106
clinical manifestations of, 105
diagnosis of, 106
disease prophylaxis/prevention of, 105
epidemiology of, 105
infection prevention for children with, 106
risk factors of, 105
treatment of, 106
Legionellosis, 105
Legionnaires' disease (LD), 105
Letermovir, for cytomegalovirus, 121t
Leukemia, 23–24t, 26
acute lymphoblastic, 22, 23–24t, 26–27
acute myelogenous, 23–24t, 27
chronic myeloid, 23–24t, 27
infant, 27
Linezolid, for nocardiosis, 238
Liposomal amphotericin B
for blastomycosis, 223
for histoplasmosis, 220
Live attenuated vaccines
influenza, 63–64
for solid organ transplantation, 66
Live vaccines
for hematopoietic stem cell transplantation, 68–69
for oncology patients, 67–68
Liver, transplant recipients, 98
Liver transplantation, deep space infection after, 2
Lomentospora, 189
Low-osmolarity oral rehydration solution, for norovirus, 254
Lung, transplant recipients, 97–98
Lung transplantation, deep space infection after, 2
Lymphadenopathy, 103–104
Lymphoma, 23–24t, 27–28
cryptococcosis with, 207

M

Magnetic resonance imaging
for blastomycosis, 221–222
for cerebral aspergillosis, 175
Major histocompatibility complex (MHC), 2–3
Malignancies, cryptococcosis in, 207
Mamastrovirus, 255
Mammalian target of rapamycin (mTOR) inhibitor, 8
Matrix-assisted laser desorption/ionization time-of-flight mass spectrometry (MALDI-TOF), for cryptococcosis, 208
MDROs. *see* Multidrug-resistant organisms
Measles-mumps-rubella vaccines, for solid organ transplantation, 66
Medical imaging, for histoplasmosis, 217, 217f
Meningococcal vaccines
for hematopoietic stem cell transplantation, 68
for solid organ transplantation, 66
Meningoencephalitis, cryptococcal, 207, 207f
Meropenem-vaborbactam, for carbapenem-resistant enterobacteriaceae, 101
Methicillin-resistant *S. aureus* (MRSA), 83
Metronidazole, for intestinal parasites, 252
MHC. *see* Major histocompatibility complex
Miami Transplant Institute, 247–248
Microbiome implications
effects of, 73f
hematopoietic stem cell transplantation and, 73–75
graft-versus-host disease, 73–74, 73f
infections, 74
therapeutics, 74–75
knowledge limitation of, 76–77
oncology and, 75–76
solid organ transplantation and, 76
Microbiome therapeutics, 76
Monocytes, 12
Morbidity, with varicella-zoster virus, 138
Mortality, with varicella-zoster virus, 138
Mouse polyomavirus (PyV), 162
MRSA. *see* Methicillin-resistant *S. aureus*
Mucormycosis, 181–188
adjunctive and emerging diagnostic tests of, 185
clinical manifestations of, 182, 183t
diagnosis of, 184–185, 184f
diagnostic sampling of, 184–185
disease prophylaxis for, 182–184
epidemiology and risk factors of, 181–182
genera of organisms causing, 182b
increasing incidence and breakthrough infections in, 181, 182t

Mucormycosis *(Continued)*
  infection prevention and anticipatory guidance for, 188
  other forms of, 182
  primary diagnostic tests of, 185
  prognosis and modifying factors of, 181–182
  reversal of predisposing conditions and adjunctive therapy of, 188
  step-down therapy and duration of, 188
  surgical management of, 188
  treatment of, 185–188, 186f
Mucosal barrier integrity, 75
Mucosal infections, candidiasis and, 196–197
Multidrug-resistant gram-negative infections
  clinical manifestations of, 98–102
  in transplant and oncology patients, 97
    anticipatory guidance, 102
    diagnosis of, 99, 100f
    epidemiology of, 97–98
    infection prevention of, 102
    risk factors of, 97–98
    treatment of, 99–101
Multidrug-resistant gram-negative organisms, 84
Multidrug-resistant organisms (MDROs), 55
Multiple infections, concerns for, 79
Multiplex PCR assays, for rotavirus, 255
Multivisceral and intestinal transplantation, deep space infection after, 2
Mycobacteria, 84
Mycobacterium infection
  nontuberculous, 109, 114–117
    clinical manifestations of, 115
    diagnosis of, 115–116, 116f
    disease prophylaxis for, 117
    epidemiology of, 114–115
    pathogenesis of, 114–115, 115t
    prevention of, 117
    risk factors of, 114–115
    treatment of, 116–117, 117f
  tuberculous, 109–117
    clinical manifestations of, 110
    diagnosis of, 110–112, 111f
    epidemiology of, 109–110
    pathogenesis of, 109–110
    prevention of, 113–114
    risk factors of, 109–110
    screening practices of, 113–114, 114f
    treatment of, 112
Mycophenolate mofetil (MMF or CellCept), 8
Mycoplasma, 106–108
  anticipatory guidance for children with, 108
  clinical manifestations of, 107
  diagnosis of, 107–108
  disease prophylaxis/prevention of, 107
  epidemiology of, 106–107
  infection prevention for children with, 108
  risk factors of, 106–107
  treatment of, 108
Myocarditis, CMV, 120t

N

National Cord Blood Inventory (NCBI), 41
National Healthcare Safety Network (NHSN), 82
Natural killer (NK) cells, 12, 13
Natural product, for pediatric cancer, 25–26t, 30
NCBI. *see* National Cord Blood Inventory
Necrotizing wound infections, 1–2
Nephritis, CMV, 120t
Nephropathy, polyomavirus and, 166
  diagnosis of, 167–168
Neuroblastoma, 28
Neutropenia
  candidiasis and, 200
  prolonged, *Geotrichum* spp. infections and, 213
Neutropenic patients, management principles of, 56
  bacterial infections, 59–61
    empiric antibacterial therapy for, 60
    with high-risk fever and neutropenia, 59–60
    initial antibiotic therapy for, 59
    with low-risk fever and neutropenia, 60
  epidemiology of, 56–58
    bacterial pathogens, 56–57, 57t
    fungal pathogens, 57
    viral pathogens, 57–58, 58t
  evaluation of, 58–59
    initial investigations, 58–59
    initial risk stratification, 58
  invasive fungal disease, 61
    empiric antifungal therapy for, 61
    evaluation of, 61
  prophylactic strategies for, 61–62
    antibacterial prophylaxis, 61–62
    antifungal Prophylaxis, 62
NHSN. *see* National Healthcare Safety Network
Nifurtimox, for Chagas disease, 251
Nitazoxanide
  for adenoviruses, 161
  for *Cryptosporidium* species, 249
  for norovirus, 254
  for rotavirus, 255
  for sapovirus, 257
Nocard, Edmond, 233
Nocardia, 233–238
  clinical presentation of, 234
  diagnosis of, 235, 236f
  epidemiology and risk factors of, 233
  infection prevention and anticipatory guidance for, 238
  microbiology of, 233
  prevention and prophylaxis for, 234–235
Nocardia asteroides complex, 233
Nocardiosis
  CNS, 234
  cutaneous, 234
  extrapulmonary, 234
  in hematologic malignancy and stem cell transplant, 234
  pulmonary, 234
  soft tissue, 234
  in solid organ transplant recipients, 233–234
  treatment of, 235–238, 237f, 237t
Non-Hodgkin lymphoma, 23–24t, 28
Nonrenal solid organ transplantation, polyomavirus and, 165
Nonrespiratory viruses, 85
Nontuberculous mycobacteria, 84
Nontuberculous *Mycobacterium* infection, 109, 114–117
  clinical manifestations of, 115
  diagnosis of, 115–116, 116f
  disease prophylaxis for, 117
  epidemiology of, 114–115
  pathogenesis of, 114–115, 115t
  prevention of, 117
  risk factors of, 114–115
  treatment of, 116–117, 117f
Norovirus infection, 253–254
Novel chemotherapeutics, 30–33
Nucleic acid amplification tests (NAAT), for *Clostridioides difficile* infection, 261
Nucleic acid detection, for respiratory virus, 151

O

Ocular candidiasis, 198
Oncology
  aspergillosis in, 171
  candidiasis and, 196, 199
  cytomegalovirus and, 121
  fusariosis and scedosporiasis and, 189
  hematopoietic stem cell transplant patients and, 99
  herpes simplex virus in, 134–138
  histoplasmosis and, 216
  human herpesvirus and, 144
  in immunocompromised pediatric populations, 88–89
  invasive mold diseases and, 192
  microbiome and, 75–76
  mucormycosis and, 181
  patients, 98
  varicella-zoster virus in, 138–141
Oncology patients
  hospital infection prevention for, 82
  respiratory viruses in
    clinical manifestations of, 150
    diagnosis of, 151
    disease prophylaxis/prevention for, 150
    epidemiology and risk factors for, 148
    treatment for, 151–153, 152t, 153t
Ondansetron, for norovirus, 254
Opportunistic mold, 84
OPTN. *see* Organ Procurement and Transplantation Network
Oral human immunoglobulin, for *Cryptosporidium* species, 250
Oral nystatin, for oropharyngeal candidiasis, 202
Organ Procurement and Transplantation Network (OPTN), 41
Organs, laboratory screening of, 41, 42–43t
Oropharyngeal candidiasis (thrush), 196
Osteoarticular candidiasis, 197

P

P. jirovecii pneumonia (PJP), 241
Parainfluenza, antiviral treatment for, 153
Parainfluenza viruses (PIVs), 148
Parasitic infections, 247
Paromomycin, for *Cryptosporidium* species, 250
Passive immunization, for herpes simplex virus, 138
Passive immunoprophylaxis, for Epstein-Barr virus, 128
Pathogens, in neutropenic patients
  bacterial, 56–57, 57t
  fungal, 57
  viral, 57–58, 58t
Pathogen-specific infection prevention strategies, 83–85, 83t
  Clostridium difficile, 84
  Legionella, 83
  multidrug-resistant gram-negative organisms, 84
  mycobacteria, 84
  opportunistic mold, 84
  Staphylococcus aureus and vancomycin-resistant enterococci, 83–84
  viruses, 84–85
PCR. *see* Polymerase chain reaction

PCV13. *see* Protein-conjugate vaccine
PDDTEs. *see* Potential donor-derived transmission events
Pediatric actinomycosis, 239
Pediatric cancer patient, infectious risk in, 22
  anticancer therapies for, 29–33
    conventional chemotherapeutic agents, 29–30, 31t
    immunotherapy, 30–32
  assessment of, 22–26, 23–24t, 25–26t
  autologous stem cell transplant for, 30
  disease-specific, 26–29
    hematologic malignancies, 26–28
    solid tumors, 28–29
Pediatric HSCT recipients, *Clostridioides difficile* infection in, 259
Pediatric oncologic patients, *Clostridioides difficile* infection in, 259
Pediatric renal transplant patients, *Candida* infections in, 196
Pediatric SOT
  recipients, *Clostridioides difficile* infection in, 258–259
  viral infections in, 88
Pediatric-specific invasive aspergillosis, 171–172
Pediatric transplant recipients, hospital infection prevention for, 82
Pentamidine, for *Pneumocystis* pneumonia, 242, 245
Pentavalent human-bovine rotavirus reassortant vaccine, 255
Perioperative antimicrobial prophylaxis, for solid organ transplantation recipient, 54–55
Peripheral blood stem cells, 16
Personal hygiene, 85
Personal protective equipment (PPE), infection prevention strategies, 82
Pertussis vaccine
  for hematopoietic stem cell transplantation, 68
  for solid organ transplantation, 66
Pet care hygiene, 95
Pet care practices, 95
Pet consideration, 94–95
Pet safety, 94–95
Phaeohyphomycosis, 192
PIVs. *see* Parainfluenza viruses
PJP. *see P. jirovecii* pneumonia
Platinum analogs, 25–26t, 29
PML. *see* Progressive multifocal leukoencephalopathy
Pneumococcal vaccines
  for hematopoietic stem cell transplantation, 68
  for oncology patients, 67
  for solid organ transplantation, 64–65
Pneumococcus, vaccinations for, 67
Pneumocystis carinii, 241
Pneumocystis jirovecii, 241
  pneumonia, 52
Pneumocystis pneumonia, 241
  alternative agents for, 242–243
  clinical manifestations of, 241
  diagnosis of, 243
  disease prophylaxis and prevention of, 241–243, 242t
  duration of prophylaxis for, 243
  epidemiology and risk factors of, 241
  imaging of, 241
  infection prevention and anticipatory guidance for, 246
  treatment of, 243–246, 244f, 244t, 245f
Pneumonia
  CMV, 120t
  cryptococcosis and, 207–208, 208f
  Legionella and, 106
  Mycoplasma and *Ureaplasma* and, 107
  P. jirovecii, 241
  Pneumocystis, 241
    alternative agents for, 242–243
    clinical manifestations of, 241
    diagnosis of, 243
    disease prophylaxis and prevention of, 241–243, 242t
    duration of prophylaxis for, 243
    epidemiology and risk factors of, 241
    imaging of, 241
    infection prevention and anticipatory guidance for, 246
    treatment of, 243–246, 244f, 244t, 245f
  secondary to *Blastomyces dermatitidis,* 222f
Pneumothorax, in *P. jirovecii* pneumonia, 241
Poliovirus vaccine, for hematopoietic stem cell transplantation, 68
Polymerase chain reaction (PCR)
  for aspergillosis, 176
  for candidiasis, 200
  for norovirus, 254
  for *Pneumocystis* pneumonia, 243
  for rotavirus, 255
  for strongyloidiasis, 248
Polymerase chain reaction (PCR) assay, for *T. gondii* infection, 230–231
Polymerase chain reaction (PCR) methodology, for histoplasmosis, 219
Polymicrobial infections, concerns for, 79
Polymyxin antibiotics, for carbapenem-resistant enterobacteriaceae, 101
Polyomavirus, 162
  anticipatory guidance for, 169
  associated with disease in immunocompromised patients, 163t
  clinical manifestations of, 163t, 165–166
  diagnosis of, 167–169
  disease prophylaxis/prevention for, 167, 168f
  epidemiology and risk factors of, 162–165
  in general populations, 162–163
  hematopoietic cell transplantation and, 165
  hemorrhagic cystitis and, 166
  infection prevention for, 169
  kidney transplantation and, 163–165, 164f
  life cycle of, 162
  nephropathy and, 166
  nonrenal solid organ transplantation and, 165
  treatment of, 169
  viral structure of, 162
Polysaccharide vaccine (PPV23), 64
Posaconazole
  for fusariosis, 191
  for histoplasmosis, 221
  for mucormycosis, 187–188
Postbiotics, microbiome therapeutics and, 74
Posttransplant lymphoproliferative disorder (PTLD), 40–41
  exceptional clinical situations in, 133
  in HSCT, 133
  infection prevention and anticipatory guidance, 133
  prognostic indicators of, 133
  in solid organ transplant recipients, 130–132
Posttransplant lymphoproliferative disorder *(Continued)*
    local disease control, 131
    reduction of immunosuppression, 130–131
    systemic therapy, 132
  therapy for, 130–133, 131f, 132f
  of "true" lymphoma, 132–133
Posttransplantation screening, for polyomavirus, 167, 168f
Potential donor-derived transmission events (PDDTEs), 43–44
PPE. *see* Personal protective equipment
PPV23. *see* Polysaccharide vaccine
Prebiotics, microbiome therapeutics and, 74
Pre-engraftment period, after HSCT, 10
Pretransplant serology screening, for *T. gondii* infection, 229
Probiotics, microbiome therapeutics and, 74
"Progressive disseminated histoplasmosis," 216
Progressive multifocal leukoencephalopathy (PML), 162
Prophylaxis, disease, prevention and, 99
Protective immunity, *T. gondii* infection and, 227
Protective titer levels, 63
Protein-conjugate vaccine (PCV13), 64
Pseudomembranous colitis, 260
PTLD. *see* Posttransplant lymphoproliferative disorder
Pulmonary candidiasis, 198
Pulmonary cryptococcosis, 207–208, 208f
Pulmonary fungal disease, in pediatric lung transplant recipients, 196
Pulmonary imaging, for aspergillosis, 173–175
Pulmonary infection, herpes simplex virus and, 135
Pulmonary mucormycosis, 182, 183f
Pulmonary nocardiosis, 234
Pulsed-field gel electrophoresis, of organism, 92
Pyrimethamine, with sulfadiazine, for *T. gondii* infection, 231, 231t

Q

QOL. *see* Quality of life
Quality of life (QOL), 56

R

Radiology, for aspergillosis, 173–175
Recipient age, HSCT and, 17
Recipient evaluation, of hematopoietic stem cell transplantation, 46–47, 47b
  additional evaluations in, 47
  history in, 46
  imaging in, 47
  pathogen-specific testing in, 47, 48t
  physical examination in, 47
  transplant information, 46–47
Recreational water, 92t
Rejection, after solid organ transplant, 4–5
  acute, 4
  chronic, 4–5
  hyperacute, 4
  therapies, 8–9
Renal candidiasis, 197
Renal transplant recipients, 98
Respiratory infections, prevention of, 90–91
Respiratory syncytial virus, antiviral treatment for, 151–152, 152t
Respiratory tract, aspergillosis in, 172

Respiratory virus, 148
anticipatory guidance for, 154
clinical manifestations of, 148–150
diagnosis of, 151
disease prophylaxis/prevention for, 150–151
epidemiology and risk factors for, 148, 149f
infection prevention in, 154
influenza chemoprophylaxis in, 150
influenza prophylaxis in, 150
new therapeutics for, 153
nucleic acid detection for, 151
sample type and handling for, 151
treatment for, 151–153
vaccines in development for, 150
Retinitis, CMV, 120t
Reverse halo sign, in pulmonary mucormycosis, 182, 183f
Reverse transcription PCR, for sapovirus, 257
Rhinocerebral mucormycosis, 182
Rhodotorula species infections, 212
Ribavirin, for adenoviruses, 160–161
Ring-enhancing lesions, in *Nocardia,* 235, 236f
Rituximab (Rituxan), 8–9
Rotavirus, 254–255
vaccine, 255
for solid organ transplantation, 67

S

Saccharomyces species infections, 212–213
Safe living, after transplantation/chemotherapy, 90
animal contact and pet safety, 94–95
food safety, 93
prevention of infections by direct contact, 90
recreational activities including travel, 95–96
returning to school, 95
water safety/exposure to *Cryptosporidium,* 91–93
Salvage antifungal therapy, for mucormycosis, 187–188
Sapovirus, 256–257
Sapovirus gastroenteritis, 256–257
Sarcoma, 23–24t, 28–29
Scedosporiasis, 188–191
adjunctive therapy of, 191
clinical manifestations of, 190
diagnosis of, 190
disease prophylaxis for, 190
epidemiology and risk factors of, 188–189
infection prevention and anticipatory guidance for, 191
prognosis and modifying factors of, 189
surgical management of, 191
treatment of, 191
Scedosporium, 188
Serology, for histoplasmosis, 218
Serology assays, for *T. gondii* infection, 230–231
Serum (1, 3)-β-D-glucan, for *Pneumocystis* pneumonia, 243
Serum galactomannan testing, for aspergillosis, 175
Sex and parity, HSCT and, 17
Sexual activity, after transplantation and chemotherapy, 96
Sinus imaging, for aspergillosis, 175
Sinusitis, invasive *Aspergillus,* 172
Sirolimus, 8
Skin infections, nocardiosis in, 234
Skin injury, aspergillosis and, 172
Smoking, as risk factor for fusariosis, 189
Soft tissue infections, nocardiosis in, 234
Soft tissue nocardiosis, 234
Solid organ transplant (SOT)
adenoviruses and, 155–156, 156t, 157
aspergillosis in, 171
candidiasis in, 195–196, 198–199
cytomegalovirus and, 120
endemic mycoses in, 214
fusariosis and scedosporiasis in, 189
human herpesvirus and, 143–144
in immunocompromised pediatric populations, 88
infectious disease evaluation of infants and children awaiting, 34
additional screening measures for, 37–38, 37b
candidate, screening of, 35, 35b
extremes of age, considerations for, 38–39
future directions of, 38–39
herpesvirus screening in, 36, 36t
HIV and hepatitis screening in, 35–36
immunization, pretransplant, 38
pretransplant, principles of, 34–38
tuberculosis screening in, 37
invasive mold diseases in, 192
microbiome implications and, 76
mucormycosis in, 181
patients, 98–99
in *Pneumocystis* pneumonia, 241
polyomavirus and, 165
T. gondii infection in, 228t, 229
Solid organ transplant pediatric recipient, surgical and immunosuppressive basis for infections in, 1
considerations of, 1–2
deep surgical site infections, 2
superficial surgical site infections, 1–2
current outcomes of, 6
immune system
components of, 2–4, 3f
evolution of, 3–4, 5f
immunologic overview of, 2
immunosuppressive medications for, 6–9, 7t
induction therapies, 6–7
maintenance therapies, 7–8
rejection therapies, 8–9
rejection after, 4–5
acute, 4
chronic, 4–5
hyperacute, 4
Solid organ transplant recipients
actinomycosis in, 239
Epstein-Barr virus in, 126
nocardiosis in, 233–234
prevention of infections in, 54
perioperative antimicrobial prophylaxis for, 54–55
posttransplant prophylaxis and monitoring of, 55
pretransplant evaluation of, 54
vaccination for, 54
respiratory viruses in
clinical manifestations of, 150
diagnosis of, 151
disease prophylaxis/prevention for, 150
epidemiology and risk factors for, 148
infection prevention in, 154
treatment for, 151–153, 152t, 153t
Solid tumors, 23–24t, 28–29
central nervous system tumors, 28
hepatoblastoma, 29
neuroblastoma, 28
sarcoma, 28–29
Wilms tumor, 29
SOT. *see* Solid organ transplant
SOT recipients, donor-derived infections in, 43
SPLIT. *see* Studies of Pediatric Liver Transplantation
Sporozoites, 227
Sports, after transplantation and chemotherapy, 95
Sputum culture, for aspergillosis, 173
Standardizing infection prevention practices, future areas of research in, 89
Staphylococcus aureus, 83–84
Stem cell transplant, nocardiosis in, 234
Stem cells
dose, 16
peripheral blood, 16
source, 16
Stewardship
goals of, in immunocompromised hosts, 78–79
metrics in transplant population, 80–81
strategies and tactics, for in immunocompromised hosts, 80
team, provider autonomy and, 79
Strongyloides rhabditiform, 247
Strongyloides stercoralis, 53, 247
Strongyloidiasis, 247–248
clinical manifestations of, 247
diagnosis of, 248, 248f
disease prophylaxis and prevention of, 247–248
epidemiology and risk factors of, 247
infection prevention and anticipatory guidance for, 248
treatment of, 248, 248t
Studies of Pediatric Liver Transplantation (SPLIT), 6
Sulfadiazine, pyrimethamine with, for *T. gondii* infection, 231, 231t
Superficial candidiasis, definitive therapy for, 202
Superficial surgical site infections, 1–2
Supportive treatment, for respiratory virus, 151
Suppressive therapy, for herpes simplex virus, 135–136, 136t
Surgery
for fusariosis and scedosporiasis, 191
for invasive mold diseases, 194
Surgical drainage, for actinomycosis, 239–240
Surgical site infections
deep, 2
superficial, 1–2
Symptomatic candiduria, 197
Symptomatic extrapulmonary disease, 214
Systemic therapy, for PTLD treatment, 132

T

T-cell mediated immunity, in adenoviruses, 161
T-cell-depleting biologic agents, 6
T cells, 2–3, 3f
T regulatory cells (Tregs), 14
T2Candida, 200–201
Tachyzoites, 227
TCR excision circles (TRECs), 14
TDM. *see* Therapeutic drug monitoring
Tedizolid, for nocardiosis, 238

Tetanus toxoid vaccine, for hematopoietic stem cell transplantation, 68
Therapeutic drug monitoring (TDM), for candidiasis, 205
Thoracic actinomycosis, 239
Thrush. *see* Oropharyngeal candidiasis
Tinidazole, for intestinal parasites, 252
Tissue cysts, in *Toxoplasma gondii*, 227
TMP/SMX. *see* Trimethoprim-sulfamethoxazole
Toxoplasma gondii, 53, 227
  transmission of, 227, 228f
Toxoplasma gondii infection, 227
  active, 53
  clinical manifestations of, 228–229, 228t
  diagnosis of, 230–231, 230t
  disease prophylaxis and prevention of, 229–230
    chemoprophylaxis, 229–230t, 229–230
    posttransplant monitoring, 229
    pretransplant monitoring, 229
  epidemiology and risk factors of, 227–229, 228t
  infection prevention and anticipatory guidance for, 231–1, 232t
  prevention, 53
  treatment of, 231, 231t
Transplant
  herpes simplex virus in, 134–138
  with histoplasmosis, 214
  varicella-zoster virus in, 138–141
Transplant population, stewardship metrics in, 80–81
Transplant recipients
  cryptococcosis in, 206–207
  T. gondii infection in, 227–228
Transplant-Associated Infection Surveillance Network (TRANSNET), 216, 221
  study, aspergillosis and, 170
Transplantation
  hematopoietic cell, polyomavirus and, 165
  kidney, polyomavirus and, 163–165, 164f
  microbiome implications in, 71
    effects of, 73f
    graft-versus-host disease, 73–74, 73f
    hematopoietic stem cell transplantation and, 73–75
    infections, 74
    knowledge limitation of, 76–77
    oncology and, 75–76
    solid organ transplantation and, 76
    therapeutics, 74–75
    in transplantation, 71
  nonrenal solid organ, polyomavirus and, 165
  safe living after, 90
    animal contact and pet safety, 94–95
    food safety, 93
    prevention of infections by direct contact, 90
    recreational activities including travel, 95–96
    returning to school, 95
    water safety/exposure to *Cryptosporidium*, 91–93
  vaccination issues for, 63
Travel, after transplantation and chemotherapy, 96
  water safety during, 92t
TRECs. *see* TCR excision circles
Triazole monotherapy, for mucormycosis, 186–187
Triazoles, for *Trichosporon* species infection, 212
Trichosporon species infection
  clinical manifestations of, 211
  diagnosis of, 211–212
  epidemiology and risk factors for, 210–212
  treatment of, 212
Trimethoprim-sulfamethoxazole (TMP/SMX)
  for *Nocardia*, 234–235
  for *Pneumocystis* pneumonia, 241–242, 243–245
  for *T. gondii* infection, 229
Tuberculosis, 52–53
  active infection, 52
  infection, preventing, 52–53
Tuberculosis screening, in infectious disease evaluation, 37
Tuberculous *Mycobacterium* infection, 109
  clinical manifestations of, 110
  diagnosis of, 110–112, 111f
  epidemiology of, 109–110
  pathogenesis of, 109–110
  prevention of, 113–114
  risk factors of, 109–110
  screening practices of, 113–114, 114f
  treatment of, 112

U

U. urealyticum, 107
Umbilical cord blood, 16
Unanticipated donor-derived infections, 40–41
Ureaplasma, 106–108
  anticipatory guidance for children with, 108
  clinical manifestations of, 107
  diagnosis of, 107–108
  disease prophylaxis/prevention of, 107
  epidemiology of, 106–107
  infection prevention for children with, 108
  risk factors of, 106–107
  treatment of, 108
Urinary tract infections (UTIs), 59
UTIs. *see* Urinary tract infections

V

Vaccination
  administration before immunosuppression, 63
  of health care workers and close contacts, 85
  history, 63
  posttransplant, 64
  pretransplantation, 64
  timing to start, 68, 68f, 69f
  transplantation and chemotherapy issues, 63
    general considerations, 63–64
    hematopoietic stem cell transplantation, 68–70
    oncology patients, 67–68
    solid organ transplantation, 64–67
  for varicella-zoster virus, 140–141
Vaccine
  administration, window of time between, 63
  for norovirus, 254
  in special circumstances, 69–70
Vaccine-preventable diseases, 64
Valacyclovir, for herpes simplex virus, 136
Valganciclovir, for cytomegalovirus, 121t
Vancomycin, for *Clostridioides difficile* infection, 261
Vancomycin-resistant enterococci, 83–84
Varicella vaccine, 64
Varicella-zoster vaccine (VZV), for solid organ transplantation, 66–67
Varicella-zoster virus
  clinical manifestations of, 138
  diagnosis of, 138
  epidemiology of, 138
  exposure avoidance, 139–140
  future directions for, 141
  immunization of contacts for, 139–140
  infection prevention for, 139–140
  in oncology, 138–141
  prophylaxis for, 139
  risk factors for, 138
  in transplant, 138–141
  treatment of, 138–139, 139t
  vaccination for, 140–141
    after chemotherapy or transplant, 140
    pretransplant, 140
    zoster, 140–141
Ventriculitis, CMV, 120t
Viral gastroenteritis, 253
Viral infections, prevention of, 50–52
  active, 50
  disease, 50–52
  exposure, 50
Viral pathogens, 57–58, 58t
Viruses, 84–85
Visitation policies, 85
Voriconazole
  for aspergillosis, 178
  for fusariosis, 191
  for histoplasmosis, 221
VZV. *see* Varicella-zoster vaccine

W

Water quality, good practice recommendations and, 87
Water safety
  recommendations, 92t
  during travel, after transplantation and chemotherapy, 92t
Waterborne infections, pathogens associated with, 91–92t
Wilms tumor, 29

Y

Young adults, CMV in, 125